AF595562

Respiratory and Critical Care

Respiratory and Critical Care

Editors

Ioannis Pantazopoulos
Ourania S. Kotsiou

MDPI • Basel • Beijing • Wuhan • Barcelona • Belgrade • Manchester • Tokyo • Cluj • Tianjin

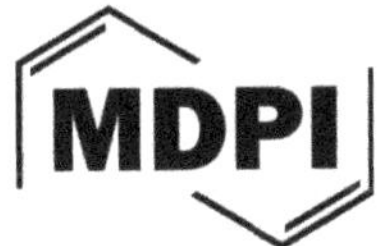

Editors

Ioannis Pantazopoulos
Department of Emergency Medicine
University of Thessaly, Faculty of Medicine
Larissa
Greece

Ourania S. Kotsiou
Department of Human Pathophysiology
University of Thessaly, Faculty of Nursing
Larissa
Greece

Editorial Office
MDPI
St. Alban-Anlage 66
4052 Basel, Switzerland

This is a reprint of articles from the Special Issue published online in the open access journal *Journal of Personalized Medicine* (ISSN 2075-4426) (available at: www.mdpi.com/journal/jpm/special_issues/respiratory_critical_care).

For citation purposes, cite each article independently as indicated on the article page online and as indicated below:

LastName, A.A.; LastName, B.B.; LastName, C.C. Article Title. *Journal Name* **Year**, *Volume Number*, Page Range.

ISBN 978-3-0365-6375-6 (Hbk)
ISBN 978-3-0365-6374-9 (PDF)

Contents

About the Editors

Ioannis Pantazopoulos

Dr. Ioannis Pantazopoulos is an Assistant Professor of Emergency Medicine at the University of Thessaly in Greece and Adjunct Professor both at the University of Bern in Switzerland and the European University of Cyprus. He is both a Respiratory Medicine and Intensive Care Specialist with two Master of Science degrees and a PhD in Resuscitation from the University of Athens, Greece. His extensive field of expertise includes the European Diploma in Adult Respiratory Medicine (HERMES) and the Diploma in Prehospital Emergency Medicine. He participates as a member of the organizing committee and as an active instructor in four Master of Science courses at the University of Athens and the University of Thessaly focusing in Respiratory, Intensive Care and Emergency Medicine. Director of the "Emergency Medicine and Resuscitation"course as well as in Life Support courses and Head of the Department of Emergency Medicine at the University of Thessaly. An avid researcher, he co-authored various book chapters, has published dozens of research articles in international medical journals and conferences, having been awarded twelve times for his work to this day. His research work has focused mainly on respiratory failure and resuscitation.

Ourania S. Kotsiou

Ourania S. Kotsiou is an Assistant Professor of Human Pathophysiology in the Faculty of Nursing at the University of Thessaly, Greece. She was licensed as a respiratory physician in 2017. Since then, she has served as principal, co-chief, or sub-investigator in several research programs and clinical trials in the Department of Respiratory Medicine at the University of Thessaly, in Greece. Ourania S. Kotsiou holds a Ph.D. in Pleural Pathophysiology from the University of Thessaly. With a background comprising many years of teaching, academic advising, and research, Ourania S. Kotsiou has gained considerable project management experience, communication skills, and expertise in identifying gaps in scientific knowledge and clinical research priorities.

Preface to "Respiratory and Critical Care"

The COVID-19 pandemic has affected health care across the world, with respiratory and critical care medicine being affected the most. The response of clinicians and researchers who have provided care and research not only for patients with COVID-19, but in all areas of respiratory and critical care medicine in extraordinary circumstances, has been impressive. In this Special Issue of the *Journal of Personalized Medicine*, we invited scholars to contribute manuscripts that highlight and further the knowledge in the abovementioned challenging disciplines.

The target readership encompasses respiratory and critical care physicians, rehabilitation practitioners, nurses, and technicians, in addition to all respiratory and critical care fellows and aims to provide important scientific information across all areas of respiratory research including COVID-19, COPD, asthma, pulmonary embolism, pneumonia, sleep medicine and respiratory critical care.

This reprint is the product of a collaborative effort by a dedicated team of physicians from the University of Thessaly whose specialties span the entire field of respiratory and critical care, along with contributions from around the world.

Many thanks to Professor Konstantinos Gourgoulianis for his support, encouragement and inspiration.

Ioannis Pantazopoulos and Ourania S. Kotsiou
Editors

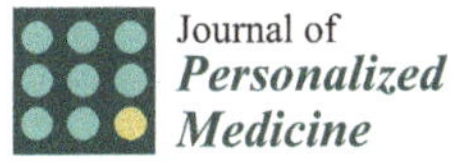
Journal of *Personalized Medicine*

MDPI

Editorial

Cutting-Edge Approaches in Respiratory and Critical Care Medicine

Ioannis Pantazopoulos [1,*] and Ourania S. Kotsiou [2]

[1] Department of Emergency Medicine, Faculty of Medicine, University of Thessaly, 41500 Larissa, Greece
[2] Department of Human Pathophysiology, Faculty of Nursing, University of Thessaly, 41110 Larissa, Greece
* Correspondence: pantazopoulosioannis@yahoo.com; Tel.: +30-6945661525

The COVID-19 pandemic has affected health care across the world, with respiratory and critical care medicine being affected the most. The response of clinicians and researchers who have provided care and research not only for patients with COVID-19, but in all areas of respiratory and critical care medicine in extraordinary circumstances has been impressive. In this Special issue of the *Journal of Personalized Medicine,* we invited scholars to contribute manuscripts that highlight and further the knowledge in the abovementioned challenging disciplines.

From the beginning of the pandemic, many nations introduced the use of face masks and respirators in the community to protect people against SARS-CoV-2 transmission. However, masks and respirators can provide different levels of protection depending on the type of the mask. Cloth masks provide the least protection, while surgical masks are safer and FFP/(K)N95 masks provide the highest protection [1]. On the other hand, prolonged mask use has been associated with a higher likelihood of a frequent cough, sputum production, dyspnea and panic attacks [1,2]. Given that the emergency phase of the pandemic is over, masks and respirators are recommended only for patients with a high mortality risk [3]. An increased mortality risk from COVID-19 has been observed for patients with the following factors: older age, male sex, β-thalassemia heterozygosity and respiratory disease [4]. Moreover, acute kidney injury, diabetes, hypertension, cardiovascular disease, cancer and obesity have also been reported as risk factors for a fatal outcome associated with SARS-CoV-2 [5].

The swift development of effective vaccines against COVID-19 was an unprecedented scientific achievement. In spite of this, the immunization of a critical proportion of the community proved to be very challenging mostly after the appearance of new strains of the virus that questioned the effectiveness of the vaccines and increased hesitancy. However, a large study from central Greece after the prevalence of new variants of the virus (Delta and Omicron) demonstrated that vaccination was still effective and provided high protection in terms of mortality and the clinical severity of COVID-19 [6]. Nevertheless, even in fully vaccinated patients, older age, higher viral load and a shorter period between symptom onset and hospital admission were associated with absence of anti-S SARS-CoV-2 antibodies upon hospital admission and poor clinical outcomes [7]. On the other hand, individuals vaccinated against COVID-19, but who were still infected by the virus, showed an "excellent boost" in their immune response [8].

For hospitalized patients, in addition to remdesivir, dexamethasone, immunomodulatory agents and monoclonal antibodies that have been approved for various severity stages of COVID-19, efforts for more largely available and safe drugs were continuous over the first two years of the pandemic. Among other methods, the administration of vitamin D was proposed mainly due to its immunomodulatory activity. However, no absolute conclusions could be drawn from a recent systematic review of the literature, due to the large variation in vitamin D supplementation schemes [9].

Citation: Pantazopoulos, I.; Kotsiou, O.S. Cutting-Edge Approaches in Respiratory and Critical Care Medicine. *J. Pers. Med.* **2023**, *13*, 105. https://doi.org/10.3390/jpm13010105

Received: 23 December 2022
Accepted: 26 December 2022
Published: 3 January 2023

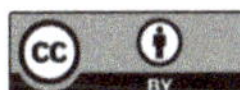

The incidence of pulmonary embolism (PE) has been reported to be around 2.6–8.9% in hospitalized COVID-19 patients, which is approximately nine-fold higher than in the general population [10]. Nevertheless, the prevalence of anticoagulant therapy-associated hemorrhagic complications in hospitalized patients with PE has been scarcely investigated. Pagkratis et al. retrospectively investigated the prevalence of hemorrhages in hospitalized PE patients during a 7-year period and found that one fifth of the patients hospitalized for PE suffered a non-fatal hemorrhage. The hemorrhages were mainly minor and lasted for 3 ± 2 days. Among low-molecular-weight heparins (LMWHs), nadroparin was related to a higher percentage of hemorrhages [11].

In the post-hospitalization period, pre-hospitalization methodical physical activity was associated with less dyspnea and a shorter recovery period, highlighting the importance of avoiding a sedentary life and engaging in exercise. On the other hand, in-hospital weight loss, comorbidities and dyspnea upon admission predicted a longer post-hospitalization recovery time [12].

The role of skeletal muscle mass in modulating immune response and supporting metabolic stress has been increasingly confirmed. Based on empirical data, patients with sarcopenia are speculated to have increased infection rates and poor prognoses amid the current COVID-19 pandemic [12]. In this context, this Special Issue aimed to shed light on the impact of less discussed comorbidities, such as the progressive loss of skeletal muscle mass and loss of muscle function, broadly known as sarcopenia in patients with chronic respiratory disease, such as bronchial asthma and/or COPD. Sarcopenia has been related to reduced lung function, a higher mortality risk, and higher risk of osteopenia and osteoporosis progression, leading to an increased risk of fractures, immobilization, and disability. Thus, physicians who examine sarcopenic patients with chronic airway diseases such as bronchial asthma or COPD should be able to appropriately collaborate with specialists who deal with nutrition and exercise, giving their patients a multimodal approach concerning these entities' interplay and the optimum treatment [13].

The importance of exercise training was not only highlighted in COVID-19 patients. It is widely regarded as the cornerstone of pulmonary rehabilitation in patients with chronic airway diseases such as COPD. The COVID-19 pandemic has given telemedicine and telemonitoring a significant boost. Accordingly, the study of Barata et al. showed that the online pulmonary rehabilitation programs are not inferior to the traditional method in COPD patients [14]. Moreover, the use of rehabilitation programs for patients who have successfully completed anti-tuberculosis treatment has been highlighted as a potent multi-faceted measure in preventing the increase in mortality rates, as researchers concluded that a patient with a TB diagnosis, even after fully completing pharmacotherapy, is threatened by a potential life loss of 4 years, in comparison to healthy individuals [15]. Moreover, there is evidence that an eight-week course of a respiratory muscle training (RMT) program was helpful in increasing diaphragmatic thickness in COPD patients with an FEV1% of $\geq 30\%$, in addition to lung function and cognition [16].

Exercise itself may be classified as a fundamental therapeutic approach in that it restabilizes sleep architecture and quality. The sleep state has been associated with significant changes in respiratory physiology, including ventilatory responses to hypoxia and hypercapnia, upper airway and intercostal muscle tone, tidal volume and minute ventilation. In addition, sleep disruption may induce a pro-inflammatory state that is associated with an impairment of immune system function [17]. On the other hand, inspiratory muscle strength training (IMT) has shown promising results in managing both sleep apnea and arterial hypertension. The review of Papanikolaou et al. suggested that training inspiratory strength in athletes could prove to be beneficial in counteracting the detrimental effects of the aforementioned sleep disturbances [17]. Furthermore, a recent meta-analysis showed that mandibular advancement devices (MADs), instead of continuous positive airway pressure (CPAP), support the mandible in order to increase the airway space and reduce pharyngeal collapsibility [18].

An increase in particulate matter (PM2.5) levels due to environmental pollution has been associated with the increased incidence of COVID-19 and risk of mortality [19]. Moreover, an increase in PM2.5 levels above the daily limit has been significantly associated with an increase in emergency department visits due to exacerbation of asthma and COPD, upper respiratory tract infections and pneumonia [20]. Biomarkers are recognized as essential tools for the diagnosis and management of all the above-mentioned respiratory diseases. It has been previously suggested that suPAR, the soluble form of urokinase plasminogen activator receptor (uPAR), which is a glycosyl-phosphatidylinositol (GPI)-linked membrane protein, can be used as a marker of both inflammation and disease severity [21]. A recent study that investigated the effectiveness of suPAR as an indicator of the severity of asthma, a chronic inflammatory disease of the airways, demonstrated that suPAR levels could discriminate moderate uncontrolled asthma from severe asthma [22]. Its use was also studied in patients with pulmonary embolism, since suPAR is an integral part of the fibrinolytic system. However, its role is still unclear and needs further examination before definite conclusions can be drawn [23]. Interestingly, CRP, a traditional marker of inflammation, was identified as a predictor of 30-day survival and length of hospital stay in community-acquired pneumonia. Indeed, CRP with a cut-off point of 9 mg/dL on day 4 and 7 of hospitalization could predict survival with an area under the curve of 0.765 (0.538–0.992) and 0.784 (0.580–0.989), respectively. Moreover, a reduction in CRP above 50% by the fourth day of hospitalization could predict a shorter hospital stay [24]. Many biomarkers have also been studied in COPD patients. However, due to disease heterogeneity, especially at the level of COPD severity, progression, patients' comorbidities and clinical status, there is a need for more personalized management. Specifically, the measurement and evaluation of each patient's unique biomarker panel, rather than one unique biomarker, are expected in the coming years [25]. Furthermore, preliminary data from Ortakoylu et al. suggested the impressive performance of interferon (IFN)-gamma-inducible protein 10 (IP-10) as a marker to detect latent tuberculosis infection (LTBI) in patients with inflammatory rheumatic diseases (IRD). At the cut-off point of 2197 pg/mL, IP-10 showed 89% specificity with a sensitivity of 91% (AUC: 0.950; 95% CI 0.906–0.994) [26].

Nowadays, researchers warn that a tripledemic is heading our way this winter. This triple viral threat includes respiratory syncytial virus (RSV), influenza and COVID-19. All these viruses can cause cardiovascular manifestations, including arrhythmia, acute coronary syndrome, acute myocarditis, or acute heart failure, increasing cardiovascular morbidity and mortality. Researchers from Spain identified that high-sensitivity troponin T could predict mortality in influenza patients. In fact, patients with levels below 24 ng/L could be safely discharged from the emergency department, since at this cut-off point, high-sensitivity troponin T demonstrated both high sensitivity and a negative predictive value of 100% [27]. Future studies aimed at consolidating this result and examining its usefulness in patients with COVID-19 and RSV infection will be useful.

This Special Issue also presents significant scientific advances in non-COVID-19 critical care medicine. In a landmark article by Chalkias et al. who investigated the dynamic changes in determinants of venous return during hyperdynamic septic shock, the authors used two translational models (hemorrhagic and septic shock) to assess the decrease in stressed volume in severe septic conditions [28]. Most importantly, they identified for the first time the existence of another circulatory volume, the rest volume (Vr), that seems to have dual main functions in the steady state, i.e., to prevent an increase in venous resistance and maintain critical closing pressure. The maintenance of Vr may be a key factor for the cardiovascular stability reported during selective iloprost nebulization by Lee et al. [29], suggesting that Vr may have a key role in the prevention of V/Q mismatch. These conditions are important for maintaining (or improving) hemodynamic coherence, i.e., the translation of macrohemodynamics to effective cellular oxygenation, and thus a low endothelial inflammatory status. Inflammation and increased reactive oxygen species formation may affect all organ systems, including the lungs. Thus, the attenuation of NO exhalation by propofol and sevoflurane reported by Vekrakou et al. may imply the preservation of bronchial microcirculatory perfusion and decreased NO synthesis, due to the immunomodulatory effects and the effects on microcirculation mediated by anesthetics in steady states [30,31] and in disease [32,33]. All the aforementioned factors can improve heart–lung interactions and facilitate the application of lung-protective ventilation strategies, preventing injurious mechanical stretching of lung parenchyma, and subsequent progression to fibrosis in patients with ARDS [34].

In conclusion, the research findings provided in this Special Issue contributed to different areas of research by offering new knowledge and mapping out the research field of all areas of respiratory and critical care medicine.

Author Contributions: Conceptualization, I.P. and O.S.K.; writing—original draft preparation, I.P. and O.S.K.; writing—review and editing, I.P. and O.S.K. All authors have read and agreed to the published version of the manuscript.

Conflicts of Interest: The authors declare no conflict of interest.

References

1. Mouliou, D.S.; Pantazopoulos, I.; Gourgoulianis, K.I. Medical/Surgical, Cloth and FFP/(K)N95 Masks: Unmasking Preference, SARS-CoV-2 Transmissibility and Respiratory Side Effects. *J. Pers. Med.* **2022**, *12*, 325. [CrossRef] [PubMed]
2. Perna, G.; Cuniberti, F.; Daccò, S.; Nobile, M.; Caldirola, D. Impact of Respiratory Protective Devices on Respiration: Implications for Panic Vulnerability during the COVID-19 Pandemic. *J. Affect. Disord.* **2020**, *277*, 772–778. [CrossRef] [PubMed]
3. Ioannidis, J.P.A. The End of the COVID-19 Pandemic. *Eur. J. Clin. Investig.* **2022**, *52*, e13782. [CrossRef] [PubMed]
4. Sotiriou, S.; Samara, A.A.; Lachanas, K.E.; Vamvakopoulou, D.; Vamvakopoulos, K.-O.; Vamvakopoulos, N.; Janho, M.B.; Perivoliotis, K.; Donoudis, C.; Daponte, A.; et al. Vulnerability of β-Thalassemia Heterozygotes to COVID-19: Results from a Cohort Study. *J. Pers. Med.* **2022**, *12*, 352. [CrossRef] [PubMed]
5. Dessie, Z.G.; Zewotir, T. Mortality-Related Risk Factors of COVID-19: A Systematic Review and Meta-Analysis of 42 Studies and 423,117 Patients. *BMC Infect. Dis.* **2021**, *21*, 855. [CrossRef]
6. Samara, A.A.; Boutlas, S.; Janho, M.B.; Gourgoulianis, K.I.; Sotiriou, S. COVID-19 Severity and Mortality after Vaccination against SARS-CoV-2 in Central Greece. *J. Pers. Med.* **2022**, *12*, 1423. [CrossRef]
7. Livanou, E.; Rouka, E.; Sinis, S.; Dimeas, I.; Pantazopoulos, I.; Papagiannis, D.; Malli, F.; Kotsiou, O.; Gourgoulianis, K.I. Predictors of SARS-CoV-2 IgG Spike Antibody Responses on Admission and Clinical Outcomes of COVID-19 Disease in Fully Vaccinated Inpatients: The CoVax Study. *J. Pers. Med.* **2022**, *12*, 640. [CrossRef]
8. Kotsiou, O.S.; Karakousis, N.; Papagiannis, D.; Matsiatsiou, E.; Avgeri, D.; Fradelos, E.C.; Siachpazidou, D.I.; Perlepe, G.; Miziou, A.; Kyritsis, A.; et al. The Comparative Superiority of SARS-CoV-2 Antibody Response in Different Immunization Scenarios. *J. Pers. Med.* **2022**, *12*, 1756. [CrossRef]
9. Bania, A.; Pitsikakis, K.; Mavrovounis, G.; Mermiri, M.; Beltsios, E.T.; Adamou, A.; Konstantaki, V.; Makris, D.; Tsolaki, V.; Gourgoulianis, K.; et al. Therapeutic Vitamin D Supplementation Following COVID-19 Diagnosis: Where Do We Stand?—A Systematic Review. *J. Pers. Med.* **2022**, *12*, 419. [CrossRef]
10. Sakr, Y.; Giovini, M.; Leone, M.; Pizzilli, G.; Kortgen, A.; Bauer, M.; Tonetti, T.; Duclos, G.; Zieleskiewicz, L.; Buschbeck, S.; et al. Pulmonary Embolism in Patients with Coronavirus Disease-2019 (COVID-19) Pneumonia: A Narrative Review. *Ann. Intensive Care* **2020**, *10*, 124. [CrossRef]
11. Pagkratis, N.; Matsagas, M.; Malli, F.; Gourgoulianis, K.I.; Kotsiou, O.S. Prevalence of Hemorrhagic Complications in Hospitalized Patients with Pulmonary Embolism. *J. Pers. Med.* **2022**, *12*, 1133. [CrossRef] [PubMed]
12. Kontopoulou, S.; Daniil, Z.; Gourgoulianis, K.I.; Kotsiou, O.S. Exercise Preferences and Benefits in Patients Hospitalized with COVID-19. *J. Pers. Med.* **2022**, *12*, 645. [CrossRef] [PubMed]
13. Karakousis, N.D.; Kotsiou, O.S.; Gourgoulianis, K.I. Bronchial Asthma and Sarcopenia: An Upcoming Potential Interaction. *J. Pers. Med.* **2022**, *12*, 1556. [CrossRef] [PubMed]
14. Barata, P.I.; Crisan, A.F.; Maritescu, A.; Negrean, R.A.; Rosca, O.; Bratosin, F.; Citu, C.; Oancea, C. Evaluating Virtual and Inpatient Pulmonary Rehabilitation Programs for Patients with COPD. *J. Pers. Med.* **2022**, *12*, 1764. [CrossRef]
15. Meca, A.-D.; Mititelu-Tarțău, L.; Bogdan, M.; Dijmarescu, L.A.; Pelin, A.-M.; Foia, L.G. Mycobacterium Tuberculosis and Pulmonary Rehabilitation: From Novel Pharmacotherapeutic Approaches to Management of Post-Tuberculosis Sequelae. *J. Pers. Med.* **2022**, *12*, 569. [CrossRef]
16. Cheng, Y.-Y.; Lin, S.-Y.; Hsu, C.-Y.; Fu, P.-K. Respiratory Muscle Training Can Improve Cognition, Lung Function, and Diaphragmatic Thickness Fraction in Male and Non-Obese Patients with Chronic Obstructive Pulmonary Disease: A Prospective Study. mboxemphJ. Pers. Med. **2022**, *12*, 475. [CrossRef]
17. Papanikolaou, D.D.; Astara, K.; Vavougios, G.D.; Daniil, Z.; Gourgoulianis, K.I.; Stavrou, V.T. Elements of Sleep Breathing and Sleep-Deprivation Physiology in the Context of Athletic Performance. *J. Pers. Med.* **2022**, *12*, 383. [CrossRef]

18. Tsolakis, I.A.; Palomo, J.M.; Matthaios, S.; Tsolakis, A.I. Dental and Skeletal Side Effects of Oral Appliances Used for the Treatment of Obstructive Sleep Apnea and Snoring in Adult Patients—A Systematic Review and Meta-Analysis. *J. Pers. Med.* **2022**, *12*, 483. [CrossRef]
19. Meo, S.A.; Al-Khlaiwi, T.; Ullah, C.H. Effect of Ambient Air Pollutants PM2.5 and PM10 on COVID-19 Incidence and Mortality: Observational Study. *Eur. Rev. Med. Pharmacol. Sci.* **2021**, *25*, 7553–7564. [CrossRef]
20. Mermiri, M.; Mavrovounis, G.; Kanellopoulos, N.; Papageorgiou, K.; Spanos, M.; Kalantzis, G.; Saharidis, G.; Gourgoulianis, K.; Pantazopoulos, I. Effect of PM2.5 Levels on ED Visits for Respiratory Causes in a Greek Semi-Urban Area. *J. Pers. Med.* **2022**, *12*, 1849. [CrossRef]
21. Chalkias, A.; Skoulakis, A.; Papagiannakis, N.; Laou, E.; Tourlakopoulos, K.; Pagonis, A.; Michou, A.; Ntalarizou, N.; Mermiri, M.; Ragias, D.; et al. Circulating SuPAR Associates with Severity and In-Hospital Progression of COVID-19. *Eur. J. Clin. Investig.* **2022**, *52*, e13794. [CrossRef] [PubMed]
22. Kotsiou, O.S.; Pantazopoulos, I.; Mavrovounis, G.; Marsitopoulos, K.; Tourlakopoulos, K.; Kirgou, P.; Daniil, Z.; Gourgoulianis, K.I. Serum Levels of Urokinase Plasminogen Activator Receptor (SuPAR) Discriminate Moderate Uncontrolled from Severe Asthma. *J. Pers. Med.* **2022**, *12*, 1776. [CrossRef] [PubMed]
23. Gkana, A.; Papadopoulou, A.; Mermiri, M.; Beltsios, E.; Chatzis, D.; Malli, F.; Adamou, A.; Gourgoulianis, K.; Mavrovounis, G.; Pantazopoulos, I. Contemporary Biomarkers in Pulmonary Embolism Diagnosis: Moving beyond D-Dimers. *J. Pers. Med.* **2022**, *12*, 1604. [CrossRef]
24. Travlos, A.; Bakakos, A.; Vlachos, K.F.; Rovina, N.; Koulouris, N.; Bakakos, P. C-Reactive Protein as a Predictor of Survival and Length of Hospital Stay in Community-Acquired Pneumonia. *J. Pers. Med.* **2022**, *12*, 1710. [CrossRef] [PubMed]
25. Pantazopoulos, I.; Magounaki, K.; Kotsiou, O.; Rouka, E.; Perlikos, F.; Kakavas, S.; Gourgoulianis, K. Incorporating Biomarkers in COPD Management: The Research Keeps Going. *J. Pers. Med.* **2022**, *12*, 379. [CrossRef] [PubMed]
26. Ortakoylu, M.G.; Bahadir, A.; Iliaz, S.; Soy Bugdayci, D.; Uysal, M.A.; Paker, N.; Tural Onur, S. Interferon-Inducible Protein-10 as a Marker to Detect Latent Tuberculosis Infection in Patients with Inflammatory Rheumatic Diseases. *J. Pers. Med.* **2022**, *12*, 1027. [CrossRef]
27. Tazón-Varela, M.A.; Ortiz de Salido-Menchaca, J.; Muñoz-Cacho, P.; Iriondo-Bernabeu, E.; Martos-Almagro, M.J.; Lavín-López, E.; Vega-Zubiaur, A.; Escalona-Canal, E.J.; Alcalde-Díez, I.; Gómez-Vildosola, C.; et al. High-Sensitivity Troponin T: A Potential Safety Predictive Biomarker for Discharge from the Emergency Department of Patients with Confirmed Influenza. *J. Pers. Med.* **2022**, *12*, 520. [CrossRef]
28. Chalkias, A.; Laou, E.; Papagiannakis, N.; Spyropoulos, V.; Kouskouni, E.; Theodoraki, K.; Xanthos, T. Assessment of Dynamic Changes in Stressed Volume and Venous Return during Hyperdynamic Septic Shock. *J. Pers. Med.* **2022**, *12*, 724. [CrossRef]
29. Lee, K.; Kim, M.; Kim, N.; Kang, S.J.; Oh, Y.J. Effects of Iloprost on Arterial Oxygenation and Lung Mechanics during One-Lung Ventilation in Supine-Positioned Patients: A Randomized Controlled Study. *J. Pers. Med.* **2022**, *12*, 1054. [CrossRef]
30. Vekrakou, A.; Papacharalampous, P.; Logotheti, H.; Valsami, S.; Argyra, E.; Vassileiou, I.; Theodoraki, K. Effect of General Anesthesia Maintenance with Propofol or Sevoflurane on Fractional Exhaled Nitric Oxide and Eosinophil Blood Count: A Prospective, Single Blind, Randomized, Clinical Study on Patients Undergoing Thyroidectomy. *J. Pers. Med.* **2022**, *12*, 1455. [CrossRef]
31. Chalkias, A.; Xenos, M. Relationship of Effective Circulating Volume with Sublingual Red Blood Cell Velocity and Microvessel Pressure Difference: A Clinical Investigation and Computational Fluid Dynamics Modeling. *J. Clin. Med.* **2022**, *11*, 4885. [CrossRef] [PubMed]
32. Chalkias, A.; Spyropoulos, V.; Georgiou, G.; Laou, E.; Koutsovasilis, A.; Pantazopoulos, I.; Kolonia, K.; Vrakas, S.; Papalois, A.; Demeridou, S.; et al. Baseline Values and Kinetics of IL-6, Procalcitonin, and TNF-α in Landrace-Large White Swine Anesthetized with Propofol-Based Total Intravenous Anesthesia. *BioMed Res. Int.* **2021**, *2021*, 6672573. [CrossRef] [PubMed]
33. Chalkias, A.; Laou, E.; Mermiri, M.; Michou, A.; Ntalarizou, N.; Koutsona, S.; Chasiotis, G.; Garoufalis, G.; Agorogiannis, V.; Kyriakaki, A.; et al. Microcirculation-Guided Treatment Improves Tissue Perfusion and Hemodynamic Coherence in Surgical Patients with Septic Shock. *Eur. J. Trauma Emerg. Surg.* **2022**, *48*, 4699–4711. [CrossRef] [PubMed]
34. Li, H.-H.; Wang, C.-W.; Chang, C.-H.; Huang, C.-C.; Hsu, H.-S.; Chiu, L.-C. Relationship between Mechanical Ventilation and Histological Fibrosis in Patients with Acute Respiratory Distress Syndrome Undergoing Open Lung Biopsy. *J. Pers. Med.* **2022**, *12*, 474. [CrossRef]

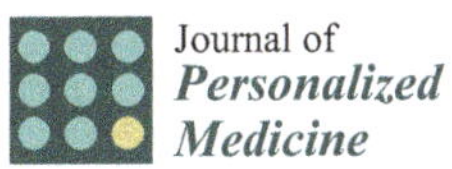

Journal of *Personalized Medicine*

MDPI

Article

Medical/Surgical, Cloth and FFP/(K)N95 Masks: Unmasking Preference, SARS-CoV-2 Transmissibility and Respiratory Side Effects

Dimitra S. Mouliou [1,2,*], Ioannis Pantazopoulos [1,2] and Konstantinos I. Gourgoulianis [1]

1 Department of Respiratory Medicine, Faculty of Medicine, University of Thessaly, BIOPOLIS, 41110 Larissa, Greece; pantazopoulosioannis@yahoo.com (I.P.); kgourg@uth.gr (K.I.G.)

2 Department of Emergency Medicine, Faculty of Medicine, University of Thessaly, BIOPOLIS, 41110 Larissa, Greece

* Correspondence: demymoole@gmail.com

Abstract: Background: Social distancing and mask-wearing were recommended and mandatory for people during the COVID-19 pandemic. Methods: A web-based questionnaire was disseminated through social media assessing mask type preference and COVID-19 history amongst tertiary sector services and the rates of the triad of respiratory symptoms in each mask type, along with other respiratory-related parameters. Results: Amongst 4107 participants, 63.4% of the responders, mainly women, preferred medical/surgical masks; 20.5%, mainly men, preferred cotton cloth masks; and 13.8% preferred FFP/(K)N95 masks. COVID-19 history was less common in FFP/(K)N95 compared to medical/surgical (9.2% vs. 15.6%, $p < 0.001$) or cloth masks (9.2% vs. 14.4%, $p = 0.006$). Compared to the control group (rare mask-wearing, nonsmokers and without lung conditions), those wearing one medical mask were more likely to report frequent sputum production (4.4% vs. 1.9%, $p = 0.026$) and frequent cough (4.4% vs. 1.6%, $p = 0.013$), and those wearing FFP/(K)N95 masks were more likely to report frequent cough (4.1% vs. 1.6%, $p = 0.048$). Compared to the control group, those preferring cotton cloth masks were more likely to report a frequent cough (7.3% vs. 1.6%, $p = 0.0002$), sputum production (6.3% vs. 1.9%, $p = 0.003$) and dyspnea (8% vs. 1.3%, $p = 0.00001$). Conclusions: Safe mask-wearing should be in parallel with a more personalized and social interaction approach.

Keywords: SARS-CoV-2; transmission; masks; medical masks; FFP masks; N95 masks; cloth masks; respiratory side effects; cough; dyspnea; sputum

Citation: Mouliou, D.S.; Pantazopoulos, I.; Gourgoulianis, K.I. Medical/Surgical, Cloth and FFP/(K)N95 Masks: Unmasking Preference, SARS-CoV-2 Transmissibility and Respiratory Side Effects. *J. Pers. Med.* **2022**, *12*, 325. https://doi.org/10.3390/jpm12030325

Academic Editor: Bruno Mégarbané

Received: 23 January 2022
Accepted: 20 February 2022
Published: 22 February 2022

1. Introduction

Coronaviruses have globally affected populaces since the early beginning of the 21st century. In December 2019, the novel severe acute respiratory syndrome coronavirus 2 (SARS-CoV-2) was identified from a cluster of cases of pneumonia in Wuhan, China [1]. On 30 January 2020, the World Health Organization (WHO) announced the coronavirus disease 19 (COVID-19) as a Public Health Emergency of International Concern, and a month and a half later, the COVID-19 epidemic was portrayed as a pandemic [2]. In the following two years, it seems that societies have acculturated SARS-CoV-2 and its mutants and that COVID-19 is likely to become an endemic disease.

Heretofore, scientific communities have made multifarious endeavors to monitor SARS-CoV-2 spread and to manage the COVID-19 pandemic. In particular, rapid testing, performed by qualified personnel, experts or even for self-diagnosis purposes, has been prevalent in populaces the last year, despite the fact that no method is completely foolproof [3,4]. Undeniably, the risk factors for a likely severe COVID-19 are prevalent, and, therefore, prevention against SARS-CoV-2 infection is highly required, especially for vulnerable cases, whereas vaccination strategies have been implemented for over a year now [5,6]. The WHO has recommended several ways for people to be protected against COVID-19, including vaccination, physical distancing, self-isolation of SARS-CoV-2 identified carriers, hand washing and the use of masks when physical distancing is not possible and in poorly ventilated settings [7].

Doubtlessly, masks are a key measure to suppress viral transmission and save lives, and depending on the type, masks can be used for either protection of healthy persons or to prevent onward transmission [8]. The WHO has also recommended the usage of medical masks predominantly for healthcare workers in clinical settings, symptomatic people, confirmed SARS-CoV-2 carriers, people with close contacts with COVID-19 cases, people over 60 and people with preexisting medical conditions that could place them at a risk for a likely severe COVID-19, whereas nonmedical masks can be used by the public under 60 and without underlying medical conditions [8].

Literature data also support that there is an association between mask use and SARS-CoV-2 transmission and that wearing a mask could reduce the risk of the infection [9,10]. Community mask use by healthy people could be beneficial, particularly for SARS-CoV-2, since transmission may occur in presymptomatic stage [11]. Moreover, given the current shortages of medical masks, the adoption of the public wearing of cloth masks is also recommended as an effective form of source control, in conjunction with existing hygiene, distancing and contact tracing strategies [12]. A review has stated that despite the lower efficiency of cloth masks compared to medical masks, laboratory results may underestimate the efficiency of cloth masks in real life [13]. A prepandemic article cautioned against the use of cloth masks in healthcare workers, since they may have an increased risk of infection [14]. However, the extended mask-wearing by the general population could lead to adverse effects and consequences in many medical fields [15].

The aim of this study is to present the mask type preferences amongst tertiary sector services and to monitor SARS-CoV-2 transmissibility in the wearing of specific mask types. Furthermore, the presence of the basic triad of respiratory symptoms is assessed for potential side effects in each mask type, and, finally, some future directions and aspects regarding future mask-wearing are well discussed.

2. Materials and Methods

2.1. WBQ Design

Although WBQs are currently being considered as a fluid form of observational, descriptive and analytical studies, they bespeak an upcoming propitious tool, enabling experts to combine ontological, ethical and epistemological principles to surveil society. WBQs enable motivated individuals to provide their answers, rapidly, at the touch of a button; they are automated, cost-effective and error-free [5–7]. The traditional closed-ended WBQs, structured with qualitative categorical or dichotomous questions, seem to be advantageous psychometric attempts and are desirable options for participation, contrary to open-ended questions requiring written answers [5–7].

Primarily, the WBQ of this study consisted of a binary question regarding gender. The occupation-related question was based on the sectors of classical economy, with further analysis in the tertiary sector, and included the following subgroups: (i) primary sector; (ii) secondary sector; (iii) tertiary sector with further subgrouping in public/private services, healthcare providers, food services, education, uniformed/military/policemen, freelancers and some other extra subgroups (for retirees, unemployed and university students). Considering the qualitative WBQ type for a better e-sample response, in addition to the fact that European countries are mainly aging, the concept of age-related questions was to follow a generation-based model with age ranges to reveal each generation's criticism and attitudes. Generation categories included (i) Generation A, (ii) Baby Boomers, (iii) Generation X, (iv) Millennials, (v) Generation Z restricted in adults and (vi) Silent Generation (all labeled with age ranges as seen in 2021, i.e., <18, 18–24, 25–40, 41–56, 57–75, >75) [5–7]. Unemployed and retirees were included in the survey.

The exclusion criteria for the survey, regarding the parameter of age, were those aged under 18 and over 75. Furthermore, the study was solely designed for the tertiary sector services where social interactions are required, as aerosols and droplets may be controlled naturally in the primary sector and secondary sector industries are closed structures. Moreover, in the primary and secondary sectors, respiratory symptoms could be present due to inhalation of dust, particulate matters or heavy metals, and thus, respiratory symptom monitoring would not be precise.

Two questions regarding the frequency of mask-wearing were included, one for days per week and the other for hours per day, and individuals with at least 3 h of continuous daily mask use were analyzed for the third part of the survey since it is more accurate to monitor SARS-CoV-2 transmissibility for each mask type amongst those with frequent daily mask use rather than in those with spontaneous mask use. Another categorical question was included for the mask type, referring to (i) medical/surgical mask, (ii) two medical/surgical masks, (iii) FFP/(K)N95, (iv) cotton cloth masks and (v) other type cloth masks. Questions were also included for the frequency of cough, dyspnea and sputum, with three answers, (i) rarely, (ii) middle and (iii) frequently, and the last responses were considered for the study.

Apart from these basic questions, some other binary questions regarding COVID-19 status, smoking and chronic lung disease (CLD) status were included. The questionnaire also included questions regarding home geographical location, as well as outdoor and indoor air pollution, with the last one referring to fireplace/indoor pet since, generally, all people living in a house are somewhat exposed to indoor cleaning chemicals and kitchen pollution.

The control group of the fourth part of this study was the responders with rare nondaily mask use for no more than half an hour, nonsmokers and without CLD, whereas the mask-wearing group was those with at least 3 h of continuous daily mask use, with no smoking or CLD status, so as to be more accurate and precise with mask side effects.

2.2. Population-Based Sample and WBQ Administration

The survey was conducted in the Greek mainland, where strict lockdown policies were imposed the previous year and strict social distancing and mask use are presently implemented. Greece has also imposed strict limitations on nonvaccinated people in parallel with the ongoing financial crisis that the country is facing. The WBQ was disseminated around late November (18–27 November 2021), and adults were randomly invited to participate in the survey through social media shares in profiles and Facebook teams. Informed consent was obtained from all subjects during accepting participation in the study. WBQs were submitted in Google forms, and data were saved in an Excel spreadsheet.

2.3. Statistical Analysis

Statistical analyses were effectuated via the statistical software IBM SPSS Statistics for Windows, Version 26.0 (headquartered in Chicago). Data normality was assessed with Kolmogorov–Smirnov test. Tests were two-tailed, and the level of statistical significance was established at $p \leq 0.05$. Chi-square test was applied for comparisons of frequencies, and Bonferroni correction was used for comparisons between subgroups. Spearman or Pearson/phi coefficients were used to evaluate correlations between variables.

3. Results

3.1. The Distribution of Genders and Generations by Tertiary Sector Services

The population-based sample consisted of 4107 participants, including 1129 (27.5%) men and 2978 (72.5%) women. Generation Z consisted of 623 (15.2%) participants, Millennials were about 2383 (58%) individuals, Generation X included 1000 (24.3%) individuals and 101 (2.5%) of the population-based sample were Baby Boomers. Table 1 illustrates the distribution of the responders in each service amongst genders and generations.

Table 1. Distribution of genders and generations by tertiary sector services.

Tertiary Sector Services	n	Gender		p-Value	Generations			
		Male (% out of n)	Female (% out of n)		Generation Z (% out of n)	Millennials (% out of n)	Generation X (% out of n)	Baby Boomers (% out of n)
Healthcare providers	381	65 (17.1)	316 (82.9)	<0.001	38 (10) [a]	249 (65.4) [b]	88 (23) [a,b]	6 (1.6) [a]
Food Services	300	93 (31)	207 (69)	0.157	66 (22) [a]	188 (62.7) [a,b]	45 (15) [a,b]	1 (0.3) [c]
Public education	194	33 (17)	161 (83)	<0.001	10 (5.2) [a]	113b (58.2) [a]	65 (33.5) [a,b]	6 (3.1) [a]
Private education	188	23 (12.2)	165 (87.8)	<0.001	19 (10.1) [a]	132 (70.2) [b]	35 (18.6) [a,b]	2 (1.1) [a]
Uniformed	74	54 (73)	20 (27)	<0.001	5 (6.8) [a]	42 (56.7) [b]	27 (36.5) [a,b]	-
Freelancers	363	140 (38.6)	223 (61.4)	<0.001	10 (2.8) [a]	224 (61.7) [b]	121 (33.3) [b]	8 (2.2) [a]
University students	399	107 (26.8)	292 (73.2)	<0.001	326 (81.7) [a]	73 (18.3) [b]	-	-
Other public services	222	66 (29.7)	156 (70.3)	0.442	14 (6.3) [a]	87 (39.2) [a,b]	111 (50) [b]	10 (4.5) [a]
Other private services	1570	467 (29.7)	1103 (70.3)	0.010	114 (7.3) [a]	1057 (67.2) [b]	384 (24.5) [c]	15 (1) [a]
Retirees	63	16 (25.4)	47 (74.6)	0.707	-	-	19 (30.1) [a]	44 (69.9) [b]
Unemployed	353	65 (18.4)	288 (81.6)	<0.001	21 (5.9) [a]	219 (62) [b]	104 (29.5) [a,b]	9 (2.5) [a]

* Each subscript letter denotes a subset of generation categories whose column proportions do not differ significantly from each other at the 0.05 level.

3.2. The Mask Types and Preference amongst Service Subgroups

In the whole population-based sample, 63.4% of the responders reported using medical/surgical masks, 20.5% reported wearing a cotton cloth mask and 13.8% reported a preference for FFP/(K)N95 masks. Women were more likely to prefer medical masks (65.5% vs. 57.8%, $p < 0.05$) while men were more likely to prefer cloth masks (29.4% vs. 20.4%, $p < 0.05$). Cotton cloth masks were mostly reported amongst Millennials (57.3%) and Generation X (28.9%), and medical/surgical masks were highly reported in the youth. Table 2 demonstrates the use of each mask type by job.

Table 2. Mask type preference/wearing by job.

Tertiary Sector Services	n	Mask Type				
		One Medical/Surgical Mask (% out of n)	Two Medical/Surgical Masks (% out of n)	FFP/(K)N95 Mask (% out of n)	Cotton Cloth Mask (% out of n)	Other Cloth Mask (% out of n)
Healthcare providers	381	243 (63.8) [a]	28 (7.3) [b]	82 (21.5) [b]	25 (6.6) [c]	3 (0.8) [a,c]
Food services	300	188 (62.7) [a]	4 (1.3) [a,b]	14 (4.7) [b]	76 (25.3) [a]	18 (6) [c]
Public education	194	108 (55.7) [a]	6 (3.1) [a]	41 (21.1) [b]	37 (19.1) [a,b]	2 (1)
Private education	188	108 (57.4) [a]	7 (3.7) [a]	34 (18.1) [a]	34 (18.1) [a]	5 (2.7) [a]
Uniformed	74	33 (44.6) [a]	1 (1.4) [a,b]	8 (10.8) [a,b]	27 (36.5) [b]	5 (6.8) [b]
Freelancers	363	216 (59.5) [a]	6 (1.7) [a]	60 (16.5) [a]	68 (18.7) [a]	13 (3.6) [a]
University students	399	270 (67.7) [a]	14 (3.5) [a,b]	48 (12) [a,b]	63 (15.8) [b]	4 (1) [a,b]
Other public services	222	135 (60.8) [a]	9 (4.1) [a]	31 (14) [a]	43 (19.4) [a]	4 (1.8) [a]
Other private services	1570	949 (60.4) [a]	36 (2.3) [a]	201 (12.8) [a]	351 (22.4) [a]	33 (2.1) [a]
Retirees	63	40 (63.5) [a]	1 (1.6) [a]	7 (11.1) [a]	12 (19) [a]	3 (4.8) [a]
Unemployed	353	193 (54.7) [a]	7 (2) [a,b]	39 (11) [a]	107 (30.3) [b]	7 (2) [a,b]

* Each subscript letter denotes a subset of mask categories whose column proportions do not differ significantly from each other at the 0.05 level.

3.3. Mask Preference and SARS-CoV-2 Infection

Of the population-based sample, 80.4% reported daily mask-wearing for at least 3 h, and also 14.4% of them reported they had passed COVID-19. Amongst the responders with a frequent mask-wearing but who disclosed a history of SARS-CoV-2 infection, there was a significant difference for the FFP/(K)N95 masks compared to one medical/surgical mask (9.2% vs. 15.6%, $p < 0.001$) or cloth masks (9.2% vs. 14.4%, $p = 0.006$), whereas there was no significant difference for those reported the use of two medical/surgical masks (9.2% vs. 11.9%, $p = 0.378$). Table 3 shows the SARS-CoV-2 infection history in each job among each mask subtype.

Table 3. History of SARS-CoV-2 infection amongst services by mask type.

Tertiary Sector Services	n	History of SARS-CoV-2 Infection (% out of n)	Mask Type		
			Medical/Surgical Mask (%) *	FFP/(K)N95 Mask (%) *	Cloth Mask (%) *
Healthcare providers	353	42 (11.9)	28 (11.2) [a]	9 (11) [a]	5 (22.7) [b]
Food services	251	48 (19.1)	34 (21.1) [a]	2 (15.4) [b]	12 (15.6) [b]
Public education	181	33 (18)	20 (18.7) [a]	8 (1.5) [a]	5 (14.3) [b]
Private education	177	22 (12.4)	14 (13) [a]	2 (5.9) [b]	6 (17.1) [a]
Uniformed	52	12 (23.1)	5 (20.8) [a]	-	7 (35) [b]
Freelancers	251	29 (11.6)	17 (11.6) [a]	6 (11.1) [a]	6 (12) [a]
University students	355	63 (17.7)	47 (18.8) [a]	3 (6.4) [b]	13 (22.4) [c]
Other public services	199	27 (13.6)	19 (14.4) [a]	2 (6.6) [b]	6 (14.6) [a]
Other private services	1301	173 (13.3)	128 (15.3) [a]	14 (7.4) [b]	31 (11.9) [a]
Retirees	17	2 (11.8)	1 (9) [a]	-	1 (50) [b]
Unemployed	163	24 (14.7)	19 (19.2) [a]	3 (10.3) [b]	2 (5.7) [c]

* Each subscript letter denotes a subset of mask type categories in each row whose column proportions do not differ significantly from each other at the 0.05 level, and percentages refer to the number of COVID-19 cases in each mask subgroup of each row.

3.4. Masks and Respiratory Side Effects

Of the responders, 45.8% reported being smokers and 8.6% reported a CLD status, and they were excluded from this part of the study. Thus, the control group consisted of 375 responders and the mask-wearing group consisted of 1673 responders, of whom 58.1% reported a preference for wearing one medical/surgical mask, 18% reported a preference for FFP/(K)N95 and 19% reported a preference for wearing a cotton cloth mask. Compared to the control group, those wearing one medical mask were more likely to report frequent sputum production (4.4% vs. 1.9%, $p = 0.026$) and frequent cough (4.4% vs. 1.6%, $p = 0.013$), but dyspnea showed no significant difference (3.1% vs. 1.3%, $p = 0.069$). Compared to the control group, those wearing FFP/(K)N95 masks were more likely to report frequent cough (4.1% vs. 1.6%, $p = 0.048$), while dyspnea and sputum production had no significant difference (2.4% vs. 1.3%, $p = 0.308$, and 2% vs. 1.9%, $p = 0.866$). Compared to the control group, those preferring cotton cloth masks were more likely to report a frequent cough (7.3% vs. 1.6%, $p = 0.0002$), sputum production (6.3% vs. 1.9%, $p = 0.003$) and dyspnea (8% vs. 1.3%, $p = 0.00001$).

Generally, no significant differences were observed for genders' respiratory symptoms and each mask type, except for cough and dyspnea that were absent in men preferring FFP(K)N95 masks. In addition, the younger generations were more likely to report respiratory symptoms compared to the older ones. Additionally, smokers showed higher rates of respiratory symptoms but showed the same variations as the mask-wearing group for each mask type, and responders with CLDs were more likely to report cough and dyspnea when wearing one medical/surgical mask rather than FFP/(K)N95 masks.

4. Discussion

In our study, more than half of the responders reported a preference for medical/surgical masks and one-fifth reported FFP/(K)N95 mask-wearing, and healthcare professionals highly shaped this rate. Medical/surgical masks were mostly preferred by women and youth, and healthcare providers showed the highest rate in wearing two medical/surgical masks, whereas mainly men, half of the Millennials, uniformed and unemployed preferred cotton cloth masks. The overall history of SARS-CoV-2 infection was less common amongst those with daily FFP/(K)N95 mask-wearing, but public education and food services showed the highest rates of infection compared to other tertiary sector services with that type of daily mask-wearing. The highest rates of SARS-CoV-2 infection were seen for cloth masks in healthcare providers, uniformed and university students, and, regarding medical/surgical masks, high rates were observed especially in food services and uniformed. Regarding respiratory side effects, the FFP/(K)N95 mask-wearing group was free of frequent sputum production and dyspnea compared to the control group, but frequent cough was statistically significantly more prevalent in this group than the control group but without any difference compared to medical/surgical masks, while frequent dyspnea showed no difference but frequent sputum and cough were significant compared to those with rare mask-wearing. Cotton cloth mask-wearing showed the highest percentages in all the analyzed respiratory symptoms, being significant compared to those without frequent mask-wearing and even amongst the other mask types. As expected, smokers showed higher rates in frequencies of all respiratory symptoms, but frequent cough and dyspnea in people with CLDs were more common in medical/surgical masks rather than FFP(K)N95 masks; thus, this mask type may be appropriate specifically for those with lung conditions.

On the whole, FFP/(K)N95 mask-wearing responders were significantly less likely to have a COVID-19 history. Women were more likely to prefer medical/surgical masks; they are more sensitive than men in health issues, and men mostly preferred cotton cloth masks. The WHO has recommended that healthcare providers should wear medical and FFP/(K)N95 masks, but, on the contrary, we revealed that some healthcare providers prefer cloth mask-wearing [8]. Doubtlessly, this fact is unacceptable for the health field during the COVID-19 pandemic. Fortunately, two medical/surgical mask-wearing was mostly seen in healthcare services. Sadly, a study revealed that less than half of healthcare professionals were informed about mask types against SARS-CoV-2 [16]. Doubtlessly, the percentage of penetration in cloth masks is higher than that in surgical masks or N95 respirators [17]. In our study, healthcare providers that are highly exposed to SARS-CoV-2 carriers were more likely to report a COVID-19 history with cloth mask-wearing, and public education teachers were more likely to catch the virus with cloth mask-wearing; teachers are in schools with children that easily transmit the virus and can pass it with mild symptoms without understanding it. In addition, university students showed high rates of COVID-19 history with cloth mask types since, undeniably, close contacts in the youth cannot be fully amended. Most uniformed work in closed structures in which it is easy for the virus to be transmitted, and they preferred cloth masks; unemployed responders preferred them too, which may be due to the cost compared to the others and the ability to wash and reuse them—a method being cost-free. Food services also showed high rates in cloth masks, but it is easy for delivery workers to catch and transmit the virus by contacting many people daily, and maybe that is why both medical/surgical and cloth mask-wearers reported high rates of COVID-19 history. Despite the fact that uniformed can transmit the virus in their closed structures, partially explaining their higher rates of COVID-19 history, another study revealed that those working in food services were more vulnerable to SARS-CoV-2 infection [18]. The WHO also recommended people with health risks to be well protected, but in our study, smokers and people with CLDs showed various preferences for mask types, even cloth masks. Regarding freelancers, there was no difference for COVID-19 history in various mask types, but some of their work includes vigorous physical activity, and it should be further discussed to what extent should they wear a mask during work since the WHO recommended that even in an area of SARS-CoV-2 transmission masks should not be worn because of the risk of reducing breathing capacity [8]. However, generally speaking, the efficacy of medical masks is not the same as that of cloth masks for respiratory viral transmission [19]. Since a sole cloth fabric is not a material designed solely to be a face mask and protect against pathogen transmission, we highlight the need for cloth masks to be disallowed in specific services.

To our knowledge, this is the first study to evaluate the triad of respiratory symptoms amongst the wearing of various mask types. In our study, the daily medical/surgical mask-wearing was more likely to show frequent sputum production and cough in comparison with rare/spontaneous mask-wearing. Several effects of mask-wearing have been discussed, such as physiological adverse effects in cardiopulmonary exercise capacity, including increased rebreathing of expelled carbon dioxide, significant increased respiratory rate, hyperventilation, increase in CO_2 in the blood, hypoxemia and hypercapnia [20]. Cotton cloth mask-wearing showed the highest rates in the triad of respiratory symptoms in our population-based sample. However, no further nonrespiratory symptoms were evaluated in this study, and another study revealed adverse skin reactions due to medical masks compared to cloth masks [21]. More targeted studies, in the future, should analyze the possibility of the prolonged wearing of cotton cloth masks leading to early byssinosis signs, since it is an evident lung condition among cotton workers due to fiber inhalation [22]. Nevertheless, cotton cloth masks not only were not such effective in preventing SARS-CoV-2 transmission, but also had the highest levels of respiratory side effects; additionally, daily FFP/(K)N95 mask-wearing responders were less likely to have COVID-19 history and also had lower levels of respiratory side effects. Frequent dyspnea and sputum production were not significantly seen in FFP/(K)N95 mask-wearing, and cough rates (only women reported cough) were not much different from those seen in medical/surgical mask-wearing, yet significantly different compared to the control group. Even if cough was the only respiratory symptom seen in this mask type, a study studying healthcare professionals showed that prolonged use of medical and N95 masks had caused headaches, rash, acne, skin breakdown and impaired cognition in most of those surveyed [23]. The authors suggest frequent breaks, improved hydration and rest and skin care for healthcare professionals with prolonged mask-wearing [23]. We also highlight the need for FFP/(K)N95 masks to be thoroughly studied for other potential adverse effects since, in this study, we have assessed only some basic respiratory issues.

Further studies are needed to finally evaluate if mask-wearing is effective or if the effectiveness is attributable to the social distancing and other personal care and protection strategies and the overall psychology amongst people, as several side effects of mask-wearing have been reported in current literature. Some variations in COVID-19 history amongst healthcare professionals, unemployed or food services—comparing rates of infection of each mask type—could show that in specific services where viral transmission is high, mask type efficacy may not be efficiently monitored, or that social distancing and personalized protection strategies may play a more important role in preventing transmission. Public health strategies may have overreacted in this pandemic, and the medical motto "primum non nocere" ("first, do no harm"), a moral principle everyone should at least consider following, was evidently not observed during the pandemic [20]. Moreover, presymptomatic carriers may transmit the virus, but false positives are evident, and a current perspective doubted the realistic existence of asymptomatic patients in COVID-19 [3,24]. As a result, maybe it is healthier for symptomatic patients to wear masks so as not to transmit the virus to others and for all the others being at risk for a likely severe COVID-19 to wear them only in crowded places with high social interactions or in places with a high risk of SARS-CoV-2 transmission. However, vaccinated people should follow the same path since, even if they will likely pass COVID-19 with mild symptoms, they can still transmit the virus to others [6,25]. Finally, there may be a need for some more safe mask designs for future epidemics, and it is required that safe mask-wearing be acculturated in society, especially in environmental pollution such as during summer fires in some Mediterranean cities or even in extreme air pollution due to cars or because of fireplace smoke in winter.

No study is completely foolproof. Besides healthcare professionals to some extent, we do not know if all the others were equally exposed to the virus; in what conditions they caught the virus; and if it happened during work, on transportation, at a friend or family level of transmission or elsewhere. People started wearing N95 masks later due to limited availability at the beginning of the pandemic, and we do not know when the participants contracted the virus. However, respiratory side effects are irrelevant to this parameter, but we did not exclude those with allergies as no related question was included in our WBQ. In addition, the FFP/(K)N95 mask-wearing group could be larger so as to analyze more accurately respiratory symptoms and their potential respiratory safety.

5. Conclusions

FFP/(K)N95 mask-wearing responders were less likely to have a COVID-19 history and were less likely to report respiratory symptoms, compared to the other mask types. Cotton cloth masks not only did not prevent SARS-CoV-2 transmission but also were more likely to cause frequent cough, dyspnea and sputum production. Public health strategies may have overreacted during the pandemic; mask-wearing but with safe mask-types should follow a more personalized and social interaction approach, and safe mask-wearing should also be recommended in future epidemics or environmental issues.

Author Contributions: Conceptualization, D.S.M.; methodology, I.P. and K.I.G.; formal analysis, D.S.M.; investigation, K.I.G., D.S.M. and I.P.; writing—original draft preparation, D.S.M. and I.P.; writing—review and editing, K.I.G.; supervision, K.I.G. All authors have read and agreed to the published version of the manuscript.

Funding: This research received no external funding.

Institutional Review Board Statement: The study was conducted according to the guidelines of the Declaration of Helsinki and approved by the Ethics Committee of the University of Thessaly (No. 2800-01/11/2021).

Informed Consent Statement: Informed consent was obtained from all subjects involved in the study.

Data Availability Statement: Data sharing is not applicable to this article. The data are not publicly available due to restrictions. They contain information that could compromise the privacy of the participants.

Conflicts of Interest: The authors declare no conflict of interest.

References

1. Zhu, N.; Zhang, D.; Wang, W.; Li, X.; Yang, B.; Song, J.; Zhao, X.; Huang, B.; Shi, W.; Lu, R.; et al. A Novel Coronavirus from Patients with Pneumonia in China, 2019. *N. Engl. J. Med.* **2020**, *382*, 727–733. [CrossRef] [PubMed]
2. WHO. Director-General's Opening Remarks at the Media Briefing on COVID-19—11 March 2020. Available online: https://www.who.int/director-general/speeches/detail/who-director-general-s-opening-remarks-at-the-media-briefing-on-covid-19---11-march-2020 (accessed on 2 December 2021).
3. Mouliou, D.S.; Gourgoulianis, K.I. False-Positive and False-Negative COVID-19 Cases: Respiratory Prevention and Management Strategies, Vaccination, and Further Perspectives. *Expert Rev. Respir. Med.* **2021**, *15*, 993–1002. [CrossRef] [PubMed]
4. Mouliou, D.S.; Pantazopoulos, I.; Gourgoulianis, K.I. Societal Criticism towards COVID-19: Assessing the Theory of Self-Diagnosis Contrasted to Medical Diagnosis. *Diagnostics* **2021**, *11*, 1777. [CrossRef] [PubMed]
5. Mouliou, D.S.; Kotsiou, O.S.; Gourgoulianis, K.I. Estimates of COVID-19 Risk Factors among Social Strata and Predictors for a Vulnerability to the Infection. *Int. J. Environ. Res. Public Health* **2021**, *18*, 8701. [CrossRef] [PubMed]
6. Mouliou, D.S.; Pantazopoulos, I.; Gourgoulianis, K.I. Social Response to the Vaccine against COVID-19: The Underrated Power of Influence. *JPM* **2021**, *12*, 15. [CrossRef]

7. Advice for the Public on COVID-19—World Health Organization. Available online: https://www.who.int/emergencies/diseases/novel-coronavirus-2019/advice-for-public (accessed on 17 December 2021).
8. Coronavirus Disease (COVID-19): Masks. Available online: https://www.who.int/news-room/questions-and-answers/item/coronavirus-disease-covid-19-masks (accessed on 17 December 2021).
9. Li, Y.; Liang, M.; Gao, L.; Ayaz Ahmed, M.; Uy, J.P.; Cheng, C.; Zhou, Q.; Sun, C. Face Masks to Prevent Transmission of COVID-19: A Systematic Review and Meta-Analysis. *Am. J. Infect Control* **2021**, *49*, 900–906. [CrossRef]
10. Tabatabaeizadeh, S.-A. Airborne Transmission of COVID-19 and the Role of Face Mask to Prevent It: A Systematic Review and Meta-Analysis. *Eur. J. Med. Res.* **2021**, *26*, 1. [CrossRef]
11. MacIntyre, C.R.; Chughtai, A.A. A Rapid Systematic Review of the Efficacy of Face Masks and Respirators against Coronaviruses and Other Respiratory Transmissible Viruses for the Community, Healthcare Workers and Sick Patients. *Int. J. Nurs. Stud.* **2020**, *108*, 103629. [CrossRef]
12. Howard, J.; Huang, A.; Li, Z.; Tufekci, Z.; Zdimal, V.; van der Westhuizen, H.-M.; von Delft, A.; Price, A.; Fridman, L.; Tang, L.-H. An Evidence Review of Face Masks against COVID-19. *Proc. Natl. Acad. Sci. USA* **2021**, *118*, e2014564118. [CrossRef]
13. Santos, M.; Torres, D.; Cardoso, P.C.; Pandis, N.; Flores-Mir, C.; Medeiros, R.; Normando, A.D. Are Cloth Masks a Substitute to Medical Masks in Reducing Transmission and Contamination? A Systematic Review. *Braz. Oral Res.* **2020**, *34*, e123. [CrossRef]
14. MacIntyre, C.R.; Seale, H.; Dung, T.C.; Hien, N.T.; Nga, P.T.; Chughtai, A.A.; Rahman, B.; Dwyer, D.E.; Wang, Q. A Cluster Randomised Trial of Cloth Masks Compared with Medical Masks in Healthcare Workers. *BMJ Open* **2015**, *5*, e006577. [CrossRef] [PubMed]
15. Kisielinski, K.; Giboni, P.; Prescher, A.; Klosterhalfen, B.; Graessel, D.; Funken, S.; Kempski, O.; Hirsch, O. Is a Mask That Covers the Mouth and Nose Free from Undesirable Side Effects in Everyday Use and Free of Potential Hazards? *Int. J. Environ. Res. Public Health* **2021**, *18*, 4344. [CrossRef] [PubMed]
16. Aladul, M.I.; Kh Al-Qazaz, H.; Allela, O.Q.B. Healthcare Professionals' Knowledge, Perception and Practice towards COVID-19: A Cross-Sectional Web-Survey. *J. Pharm. Health Serv. Res.* **2020**, *11*, 355–363. [CrossRef] [PubMed]
17. Jain, M.; Kim, S.T.; Xu, C.; Li, H.; Rose, G. Efficacy and Use of Cloth Masks: A Scoping Review. *Cureus* **2020**, *12*, e10423. [CrossRef] [PubMed]
18. Kotsiou, O.S.; Pantazopoulos, I.; Papagiannis, D.; Fradelos, E.C.; Kanellopoulos, N.; Siachpazidou, D.; Kirgou, P.; Mouliou, D.S.; Kyritsis, A.; Kalantzis, G.; et al. Repeated Antigen-Based Rapid Diagnostic Testing for Estimating the Coronavirus Disease 2019 Prevalence from the Perspective of the Workers' Vulnerability before and during the Lockdown. *Int. J. Environ. Res. Public Health* **2021**, *18*, 1638. [CrossRef] [PubMed]
19. Szarpak, L.; Smereka, J.; Filipiak, K.J.; Ladny, J.R.; Jaguszewski, M. Cloth Masks versus Medical Masks for COVID-19 Protection. *Cardiol. J.* **2020**, *27*, 218–219. [CrossRef]
20. Lansiaux, E.; Tchagaspanian, N.; Arnaud, J.; Durand, P.; Changizi, M.; Forget, J. Side-Effects of Public Health Policies against Covid-19: The Story of an Over-Reaction. *Front. Public Health* **2021**, *9*, 792. [CrossRef]
21. Techasatian, L.; Lebsing, S.; Uppala, R.; Thaowandee, W.; Chaiyarit, J.; Supakunpinyo, C.; Panombualert, S.; Mairiang, D.; Saengnipanthkul, S.; Wichajarn, K.; et al. The Effects of the Face Mask on the Skin Underneath: A Prospective Survey During the COVID-19 Pandemic. *J. Prim. Care Community Health* **2020**, *11*, 2150132720966167. [CrossRef]
22. Hinson, A.V.; Schlünssen, V.; Agodokpessi, G.; Sigsgaards, T.; Fayomi, B. The Prevalence of Byssinosis among Cotton Workers in the North of Benin. *Int. J. Occup. Environ. Med.* **2014**, *5*, 194–200.
23. Rosner, E. Adverse effects of prolonged mask use among healthcare professionals during COVID-19. *J. Infect Dis. Epidemiol.* **2020**, *6*, 130. [CrossRef]
24. Mouliou, D.S.; Gourgoulianis, K.I. COVID-19 "Asymptomatic" Patients: An Old Wives' Tale. *Expert Rev. Respir. Med.* **2022**. [CrossRef] [PubMed]
25. Bleier, B.S.; Ramanathan, M.; Lane, A.P. COVID-19 Vaccines May Not Prevent Nasal SARS-CoV-2 Infection and Asymptomatic Transmission. *Otolaryngol. Head Neck Surg.* **2021**, *164*, 305–307. [CrossRef] [PubMed]

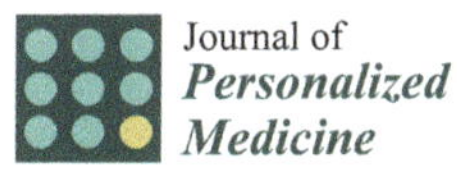
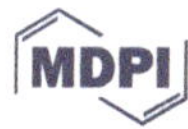

Article

Vulnerability of β-Thalassemia Heterozygotes to COVID-19: Results from a Cohort Study

Sotirios Sotiriou [1], Athina A. Samara [1,*], Konstantinos E. Lachanas [2], Dimitra Vamvakopoulou [3], Konstantinos-Odysseas Vamvakopoulos [1], Nikolaos Vamvakopoulos [4], Michel B. Janho [1], Konstantinos Perivoliotis [1], Christos Donoudis [5], Alexandros Daponte [5], Konstantinos I. Gourgoulianis [6] and Stylianos Boutlas [6]

1 Department of Embryology, Faculty of Medicine, School of Health Sciences, University of Thessaly, 41110 Larissa, Greece; sotiriousoti@yahoo.gr (S.S.); kostantinos753@gmail.com (K.-O.V.); micheljanho@live.co.uk (M.B.J.); kperi19@gmail.com (K.P.)
2 Department of Public Health and Social Medicine, Koutlimpanio General Hospital, 41221 Larissa, Greece; klachanas@hotmail.com
3 1st Neonatal Intensive Care Unit, "Agia Sophia" Children's Hospital, 11527 Athens, Greece; gina_dimitra@hotmail.com
4 Department of Biology, Faculty of Medicine, University of Thessaly, 41110 Larissa, Greece; nvamvak@yahoo.com
5 Department of Obstetrics and Gynaecology, Faculty of Medicine, University of Thessaly, 41110 Larissa, Greece; xdonoudis@gmail.com (C.D.); daponte@uth.gr (A.D.)
6 Department of Respiratory Medicine, Faculty of Medicine, University of Thessaly, 41110 Larissa, Greece; kgourg@med.uth.gr (K.I.G.); sboutlas@gmail.com (S.B.)
* Correspondence: at.samara93@gmail.com; Tel.: +30-697-737-9540

Citation: Sotiriou, S.; Samara, A.A.; Lachanas, K.E.; Vamvakopoulou, D.; Vamvakopoulos, K.-O.; Vamvakopoulos, N.; Janho, M.B.; Perivoliotis, K.; Donoudis, C.; Daponte, A.; et al. Vulnerability of β-Thalassemia Heterozygotes to COVID-19: Results from a Cohort Study. *J. Pers. Med.* **2022**, *12*, 352. https://doi.org/10.3390/jpm12030352

Academic Editors: Ioannis Pantazopoulos and Ourania S. Kotsiou

Received: 17 January 2022
Accepted: 24 February 2022
Published: 25 February 2022

Abstract: Background: The assignment of mortality risk from SARS-CoV-2 virus (COVID-19) to vulnerable patient groups is an important step toward containment of the pandemic. **Methods:** A total of 760 patients with a positive molecular test for SARS-CoV-2 who were unvaccinated against COVID-19 were recruited between 1 January and 30 June 2021. Patients were grouped by age; sex; and common morbidities, such as atrial fibrillation, chronic respiratory disease, coronary disease, diabetes type II, neoplasia, hypertension and β-Thalassemia heterozygosity. As a primary endpoint, we assessed mortality risk from COVID-19, and as secondary endpoints, we considered clinical severity and need for Intense Care Unit (ICU) admission. **Results:** In multivariate analysis, male sex ($p < 0.001$, OR = 2.59), increasing age ($p < 0.001$, OR = 1.049), β-Thalassemia heterozygosity ($p = 0.001$, OR = 2.41) and chronic respiratory disease ($p = 0.018$, OR = 1.84) were identified as risk factors associated with mortality due to COVID-19. Moreover, male sex ($p < 0.001$, OR = 1.98), increasing age ($p < 0.001$, OR = 1.052) and β-Thalassemia heterozygosity ($p = 0.001$, OR = 2.59) were associated with clinical severity in logistic regression. Regarding ICU admission, the risk factors were identified as male sex ($p = 0.002$, OR = 1.99), chronic respiratory disease ($p = 0.007$, OR = 2.06) and hypertension ($p < 0.001$, OR = 5.81). **Conclusions:** An increased mortality risk from COVID-19 was observed for older age, male sex, β-Thalassemia heterozygosity and respiratory disease. Carriers of β-Thalassemia were identified as more vulnerable for severe clinical symptomatology, but there was no increased possibility for ICU admission. Readjustment of these findings to consider impacts of variant strains prevailing during the latest viral outbreak among vulnerable patient groups may offer timely relief from the pandemic.

Keywords: COVID-19; β-Thalassemia; mortality; critical care; pandemic

1. Introduction

Over the last two years, the SARS-CoV-2 virus (COVID-19) pandemic has spread globally, affecting every country worldwide [1]. The identification of common comorbidities that increase the mortality risk by severe acute respiratory syndrome–coronavirus 2

(COVID-19) is an important first step toward morbidity and mortality risk containment from the pandemic. Early identification, consultation and intervention practices among vulnerable groups could reduce the morbidity rates and mortality risk from COVID-19.

Several risk factors attributing to mortality due to COVID-19, including patients' demographic characteristics and common comorbidities, have been identified since the beginning of the pandemic. More specifically, increasing age and male sex increase the severity and mortality risk [2,3]. Furthermore, common comorbidities, including hypertension, diabetes mellitus and chronic obstructive lung disease, have also been reported as factors associated with an increased mortality in infected patients [4,5].

β-Thalassemia is the most common inherited single gene disorder in the world, with approximately 1.5% of the global population being heterozygous for β-Thalassemia [6]. In a recently published pilot study during the second wave of the pandemic, β-Thalassemia heterozygotes were identified as a group of patients vulnerable to COVID-19, with an increased mortality risk [7]. These findings have to be updated during the next pandemic waves with novel variants of the virus being dominant.

Herein, to consolidate our pilot observations [7], we analyzed considerably more COVID-19-positive and unvaccinated cases among these vulnerable groups, spanning a longer time period. Mortality risk, clinical severity and need for Intense Care Unit (ICU) admission were assessed as endpoints.

2. Methods

2.1. Settings

The present retrospective cohort study includes 760 consecutive patients unvaccinated against COVID-19 with a positive SARS-CoV-2 Real-Time Polymerase Chain Reaction (RT-PCR) molecular test. All participants were registered in the emergency department (ER) of the tertiary referral center in central Greece (University Hospital of Larisa), between 1 January and 30 June 2021.

2.2. Participants and Study Design

A retrospective analysis was conducted of medical and laboratory records from consecutive patients registered in the ER of a tertiary referral hospital. A database was created based on medical history and laboratory tests of confirmed COVID-19-positive subjects. We examined the mortality risk of vulnerable patient groups with common morbidity symptoms, including β-Thalassemia heterozygotes. The course of non-hospitalized participants was followed by telephone interviews.

The primary outcome of this study was the association of clinical and demographic variants with mortality due to COVID-19 in infected individuals. COVID-19 infection was the single common official cause of death for our study participants, as registered in hospital archives. Furthermore, clinical severity of symptomatology and need for Intense Care Unit (ICU) admission were considered as secondary endpoints.

Patient demographic characteristics of age; sex; and common morbidities, including atrial fibrillation, chronic respiratory disease, coronary disease, diabetes, neoplasia and hypertension were recorded. In addition, β-Thalassemia heterozygosity was assessed through laboratory tests and known medical history. We excluded the current smoking-status parameter from patient characteristics being studied, based on preliminary indications of notable absence of statistically significant correlations between smoking and mortality from COVID-19.

2.3. Ethical Considerations

Experimental therapeutic protocols were not applicable in this study. All data were analyzed anonymously, using code numbers with respect to the patient's privacy, and collected in the context of routine diagnostic and therapeutic procedures. Nevertheless, the study conformed to the Research and Ethical Committee guidelines of the University Hospital of Larisa.

2.4. Sample Estimation

Considering an estimated prevalence of 8% in our entire study population, a precision of ±3.5% and 95% confidence interval (CI), the minimum sample size required was calculated by a precision analysis, using Epi Info 7 [8]. A minimum study sample was set at 231 patients.

2.5. Statistical Analysis

Analysis was carried out by using SPSS version 26.0 (IBM, Chicago, IL, USA). Categorical variables are described by using frequency and relative frequency. Continuous variables are described with means and standard deviation. Analysis of continuous variables was conducted by using the Mann–Whitney U test and Kruskal–Wallis test, since the assumption of normal distribution was violated. Data were checked for deviation from normal distribution, using the Shapiro–Wilk normality test. Categorical data were analyzed with the use of Chi-square test or Fisher's exact test. Multivariate analysis was performed in the form of binary logistic regression. For all the analyses, a 5% significance level was set.

3. Results

A total of 760 patients were included in the study, of which 448 (58.9%) were male and 312 (41.1%) female, with a mean age of 62.21 (±16.42) years, ranging from 20 to 93. A total of 448 (58,9%) patients were male and 312 (41.1%) female. Overall, 189 study participants died, resulting in a mortality rate of 24.86%.

Regarding mortality, in univariate analysis, male sex ($p < 0.001$, OR = 2.44), increased age ($p < 0.001$), atrial fibrillation ($p < 0.001$, OR = 2.44), chronic respiratory disease ($p < 0.001$, OR = 2.71), coronary disease ($p < 0.001$, OR = 2.11), hypertension ($p < 0.001$, OR = 2.77) and β-Thalassemia heterozygosity ($p < 0.001$, OR = 2.26) were associated with increased mortality due to COVID-19 (Table 1).

Table 1. Assessing mortality risk of study groups from COVID-19 by univariate and multivariate statistical analysis.

		Outcome: Mortality	Univariate			Multivariate Binary Logistic Regression	
		Yes (%)	Sig.	OR with 95% CI	RR with 95% CI	Sig.	aOR with 95% CI
Sex (M/F)	M: F:	140 (31.3) 49 (15.7)	**<0.001 (C)**	2.44 (1.69–3.51)	1.99 (1.49–2.66)	**<0.001 (C)**	2.59 (1.73–3.90)
Age (median, IQR)		Dead: 73 (16) Alive: 62 (23)	**<0.001 (M–W)**	-	-	**<0.001 (C)**	1.049 (1.031–1.066)
β-Thalassemia heterozygosity	Yes: No:	53 (38.7) 136 (21.8)	**<0.001 (C)**	2.26 (1.53–3.35)	1.77 (1.37–2.29)	**0.001**	2.41 (1.55–3.74)
Chronic respiratory disease	Yes: No:	41 (43.6) 148 (22.2)	**<0.001 (C)**	2.71 (1.73–4.23)	1.96 (1.50–2.57)	**0.018**	1.84 (1.11–3.05)
Atrial fibrillation	Yes: No:	84 (37.0) 103 (19.4)	**<0.001 (C)**	2.44 (1.73–3.45)	1.91 (1.50–2.43)	0.058	1.50 (0.99– 2.28)
Hypertension	Yes: No:	138 (32.9) 51 (15.0)	**<0.001 (C)**	2.77 (1.93–3.98)	2.19 (1.64–2.92)	0.243	1.31 (0.83–2.04)
Coronary disease	Yes: No:	53 (37.3) 136 (22.0)	**<0.001 (C)**	2.11 (1.43–3.12)	1.70 (1.31–2.20)	0.617	0.89 (0.55–1.42)
Diabetes mellitus type II	Yes: No:	48 (30.8) 141 (23.3)	0.056 (C)	1.46 (0.99–2.15)	1.32 (1.00–1.74)	0.439	0.84 (0.54–1.30)
Neoplasia	Yes: No:	27 (31.8) 162 (24.1)	0.122 (C)	1.47 (0.90–2.40)	1.32 (0.94–1.85)	0.653	0.88 (0.52–1.51)

C, Chi-square test; F, Fisher's exact test; M–W, Mann–Whitney U test.

In logistic regression analysis, male patients were 2.6 times more likely to die than female patients ($p < 0.001$, OR = 2.59). Furthermore, older participants were more likely to die from COVID-19; moreover, every year of age increased the possibility to die by 4.9% ($p < 0.001$, OR = 1.049). Patients with underlying chronic respiratory disease had a 1.8-times increased mortality possibility than patients without respiratory disease history ($p = 0.018$,

OR = 1.84). Interestingly, β-Thalassemia heterozygotes had a 2.4-times increased possibility of mortality compared to patients without the trait ($p < 0.001$, OR = 2.41) (Figure 1). There was no statistically significant association between COVID-19 attributed mortality and other comorbidities, such as atrial fibrillation ($p = 0.058$), hypertension ($p = 0.243$), coronary disease ($p = 0.617$), diabetes type II ($p = 0.439$) and neoplasia ($p = 0.653$) (Table 1).

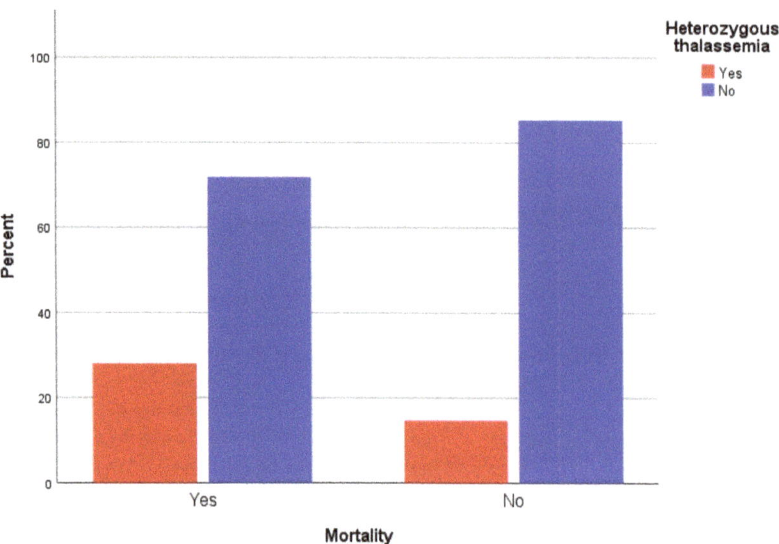

Figure 1. Mortality of β-Thalassemia heterozygotes from COVID-19: distribution of SARS-CoV-2 infected β-Thalassemia trait carriers (red box) among study participants who died (Yes), or survived (No) from COVID-19, relative to non-carriers (blue box).

Regarding severity of clinical symptoms, in univariate analysis, male sex ($p < 0.001$), increased age ($p < 0.001$), atrial fibrillation ($p < 0.001$), chronic respiratory disease ($p < 0.001$), coronary disease ($p < 0.001$), hypertension ($p < 0.001$) and β-Thalassemia heterozygosity ($p < 0.001$) were associated with increased severity of clinical symptoms attributed to COVID-19 (Table 2). Moreover, in logistic regression, there was almost double the possibility of severe clinical disease for male patients than female ones ($p < 0.001$, OR = 1.98). Older participants were more likely to have symptoms with increased severity ($p < 0.001$, OR = 1.052), with every year of age increasing the possibility of severe disease by 5.2%. β-Thalassemia heterozygosity was also identified as an independent risk factor for severe clinical symptoms of COVID-19 ($p < 0.001$, OR = 2.59) (Figure 2).

When assessing ICU admission, in univariate analysis, male sex ($p = 0.001$), increased age ($p = 0.005$), chronic respiratory disease ($p < 0.001$), coronary disease ($p < 0.001$) and hypertension ($p < 0.001$) were associated with the need for ICU admission. In logistic regression, male patients had double the possibility for ICU stay than female ones ($p = 0.002$, OR = 1.99). Furthermore, chronic respiratory disease and hypertension were identified as independent risk factors for ICU admission due to COVID-19 ($p = 0.007$, OR = 2.06 and $p < 0.001$, OR = 5.81 respectively), with patients with hypertension being 5.8 times more possible to need ICU.

Table 2. Assessing clinical severity of COVID-19 by univariate and multivariate statistical analysis.

	Outcome: Severity			Univariate	Multivariate Ordinal Logistic Regression	
	Asymptomatic-Mild (%)	Moderate (%)	Severe-Critical (%)	Sig.	Sig.	aOR with 95% CI
Sex (Male)	94 (49.5)	210 (56.3)	144 (73.1)	**<0.001 (C)**	**<0.001**	1.98 (1.47–2.66)
Age (median, IQR)	52 (32)	65 (18)	72 (16)	**<0.001 (K-W)**	**<0.001**	1.052 (1.040–1.064)
Atrial Fibrillation	51 (26.8)	93 (24.9)	83 (42.6)	**<0.001 (C)**	0.373	0.85 (0.60–1.21)
Chronic respiratory disease	15 (7.9)	38 (10.2)	41 (20.8)	**<0.001 (C)**	0.098	1.45 (0.93–2.26)
Coronary disease	20 (10.5)	69 (18.5)	53 (26.9)	**<0.001 (C)**	0.634	1.10 (0.73–1.67)
Diabetes mellitus Type II	29 (15.3)	79 (21.2)	48 (24.4)	0.078 (C)	0.331	0.83 (0.58–1.20)
Neoplasia	20 (10.5)	35 (9.4)	30 (15.2)	0.108 (C)	0.173	0.73 (0.47–1.15)
Hypertension	69 (36.3)	204 (54.7)	147 (74.6)	**<0.001 (C)**	0.104	1.34 (0.94–1.91)
β-Thalassemia heterozygosity	15 (7.9)	66 (17.7)	56 (28.4)	**<0.001 (C)**	**<0.001**	2.59 (1.78–3.77)

C, Chi-square test; K-W, Kruskal–Wallis Test.

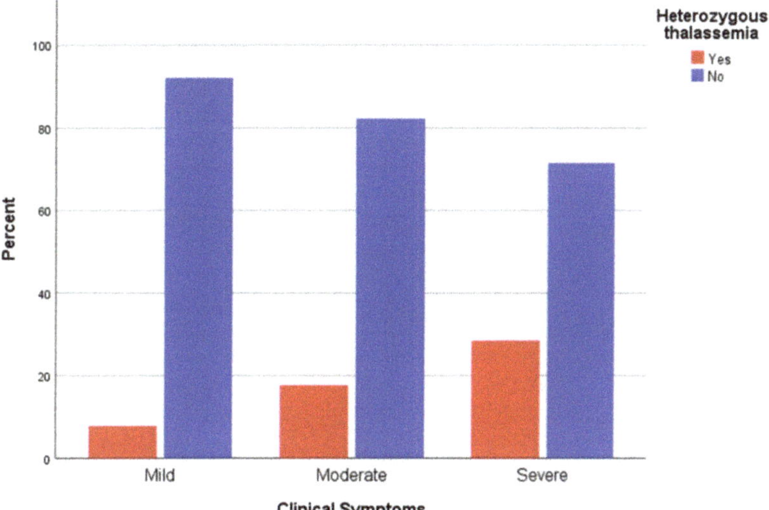

Figure 2. Clinical symptoms of COVID-19 in β-Thalassemia heterozygotes patients and control: distribution of clinical symptoms of SARS-CoV-2-infected β-Thalassemia trait carriers (red box) and non-carriers (blue box).

4. Discussion

In the present study, we assessed the role of common comorbidities as independent risk factors for COVID-19 attributed mortality among 760 unvaccinated patients against SARS-CoV-2 during the first half of 2021. The current findings support earlier observations of strong statistical association between mortality due to COVID-19 and male sex, increased age, chronic respiratory disease and β-Thalassemia heterozygosity [3,5–8]. Patients with underlying chronic respiratory disease were included in the high-mortality-risk group of patients from the beginning of the pandemic [9].

β-Thalassemias are a group of hereditary autosomal recessive anemias caused by either reduced or complete absence of production of β-globin chains of the hemoglobin tetramer [10]. Data regarding potential effects of associated comorbidities in thalassemic patients with COVID-19 are limited. Recent studies reported that patients with β-Thalassemia have a chronic condition which may contribute to an increase in susceptibility to SARS-CoV-2 infection [11,12]. The underlying disease is associated with several comorbidities and complications of chronic transfusions, including heart failure, pulmonary hypertension, hypogonadism and diabetes, that may attribute to the susceptibility of this group of patients to COVID-19 infection [11].

In this context, it is necessary to investigate the potential role of the β-Thalassemia trait as a risk factor for morbidity and mortality by COVID-19. The compromised nature of response to stress that is inherent to asymptomatic or mildly anemic β-Thalassemia heterozygotes facilitates collective induction of innate immune receptor CD45, Toll-like receptor 4 and CD32 expression; reduces ability to produce oxidative bursts; and elevates membrane lipid peroxidation [13]. Borderline resistance of β-Thalassemia trait carriers to stress may explain the low threshold of COVID-19 symptoms required to begin treatment that appear with considerable time lag, require longer periods of hospitalization and ICU care and result in over twice the possibility of mortality due to COVID-19.

The vascular nature of COVID-19 symptoms leads to mortality from cardiovascular (CVS) failure [14], rendering CVS control a primary target during the pandemic. CVS control is exerted through classical renin-angiotensin system (RAS)-inducing vasoconstriction via renin processed angiotensin II (ATII) vasoconstrictors, and counter-balancing non-classical RAS-inducing vasodilation via ACE2 conversion of ATII or processing of ATI to AT 1–7 vasodilators [15,16]. SARS-CoV-2 inhibits ACE2 expression and deranges CVS homeostasis [16]. Current COVID-19 treatment strategies aim to suppress SARS-CoV-2 main protease activity, required to release active viral protein products [17] and induce ACE2 expression [16]. Thus, CVS control of COVID-19 positive vulnerable patient groups by statins, merits thorough consideration as a potential first-line treatment option.

Updated data of patients with adaptive evolutionary viral alterations may improve the representability of data collection and enhance the reliability of associated clinical findings. Future studies on COVID-19 mortality risk should address pregnancy and high-risk pregnancy, particularly for women with genotypic variations associated with early onset preeclampsia, such as variant TLR-4 alleles [18], and mutant angiotensin type I and type II receptor combination genotypes [19].

This new addition may have not only statistical explanations (more participants analyzed), but mainly biological explanations (longer time period of data collection). A possible biological explanation for the observed mortality boost of this new subgroup may rely on the enriched blend of viral variants that prevailed during the first half of 2021, rather than during its narrower last quarter of 2020 previously examined [3]. According to this explanation, the reliability of clinical observations related to mortality impact from COVID-19 depends on timing of participant data collection during the course of the pandemic.

The present study identified independent risk factors associated with mortality due to COVID-19. The most noteworthy association is confirmation of the susceptibility of individuals heterozygous for β-Thalassemia to COVID-19. However, prior to the appraisal of these results, several limitations should be considered. Data were collected retrospectively, depending on the availability and accuracy of data records, and information bias may have occurred. Furthermore, data were collected from a single tertiary hospital, and the generalization of our findings is limited.

Analogous studies on the distribution of mortality risk from COVID-19 among heterozygotes of less frequent abnormal hemoglobins [20] may help elucidate key mortality factors of this vulnerable asymptomatic group and are worth pursuing on both clinical and academic grounds.

5. Conclusions

We conclude that COVID-19 mortality is affected primarily by male sex, aging, β-Thalassemia trait and chronic respiratory disease/asthma, followed by atrial fibrillation, hypertension, coronary disease, diabetes and neoplasia. Timely accounts of these observations with vaccination against SARS-CoV-2 will assess the effect of vaccination status on mortality risk and facilitate early identification, consultation and treatment of COVID-19-susceptible cases for optimal pandemic control.

Author Contributions: Conceptualization, S.S., S.B. and A.A.S.; methodology, K.E.L.; formal analysis, K.P.; investigation, M.B.J., D.V., K.-O.V. and C.D.; writing—original draft preparation, S.S. and A.A.S.; writing—review and editing, K.I.G. and A.D.; supervision, S.B., K.I.G., N.V. and A.D. All authors have read and agreed to the published version of the manuscript.

Funding: This research received no external funding.

Institutional Review Board Statement: The study was conducted according to the guidelines of the Declaration of Helsinki, and approved by the Institutional Review Board of University Hospital of Larissa.

Data Availability Statement: Data are available upon reasoning request.

Acknowledgments: Special thanks to Lemonia Anagnostopoulos for language editing.

Conflicts of Interest: The authors declare that there is no conflict of interest.

References

1. World Health Organization. WHO Coronavirus (COVID-19) Dashboard. Available online: https://covid19.who.int/ (accessed on 8 January 2022).
2. Ramírez-Soto, M.C.; Arroyo-Hernández, H.; Ortega-Cáceres, G. Sex differences in the incidence, mortality, and fatality of COVID-19 in Peru. *PLoS ONE* **2021**, *16*, e0253193. [CrossRef] [PubMed]
3. Shakor, J.K.; Isa, R.A.; Babakir-Mina, M.; Ali, S.I.; Hama-Soor, T.A.; Abdulla, J.E. Health related factors contributing to COVID-19 fatality rates in various communities across the world. *J. Infect. Dev. Ctries* **2021**, *15*, 1263–1272. [CrossRef] [PubMed]
4. Seong, G.M.; Baek, A.R.; Baek, M.S.; Kim, W.Y.; Kim, J.H.; Lee, B.Y.; Na, Y.S.; Lee, S.I. Comparison of Clinical Characteristics and Outcomes of Younger and Elderly Patients with Severe COVID-19 in Korea: A Retrospective Multicenter Study. *J. Pers. Med.* **2021**, *11*, 1258. [CrossRef] [PubMed]
5. Gao, Y.D.; Ding, M.; Dong, X.; Zhang, J.J.; Kursat Azkur, A.; Azkur, D.; Gan, H.; Sun, Y.L.; Fu, W.; Li, W.; et al. Risk factors for severe and critically ill COVID-19 patients: A review. *Allergy* **2021**, *76*, 428–455. [CrossRef] [PubMed]
6. Whetheral, D.J. The thalassemias. In *Williams Hematology*, 5th ed.; Beutler, E., Lichtman, M.A., Coller, B.S., Kipps, T.J., Eds.; McGraw-Hill: New York, NY, USA, 1995.
7. Sotiriou, S.; Samara, A.A.; Vamvakopoulou, D.; Vamvakopoulos, K.-O.; Sidiropoulos, A.; Vamvakopoulos, N.; Janho, M.B.; Gourgoulianis, K.I.; Boutlas, S. Susceptibility of β-thalassemia heterozygotes to COVID-19. *J. Clin. Med.* **2021**, *10*, 3645. [CrossRef] [PubMed]
8. Dean, A.; Arner, T.; Sunki, G.; Friedman, R.; Lantinga, M.; Sangam, S.; Zubieta, J.C.; Sullivan, K.M.; Brendel, K.A.; Gao, Z.; et al. *Epi Info. (TM), a Database and Statistics Program for Public Health Professionals*, 7.2.3.1 ed.; CDC: Atlanta, GA, USA, 2011.
9. Cho, K.H.; Kim, S.W.; Park, J.W.; Do, J.Y.; Kang, S.H. Effect of Sex on Clinical Outcomes in Patients with Coronavirus Disease: A Population-Based Study. *J. Clin. Med.* **2020**, *10*, 38. [CrossRef] [PubMed]
10. O'Brien, J.; Du, K.Y.; Peng, C. Incidence, clinical features, and outcomes of COVID-19 in Canada: Impact of sex and age. *J. Ovarian Res.* **2020**, *13*, 137. [CrossRef] [PubMed]
11. Wang, M.; Jiang, N.; Li, C.; Wang, J.; Yang, H.; Liu, L.; Tan, X.; Chen, Z.; Gong, Y.; Yin, X.; et al. Sex-Disaggregated Data on Clinical Characteristics and Outcomes of Hospitalized Patients With COVID-19: A Retrospective Study. *Front. Cell. Infect. Microbiol.* **2021**, *11*, 680422. [CrossRef] [PubMed]
12. Peckham, H.; de Gruijter, N.M.; Raine, C.; Radziszewska, A.; Ciurtin, C.; Wedderburn, L.R.; Rosser, E.C.; Webb, K.; Deakin, C.T. Male sex identified by global COVID-19 meta-analysis as a risk factor for death and ITU admission. *Nat. Commun.* **2020**, *11*, 6317. [CrossRef] [PubMed]
13. Seltzer, S. Linking ACE2 and angiotensin II to pulmonary immunovascular dysregulation in SARS-CoV-2 infection. *Int. J. Infect. Dis.* **2020**, *101*, 42–45. [CrossRef] [PubMed]
14. Galanello, R.; Origa, R. Beta-thalassemia. *Orphanet J. Rare Dis.* **2010**, *5*, 11. [CrossRef] [PubMed]
15. Karimi, M.; Haghpanah, S.; Zarei, T.; Azarkeivan, A.; Shirkavand, A.; Matin, S.; Tavakoli, M.A.; Zahedi, Z.; De Sanctis, V. Prevalence and severity of Coronavirus disease 2019 (COVID-19) in Transfusion Dependent and Non-Transfusion Dependent β-thalassemia patients and effects of associated comorbidities: An Iranian nationwide study. *Acta Biomed.* **2020**, *91*, e2020007. [CrossRef] [PubMed]
16. Karimi, M.; Haghpanah, S.; Azarkeivan, A.; Zahedi, Z.; Zarei, T.; Akhavan Tavakoli, M.; Bazrafshan, A.; Shirkavand, A.; De Sanctis, V. Prevalence and mortality in β-thalassaemias due to outbreak of novel coronavirus disease (COVID-19): The nationwide Iranian experience. *Br. J. Haematol.* **2020**, *190*, e137–e140. [CrossRef] [PubMed]
17. Ondei, L.D.S.; Estevão, I.D.F.; Rocha, M.I.P.; Percário, S.; Souza, D.R.S.; Pinhel, M.A.D.S.; Bonini-Domingos, C.R. Oxidative stress and antioxidant status in beta-thalassemia heterozygotes. *Rev. Bras. Hematol. Hemoter.* **2013**, *35*, 409–413. [CrossRef] [PubMed]

18. Chung, M.K.; Zidar, D.A.; Bristow, M.R.; Cameron, S.J.; Chan, T.; Harding, C.V., III; Kwon, D.H.; Singh, T.; Tilton, J.C.; Tsai, E.J.; et al. COVID-19 and Cardiovascular Disease. *Circ. Res.* **2021**, *128*, 1214–1236. [CrossRef] [PubMed]
19. Li, X.C.; Zhang, J.; Zhuo, J.L. The vasoprotective axes of the renin-angiotensin system: Physiological relevance and therapeutic implications in cardiovascular, hypertensive and kidney diseases. *Pharmacol. Res.* **2017**, *125*, 21–38. [CrossRef] [PubMed]
20. Aleksova, A.; Gagno, G.; Sinagra, G.; Beltrami, A.; Janjusevic, M.; Ippolito, G.; Zumla, A.; Fluca, A.; Ferro, F. Effects of SARS-CoV-2 on Cardiovascular System: The Dual Role of Angiotensin-Converting Enzyme 2 (ACE2) as the Virus Receptor and Homeostasis Regulator-Review. *Int. J. Mol. Sci.* **2021**, *22*, 4526. [CrossRef] [PubMed]

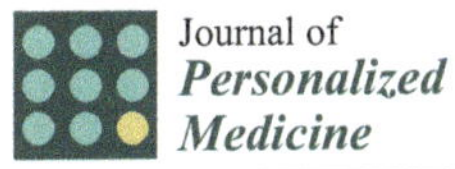

Journal of *Personalized Medicine*

MDPI

Article

COVID-19 Severity and Mortality after Vaccination against SARS-CoV-2 in Central Greece

Athina A. Samara [1,*], Stylianos Boutlas [2], Michel B. Janho [1], Konstantinos I. Gourgoulianis [2] and Sotirios Sotiriou [1]

1 Department of Embryology, Faculty of Medicine, School of Health Sciences, University of Thessaly, 41110 Larissa, Greece

2 Department of Respiratory Medicine, Faculty of Medicine, University of Thessaly, 41110 Larissa, Greece

* Correspondence: at.samara93@gmail.com; Tel.: +30-241-350-1701

Abstract: Background: Vaccination against SARS-CoV-2 (COVID-19) has become crucial for limiting disease transmission and reducing its severity, hospitalizations and mortality; however, despite universal acceptance, vaccine hesitancy is still significant. In the present manuscript, we aim to assess COVID-19-attributed mortality after the prevalence of new variants of the virus (Delta and Omicron viral strains) and to evaluate the vaccination effect. Methods: All patients that were hospitalized due to COVID-19 infection in the Respiratory Department of a tertiary referral center in central Greece between 1st of June 2021 and 1st of February 2022 were included in the present study. Results: 760 consecutive patients were included in the study; 89 (11.7%) were diagnosed with severe COVID-19 and 220 (38.7%) patients were fully vaccinated. In logistic regression, increased age (aOR = 1.12, $p < 0.001$), male gender (aOR = 2.29, $p = 0.013$) and vaccination against SARS-CoV-2 virus (aOR = 0.2, $p < 0.001$) were associated with mortality attributed to COVID-19 with a statistically significant association. Moreover, increased age (aOR = 1.09, $p < 0.001$), male gender (aOR = 1.92, $p = 0.025$) and vaccination against SARS-CoV-2 virus (aOR = 0.25, $p < 0.001$) were statistically significantly associated with clinical severity of COVID-19 infection. However, when comparing the length of hospitalization between vaccinated and unvaccinated patients, the difference was not statistically significant between the two groups ($p = 0.138$). Conclusions: Vaccination against SARS-CoV-2 virus had a protective effect in terms of mortality and clinical severity of COVID-19 during the fourth wave of the pandemic in Central Greece. The national vaccination policy has to focus on vulnerable populations that are expected to benefit the most from the vaccine's protection.

Keywords: COVID-19; vaccination; risk factors; effectiveness; mortality

Citation: Samara, A.A.; Boutlas, S.; Janho, M.B.; Gourgoulianis, K.I.; Sotiriou, S. COVID-19 Severity and Mortality after Vaccination against SARS-CoV-2 in Central Greece. *J. Pers. Med.* **2022**, *12*, 1423. https://doi.org/10.3390/jpm12091423

Academic Editor: Eumorfia Kondili

Received: 12 July 2022
Accepted: 27 August 2022
Published: 31 August 2022

1. Introduction

SARS-CoV-2 is a member of the coronavirus family, a group of enveloped single-stranded RNA viruses. Over the last two years, the SARS-CoV-2 virus (COVID-19) pandemic has spread globally, affecting almost every country worldwide [1]. Clinical signs of COVID-19 differ from mild illness to very severe disease requiring hospitalization with an often fatal outcome [2]. In persons with critical clinical illness due to SARS-CoV-2, the respiratory system is the most commonly affected. However, the virus can affect all systems [3].

The virus binds to angiotensin-converting enzyme 2 (ACE2) receptors present in almost all vascular endothelial cells [4]. COVID-19 mortality and morbidity are affected by many different factors, i.e., gender, aging and several chronic diseases such as chronic respiratory disease/asthma, heart arrhythmias, hypertension, coronary disease, diabetes and neoplasia [5]. Inherited diseases and genetic predispositions such as hemoglobinopathies in homozygous or heterozygous status can also alter disease outcome [6].

Vaccination against SARS-CoV-2 has become crucial for limiting disease transmission and reducing its severity, hospitalization and mortality [7]. More specifically, data from systematic reviews underline the efficacy of vaccination in terms of clinical severity and mortality [8,9]. Despite universal acceptance, vaccine hesitancy is still significant [10]. Finally, the prevalence of the Omicron variant changed the data in relation to previous emerging virus strains [11]. In this context, analysis of real-world data regarding the clinical severity and mortality of COVID-19 during the next stages of the pandemic is essential in order to guide the national health policy.

The first Omicron sequence available, however, was from a specimen collected on 11 November 2021 in Botswana. Ever since the identification of Omicron, the variant appears to have rapidly spread. The early doubling time of the Beta, Delta and Omicron variants was calculated to be about 1.7, 1.5 and 1.2 days, respectively [12]. These data indicate that the Omicron variant is probably more infectious than the Delta and Beta variants. Analysis of the genomic sequences of the Omicron variant has revealed a high number of nonsynonymous mutations, including several ones in spike that have been proven to be involved in transmissibility, disease severity and immune escape [13].

In the present manuscript, we aim to assess COVID-19-attributed mortality and clinical severity after the prevalence of new variants of the virus (Delta and Omicron viral strains), to identify common risk factors and to evaluate the vaccination effect in fully vaccinated patients.

2. Materials and Methods

2.1. Settings

All consecutive patients that were hospitalized due to COVID-19 infection in the Respiratory Department of a tertiary referral center in Central Greece (University Hospital of Larisa) between 1 June 2021 and 1 February 2022 were included in the present study. Final diagnosis was established with a positive SARS-CoV-2 real-time polymerase chain reaction (RT-PCR) molecular test.

2.2. Participants and Study Design

A retrospective analysis of medical and laboratory records was conducted. An anonymous database of all patients that needed hospitalization due to COVID-19 infection was created and included both the medical history of common morbidities and clinical records during their hospitalization. Basic demographic characteristics of age and gender and common morbidities, including atrial fibrillation, chronic respiratory disease, coronary disease, diabetes, malignancy and hypertension were recorded. Moreover, vaccination status was recorded from the national vaccination registry.

As primary outcome of the present study was the association of clinical and demographic factors with mortality due to COVID-19 in infected individuals. Furthermore, clinical severity of symptomatology, classified according to the World Health Organization [14], and the length of hospitalization were considered as secondary endpoints.

Current smoking-status parameter was excluded from multivariate analysis due to insufficient data in the patients' records, and based on the univariate analysis, no statistically significant correlations between smoking and mortality attributed to COVID-19 were found. Furthermore, patients <18 years of age were excluded from the present study.

2.3. Ethical Considerations

Experimental therapeutic protocols were not applicable in this study. All data were analyzed anonymously, using code numbers with respect to the patient's privacy, and collected in the context of routine diagnostic and therapeutic procedures. The study conformed to the Research and Ethical Committee guidelines of the University Hospital of Larissa.

2.4. Statistical Analysis

Analysis was carried out with SPSS version 26.0. Categorical variables are described with the use of frequency and relative frequency. Continuous variables are described with means and standard deviation. The analysis of continuous variables was conducted using the Mann–Whitney U test since the assumption of normal distribution was violated. Data were checked for deviation from normal distribution using Shapiro–Wilk normality test. Categorical data were analyzed with the use of Chi-square test or Fisher's exact test; multivariate analysis was performed in the form of binary logistic regression. For all analyses, a 5% significance level was set.

3. Results

In total, 760 consecutive patients were hospitalized in a 7-month period in our department and included in the present study. A total of 671 (88.3%) of patients were diagnosed with moderate symptomatology of COVID-19, and 89 (11.7%) experienced severe symptoms. Furthermore, 220 (38.7%) patients were fully vaccinated against SARS-CoV-2 with two doses of one of the four vaccines licensed in Greece (Pfizer/BioNTech Comirnaty, AstraZeneca/AZD1222, Janssen/Ad26.COV 2.S Johnson & Johnson, Moderna COVID-19-mRNA 1273 vaccines). COVID-19 infection was the single most common official cause of death for our study participants, as registered in hospital archives. The fatality rate was calculated at 10.1% (77/760).

In Table 1 are displayed the results of univariate and multivariate statistical analysis regarding mortality risk due to COVID-19 infection. In univariate analysis, increased age ($p < 0.001$), atrial fibrillation (OR = 3.47, $p < 0.001$), chronic respiratory disease (OR = 2.59, $p = 0.004$), coronary disease (OR = 3.83, $p < 0.001$), diabetes type II (OR = 2.5, $p < 0.001$), dyslipidemia (OR = 2.94, $p < 0.001$) and hypertension (OR = 3.41, $p < 0.001$) have been associated with increased mortality attributed to COVID-19. More specifically, regarding the cardiovascular system, patients with atrial fibrillation, coronary disease and hypertension had almost 3.5, 4 and 3.5 times increased mortality risk, respectively, compared with patients without these comorbidities. Moreover, diabetic patients were associated with 2.5 times increased possibility of mortality, while patients with chronic respiratory diseases were 2.6 times more likely to decease after the COVID-19 infection.

Table 1. Assessment of mortality risk due to COVID-19 by univariate and multivariate statistical analysis.

	Mortality	Univariate			Multivariate Binary Logistic Regression	
	Yes (%)	Significance	OR with 95% CI	RR with 95% CI	Significance	aOR with 95% CI
Male gender	45 (13.9)	0.805 (C)	1.09 (0.67–1.78)	1.08 (0.71–1.65)	0.013	2.29 (1.19–4.39)
Age (median, IQR)	Dead: 83 (13) Alive: 61 (26)	<0.001 (M-W)	–		<0.001	1.12 (1.09–1.16)
Smoking *	2 (3.6)	0.521 (F)	0.48 (0.10–2.24)	0.50 (0.11–2.19)	Insufficient data	
Vaccination	24 (10.9)	0.169 (C)	0.70 (0.42–1.17)	0.73 (0.46–1.15)	<0.001	0.20 (0.10–0.39)
Atrial fibrillation	23 (29.9)	<0.001 (C)	3.47 (1.98–6.10)	2.73 (1.79–4.18)	0.500	1.27 (0.63–2.56)
Chronic respiratory fisease	14 (26.4)	0.004 (C)	2.59 (1.33–5.04)	2.17 (1.31–3.60)	0.437	1.40 (0.60–3.24)
Coronary disease	27 (30.7)	<0.001 (C)	3.83 (2.24–6.57)	2.96 (1.97–4.46)	0.549	1.24 (0.62–2.47)
Diabetes type II	23 (24.2)	0.001 (C)	2.50 (1.44–4.32)	2.13 (1.38–3.30)	0.218	1.56 (0.77–2.18)
Malignancy	7 (14.9)	0.768 (C)	1.14 (0.49–2.63)	1.12 (0.54–2.28)	0.803	1.14 (0.42–3.09)
Dyslipidemia	39 (23.4)	<0.001 (C)	2.94 (1.80–4.79)	2.48 (1.65–3.74)	0.090	1.75 (0.92–3.35)
Hypertension	57 (20.2)	<0.001 (C)	3.41 (1.99–5.84)	2.92 (1.80–4.73)	0.692	1.16 (0.56–2.38)

C: Chi-square test; F: Fisher's exact test M-W: Mann-Whitney U test

* Insufficient data.

In logistic regression of our primary outcome, only increased age (aOR = 1.12, $p < 0.001$), male gender (aOR = 2.29, $p = 0.013$) and vaccination against SARS-CoV-2 virus (aOR = 0.2, $p < 0.001$) were associated with mortality attributed to COVID-19 with a statistically significant association. More precisely, every additional year of age increased the possibility of death by 12% and male patients had almost 2.5 times increased mortality risk compared to females. Moreover, vaccinated patients were associated with a 5 times decreased mortality risk (Figure 1). A result that is worth being underlined is the fact that after the vaccination effect, in multivariate analysis, severe and common comorbidities were not associated with increased mortality risk.

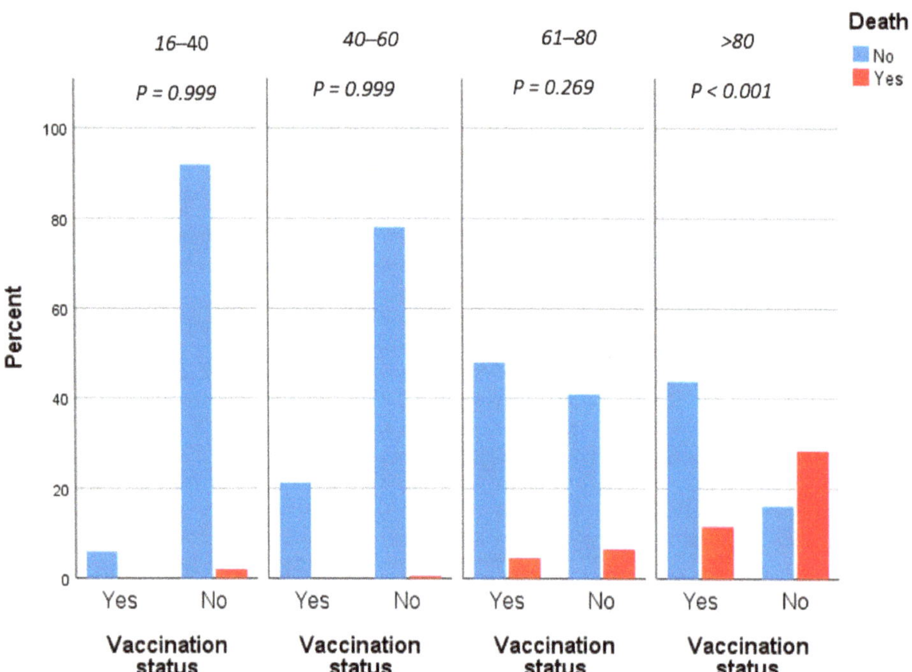

Figure 1. Fatality rates grouped by vaccination status and adjusted by age.

Table 2 displays the results of univariate and multivariate statistical analysis regarding the clinical severity of COVID-19. Increased age ($p < 0.001$), atrial fibrillation (OR = 2.76, $p < 0.001$), chronic respiratory disease (OR = 2.37, $p = 0.007$), coronary disease (OR = 3.01, $p < 0.001$), diabetes type II (OR = 2.3, $p = 0.002$), dyslipidemia (OR = 2.85, $p < 0.001$) and hypertension (OR = 2.91, $p < 0.001$) have been associated with increased mortality attributed to COVID-19. However, similar to the mortality risk assessment, in logistic regression, only increasing age (aOR = 1.09, $p < 0.001$), male gender (aOR = 1.92, $p = 0.025$) and vaccination against SARS-CoV-2 virus (aOR = 0.25, $p < 0.001$) were statistically significantly associated with clinical severity of COVID-19 infection. In this context, every additional year of age increased the risk of severe disease by 9%, while male patients had almost double the risk of severe COVID-19. Similar to the mortality risk, unvaccinated individuals had four times a greater risk of severe infection compared to vaccinated patients (Figure 2).

However, when comparing the length of hospitalization between vaccinated and unvaccinated patients, the difference was not statistically significant between the two groups ($p = 0.138$) (Figure 3).

Table 2. Assessment of clinical severity of COVID-19 by univariate and multivariate statistical analysis.

	Severe COVID-19 (N = 89)	Univariate			Multivariate Binary Logistic Regression	
		Significance	**OR with 95% CI**	**RR with 95% CI**	**Significance**	**aOR with 95% CI**
Male gender	51 (15.8)	0.879 (C)	1.04 (0.66–1.64)	1.03 (0.70–1.52)	0.025	1.92 (1.09–3.41)
Age (median, IQR)	Moderate: 61 (13) Severe: 83 (26)	<0.001 (M-W)	–		<0.001	1.09 (1.06–1.11)
Smoking *	5 (8.9)	0.789 (F)	1.16 (0.39–3.46)	1.15 (0.42–3.11)	Insufficient data	
Vaccination	27 (12.3)	0.109 (C)	0.67 (0.41–1.10)	071 (0.47–1.09)	<0.001	0.25 (0.14–0.45)
Atrial fibrillation	23 (29.9)	<0.001 (C)	2.76 (1.59–4.80)	2.24 (1.49–3.37)	0.712	1.13 (0.59–2.19)
Chronic respiratory disease	15 (28.3) 74 (14.3)	0.007 (C)	2.37 (1.24–4.52)	1.98 (1.23–3.19)	0.406	1.39 (0.64–3.04)
Coronary disease	27 (30.7) 62 (12.8)	<0.001 (C)	3.01 (1.78–5.08)	2.39 (1.62–3.53)	0.892	1.05 (0.55–2.00)
Diabetes type II	25 (26.3) 64 (13.4)	0.002 (C)	2.30 (1.36–3.90)	1.96 (1.30–2.94)	0.272	1.44 (0.75–2.78)
Malignancy	11 (23.4) 78 (14.9)	0.123 (C)	1.75 (0.85–3.58)	1.57 (0.90–2.74)	0.142	1.85 (0.81–4.23)
Dyslipidemia	44 (26.3) 45 (11.1)	<0.001 (C)	2.85 (1.80–4.54)	2.37 (1.63–3.44)	0.056	1.76 (0.99–3.12)
Hypertension	63 (22.3) 26 (9.0)	<0.001 (C)	2.91 (1.78–4.75)	2.48 (1.62–3.80)	0.748	1.11 (0.59–2.07)

C: Chi-square test; F: Fisher's exact test M-W: Mann-Whitney U test

* Insufficient data.

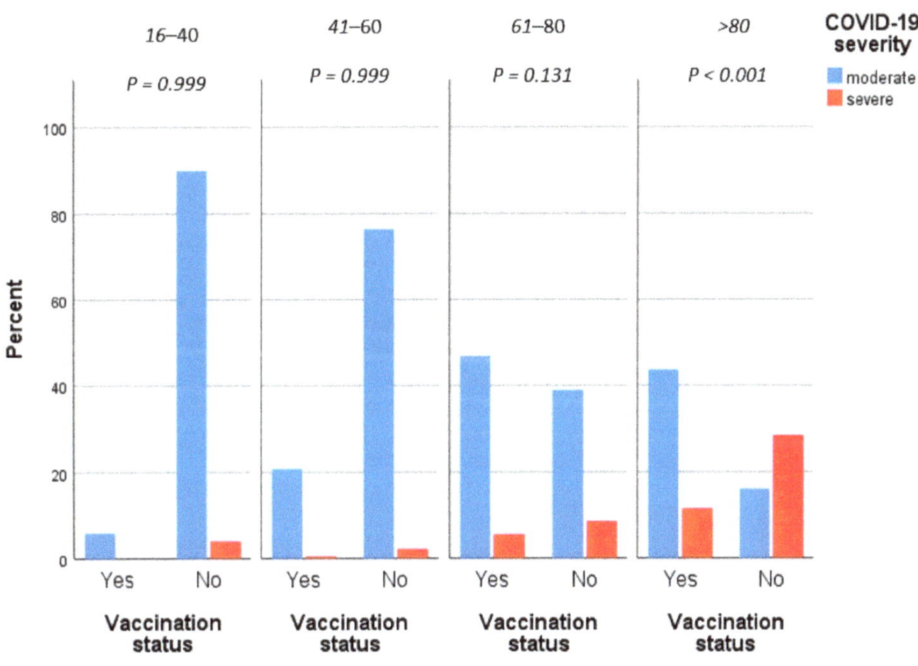

Figure 2. Severity grouped by vaccination status.

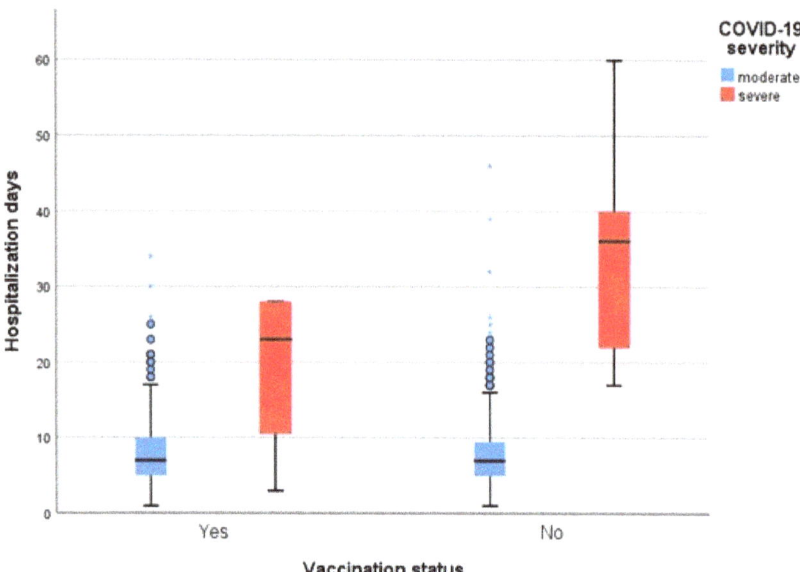

Figure 3. Length of hospitalization grouped by vaccination status and adjusted by clinical severity.

4. Discussion

The present study confirmed the protective effect of vaccination against the SARS-CoV-2 virus in terms of mortality and clinical severity of COVID-19 during the fourth wave of the pandemic in Central Greece. More specifically, vaccinated patients were associated with a 5 times decreased mortality risk and 4 times decreased risk of severe infection compared to unvaccinated individuals. Furthermore, the vaccination coverage between the hospitalized due to COVID-19 infection patient was relatively low at 28.9%, compared with the national vaccination coverage during the same time period. Additionally, in multivariate analysis, except for vaccination, male gender and aging were also identified as independent risk factors for mortality and increased clinical severity of COVID-19 infection.

Identifying mutations of SARS-CoV-2 is crucial, especially those with significant clinical impact and variants of concern (VOC), as they can modify public health policies, surveillance and immunization strategies [15,16]. Delta was the predominant SARS-CoV-2 variant during the fourth COVID-19 wave in many countries worldwide, including Greece; however, the novel Omicron variant rapidly spread due to the increased transmissibility of the variant [17,18]. Early observations suggest that the Omicron outbreak occurred more quickly and with larger magnitude, and despite substantial increases in vaccinations and prior infections, may be less severe than those caused by other virus strains [19,20]. In line with these observations, the fatality rate of the present study was 10.1% compared to the 24.9% that was observed during the second and third waves of the pandemic in Central Greece [6].

Developing COVID-19 vaccines within a short timeframe has raised several concerns about the safety and efficacy of the vaccines, which have been assessed by many studies. A recently published systematic review [21] analyzed the efficacy of different licensed vaccines based on 42 original studies and concluded that COVID-19 vaccines successfully reduced the rates of infections, severity, hospitalization and mortality. More specifically, the Pfizer/BioNTech vaccine was the most extensively studied among the COVID-19 vaccines with >90% effectiveness, followed by the Moderna vaccine with >80% effectiveness against infection, the AstraZeneca vaccine with 80.7% effectiveness against infection after the second dose and 74% effectiveness against infection after the first dose, and a single dose of the Johnson & Johnson vaccine with >60% effectiveness against infection [22].

The determinants of effectiveness of the approved vaccine against SARS-CoV-2 virus and breakthrough rates are yet to be determined, especially in light of the emergence of viral VOC [23]. In a recently published prospective study of fully vaccinated COVID-19 patients needing hospitalization due to COVID-19 infection, older age, lower real-time PCR cycle threshold values and a shorter duration between symptom onset and hospital admission were associated with a lack of anti-S SARS-CoV-2 antibodies and poor clinical outcomes of COVID-19 disease [23]. Moreover, published data from the COVAX study revealed that diabetic patients had significantly higher possibilities to have undetectable antibodies on hospital admission due to COVID-19 [24].

The beneficial role of the national vaccination campaign in Greece in terms of SARS-CoV-2 cases, ICU admissions and mortality is well-documented [25]. Another recent study by Lytras et al. [24] documented the high and durable effectiveness of COVID-19 vaccination in preventing severe disease and mortality in all age groups, both against Delta and older SARS-CoV-2 variants; however, the study lacks data regarding the Omicron strain. It is estimated that vaccination prevented approximately 19,691 COVID-19 deaths during 2021 in Greece [26].

Several studies reported a reduction in effectiveness of COVID-19 vaccination against variants of the virus compared to the original strain [27–30]. The accumulation of mutations in these VOCs and others demonstrates the quantifiable risk of antigenic drift and subsequent reduction in vaccine efficacy [31]. Neutralization titers against VOCs were 3-fold lower when analyzing convalescent sera and 3.3-fold and 2.5-fold lower for Pfizer and AstraZeneca vaccinees, respectively [27]. Moreover, Kodera et al. [32] estimated the effectiveness of vaccination at 62.1% (95% CI: 48–66%) compared to the Delta variant. However, the impact of this reduction of the vaccination's effectiveness in molecular level with waning antibody levels remains unclear. Our study confirms the protective role of vaccination from severe disease caused by mutated virus strains.

A finding of a great interest is the fact that vaccination modifies common risk factors that had been strongly associated with COVID-19-attributed mortality and morbidity. Underlying comorbidities including hypertension, diabetes, chronic respiratory diseases, cardiac disease and malignancy have been previously associated with severe infection [33,34]. According to the results of several studies, acute and chronic kidney disease, COPD, diabetes, hypertension, cardiovascular disease, cancer, increased D-dimer, male gender, older age, being a current smoker and obesity are clinical risk factors associated with mortality due to COVID-19 [35–37]. In univariate analysis of our data, atrial fibrillation, coronary disease and hypertension were associated with 3.5, 4 and 3.5 times increased mortality risk, respectively, compared with patients without these comorbidities. Moreover, diabetic patients were associated with 2.5 times increased possibility of mortality, while patients with chronic respiratory diseases were 2.6 times more likely to decease after the COVID-19 infection. The modification of these possibilities in multivariate analysis indicates the crucial protective role of vaccination in high-risk patients. In line with these observations, national vaccination campaigns have to focus on vulnerable populations that are expected to be benefited the most by vaccination's protection. Campaigns informing the general population regarding the safety and efficacy of the new COVID-19 vaccines could reinforce the acceptability of vaccination [38,39].

Prior to the appraisal of our results, several limitations should be considered. Data were collected from a database of consecutive patients, eliminating the possibility of selection bias. However, information bias may have occurred due to the retrospective design of the present study, depending on the availability and accuracy of data records. Moreover, missing data regarding current smoking status and the lack of data regarding obesity profile remain two major limitations of our study. Furthermore, data were collected from a single tertiary hospital including only hospitalized patients, and the generalization of our findings is limited.

5. Conclusions

Vaccination against the SARS-CoV-2 virus had a protective effect on terms of mortality and clinical severity of COVID-19 during the fourth wave of the pandemic in Central Greece. Moreover, vaccination modified common risk factors, including hypertension, diabetes, chronic respiratory diseases, cardiac disease and malignancy, that had been strongly associated with COVID-19-attributed mortality. The national vaccination policy has to focus on vulnerable populations that are expected to benefit the most from the vaccine's protection.

Author Contributions: Conceptualization, A.A.S., S.B., K.I.G. and S.S.; data curation, M.B.J.; formal analysis, A.A.S.; investigation, S.B. and M.B.J.; methodology, M.B.J., K.I.G. and S.S.; supervision, K.I.G. and S.S.; writing—original draft, A.A.S. and S.B.; writing—review and editing, M.B.J., K.I.G. and S.S. All authors have read and agreed to the published version of the manuscript.

Funding: This research received no external funding.

Institutional Review Board Statement: The study was conducted according to the guidelines of the Declaration of Helsinki, and approved by the Ethics Committee of the University Hospital of Larissa, Greece (46943/29 November 2021).

Informed Consent Statement: Informed consent was obtained from all subjects involved in the study.

Data Availability Statement: Data are available upon reasoning request.

Conflicts of Interest: The authors declare no conflict of interest.

References

1. World Health Organization. WHO Coronavirus (COVID-19) Dashboard. Available online: https://covid19.who.int/ (accessed on 8 January 2022).
2. Wang, Y.; Wang, Y.; Chen, Y.; Qin, Q. Unique epidemiological and clinical features of the emerging 2019 novel coronavirus pneumonia (COVID-19) implicate special control measures. *J. Med. Virol.* **2020**, *92*, 568–576. [CrossRef] [PubMed]
3. Jain, U. Effect of COVID-19 on the Organs. *Cureus* **2020**, *12*, e9540. [CrossRef] [PubMed]
4. Zou, X.; Chen, K.; Zou, J.; Han, P.; Hao, J.; Han, Z. Single-cell RNA-seq data analysis on the receptor ACE2 expression reveals the potential risk of different human organs vulnerable to 2019-nCoV infection. *Front. Med.* **2020**, *14*, 185–192. [CrossRef]
5. Maximiano Sousa, F.; Roelens, M.; Fricker, B.; Thiabaud, A.; Iten, A.; Cusini, A.; Flury, D.; Buettcher, M.; Zukol, F.; Balmelli, C.; et al. Risk factors for severe outcomes for COVID-19 patients hospitalised in Switzerland during the first pandemic wave, February to August 2020: Prospective observational cohort study. *Swiss Med. Wkly.* **2021**, *151*, w20547. [CrossRef] [PubMed]
6. Sotiriou, S.; Samara, A.A.; Lachanas, K.E.; Vamvakopoulou, D.; Vamvakopoulos, K.-O.; Vamvakopoulos, N.; Janho, M.B.; Perivoliotis, K.; Donoudis, C.; Daponte, A.; et al. Vulnerability of β-Thalassemia Heterozygotes to COVID-19: Results from a Cohort Study. *J. Pers. Med.* **2022**, *12*, 352. [CrossRef]
7. Mohammed, I.; Nauman, A.; Paul, P.; Ganesan, S.; Chen, K.-H.; Jalil, S.M.S.; Jaouni, S.H.; Kawas, H.; Khan, W.A.; Vattoth, A.L.; et al. The efficacy and effectiveness of the COVID-19 vaccines in reducing infection, severity, hospitalization, and mortality: A systematic review. *Hum. Vaccines Immunother.* **2022**, *18*, 2027160. [CrossRef] [PubMed]
8. Huang, Y.Z.; Kuan, C.C. Vaccination to reduce severe COVID-19 and mortality in COVID-19 patients: A systematic review and meta-analysis. *Eur. Rev. Med. Pharmacol. Sci.* **2022**, *26*, 1770–1776. [CrossRef]
9. Lopez Bernal, J.; Andrews, N.; Gower, C.; Robertson, C.; Stowe, J.; Tessier, E.; Simmons, R.; Cottrell, S.; Roberts, R.; O'Doherty, M.; et al. Effectiveness of the Pfizer-BioNTech and Oxford-AstraZeneca vaccines on COVID-19 related symptoms, hospital admissions, and mortality in older adults in England: Test negative case-control study. *BMJ* **2021**, *373*, n1088. [CrossRef]
10. Gravelle, T.B.; Phillips, J.B.; Reifler, J.; Scotto, T.J. Estimating the size of "anti-vax" and vaccine hesitant populations in the US, UK, and Canada: Comparative latent class modeling of vaccine attitudes. *Hum. Vaccines Immunother.* **2022**, *18*, 2008214. [CrossRef]
11. Joshi, G.; Poduri, R. Omicron, a new SARS-CoV-2 variant: Assessing the impact on severity and vaccines efficacy. *Hum. Vaccines Immunother.* **2022**, *18*, 2034458. [CrossRef]
12. Karim, S.S.A.; Karim, Q.A. Omicron SARS-CoV-2 Variant: A New Chapter in the COVID-19 Pandemic. *Lancet* **2021**, *398*, 2126–2128. [CrossRef]
13. He, X.M.; Hong, W.Q.; Pan, X.Y.; Lu, G.W.; Wei, X.W. SARS-CoV-2 Omicron variant: Characteristics and prevention. *MedComm* **2021**, *2*, 838–845. [CrossRef] [PubMed]
14. World Health Organization. Living Guidance for Clinical Management of COVID-19. Available online: https://apps.who.int/iris/bitstream/handle/10665/349321/WHO-2019-nCoV-clinical-2021.2-eng.pdf (accessed on 8 July 2022).

15. Nonaka, C.K.; Franco, M.M.; Gräf, T.; de Lorenzo Barcia, C.A.; de Ávila Mendonça, R.N.; de Sousa, K.A.; Neiva, L.M.; Fosenca, V.; Mendes, A.V.; de Aguiar, R.S.; et al. Genomic Evidence of SARS-CoV-2 Reinfection Involving E484K Spike Mutation, Brazil. *Emerg. Infect. Dis.* **2021**, *27*, 1522–1524. [CrossRef] [PubMed]
16. Halvatsiotis, P.; Vassiliu, S.; Koulouvaris, P.; Chatzantonaki, K.; Asonitis, K.; Charvalos, E.; Siatelis, A.; Houhoula, D. Severe Acute Respiratory Syndrome Coronavirus 2 (SARS-CoV-2) Mutational Pattern in the Fourth Pandemic Phase in Greece. *Curr. Issues Mol. Biol.* **2022**, *44*, 329–335. [CrossRef]
17. Del Rio, C.; Omer, S.B.; Malani, P.N. Winter of Omicron—The Evolving COVID-19 Pandemic. *JAMA* **2022**, *327*, 319–320. [CrossRef]
18. Chassalevris, T.; Chaintoutis, S.C.; Koureas, M.; Petala, M.; Moutou, E.; Beta, C.; Kyritsi, M.; Hadjichristodoulou, C.; Kostoglou, M.; Karapantsios, T.; et al. SARS-CoV-2 wastewater monitoring using a novel PCR-based method rapidly captured the Delta-to-Omicron BA.1 transition patterns in the absence of conventional surveillance evidence. *Sci. Total Environ.* **2022**, *844*, 156932. [CrossRef] [PubMed]
19. Wrenn, J.O.; Pakala, S.B.; Vestal, G.; Shilts, M.H.; Brown, H.M.; Bowen, S.M.; Strickland, B.A.; Williams, T.; Mallal, S.A.; Jones, I.D.; et al. COVID-19 severity from Omicron and Delta SARS-CoV-2 variants. *Influ. Other Respir. Viruses* **2022**, *16*, 832–836. [CrossRef]
20. Lundberg, A.L.; Lorenzo-Redondo, R.; Ozer, E.A.; Hawkins, C.A.; Hultquist, J.F.; Welch, S.B.; Prasad, P.V.; Oehmke, J.F.; Achenbach, C.J.; Murphy, R.L.; et al. Has Omicron Changed the Evolution of the Pandemic? *JMIR Public Health Surveill.* **2022**, *8*, e35763. [CrossRef]
21. Di Fusco, M.; Lin, J.; Vaghela, S.; Lingohr-Smith, M.; Nguyen, J.L.; Sforzolini, T.S.; Judy, J.; Cane, A.; Moran, M.M. COVID-19 vaccine effectiveness among immunocompromised populations: A targeted literature review of real-world studies. *Expert Rev. Vaccines* **2022**, *21*, 435–451. [CrossRef]
22. Lipsitch, M.; Krammer, F.; Regev-Yochay, G.; Lustig, Y.; Balicer, R.D. SARS-CoV-2 breakthrough infections in vaccinated individuals: Measurement, causes and impact. *Nat. Rev. Immunol.* **2022**, *22*, 57–65. [CrossRef]
23. Livanou, E.; Rouka, E.; Sinis, S.; Dimeas, I.; Pantazopoulos, I.; Papagiannis, D.; Malli, F.; Kotsiou, O.; Gourgoulianis, K.I. Predictors of SARS-CoV-2 IgG Spike Antibody Responses on Admission and Clinical Outcomes of COVID-19 Disease in Fully Vaccinated Inpatients: The CoVax Study. *J. Pers. Med.* **2022**, *12*, 640. [CrossRef] [PubMed]
24. Rouka, E.; Livanou, E.; Sinis, S.; Dimeas, I.; Pantazopoulos, I.; Papagiannis, D.; Malli, F.; Kotsiou, O.; Gourgoulianis, K.I. Immune response to the severe acute respiratory syndrome coronavirus 2 vaccines: Is it sustained in the diabetes population? *J. Diabetes Investig.* **2020**, *13*, 1461–1462. [CrossRef] [PubMed]
25. Malli, F.; Lampropoulos, I.C.; Papagiannis, D.; Papathanasiou, I.V.; Daniil, Z.; Gourgoulianis, K.I. Association of SARS-CoV-2 Vaccinations with SARS-CoV-2 Infections, ICU Admissions and Deaths in Greece. *Vaccines* **2022**, *10*, 337. [CrossRef] [PubMed]
26. Lytras, T.; Kontopidou, F.; Lambrou, A.; Tsiodras, S. Comparative effectiveness and durability of COVID-19 vaccination against death and severe disease in an ongoing nationwide mass vaccination campaign. *J. Med. Virol.* **2022**, *94*, 5044–5050. [CrossRef]
27. Jabłońska, K.; Aballéa, S.; Toumi, M. The real-life impact of vaccination on COVID-19 mortality in Europe and Israel. *Public Health* **2021**, *198*, 230–237. [CrossRef]
28. Zuckerman, N.; Nemet, I.; Kliker, L.; Atari, N.; Lustig, Y.; Bucris, E.; Bar Ilan, D.; Geva, M.; Sorek-Abramovich, R.; Weiner, C.; et al. The SARS-CoV-2 Lambda variant and its neutralisation efficiency following vaccination with Comirnaty, Israel, April to June 2021. *Eurosurveillance* **2021**, *26*, 2100974. [CrossRef]
29. Lustig, Y.; Zuckerman, N.; Nemet, I.; Atari, N.; Kliker, L.; Regev-Yochay, G.; Sapir, E.; Mor, O.; Alroy-Preis, S.; Mendelson, E.; et al. Neutralising capacity against Delta (B.1.617.2) and other variants of concern following Comirnaty (BNT162b2, BioNTech/Pfizer) vaccination in health care workers, Israel. *Eurosurveillance* **2021**, *26*, 2100557. [CrossRef]
30. Trabace, L.; Pace, L.; Morgese, M.G.; Santo, I.B.; Galante, D.; Schiavone, S.; Cipolletta, D.; Rosa, A.M.; Reveglia, P.; Parisi, A.; et al. SARS-CoV-2 Gamma and Delta Variants of Concern Might Undermine Neutralizing Activity Generated in Response to BNT162b2 mRNA Vaccination. *Viruses* **2022**, *14*, 814. [CrossRef]
31. Davis, C.; Logan, N.; Tyson, G.; Orton, R.; Harvey, W.T.; Perkins, J.S.; Mollett, G.; Blacow, R.M.; The COVID-19 Genomics UK (COG-UK) Consortium; Peacock, T.P.; et al. Reduced neutralisation of the Delta (B.1.617.2) SARS-CoV-2 variant of concern following vaccination. *PLOS Pathog.* **2021**, *17*, e1010022. [CrossRef]
32. Kodera, S.; Rashed, E.A.; Hirata, A. Estimation of Real-World Vaccination Effectiveness of mRNA COVID-19 Vaccines against Delta and Omicron Variants in Japan. *Vaccines* **2022**, *10*, 430. [CrossRef]
33. Gao, Y.-D.; Ding, M.; Dong, X.; Zhang, J.-J.; Azkur, A.K.; Azkur, D.; Gan, H.; Sun, Y.-L.; Fu, W.; Li, W.; et al. Risk factors for severe and critically ill COVID-19 patients: A review. *Allergy* **2021**, *76*, 428–455. [CrossRef] [PubMed]
34. Sotiriou, S.; Samara, A.A.; Vamvakopoulou, D.; Vamvakopoulos, K.-O.; Sidiropoulos, A.; Vamvakopoulos, N.; Janho, M.B.; Gourgoulianis, K.I.; Boutlas, S. Susceptibility of β-Thalassemia Heterozygotes to COVID-19. *J. Clin. Med.* **2021**, *10*, 3645. [CrossRef]
35. Dessie, Z.G.; Zewotir, T. Mortality-related risk factors of COVID-19: A systematic review and meta-analysis of 42 studies and 423,117 patients. *BMC Infect. Dis.* **2021**, *21*, 855. [CrossRef] [PubMed]
36. Izcovich, A.; Ragusa, M.A.; Tortosa, F.; Marzio, M.A.L.; Agnoletti, C.; Bengolea, A.; Ceirano, A.; Espinosa, F.; Saavedra, E.; Sanguine, V.; et al. Prognostic factors for severity and mortality in patients infected with COVID-19: A systematic review. *PLoS ONE* **2020**, *15*, e0241955. [CrossRef]
37. Vimercati, L.; De Maria, L.; Quarato, M.; Caputi, A.; Gesualdo, L.; Migliore, G.; Cavone, D.; Sponselli, S.; Pipoli, A.; Inchingolo, F.; et al. Association between Long COVID and Overweight/Obesity. *J. Clin. Med.* **2021**, *10*, 4143. [CrossRef]

38. Davis, C.J.; Golding, M.; McKay, R. Efficacy information influences intention to take COVID-19 vaccine. *Br. J. Health Psychol.* **2022**, *27*, 300–319. [CrossRef]
39. Bianchi, F.P.; Tafuri, S.; Migliore, G.; Vimercati, L.; Martinelli, A.; Lobifaro, A.; Diella, G.; Stefanizzi, P.; on behalf of the Control Room Working Group. BNT162b2 mRNA COVID-19 Vaccine Effectiveness in the Prevention of SARS-CoV-2 Infection and Symptomatic Disease in Five-Month Follow-Up: A Retrospective Cohort Study. *Vaccines* **2021**, *9*, 1143. [CrossRef]

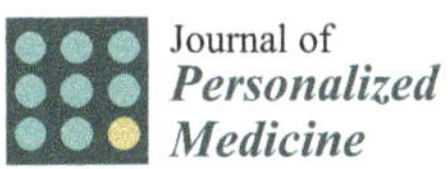
Journal of *Personalized Medicine*

MDPI

Article

Predictors of SARS-CoV-2 IgG Spike Antibody Responses on Admission and Clinical Outcomes of COVID-19 Disease in Fully Vaccinated Inpatients: The CoVax Study

Eleni Livanou [1,†], Erasmia Rouka [1,*,†], Sotirios Sinis [1], Ilias Dimeas [1], Ioannis Pantazopoulos [1], Dimitrios Papagiannis [2], Foteini Malli [2], Ourania Kotsiou [2] and Konstantinos I. Gourgoulianis [1]

1 Department of Respiratory Medicine, Faculty of Medicine, University of Thessaly, 41110 Larissa, Greece; elivanou97@gmail.com (E.L.); sinis1995@windowslive.com (S.S.); dimel13@hotmail.com (I.D.); pantazopoulosioannis@yahoo.com (I.P.); kgourg@med.uth.gr (K.I.G.)
2 Faculty of Nursing, University of Thessaly, 41500 Larissa, Greece; dpapajon@gmail.com (D.P.); mallifoteini@yahoo.gr (F.M.); raniakotsiou@gmail.com (O.K.)
* Correspondence: errouka@med.uth.gr
† These authors contributed equally to this work.

Abstract: Background: SARS-CoV-2 vaccines have shown high efficacy in protecting against COVID-19, although the determinants of vaccine effectiveness and breakthrough rates are yet to be determined. We aimed at investigating several factors affecting the SARS-CoV-2 IgG Spike (S) antibody responses on admission and clinical outcomes of COVID-19 disease in fully vaccinated, hospitalized patients. Methods: 102 subjects were enrolled in the study. Blood serum samples were collected from each patient upon admission for the semiquantitative determination of the SARS-CoV-2 IgG S levels with lateral flow assays. Factors influencing vaccine responses were documented. Results: 27 subjects had a negative antibody test upon hospital admission. Out of the 102 patients admitted to the hospital, 88 were discharged and 14 died. Both the absence of anti-S SARS-CoV-2 antibodies and poor clinical outcomes of COVID-19 disease were associated with older age, lower Ct values, and a shorter period between symptom onset and hospital admission. Ct values and time between symptom onset and hospitalization were independently associated with SARS-CoV-2 IgG S responses upon admission. The PaO2/FiO2 ratio was identified as an independent predictor of in-hospital mortality. Conclusions: Host- and disease-associated factors can predict SARS-CoV-2 IgG S responses and mortality in hospitalized patients with breakthrough SARS-CoV-2 Infection.

Keywords: breakthrough COVID-19 hospitalizations; clinical outcomes; SARS-CoV-2 IgG Spike responses; vaccine-induced immunity

Citation: Livanou, E.; Rouka, E.; Sinis, S.; Dimeas, I.; Pantazopoulos, I.; Papagiannis, D.; Malli, F.; Kotsiou, O.; Gourgoulianis, K.I. Predictors of SARS-CoV-2 IgG Spike Antibody Responses on Admission and Clinical Outcomes of COVID-19 Disease in Fully Vaccinated Inpatients: The CoVax Study. *J. Pers. Med.* **2022**, *12*, 640. https://doi.org/10.3390/jpm12040640

Academic Editor: Luisa Brussino

Received: 6 March 2022
Accepted: 11 April 2022
Published: 15 April 2022

1. Introduction

The ongoing COVID-19 pandemic, caused by the severe acute respiratory syndrome coronavirus 2 (SARS-CoV-2), has become a significant global public health issue [1]. As of 28 January 2022, there has been 364,191,494 confirmed cases of COVID-19 worldwide, with 5,631,457 deaths reported to the World Health Organization (https://covid19.who.int/, accessed: 29 January 2022). SARS-CoV-2 causes a variety of symptoms ranging from mild, flu-like symptoms to severe pulmonary damage with respiratory distress syndrome and death [2]. Subjects with pre-existing comorbidities including obesity, cardiovascular disease, type 2 diabetes mellitus (T2D), and chronic renal and lung disease are at an increased risk of developing acute respiratory distress syndrome (ARDS), requiring mechanical ventilation and admission to the intensive care unit (ICU) [3].

Vaccination is the most cost-effective medical intervention, preventing millions of deaths every year [4]. Vaccines have greatly reduced the burden of infectious diseases [5] and constitute an important tool for limiting epidemics caused by emerging pathogens [4].

Vaccine-induced immunity is mediated by the complex interaction of innate, humoral, and cell-mediated immunity [6]. Vaccines operate by inducing an immune response and, as a result, an immunological memory, which protects against infection or disease [7].

The approved SARS-CoV-2 vaccines have been highly efficient in protecting against COVID-19 [8,9], although the determinants of vaccine effectiveness and breakthrough rates are yet to be determined, especially in light of the emergence of viral variants of concern [10]. Antibody responses to SARS-CoV-2 vaccines have been shown to be affected by a variety of factors, including age [11], sex [12], central obesity [13], hypertension [11,13], cancer [14], dyslipidemia [13], and smoking habits [11,13].

However, there is a plethora of factors that influence humoral and cellular vaccine responses in humans. These include intrinsic host factors as well as extrinsic, environmental, behavioral, nutritional, and vaccine factors [6]. Variables affecting the immune response to the SARS-CoV-2 vaccination have not been extensively investigated. In this study, we examine several factors that may have an impact on SARS-CoV-2 IgG Spike (S) antibody responses and the outcome of COVID-19 disease in fully vaccinated, hospitalized patients.

2. Materials and Methods

2.1. Study Design

Within two months we prospectively studied 102 fully vaccinated adult patients (71 men, 31 women) who were admitted to the COVID-19 Department of the University Hospital of Larissa, Greece. SARS-CoV-2 infection was verified by real-time reverse-transcription polymerase chain reaction (RT-PCR). Several factors that influence vaccine responses were documented [6] (Table 1). The patients were monitored until hospital discharge or death. The study was approved by the Institutional Research Ethics Committee (46943/29.11.2021) and each participant provided written informed consent.

Table 1. The factors that were investigated in the present study in terms of their effect on SARS-CoV-2 IgG S antibody responses.

General Information	Lifestyle	Comorbidities
Age Sex BMI Number of family members Days with symptoms from onset until admission Occupation	Smoking (pack/years) Alcohol (weekly consumption) Exercise (40 min/week) Fruit and vegetable consumption (Yes/No)	Diabetes (Yes/No) Coronary artery disease (Yes/No) Arterial hypertension (Yes/No) COPD-asthma (Yes/No) Obstructive apnea syndrome (Yes/No) Renal disease (Yes/No) Neoplasia (Yes/No) Autoimmune disease (Yes/No)
Drug Consumption	**Vaccine Information**	**Antibodies**
Immunosuppressive drugs before vaccination (Yes/No) probiotics (Yes/No) Antibiotics taken one week before or after vaccination (Yes/No) Nonsteroidal anti-inflammatory drugs one week before or after vaccination (Yes/No) Vitamin intake one week before or after vaccination (Yes/No)	Anxiety about vaccination (Yes/No) Vaccine type Vaccine doses Day since last dose Symptoms after vaccination (fever > 38, hand pain, arthralgia/myalgia)	Presence of anti-S SARS-CoV-2 antibodies on admission (Yes/No)

2.2. Detection of the SARS-CoV-2 IgG S Protein-Specific Antibodies

On the first day of hospitalization, blood serum samples were collected from each patient for the semiquantitative determination of the SARS-CoV-2 IgG S protein-specific antibodies with lateral flow immunochromatographic assays (Rapid Test 2019-nCoV IgG, ProGnosis Biotech, Larissa, Greece).

5 μL of serum per sample was injected into a test tube containing dilution buffer. A strip was then immersed in the tube for 15 min. Subsequently, the strips were scanned in the S-flow reader to interpret the results. The scanner could automatically calculate the ratio (T/C) by measuring the density of the test (T) and control (C) lines of the strip. Eight standards of recombinant antibodies were used in order to create the standard/ratio curve for the anti-S Ig semiquantification. A strip in which no colored line appeared in the control band was considered invalid.

In terms of diagnostic specificity, 468 samples of pre-pandemic COVID-19 patients were analyzed, with 100% specificity. A study was conducted with 122 patients who had clinical symptoms of COVID-19 and a positive PCR result for diagnostic sensitivity. The sensitivity was calculated to be 96.72% (Rapid Test 2019-nCoV IgG, V1430, Version 24 September 2021/rev.01, ProGnosis Biotech, Larissa, Greece).

Additional blood and serum samples were collected upon hospital admission for the evaluation of the following hematological and biochemical parameters: white blood cells (WBC), lymphocytes, platelets (PLT), C-reactive protein (CRP), creatinine, urea, aspartate transaminase (SGOT), alanine transaminase (SGPT), lactate dehydrogenase (LDH), ferritin, and creatine kinase (CPK).

2.3. Statistical Analysis

The SPSS v 19.0 software (IBM) was used to conduct the statistical analysis. Data distribution was assessed using the Kolmogorov–Smirnov normality test. The independent samples *T*-Test and the Mann–Whitney test were used to determine significant differences of parametric and non-parametric data, respectively, between two groups. Associations between categorical variables were determined with the Fisher's Exact Test. Correlations between quantitative variables were measured with the Pearson (r) or the Spearman (ρ) coefficients as appropriate. Logistic regression was used for the analysis of multiple variables influencing the presence of anti-S SARS-CoV-2 antibodies upon admission and the outcome of COVID-19 disease. All the variables with significant univariate associations were entered into the analysis in a single step (method selection: Enter). Statistical significance was set at the $p < 0.05$ level.

3. Results

3.1. Baseline Characteristics of the Study Population

The mean age of participants was 72.44 ± 1.22 years. Seventy-three subjects had received the BNT162b2/Pfizer vaccine, 22 the Vaxzevria, ChAdOx1-S/AstraZeneca vaccine, and 3 the Johnson & Johnson's Janssen COVID-19 Vaccine (information regarding the type of COVID-19 vaccine was unavailable for four subjects). The mean number of days since completion of vaccination was 159.03 ± 6.35. The mean real time PCR cycle threshold (Ct) value was 20.01 ± 0.54. The baseline laboratory characteristics of the study population are presented in Table 2.

Table 2. Baseline characteristics of the study population ($N = 102$).

	Cases With A Negative Antibody Test ($N = 27$)	Cases with Detectable Antibody Levels ($N = 75$)	p Value	Deceased Patients ($N = 14$)	Non-Deceased Patients ($N = 88$)	p Value
Age, years, median ± SD *	75 ± 11.1	73 ± 12.4	0.039	82 ± 8.3	71 ± 12.2	0.003
Body mass index, median ± SD	26 ± 4.5	26.9 ± 4.1	ns	24.8 ± 3.1	27.2 ± 4.1	0.029
Male sex (%)	18	52	ns	11.9	57.4	ns
Residence, urban (ratio)	0.7	0.76	ns	0.85	0.74	ns

Table 2. *Cont.*

	Cases With A Negative Antibody Test (N = 27)	Cases with Detectable Antibody Levels (N = 75)	p Value	Deceased Patients (N = 14)	Non-Deceased Patients (N = 88)	p Value
Use of probiotics (ratio)	0	0.03	ns	0	0.02	ns
Vitamin use (ratio)	0.26	0.16	ns	0.31	0.16	ns
Weekly exercise (ratio)	0.5	0.72	ns	0.61	0.68	ns
PaO2/FiO2 (PF) ratio < 150 mm Hg (ratio)	0.48	0.22	0.014	0.93	0.2	<0.001
Corticosteroids use before vaccination (ratio)	0.08	0.03	ns	0.07	0.04	ns
COVID-19 mRNA vaccination (ratio)	0.76	0.74	ns	1	0.70	0.035
Vaccination anxiety (ratio)	0.13	0.16	ns	0.23	0.15	ns
Symptoms post vaccination (ratio)	0.22	0.41	ns	0.15	0.39	ns
Days since last vaccination dose, median ± SD	168 ± 63.1	163 ± 59.6	ns	181 ± 77.1	163 ± 58.5	ns
Days from symptom onset to admission, median ± SD	4 ± 2.3	6 ± 2.3	<0.001	5 ± 2.2	6 ± 2.45	0.007
Hospitalization days, median ± SD	6 ± 9.2	6 ± 5.2	ns	6 ± 7.8	6 ± 6.3	ns
			Laboratory testing			
SARS-CoV-2 Cycle threshold, median ± SD	15.56 ± 4.15	19.84 ± 5.5	<0.001	16.26 ± 4.2	19.25 ± 5.57	0.036
Detection of anti-S SARS-CoV-2 IgG responses (ratio)	-	1	-	0.43	0.77	0.019
anti-S SARS-CoV-2 IgG titers (A.U.), median ± SD	-	2.83 ± 3.57	-	0 ± 1.53	1.49 ± 3.6	0.001 **
White blood cells ($\times 10^9$/L), median ± SD	6100.00 ± 3758.48	7600.00 ± 3734.09	ns	7950.00 ± 3877.3	7000.00 ± 3768.4	ns

Table 2. *Cont.*

	Cases With A Negative Antibody Test (*N* = 27)	Cases with Detectable Antibody Levels (*N* = 75)	*p* Value	Deceased Patients (*N* = 14)	Non-Deceased Patients (*N* = 88)	*p* Value
Lymphocytes ($\times 10^9$/L), median ± SD	640.00 ± 340.70	740.00 ± 1312.97	ns	595.00 ± 330.6	720.00 ± 1215.1	ns
Platelets ($\times 10^9$/L), median ± SD	205000.00 ± 58002.23	219000.00 ± 83154.72	ns	201000.00 ± 85309.13	215000.00 ± 77491.78	ns
C-Reactive protein (mg/dL), median ± SD	4.72 ± 10.67	8.31 ± 6.60	ns	13.18 ± 12.9	6.63 ± 6.45	ns
Creatinine (mg/dL), median ± SD	1.19 ± 0.92	0.9 ± 0.38	0.001 **	0.97 ± 1.27	0.94 ± 0.37	ns
Urea (mg/dL), median ± SD	46.50 ± 41.80	38.00 ± 38.96	ns	44.2 ± 55.2	38.2 ± 36.27	ns
Serum glutamic-oxaloacetic transaminase (IU/L), median ± SD	27.70 ± 34.80	28.00 ± 26.10	ns	34.7 ± 31.9	27.9 ± 27.5	ns
Serum glutamic pyruvic transaminase (IU/L), median ± SD	22.00 ± 27.73	24.00 ± 30.69	ns	21.65 ± 24.7	24.1 ± 27.2	ns
Lactate Dehydrogenase (IU/L), median ± SD	314.00 ± 221.34	357.00 ± 154.93	ns	371.5 ± 275.77	335.00 ± 143.81	ns
Ferritin (ng/mL), median ± SD	619.70 ± 615.67	588.20 ± 722.72	ns	653.50 ± 1189.80	581.75 ± 546.09	ns
Creatine Kinase (U/L), median ± SD	99.00 ± 637.14	97.00 ± 133.20	ns	115.50 ± 768.43	94.50 ± 212.89	ns
			Comorbidities			
Diabetes (ratio)	0.44	0.15	0.006	0.38	0.22	ns
Coronary disease (ratio)	0.3	0.2	ns	0.3	0.2	ns
Hypertension (ratio)	0.48	0.5	ns	0.16	0.55	0.014
Asthma, Chronic obstructive pulmonary disease (ratio)	0.12	0.10	ns	0.15	0.1	ns
Obstructive Sleep Apnea Syndrome (ratio)	0	0.01	ns	0.08	0	ns
Renal disease (ratio)	0.08	0.03	ns	0	0.05	ns
Cancer (ratio)	0.08	0.07	ns	0.07	0.07	ns
Autoimmune disease (ratio)	0.13	0.07	ns	0.08	0.1	ns

* SD; Standard deviation, ** Mann-Whitney U Test.

3.2. Factors Influencing SARS-CoV-2 IgG S Antibody Responses

Twenty-seven subjects had a negative antibody test upon hospital admission. In the remaining patients, the anti-S IgG antibodies ranged from 0.09AU to >12.48AU. A strong positive correlation was observed between the SARS-CoV-2 IgG S levels (when detectable) and Ct values upon admission ($\rho = 0.592$, $p < 0.001$). Compared to cases with detectable antibody levels, cases with a negative antibody test were older ($p = 0.039$) and had a higher creatinine level on admission ($p = 0.001$). The same group of patients was also observed to have lower Ct values ($p < 0.001$) and a shorter duration between symptom onset and hospital admission ($p < 0.001$). The absence of anti-S SARS CoV-2-antibodies on the first day of hospitalization was also associated with the presence of diabetes ($p = 0.006$), PaO2/FiO2 (PF) ratio values <150 mm Hg ($p = 0.014$), and death ($p = 0.019$) (Table 2). The Ct values and time between symptom onset and hospitalization remained significant in the multiple regression analysis ($p = 0.023$ and $p = 0.025$, respectively) (Table 3).

Table 3. Results of the multiple regression analysis with respect to the variables affecting the presence of anti-S SARS-CoV-2 antibodies upon admission.

Variables in the Model	B	S.E.	Wald	df	*p* Value	Exp (B)	95% C.I. for EXP(B) **	
							Lower	Upper
age	0.006	0.027	0.047	1	0.828	1.006	0.954	1.061
Ct	0.249	0.110	5.139	1	0.023	1.283	1.034	1.591
PF atio (1)	0.758	0.668	1.288	1	0.256	2.134	0.576	7.899
Days WSBH *	0.387	0.173	4.990	1	0.025	1.472	1.049	2.067
CREATININE	−0.736	0.588	1.569	1	0.210	0.479	0.151	1.515
Diabetes (1)	0.598	0.694	0.745	1	0.388	1.819	0.467	7.083
Constant	−6.044	3.266	3.425	1	0.064	0.002		

Dependent variable: detection of anti-S SARS-CoV-2 antibodies upon admission; Parameter coding (1): non-diabetic; PF ratio > 150 mm Hg. * Days between symptom onset and hospitalization, ** B; the coefficient for the constant, S.E.; the standard error for B, Wald; the Wald chi-square test, df; the degrees of freedom for the Wald chi-square test, Exp(B); The exponentiation of the B coefficient, C.I; confidence interval.

3.3. *Factors Influencing the Outcome of COVID-19 Disease in Fully Vaccinated, Hospitalized Patients*

Out of the 102 patients admitted to the hospital, 88 were discharged and 14 died. All deceased subjects had received SARS-CoV-2 mRNA vaccines ($p = 0.035$). Poor disease outcome was associated with older age ($p = 0.003$), lower Ct values ($p = 0.036$), a shorter duration between symptom onset and hospital admission ($p = 0.007$), and lower BMI ($p = 0.029$). Non-deceased patients were more likely to have hypertension ($p = 0.014$) and PF ratio values > 150 mm Hg ($p < 0.001$) (Table 2). The PF ratio was identified by the multiple logistic regression model as an independent predictor of in-hospital mortality ($p = 0.001$) (Table 4). The "vaccine type" variable was not included in the multiple regression analysis since none of the deceased patients had received a viral vector COVID-19 vaccine.

Table 4. Results of the multiple regression analysis with respect to the variables affecting the outcome of COVID-19 disease in fully vaccinated, hospitalized patients.

Variables in the Model	B	S.E.	Wald	df	*p* Value	Exp (B)	95% C.I. for EXP(B) **	
							Lower	Upper
age	0.069	0.053	1.721	1	0.190	1.071	0.967	1.188
Ct	−0.216	0.148	2.135	1	0.144	0.806	0.603	1.077
Days_WSBH *	−0.059	0.306	0.037	1	0.847	0.943	0.517	1.718
BMI	−0.235	0.160	2.159	1	0.142	0.791	0.578	1.081
antibodies (1)	−0.275	1.194	0.053	1	0.818	0.760	0.073	7.893
PF_Ratio (1)	−4.156	1.442	8.305	1	0.004	0.016	0.001	0.265
Hypertension (1)	1.115	1.185	0.885	1	0.347	3.050	0.299	31.135
Constant	4.095	8.290	0.244	1	0.621	60.068		

Dependent variable: Mortality; Parameter coding (1): No detection of antibodies, non-hypertensive, PF ratio > 150 mm Hg. * Days between symptom onset and hospitalization, ** B; the coefficient for the constant, S.E.; the standard error for B, Wald; the Wald chi-square test, df; the degrees of freedom for the Wald chi-square test, Exp(B); The exponentiation of the B coefficient, C.I; confidence interval.

4. Discussion

To our knowledge, this is the first study to assess several factors affecting SARS-CoV-2 IgG S antibody responses in fully vaccinated COVID-19 patients needing hospitalization due to severe COVID-19 disease. We found that older age, lower Ct values, and a shorter duration between symptom onset and hospital admission were associated with a lack of anti-S SARS-CoV-2 antibodies and poor clinical outcomes of COVID-19 disease.

The available evidence suggests that humoral and cellular immune responses are impaired in aged individuals, resulting in decreased vaccine responses [15]. Age has been reported to be inversely correlated with neutralizing antibody responses following the first immunization dose of BNT162b2, a finding that was particularly evident for individuals over 80 years [16]. The investigation of humoral immunity after two doses of BNT162b2 and mRNA-1273 vaccines has indicated that adults aged 18–55 years are more responsive to vaccination and maintain humoral immunity longer compared to individuals who are older than 70 years [17]. In addition, the anti-S SARS-CoV-2 immunoglobulin G antibody titers were found to be significantly lower in elderly vaccinees over the age of 80 years, with 31.3% of them having no detectable neutralizing antibodies after the second vaccine dose [18]. These observations and our findings underline the need for prioritizing booster COVID-19 vaccination in the elderly population.

Regarding the SARS-CoV-2 viral load, it has been shown that fully vaccinated subjects with breakthrough infections have a comparable peak viral load to those who are unvaccinated [19]. However, peak viral load increased with age, highlighting the importance of adjusting for age when comparing the two groups [20]. In our cohort of fully vaccinated inpatients, lower Ct values, which are indicative of higher viral loads, were associated with the absence of anti-S SARS-CoV-2 antibodies upon admission, both in the univariate and multiple regression analysis. The shorter number of days between symptom onset and hospital admission could account for the lower Ct values in the group of cases with a negative antibody test whose disease progressed faster, requiring earlier hospitalization. Lower Ct values were also observed in the group of deceased subjects, yet this finding did not remain significant in the multiple regression analysis. With respect to the positive correlation between anti-S SARS-CoV-2 IgG levels and Ct values upon admission, it has been reported that higher Ct values following BNT162b2 vaccination are associated with higher IgG concentrations [21].

The PF ratio was identified as an independent predictive variable of mortality in our cohort of fully vaccinated COVID-19 inpatients. Both the PF ratio and the ratio between standard PaO2 over FiO2 (STP/F) have been described as accurate predictors of acute respiratory failure outcome in COVID-19 patients [22].

Despite the fact that COVID-19 is characterized by atypical pneumonia followed by severe respiratory failure, about 10% of COVID-19 inpatients have been reported to endure acute kidney injury, which is linked to a poor prognosis [23]. It has been reported that changes in serum creatinine during the early stage of admission could predict mortality during hospitalization in COVID-19 patients [23,24]. In our study, serum creatinine levels upon admission were not predictive of in-hospital mortality, but subjects with a negative anti-S SARS-CoV-2 antibody test had higher creatinine levels on the first day of hospitalization compared to participants with detectable antibody levels, albeit not independently from other factors. Of interest, a multicenter cohort study of 543 subjects on hemodialysis and 75 healthy subjects found that both the humoral and cellular immune responses to SARS-CoV-2 vaccination were significantly impaired in the patients' group [25].

Findings with respect to diabetes were recently published as sub-study results for 92 patients of the CoVax study [26]. Diabetes mellitus, particularly T2D, is a prevalent comorbidity that considerably increases the risk of mortality in COVID-19 patients [27]. The immune system is thought to cause transitory alterations in systemic metabolism as a defense against viral infection. This mechanism is impaired in subjects with T2D, reducing the antiviral immune response [28].

Comorbidities related to a metabolic syndrome such as T2D, obesity, and hypertension are also characterized by low-grade chronic inflammation, which leads to immune system dysregulation and increased susceptibility to severe COVID-19 disease [3]. Paradoxically, in our cohort, deceased patients were less likely to have hypertension and their mean BMI was lower compared to non-deceased participants. The "obesity paradox" has been described in patient cohorts with several diseases including, but not limited to, T2D, hypertension, and chronic kidney disease [29]. However, caution is needed in interpreting these data given that all possible confounding variables should be taken into account and measured prospectively [29].

The remaining factors investigated in our study were not predictive of either the SARS-CoV-2 IgG S antibody responses or the outcome of COVID-19 disease in fully vaccinated inpatients. Gender and sex-specific effects have been reported to induce different immunization and adverse events outcomes [4,30]. The recent implementation of a within-host mathematical model of vaccine dynamics from lipid nanoparticle-formulated COVID-19 mRNA vaccines found no difference between sexes in the long-term duration of humoral immunity [17]. Regarding the "place of residence" variable, it has been reported that individuals living in highly deprived areas have increased odds of post-vaccination SARS-CoV-2 infection following the first vaccine dose [31].

It would be of great importance to ensure that the positive antibody test is a resultant of immunity induced exclusively by SARS-CoV-2 vaccination. Anti-S SARS-CoV-2 antibodies are produced in response to vaccine administration and/or COVID-19 infection. Thus, our method could not distinguish between post-vaccine response and infection. We also acknowledge that this is a single center study with a relatively small sample. Future studies should evaluate the parameters that have an impact on the vaccine-induced immunity against SARS-CoV-2 in subjects with breakthrough infections not requiring hospitalization.

5. Conclusions

Host- (age) and disease-associated factors (Ct values, time between symptom onset and hospitalization, and PF ratio) can predict SARS-CoV-2 IgG S responses and clinical outcomes in hospitalized COVID-19 patients with breakthrough SARS-CoV-2 infection post vaccination.

Author Contributions: K.I.G.; Conceptualization and supervision, E.L. and E.R.; formal analysis, investigation, data curation, writing—original draft preparation, S.S. and I.D.; resources, data curation, I.P., D.P., F.M. and O.K.; writing—review and editing. All authors have read and agreed to the published version of the manuscript.

Funding: This research received no external funding.

Institutional Review Board Statement: The study was conducted in accordance with the Declaration of Helsinki and approved by the Ethics Committee of the University Hospital of Larissa, Greece (46943/29.11.2021).

Informed Consent Statement: Informed consent was obtained from all subjects involved in the study.

Data Availability Statement: The data that support the findings of this study are available upon request from the corresponding author.

Acknowledgments: The authors would like to thank Prognosis Biotech (Larissa, Greece) for providing the equipment and materials for the SARS-CoV-2 IgG Spike measurements.

Conflicts of Interest: The authors declare no conflict of interest.

References

1. Majumder, J.; Minko, T. Recent Developments on Therapeutic and Diagnostic Approaches for COVID-19. *AAPS J.* **2021**, *23*, 1–22. [CrossRef] [PubMed]
2. Lin, C.Y.; Wolf, J.; Brice, D.C.; Sun, Y.; Locke, M.; Cherry, S.; Castellaw, A.H.; Wehenkel, M.; Crawford, J.C.; Zarnitsyna, V.I.; et al. Pre-existing humoral immunity to human common cold coronaviruses negatively impacts the protective SARS-CoV-2 antibody response. *Cell Host Microbe* **2021**, *30*, 1–14. [CrossRef] [PubMed]
3. Pérez-Galarza, J.; Prócel, C.; Cañadas, C.; Aguirre, D.; Pibaque, R.; Bedón, R.; Sempértegui, F.; Drexhage, H.; Baldeón, L. Immune response to SARS-CoV-2 infection in obesity and T2D: Literature review. *Vaccines* **2021**, *9*, 102. [CrossRef]
4. Fathi, A.; Addo, M.M.; Dahlke, C. Sex Differences in Immunity: Implications for the Development of Novel Vaccines Against Emerging Pathogens. *Front. Immunol.* **2021**, *11*, 1–7. [CrossRef]

5. Andre, F.E.; Booy, R.; Bock, H.L.; Clemens, J.; Datta, S.K.; John, T.J.; Lee, B.W.; Lolekha, S.; Peltola, H.; Ruff, T.A.; et al. Vaccination greatly reduces disease, disability, death and inequity worldwide. *Bull. World Health Organ.* **2008**, *86*, 140–146. [CrossRef] [PubMed]
6. Zimmermann, P.; Curtis, N. Factors That Influence the Immune Response to Vaccination. *Clin. Microbiol. Rev.* **2019**, *32*, 1–50. [CrossRef] [PubMed]
7. Sallusto, F.; Lanzavecchia, A.; Araki, K.; Ahmed, R. Immunity Review from Vaccines to Memory and Back. *Immunity* **2010**, *33*, 451–463. [CrossRef]
8. Hadj Hassine, I. Covid-19 vaccines and variants of concern: A review. *Rev. Med. Virol.* **2021**, *2021*, e2313. [CrossRef]
9. Amanat, F.; Strohmeier, S.; Meade, P.; Dambrauskas, N.; Mühlemann, B.; Smith, D.J.; Vigdorovich, V.; Sather, D.N.; Coughlan, L.; Krammer, F. Vaccination with SARS-CoV-2 variants of concern protects mice from challenge with wild-type virus. *PLoS Biol.* **2021**, *19*, e3001384. [CrossRef]
10. Lipsitch, M.; Krammer, F.; Regev-Yochay, G.; Lustig, Y.; Balicer, R.D. SARS-CoV-2 breakthrough infections in vaccinated individuals: Measurement, causes and impact. *Nat. Rev. Immunol.* **2022**, *22*, 57–65. [CrossRef]
11. Nomura, Y.; Sawahata, M.; Nakamura, Y.; Koike, R.; Katsube, O.; Hagiwara, K.; Niho, S.; Masuda, N.; Tanaka, T.; Sugiyama, K. Attenuation of Antibody Titers from 3 to 6 Months after the Second Dose of the BNT162b2 Vaccine Depends on Sex, with Age and Smoking Risk Factors for Lower Antibody Titers at 6 Months. *Vaccines* **2021**, *9*, 1500. [CrossRef] [PubMed]
12. Wei, J.; Stoesser, N.; Matthews, P.C.; Ayoubkhani, D.; Studley, R.; Bell, I.; Bell, J.I.; Newton, J.N.; Farrar, J.; Diamond, I.; et al. Antibody responses to SARS-CoV-2 vaccines in 45,965 adults from the general population of the United Kingdom. *Nat. Microbiol.* **2021**, *6*, 1140–1149. [CrossRef] [PubMed]
13. Watanabe, M.; Balena, A.; Tuccinardi, D.; Tozzi, R.; Risi, R.; Masi, D.; Caputi, A.; Rossetti, R.; Spoltore, M.E.; Filippi, V.; et al. Central obesity, smoking habit, and hypertension are associated with lower antibody titres in response to COVID-19 mRNA vaccine. *Diabetes Metab. Res. Rev.* **2022**, *38*, 1–10. [CrossRef] [PubMed]
14. Monin, L.; Laing, A.G.; Muñoz-Ruiz, M.; McKenzie, D.R.; Del Molino Del Barrio, I.D.; Alaguthurai, T.; Domingo-Vila, C.; Hayday, T.S.; Graham, C.; Seow, J.; et al. Safety and immunogenicity of one versus two doses of the COVID-19 vaccine BNT162b2 for patients with cancer: Interim analysis of a prospective observational study. *Lancet Oncol.* **2021**, *22*, 765–778. [CrossRef]
15. Frasca, D.; Diaz, A.; Romero, M.; Landin, A.M.; Blomberg, B.B. Age effects on B cells and humoral immunity in humans. *Ageing Res. Rev.* **2011**, *10*, 330–335. [CrossRef]
16. Collier, D.A.; Ferreira, I.A.T.M.; Kotagiri, P.; Datir, R.P.; Lim, E.Y.; Touizer, E.; Meng, B.; Abdullahi, A.; Bioresource, T.C.; Elmer, A.; et al. Age-related immune response heterogeneity to SARS-CoV-2 vaccine BNT162b2. *Nature* **2021**, *596*, 417–422. [CrossRef]
17. Korosec, C.S.; Farhang-sardroodi, S.; Dick, D.W.; Gholami, S.; Ghaemi, M.S.; Moyles, I.R.; Craig, M.; Ooi, H.K.; Heffernan, J.M. Long-term predictions of humoral immunity after two doses of BNT162b2 and mRNA-1273 vaccines based on dosage, age and sex. *MedRxiv* **2021**, 1–16. [CrossRef]
18. Müller, L.; Andrée, M.; Moskorz, W.; Drexler, I.; Walotka, L.; Grothmann, R.; Ptok, J.; Hillebrandt, J.; Ritchie, A.; Rabl, D.; et al. Age-dependent Immune Response to the Biontech/Pfizer BNT162b2 Coronavirus Disease 2019 Vaccination. *Clin. Infect. Dis.* **2021**, *73*, 2065–2072. [CrossRef]
19. Singanayagam, A.; Hakki, S.; Dunning, J.; Madon, K.J.; Crone, M.A.; Koycheva, A.; Derqui-Fernandez, N.; Barnett, J.L.; Whitfield, M.G.; Varro, R.; et al. Community transmission and viral load kinetics of the SARS-CoV-2 delta (B.1.617.2) variant in vaccinated and unvaccinated individuals in the UK: A prospective, longitudinal, cohort study. *Lancet Infect. Dis.* **2021**, *22*, 183–195. [CrossRef]
20. Knol, M.J.; Backer, J.A.; de Melker, H.E.; van den Hof, S.; de Gier, B. Transmissibility of SARS-CoV-2 among fully vaccinated individuals. *Lancet Infect. Dis.* **2022**, *22*, 16–17. [CrossRef]
21. Regev-Yochay, G.; Amit, S.; Bergwerk, M.; Lipsitch, M.; Leshem, E.; Kahn, R.; Lustig, Y.; Cohen, C.; Doolman, R.; Ziv, A.; et al. Decreased infectivity following BNT162b2 vaccination: A prospective cohort study in Israel. *Lancet Reg. Health Eur.* **2021**, *7*, 100150. [CrossRef] [PubMed]
22. Prediletto, I.; Antoni, L.D.; Carbonara, P.; Daniele, F.; Dongilli, R.; Flore, R.; Pacilli, A.M.G.; Pisani, L.; Tomsa, C.; Vega, M.L.; et al. Standardizing PaO2 for PaCO2 in P / F ratio predicts in-hospital mortality in acute respiratory failure due to Covid-19 : A pilot prospective study. *Eur. J. Intern. Med.* **2021**, *92*, 48–54. [CrossRef] [PubMed]
23. Komaru, Y.; Doi, K. Does a slight change in serum creatinine matter in coronavirus disease 2019 (Covid-19) patients? *Kidney Res. Clin. Pract.* **2021**, *40*, 177–179. [CrossRef] [PubMed]
24. Alfano, G.; Ferrari, A.; Fontana, F.; Mori, G.; Ligabue, G.; Giovanella, S.; Magistroni, R.; Meschiari, M.; Franceschini, E.; Menozzi, M.; et al. Twenty-four-hour serum creatinine variation is associated with poor outcome in the novel coronavirus disease 2019 (Covid-19) patients. *Kidney Res. Clin. Pract.* **2021**, *40*, 231–240. [CrossRef]
25. Van Praet, J.; Reynders, M.; De Bacquer, D.; Viaene, L.; Schoutteten, M.K.; Caluwé, R.; Doubel, P.; Heylen, L.; De Bel, A.V.; Van Vlem, B.; et al. Predictors and dynamics of the humoral and cellular immune response to SARS-CoV-2 mRNA vaccines in hemodialysis patients: A multicenter observational study. *JASN* **2021**, *32*, 3208–3220. [CrossRef]
26. Rouka, E.; Livanou, E.; Sinis, S.; Dimeas, I.; Pantazopoulos, I.; Papagiannis, D.; Malli, F.; Kotsiou, O.; Gourgoulianis, K.I. Immune response to the severe acute respiratory syndrome coronavirus 2 vaccines: Is it sustained in the diabetes population? *J. Diabetes Investig.* **2022**. [CrossRef]

27. Cheng, X.; Liu, Y.M.; Li, H.; Zhang, X.; Lei, F.; Qin, J.J.; Chen, Z.; Deng, K.Q.; Lin, L.; Chen, M.M.; et al. Metformin Is Associated with Higher Incidence of Acidosis, but Not Mortality, in Individuals with COVID-19 and Pre-existing Type 2 Diabetes. *Cell Metab.* **2020**, *32*, 537–547. [CrossRef]
28. Turk Wensveen, T.; Gašparini, D.; Rahelić, D.; Wensveen, F.M. Type 2 diabetes and viral infection; cause and effect of disease. *Diabetes Res. Clin. Pract.* **2021**, *172*, 1–13. [CrossRef]
29. Ades, P.A.; Savage, P.D. The obesity paradox: Perception vs knowledge. *Mayo Clin. Proc.* **2010**, *85*, 112–114. [CrossRef]
30. Vassallo, A.; Shajahan, S.; Harris, K.; Hallam, L.; Hockham, C.; Womersley, K.; Woodward, M.; Sheel, M. Sex and Gender in COVID-19 Vaccine Research: Substantial Evidence Gaps Remain. *Front. Glob. Women Health* **2021**, *2*, 1–12. [CrossRef]
31. Antonelli, M.; Penfold, R.S.; Merino, J.; Sudre, C.H.; Molteni, E.; Berry, S.; Canas, L.S.; Graham, M.S.; Klaser, K.; Modat, M.; et al. Risk factors and disease profile of post-vaccination SARS-CoV-2 infection in UK users of the COVID Symptom Study app: A prospective, community-based, nested, case-control study. *Lancet Infect. Dis.* **2022**, *22*, 43–55. [CrossRef]

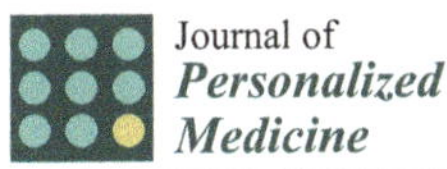
Journal of Personalized Medicine

MDPI

Brief Report

The Comparative Superiority of SARS-CoV-2 Antibody Response in Different Immunization Scenarios

Ourania S. Kotsiou [1,2,*], Nikolaos Karakousis [3], Dimitrios Papagiannis [4], Elena Matsiatsiou [1], Dimitra Avgeri [1], Evangelos C. Fradelos [1], Dimitra I. Siachpazidou [2], Garifallia Perlepe [2], Angeliki Miziou [2], Athanasios Kyritsis [2], Eudoxia Gogou [2], George D. Vavougios [2], George Kalantzis [2] and Konstantinos I. Gourgoulianis [2]

1 Faculty of Nursing, School of Health Sciences, University of Thessaly, GAIOPOLIS, 41110 Larissa, Greece
2 Department of Respiratory Medicine, Faculty of Medicine, School of Health Sciences, University of Thessaly, BIOPOLIS, 41110 Larissa, Greece
3 Primary Healthcare, Internal Medicine Department, Amarousion, 15125 Athens, Greece
4 Public Health & Vaccines Lab, Department of Nursing, School of Health Sciences, University of Thessaly, GAIOPOLIS, 41110 Larissa, Greece
* Correspondence: raniakotsiou@gmail.com or okotsiou@uth.gr

Abstract: Background: Both SARS-CoV-2 infection and/or vaccination result in the production of SARS-CoV-2 antibodies. We aimed to compare the antibody titers against SARS-CoV-2 in different scenarios for antibody production. Methods: A surveillance program was conducted in the municipality of Deskati in January 2022. Antibody titers were obtained from 145 participants while parallel recording their infection and/or vaccination history. The SARS-CoV-2 IgG II Quant method (Architect, Abbott, IL, USA) was used for antibody testing. Results: Advanced age (>56 years old) was associated with higher antibody titers. No significant differences were detected in antibody titers among genders, BMI, smoking status, comorbidities, vaccine brands, and months after the last dose. Hospitalization length and re-infection were predictors of antibody titers. The individuals who were fully or partially vaccinated and were also double infected had the highest antibody levels (25,017 ± 1500 AU/mL), followed by people who were fully vaccinated (20,647 ± 500 AU/mL) or/partially (15,808 ± 1800 AU/mL) vaccinated and were infected once. People who were only vaccinated had lower levels of antibodies (9946 ± 300 AU/mL), while the lowest levels among all groups were found in individuals who had only been infected (1124 ± 200 AU/mL). Conclusions: Every hit (infection or vaccination) gives an additional boost to immunization status.

Keywords: antibody; COVID-19; infection; immunization; vaccination

Citation: Kotsiou, O.S.; Karakousis, N.; Papagiannis, D.; Matsiatsiou, E.; Avgeri, D.; Fradelos, E.C.; Siachpazidou, D.I.; Perlepe, G.; Miziou, A.; Kyritsis, A.; et al. The Comparative Superiority of SARS-CoV-2 Antibody Response in Different Immunization Scenarios. *J. Pers. Med.* **2022**, *12*, 1756. https://doi.org/10.3390/jpm12111756

Academic Editor: Mariangela Manfredi

Received: 31 August 2022
Accepted: 21 October 2022
Published: 23 October 2022

1. Introduction

The Coronavirus disease pandemic 2019 remains an excellent concern for ethnicities. It is already well-established that the SARS-CoV-2 virus is rapidly evolving and spreading through mutagenesis, a quite threatening condition that lengthens the duration of the pandemic and might affect the efficacy of the existing vaccines and lead to the need to develop new ones in order to confront new variants of the specific viral infection [1,2].

There is a debate regarding the durability of antibody responses over time in patients infected by SARS-CoV-2, with several studies reporting stable, long-lasting antibody immunity and others showing rapidly waning antibody immunity or late appearances with low antibody levels and/or a complete lack of antibodies [3].

FDA decided on booster vaccines because the benefits of the COVID-19 vaccination far outweigh the potential risks. However, further studies are needed to demonstrate the efficacy of booster vaccinations to determine the best dosing and mix-and-match schedules of vaccinations [3]. Nevertheless, the result of the combination of infection and vaccination on the antibody levels is unknown and leads to a condition of questioning and concern.

In this study, we aimed to compare the titers of antibodies against SARS-CoV-2 in different scenarios for antibody production, which is of great importance, especially in the era of the pandemic in which we possess certain preventive tools such as vaccines.

2. Materials and Methods

A surveillance program was conducted in the semi-closed municipality of Deskati in January 2022. To assess the different scenarios for antibody production, antibody titers were obtained from participants while recording their infection and/or vaccination history since the pandemic wave initiation in the community in October 2020.

All the residents of Deskati were invited to participate in this program by the local authority and were notified of the time and place. Participants were recruited by announcing the research in the media, while local officials organized a one-month recruitment campaign. There were no exclusion criteria. The participants were analyzed to evaluate seroprevalence and antibody-response longevity to the SARS-CoV-2 infection and/or vaccination.

All subjects provided written and oral informed consent. Following consent, demographic information and data regarding past PCR-confirmed COVID-19 infection and vaccination history were recorded on questionnaire forms for all participants.

The SARS-CoV-2 IgG II Quant method (Architect, Abbott, IL, USA) was used for antibody testing. This is an automated two-step chemiluminescent microparticle immunoassay that was used for the qualitative and quantitative determination of IgG antibodies against the spike receptor-binding domain (RBD) of SARS-CoV-2 in the serum specimens, with a sensitivity of 99.9% and specificity of 100% for detecting the IgG antibodies generated by prior infection or vaccination, as previously described [4,5]. The sequence used for the receptor-binding domain was taken from the WH-Human 1 coronavirus, GenBank accession number MN908947. The analytical measurement interval is stated as 21 to 40,000 AU/mL, and the positivity cutoff as $\geq$50 AU/mL (manufacturer defined) [6].

The Pearson correlation method was used for correlation analysis between the pairs of continuous variables. Stepwise multiple linear analysis was conducted with numerical and categorical variables turned into dummy variables. It was used to analyze the correlation between antibody titers and various factors affecting the population. The mean age, gender, mean BMI, smoking status, presence of comorbidities, previous infection, hospitalization, mean length of hospitalization, re-infection, vaccination status, brand name of the vaccine, number of vaccination doses, and months after the last vaccine dose were used as independent variables in the prediction of antibody titers. To identify differences the between two independent groups, an unpaired *t*-test was used. Parametric data comparing three or more groups were analyzed with a one-way ANOVA and Tukey's multiple comparisons test, while non-parametric data were analyzed with the Kruskal–Wallis test and Dunn's multiple comparison test. Pearson's chi-squared test was used to determine whether there was a statistically significant difference between the frequencies. A result was considered statistically significant when the *p*-value was <0.05. Data were analyzed and visualized using SPSS Statistics v.23 (Armonk, NY, USA: IBM Corp.) and Tableau (Tableau Software LLC, Seattle, WA, USA), respectively.

3. Results

In this study, 145 participants were recruited. The main characteristics of the study population are presented in Table 1. As shown, females had more comorbidities than males. None of the participants were immunocompromised. Half of the population had previously been infected by SARS-CoV-2 for one year. A total amount of 8.1% of the infected population (n = 12) had a recent double infection (in the last three months) during that year, from which ten were fully vaccinated while two were not vaccinated at all.

Most of the population (93.1%, n = 135) were vaccinated. A total of 82.2% (n = 111) were fully vaccinated (with three doses), and the rest were partly vaccinated. A total of 70.3% (n = 95) of the population has been vaccinated with Pfizer/BioNTech, 29% (n = 39) by Moderna and 0.7% by Johnson & Johnson, with no difference between genders. We found no difference in antibody titers between the different brands of vaccines (Pfizer/BioNTech vs. Moderna, 14,644 ± 11,567 vs. 10,793 ± 11,596, $p = 0.084$). There was no correlation between the months after the last vaccine dose and antibody titers ($r = -0.027$, $p = 0.761$).

Table 1. Characteristics of the study population stratified by gender (N = 145).

Variable	Total (N = 145)	Males (n = 58)	Females (n = 87)	p-Value
Age (years)	56.0 ± 14.7	59.0 ± 16.0	54 ± 14	0.082
BMI (mg/kg^2)	19.0 ± 2.0	19.7 ± 2.6	19.3 ± 3.5	0.567
Comorbidities yes, n (%)	68 (46.9)	21 (36.2)	47 (54.0)	0.041
Medication yes, n (%)	74 (51.0)	24 (41.4)	50 (57.5)	0.065
Previous infection yes, n (%)	73 (50.0)	30 (51.7)	43 (49.4)	0.382
Vaccination yes, n (%)	135 (93.1)	55 (94.8)	80 (91.9)	0.364
Seropositivity yes, n (%)	135 (93.1)	55 (94.8)	80 (91.9)	0.364
Antibody titers (AU/mL)	12,663 ± 11,725	14,229 ± 11,996	11,654 ± 11,522	0.193

No difference in antibody production was observed among the genders after 27 months ($p = 0.193$). No correlation was found between BMI and antibody titers ($r = 0.92$, $p = 0.293$). No significant differences were detected in antibody titers by tobacco use (current and ex-smokers vs. nonsmokers, $p = 0.522$) and comorbidities ($p = 0.073$). Advanced age (>56 years old) was associated with higher antibody titers compared to younger adults (14,595 ± 12,869 AU/mL vs. 10,517 ± 9735 AU/mL, $p = 0.039$).

SARS-CoV-2 seropositivity was 93.1% in the study population. Seronegative ($n = 10$) were only infected but unvaccinated. More specifically, the infected and not vaccinated people had no seropositivity one year after the SARS-CoV-2 infection. The winners in antibody production were the patients who were fully or partly vaccinated and had also been infected twice (Table 2), followed by people who were fully vaccinated or partially vaccinated and were infected once, with no significant difference between the last two groups. People who were vaccinated had lower antibody levels, while individuals who had only been infected had the lowest antibody titers. A statistical analysis of the different immunization scenarios revealed a significant difference in antibody titers between the groups.

Table 2. Antibody response in different immunization scenarios during a year period in immunocompetent population (N = 145) and statistical analysis of different immunization scenarios.

Immunization Scenario	N = 145	Titers of Anti-SARS-CoV-2 Antibodies (AU/mL)	p-Value *	p-Value **	p-Value ***	p-Value #
Fully or partially vaccinated and double infected	11	25,017 ± 1500		0.023	0.015	0.012
Fully vaccinated and infected once	44	20,647 ± 500	0.023		0.042	0.004
Partially vaccinated and infected once	8	15,808 ± 1800	0.015	0.042		0.025
Only vaccinated	71	9946 ± 300	0.012	0.004	0.025	
Only infected	11	1124 ± 200	<0.001	<0.001	<0.001	0.014

Note: * One-way ANOVA compares the means of the antibody titers of fully or partially vaccinated and double infected people with all the other independent immunization scenarios; ** One-way ANOVA compares the means of the antibody titers of fully or partially vaccinated and once infected people with all the other independent immunization scenarios; *** One-way ANOVA compares the means of the antibody titers of partially vaccinated and once infected people with all the other independent immunization scenarios; # One-way ANOVA compares the means of the antibody titers of only vaccinated people with all the other independent immunization scenarios.

Stepwise multiple linear analysis was used to analyze the correlation between antibody titers and the various factors affecting the population (Table 3). The mean age, gender, mean BMI, smoking status, presence of comorbidities, previous infection, hospitalization, length of hospitalization, re-infection, vaccination status, the brand name of the vaccine, number of vaccination doses, and months after the last vaccine dose were used as independent variables in the prediction of antibody titers. The hospitalization period and re-infection were independent predictor variables of antibody titers, explaining 52% of the total variance in this regression model. There was no multicollinearity between the explanatory variables.

Table 3. Stepwise multiple linear analysis between antibody titers and significant predictors.

Coefficients [a]					
Model	Unstandardized Coefficients		Standardized Coefficients	t	*p*-Value
	B	Std. Error	Beta		
(Constant)	−4905.6	5925.1		−0.828	0.413
Re-infection (yes)	13,719.1	3768.7	0.507	3640	0.001
Length of hospitalization (days)	290.5	132.5	0.305	2192	0.034

[a] Dependent variable: antibody titers (AU/mL), R = 52.2%, R^2 = 27%, R^2 (adjusted) = 23%.

4. Discussion

In this study, for the first time, we investigated the different scenarios for antibody production among immunocompetent participants by recording their infection and/or vaccination history during a one-year period. In particular, we found that advanced age (>56 years old) was associated with higher antibody titers. No significant differences were detected in antibody titers among genders, sex, BMI, smoking status, comorbidities, vaccine brands, and months after the last shot. Hospitalization periods and re-infection were independent predictor variables of antibody titers. Individuals who were fully or partially vaccinated and were also double infected had the highest antibody levels, followed by people who were fully vaccinated or/partially vaccinated and were infected once. People who were only vaccinated had lower levels of antibodies, while the lowest levels among all the groups were found in individuals who had only been infected. A significant difference was detected between all the groups.

Interestingly, SARS-CoV-2 seropositivity was 93% in the study population. Seronegative people were only infected with the virus and remained unvaccinated. The longevity of the antibody response to the SARS-CoV-2 infection are not well defined. We have recently reported that antibody responses to the SARS-CoV-2 infection were maintained nine months after the pandemic and especially in those with severe disease leading to hospitalization [4,5]. A recent study identified the over one year duration of SARS-CoV-2 antibodies in 82.90% of 538 convalescent COVID-19 patients [7,8]. Similarly, other studies supported a long-lasting immunological memory against SARS-CoV-2 one year after mild COVID-19 [9,10]. Conversely, in this study all the people who were infected (n = 11) but not vaccinated had no seropositivity after one year [9]. One large study showed that 13% of individuals lost detectable IgG titers 10 months post-infection. Yan et al. documented that SARS-CoV-2-specific IgG persistence and titer depended on COVID-19 severity, as 74.4% of recovered asymptomatic carriers had negative anti-SARS-CoV-2 IgG test results, while many others had very low virus-specific IgG antibody titers, among a population of 473 previously infected patients [11]. Hence, further studies are needed to clarify this field.

Multiple vaccine constructs have been quite promising, with an approximately 95% protective efficacy against COVID-19 [12]. Since identifying the Omicron variant, many countries have made modifications to their vaccination programs by including the recommendation of a third and fourth injection of boosting vaccination dosages in large populations to reduce the risk of adverse effects. However, all three vaccine producers (Johnson et Johnson, BioNTech, Pfizer, and Moderna) have published statements claiming vaccines would protect against severe sickness, as well as the fact that variant-specific vaccinations and boosters are in the works [13]. Nevertheless, it is unknown how long the immunity following COVID-19 vaccinations last, and this is a quite provoking situation that leads to an increased feeling of uncertainty and disbelief. It has been supported that the antibody persistence time of the mRNA vaccine is about 180 days (six months), following the adenovirus vaccine with 90 days [14]. Moreover, a short duration of antibody persistence of about 2-months has been found after the second dose [14].

Roy et al. reported significant differences in neutralizing antibody titers after 180 days in age, sex, COVID-19 infection, tobacco use, and asthma patients [15]. Swartz et al. measured antibody titers in 4553 participants over 11 months and documented that individuals may remain antibody positive from natural infection beyond 500 days, depending on age and smoking or vaping use [15]. Conversely, in our study, no significant differences were detected in antibody titers by sex, BMI, smoking status, and comorbidities. No significant differences were also detected in antibody titers among different brands of vaccines and months after the last shot. There are supporting data that prove there is a significantly higher humoral immunogenicity of the SARS-CoV-2 mRNA-1273 vaccine (Moderna) compared with the BNT162b2 vaccine (Pfizer-BioNTech) in infected as well as uninfected participants and across age categories [16].

An interesting finding was that advanced age (>56 years old) was associated with higher antibody titers. However, age was not a predictor of antibody titers in the stepwise multiple linear analysis. Yang et al. investigated the antibody test results among 31,426 patients from a wide range of age groups and supported an age-dependent variation in antibody titers, with children having higher antibody-binding avidity compared with young adults, but the difference was not significant [17]. However, contradictory data also exist [18,19]. Although there is an expectation that COVID-19 will become endemic, the pandemic will not end with the virus disappearing, and many questions remain unanswered. Further studies are needed to clarify the arising issues.

Moreover, in this study, the hospitalization period and re-infection were independent predictor variables of antibody titers. Similarly, Klein et al. found that hospitalization for severe COVID-19 could predict greater antibody responses against SARS-CoV-2. [18]. At present, it is unclear how long serum antibodies persist after reinfection [20]. Townsend et al. supported the fact that reinfection by SARS-CoV-2 under endemic conditions would likely occur between 3months and 5.1 years after the peak antibody response, with a median of 16 months [20]. However, to identify the correlates of protection, the relationship between in vitro neutralization levels of anti-SARS-CoV-2 antibodies and protection from severe acute respiratory syndrome coronavirus 2 (SARS-CoV-2) infection by large convalescent cohorts should be tested. Khoury et al. documented that neutralizing antibody levels are highly predictive of immune protection from symptomatic SARS-CoV-2 infection and estimated the neutralization level for 50% protection against detectable SARS-CoV-2 infection to be 20.2% of the mean convalescent level, predicting that over the first 250 days after immunization a significant loss in protection from SARS-CoV-2 infection will occur, although protection from severe disease should be largely retained [21]. However, how high a titer is protective of further infection remains unclear, and we cannot provide conclusive evidence that these antibody responses protect from reinfection. However, we believe it is very likely that higher titers will decrease the odds ratio of reinfection and may attenuate disease in the case of breakthrough infection. Undoubtedly, it is imperative to swiftly perform studies to investigate and establish a correlate of protection from SARS-CoV-2 infection.

Higher antibody titers were found in cases of vaccination in previously infected subjects, according to a previous study by our scientific team [4,5]. This finding is also supported by many other studies which report that a low concentration of SARS-CoV-2 spike protein antibodies after 9–12 months indicates that re-exposure to the virus or vaccination is required to use the B-cell immunity to full capacity [22]. In the current study, we found a 15 times higher titer of anti-SARS-CoV-2 antibodies in individuals who were fully or partially vaccinated and who were double infected than previously infected patients, while fully vaccinated patients who were infected once had 25 times higher titers of anti-SARS-CoV-2 antibodies than previously infected patients. Interestingly, patients who were only vaccinated had nine times greater antibody titers than the only-infected patients. These results reflect those of Teresa Vietri et al., who also found that a booster dose resulted in a marked increase in antibody response, which then subsequently decreased over time [23].

Our study's findings should be interpreted within the context of its limitations and strengths. As such, when considering absolute numbers, our study's population is smaller compared to other studies [20,21]. It does, however, represent a specific epidemiological framework in rural Greece, reflecting remote populations differentially affected by the pandemic. Within these parameters, albeit nested, our study reports on real-world data representative of the geographical, cultural, and healthcare settings from which they stem. Furthermore, as previously mentioned, the corroboration of our findings in larger cohorts reflects that these data may be generalizable in similar settings. Another limitation was that the sample group was rather uniformly young and very lean, which limits the generalizability of our findings. It would be appealing to apply this search among individuals of a more significant number and in different geographical areas. This could give us the unique opportunity to evaluate and more profoundly assess the potential fluctuation between the titers of antibodies against SARS-CoV-2 in different scenarios in terms of antibody production and environmental conditions. In addition, it would be intriguing to study the titers of antibodies against SARS-CoV-2 in different statuses concerning the production of antibodies in various eating habits and lifestyles.

Last but not least, it would be particularly thrilling if we could develop a score or index concerning the antibody titers, the viral infection's different statuses related to the antibodies produced, and the patient's clinical image in order to have a potential prognostic tool, especially in individuals living with many comorbidities. Using scores or indices such as these, it might be possible to detect early the need for further and more specialized medical intervention and care in subjects infected with SARS-CoV-2 and vaccinated, fully or not, against the virus which has invaded our everyday routine. This could probably be beneficial not only for the infected individuals and their families but also for the healthcare system that has sustained a tremendous burden, both economically concerning every country worldwide and psychologically, especially for healthcare workers, due to the pandemic. We seem to have a long road to cross for understanding and decoding the mechanisms concerning this viral infection and its effect on human body systems.

5. Conclusions

The winners in anti-SARS-CoV-2 titers were the individuals who were fully or partially vaccinated and who were also double infected, followed by people who were fully vaccinated or/partially vaccinated and only infected once. In addition, subjects who were only vaccinated had lower levels of antibodies, whilst the lowest levels among all the groups were found in individuals who had only been infected. Overall, these results are quite promising, but the SARS-CoV-2 variant seems to be the dragon in this medical issue.

Our findings indicate that every hit (infection or vaccination) gives an additional boost in immunization status. However, the antibody response raised by vaccines is roughly affected by not only the time but also the emergence of new SARS-CoV-2 variants. The spread of new variants is associated with an escape from antibodies; therefore, to mitigate the spread of this infection in the long run, a more effective longitudinal observation of the immune response is needed.

Author Contributions: Conceptualization, K.I.G., O.S.K., D.P. and E.C.F.; methodology, K.I.G., O.S.K., D.P. and E.C.F.; formal analysis, O.S.K.; investigation, O.S.K., D.P., E.G., E.C.F., G.P., A.M., D.I.S., A.K., G.D.V., E.M., D.A., O.S.K., N.K. and G.K.; resources, D.P. and K.I.G.; writing—original draft preparation, O.S.K., G.D.V.; writing—review and editing, O.S.K.; supervision, O.S.K.; visualization, K.I.G.; project administration, K.I.G., O.S.K., D.P. and E.C.F. All authors have read and agreed to the published version of the manuscript.

Funding: This research received no external funding.

Institutional Review Board Statement: The study was conducted according to the guidelines of the Declaration of Helsinki and approved by the Institutional Review Board (or Ethics Committee) of the Ethics Committee of the University of Thessaly (No. 2800-01/11/2020; approved on 1 November 2020).

Informed Consent Statement: Informed consent was obtained from all subjects involved in the study.

Data Availability Statement: The data that support the findings of this study are available on request from the corresponding author, O.S.K.

Conflicts of Interest: The authors declare no conflict of interest.

References

1. Tatsi, E.B.; Filippatos, F.; Michos, A. SARS-CoV-2 variants and effectiveness of vaccines: A review of current evidence. *Epidemiol. Infect.* **2021**, *149*, e237. [CrossRef] [PubMed]
2. Fiolet, T.; Kherabi, Y.; MacDonald, C.J.; Ghosn, J.; Peiffer-Smadja, N. Comparing COVID-19 vaccines for their characteristics, efficacy and effectiveness against SARS-CoV-2 and variants of concern: A narrative review. *Clin. Microbiol. Infect.* **2022**, *28*, 202–221. [CrossRef] [PubMed]
3. Ali, H.; Alahmad, B.; Al-Shammari, A.A.; Alterki, A.; Hammad, M.; Cherian, P.; Alkhairi, I.; Sindhu, S.; Thanaraj, T.A.; Mohammad, A.; et al. Previous COVID-19 Infection and Antibody Levels After Vaccination. *Front. Public Health* **2021**, *9*, 778243. [CrossRef] [PubMed]
4. Kotsiou', O.S.; Vavougios, G.D.; Papagiannis, D.; Matsiatsiou, E.; Avgeri, D.; Fradelos, E.C.; Siachpazidou, D.I.; Perlepe, G.; Miziou, A.; Kyritsis, A.; et al. Lessons We Have Learned Regarding Seroprevalence in High and Low SARS-CoV-2 Contexts in Greece before the Omicron Pandemic Wave. *Int. J. Environ. Res. Public Health* **2022**, *19*, 6110. [CrossRef]
5. Kotsiou, O.S.; Papagiannis, D.; Fradelos, E.C.; Siachpazidou, D.I.; Perlepe, G.; Miziou, A.; Kyritsis, A.; Vavougios, G.D.; Kalantzis, G.; Gourgoulianis, K.I. Defining Antibody Seroprevalence and Duration of Humoral Responses to SARS-CoV-2 Infection and/or Vaccination in a Greek Community. *Int. J. Environ. Res. Public Health* **2021**, *19*, 407. [CrossRef]
6. English, E.; Cook, L.E.; Piec, I.; Dervisevic, S.; Fraser, W.D.; John, W.G. Performance of the Abbott SARS-CoV-2 IgG II Quantitative Antibody Assay Including the New Variants of Concern, VOC 202012/V1 (United Kingdom) and VOC 202012/V2 (South Africa), and First Steps towards Global Harmonization of COVID-19 Antibody Methods. *J. Clin. Microbiol.* **2021**, *59*, e0028821. [CrossRef]
7. Zeng, F.; Wu, M.; Wang, J.; Li, J.; Hu, G.; Wang, L. Over 1-year duration and age difference of SARS-CoV-2 antibodies in convalescent COVID-19 patients. *J. Med. Virol.* **2021**, *93*, 6506–6511. [CrossRef]
8. Zhang, S.; Xu, K.; Li, C.; Zhou, L.; Kong, X.; Peng, J.; Zhu, F.; Bao, C.; Jin, H.; Gao, Q.; et al. Long-Term Kinetics of SARS-CoV-2 Antibodies and Impact of Inactivated Vaccine on SARS-CoV-2 Antibodies Based on a COVID-19 Patients Cohort. *Front. Immunol.* **2022**, *13*, 829665. [CrossRef]
9. Zhan, Y.; Zhu, Y.; Wang, S.; Jia, S.; Gao, Y.; Lu, Y.; Zhou, C.; Liang, R.; Sun, D.; Wang, X.; et al. SARS-CoV-2 immunity and functional recovery of COVID-19 patients 1-year after infection. *Signal Transduct. Target Ther.* **2021**, *6*, 368. [CrossRef]
10. Choe, P.G.; Kim, K.H.; Kang, C.K.; Suh, H.J.; Kang, E.; Lee, S.Y.; Kim, N.J.; Yi, J.; Park, W.B.; Oh, M.D. Antibody Responses One Year after Mild SARS-CoV-2 Infection. *J. Korean Med. Sci.* **2021**, *36*, e157. [CrossRef]
11. Yan, X.; Chen, G.; Jin, Z.; Zhang, Z.; Zhang, B.; He, J.; Yin, S.; Huang, J.; Fan, M.; Li, Z.; et al. Anti-SARS-CoV-2 IgG levels in relation to disease severity of COVID-19. *J. Med. Virol.* **2022**, *94*, 380–383. [CrossRef]
12. Wang, P.; Nair, M.S.; Liu, L.; Iketanim, S.; Luo, Y.; Guo, Y.; Wang, M.; Yu, J.; Zhang, B.; Kwong, P.D.; et al. Antibody resistance of SARS-CoV-2 variants B.1.351 and B.1.1.7. *Nature* **2021**, *593*, 130–135. [CrossRef] [PubMed]
13. Khalid, N.; Wheeler, A.M. SARS-CoV-2 in relation to global vaccination and booster doses: What is the future of vaccination in the battle against COVID-19? *Bratisl. Lek. Listy* **2022**, *123*, 631–633. [CrossRef] [PubMed]
14. Jamshidi, E.; Asgary, A.; Shafiekhani, P.; Khajeamiri, Y.; Mohamed, K.; Esmaily, H.; Jamal Rahi, S.; Mansouri, N. Longevity of immunity following COVID-19 vaccination: A comprehensive review of the currently approved vaccines. *Hum. Vaccin. Immunother.* **2022**, *18*, 2037384. [CrossRef] [PubMed]
15. Swartz, M.D.; DeSantis, S.M.; Yaseen, A.; Brito, F.A.; Valerio-Shewmaker, M.A.; Messiah, S.E.; Leon-Novelo, L.G.; Kohl, H.W.; Pinzon-Gomez, C.L.; Hao, T.; et al. Antibody duration after infection from SARS-CoV-2 in the Texas Coronavirus Antibody Response Survey. *J. Infect. Dis.* **2022**, jiac167. [CrossRef]

16. Steensels, D.; Pierlet, N.; Penders, J.; Mesotten, D.; Heylen, L. Comparison of SARS-CoV-2 Antibody Response Following Vaccination With BNT162b2 and mRNA-1273. *JAMA* **2021**, *326*, 1533–1535. [CrossRef]
17. Yang, H.S.; Costa, V.; Racine-Brzostek, S.E.; Acker, K.P.; Yee, J.; Chen, Z.; Karbaschi, M.; Zuk, R.; Rand, S.; Sukhu, A.; et al. Association of Age With SARS-CoV-2 Antibody Response. *JAMA Netw. Open* **2021**, *4*, e214302. [CrossRef]
18. Klein, S.L.; Pekosz, A.; Park, H.-S.; Ursin, R.L.; Shapiro, J.R.; Benner, S.E.; Littlefield, K.; Kumar, S.; Naik, H.M.; Betenbaugh, M.J.; et al. Sex, age, and hospitalization drive antibody responses in a COVID-19 convalescent plasma donor population. *J. Clin. Investig.* **2020**, *130*, 6141–6150. [CrossRef]
19. Schlickeiser, S.; Schwarz, T.; Steiner, S.; Wittke, K.; Al Besher, N.; Meyer, O.; Kalus, U.; Pruß, A.; Kurth, F.; Zoller, T.; et al. Disease Severity, Fever, Age, and Sex Correlate With SARS-CoV-2 Neutralizing Antibody Responses. *Front. Immunol.* **2021**, *11*, 628971. [CrossRef]
20. Townsend, J.P.; Hassler, H.B.; Wang, Z.; Miura, S.; Singh, J.; Kumar, S.; Ruddle, N.H.; Galvani, A.P.; Dornburg, A. The durability of immunity against reinfection by SARS-CoV-2: A comparative evolutionary study. *Lancet Microbe.* **2021**, *2*, e666–e675. [CrossRef]
21. Khoury, D.S.; Cromer, D.; Reynaldi, A.; Schlub, T.E.; Wheatley, A.K.; Juno, J.A.; Subbarao, K.; Kent, S.J.; Triccas, J.A. Davenport MP. Neutralizing antibody levels are highly predictive of immune protection from symptomatic SARS-CoV-2 infection. *Nat. Med.* **2021**, *27*, 1205–1211. [CrossRef] [PubMed]
22. Kannenberg, J.; Trawinski, H.; Henschler, R.; Buhmann, R.; Hönemann, M.; Jassoy, C. Antibody course and memory B-cell response in the first year after SARS-CoV-2 infection. *J. Infect. Dis.* **2022**, *226*, jiac034. [CrossRef] [PubMed]
23. Teresa Vietri, M.; D'Elia, G.; Caliendo, G.; Passariello, L.; Albanese, L.; Maria Molinari, A.; Francesco Angelillo, I. Antibody levels after BNT162b2 vaccine booster and SARS-CoV-2 Omicron infection. *Vaccine* **2022**, *40*, 5726–5731. [CrossRef] [PubMed]

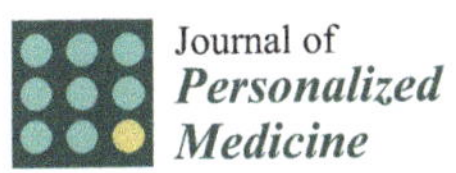
Journal of
Personalized
Medicine

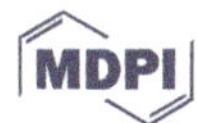

Systematic Review

Therapeutic Vitamin D Supplementation Following COVID-19 Diagnosis: Where Do We Stand?—A Systematic Review

Angelina Bania [1], Konstantinos Pitsikakis [2], Georgios Mavrovounis [3,*], Maria Mermiri [4], Eleftherios T. Beltsios [3], Antonis Adamou [5], Vasiliki Konstantaki [6], Demosthenes Makris [7], Vasiliki Tsolaki [7], Konstantinos Gourgoulianis [8] and Ioannis Pantazopoulos [3]

1 Faculty of Medicine, School of Health Sciences, University of Patras, 26504 Rion, Greece; bania.ang@gmail.com
2 School of Medicine, University of Crete, 71003 Heraklion, Greece; kpitsikakis.00@gmail.com
3 Department of Emergency Medicine, Faculty of Medicine, School of Health Sciences, University of Thessaly, 41110 Larissa, Greece; beltsioseleftherios@gmail.com (E.T.B.); pantazopoulosioannis@yahoo.com (I.P.)
4 Department of Anesthesiology, Faculty of Medicine, School of Health Sciences, University of Thessaly, 41110 Larissa, Greece; mmermiri@gmail.com
5 Department of Radiology, Faculty of Medicine, School of Health Sciences, University of Thessaly, 41110 Larissa, Greece; antonadamou@gmail.com
6 Department of Anesthesiology, General Hospital of Limassol, Limassol 4131, Cyprus; vasokonstant@yahoo.gr
7 Critical Care Department, Faculty of Medicine, School of Health Sciences, University of Thessaly, 41110 Larissa, Greece; demomakris@uth.gr (D.M.); vasotsolaki@yahoo.com (V.T.)
8 Department of Respiratory Medicine, Faculty of Medicine, School of Health Sciences, University of Thessaly, 41110 Larissa, Greece; kgourg@uth.gr
* Correspondence: gmavrovounis@gmail.com

Abstract: Vitamin D has known immunomodulatory activity and multiple indications exist supporting its potential use against SARS-CoV-2 infection in the setting of the current pandemic. The purpose of this systematic review is to examine the efficacy of vitamin D administered to adult patients following COVID-19 diagnosis in terms of length of hospital stay, intubation, ICU admission and mortality rates. Therefore, PubMed and Scopus databases were searched for original articles referring to the aforementioned parameters. Of the 1376 identified studies, eleven were finally included. Vitamin D supplements, and especially calcifediol, were shown to be useful in significantly reducing ICU admissions and/or mortality in four of the studies, but not in diminishing the duration of hospitalization of COVID-19 patients. Due to the large variation in vitamin D supplementation schemes no absolute conclusions can be drawn until larger randomized controlled trials are completed. However, calcifediol administered to COVID-19 patients upon diagnosis represents by far the most promising agent and should be the focus of upcoming research efforts.

Keywords: COVID-19; vitamin D; hospitalization; ICU admission; intubation; mortality

Citation: Bania, A.; Pitsikakis, K.; Mavrovounis, G.; Mermiri, M.; Beltsios, E.T.; Adamou, A.; Konstantaki, V.; Makris, D.; Tsolaki, V.; Gourgoulianis, K.; et al. Therapeutic Vitamin D Supplementation Following COVID-19 Diagnosis: Where Do We Stand?—A Systematic Review. *J. Pers. Med.* **2022**, *12*, 419. https://doi.org/10.3390/jpm12030419

Academic Editor: Bruno Mégarbané

Received: 18 February 2022
Accepted: 5 March 2022
Published: 8 March 2022

1. Introduction

The ongoing COVID-19 pandemic proven a major challenge both for the scientific community and society in general, resulting in millions of deaths worldwide [1]. Despite the immunization of a large percentage of the world population [1], predominantly in first-world countries, SARS-CoV-2 and its variants remain a significant cause of morbidity and mortality. In the absence of SARS-CoV-2-specific pharmacological agents, drug repurposing has emerged as the only available treatment strategy. Remdesivir plus dexamethasone, immunomodulatory agents and, more recently, monoclonal antibodies are approved under Emergency Use Authorization for various severity stages of COVID-19 [2], but efforts for more, largely available and safe drugs are continuous.

Vitamin D is a fat-soluble vitamin, regulating circulating calcium and phosphate levels with an important role in bone homeostasis. The active form of vitamin D is $1,25(OH)_2D3$

(calcitriol) and its biosynthesis includes the conversion of skin 7-dehydrocholesterol to pre-vitamin D3 and then vitamin D3 (cholecalciferol) in the presence of ultraviolet sun radiation [3,4], followed by two steps of hydroxylation to 25(OH)D3 (calcifediol) by the liver and finally to 1,25(OH)2D3 by the kidney. The vitamin D receptor (VDR) acts as a transcription factor and alongside the retinoid X receptor (RXR) binds on a DNA motif on a variety of human tissues [5], regulating the epigenome and expression of thousands of genes and gene networks [6], involved in mineral, bile acid and exogenous compound metabolism, cell differentiation and immune response [7].

Vitamin D deficiency, defined by the Endocrine Society [8] as 25(OH)D3 below 20 ng/mL and vitamin D insufficiency, defined as 25(OH)D3 of 21–29 ng/mL are highly prevalent findings among the general population, linked to rickets in children and osteomalacia and osteoporosis in adults, as well as diabetes, cardiovascular disease, auto-immune disorders, cancer, hepatitis B and C, allergies, asthma and respiratory tract infections [4,9].

In the current setting, vitamin D has been shown to exert immunomodulatory actions in SARS-CoV-2 infection [10,11]. More specifically, it increases the expression of defensins and cathelicidin (LL-37), an endogenous antimicrobial [12], as well as other antiviral agents involved in the TNF-a [13], IFN-γ [14] and NF-κB [15] pathways. It also reduces inflammation, and thus the risk to develop the potentially fatal Cytokine Storm Syndrome, by inhibiting the Th1 response and the production of inflammatory cytokines [14], while enhancing the production of anti-inflammatory cytokines [14]. Its role as a potential immunomodulatory agent is further supported by its capacity to increase regulatory T lymphocytes [16], which are significantly decreased in the setting of COVID-19 [17].

Vitamin D has been hypothesized to intervene in the mechanism by which COVID-19 infection induces a hypercoagulative state [18,19], thus increasing the risk for thrombosis, as well as results to the Acute Respiratory Distress Syndrome (ARDS). It is known that SARS-CoV-2 utilizes the angiotensin converting enzyme 2 (ACE2) receptor [20], thus downregulating it. This results in excessive accumulation of angiotensin II, the substrate of ACE2, which can lead to ARDS [21]. Serum vitamin D levels have been found to be inversely correlated with the Renin-Angiotensin-Aldosterone System activation [22,23], meaning that in COVID-19 patients with vitamin D deficiency, the increase of angiotensin may facilitate progress to ARDS. Conversely, vitamin D can protect from ARDS by lowering renin and increasing ACE2 expression [24].

Based on these data and thanks to their safety profile, availability and low cost, vitamin D supplements are currently used as an off-label pharmacological agent for the treatment of SARS-CoV-2 infection, while their efficacy has been examined in multiple studies with varying results. In this systematic review, we aim to summarize the most recent evidence regarding the therapeutic role of vitamin D on severe COVID-19 outcomes (length of hospital stay, mechanical ventilation, mortality) in adult populations.

2. Materials and Methods

2.1. Protocol

The protocol for this systematic review is registered in the International Prospective Registry of Systematic Reviews, PROSPERO, under the ID: PROSPERO2021 CRD42021281646 and is fully available online at https://www.crd.york.ac.uk/prospero/display_record.php?ID=CRD42021281646 (Last accessed: 18 February 2022; 19:01:38 EET).

2.2. Literature Search

Two investigators (A.B. and K.P.) individually performed an electronic search of the PubMed (MEDLINE) and Scopus databases to identify relevant studies, based on the predetermined inclusion and exclusion criteria. Disagreements between the two authors were resolved by discussion between them or with the help of a third investigator (G.M.), when necessary. The search algorithms, fully available in the Supplementary File Document S1, consisted of the terms 'vitamin D' and 'COVID-19' and their derivatives, as well as the Boolean operators 'AND' and 'OR'. The references of previous systematic reviews and meta-analyses were also screened for additional original studies. Only articles fully available in the English language were included in this review. The last literature search was performed on 28 September 2021.

2.3. Inclusion and Exclusion Criteria

Original articles, restricted to randomized controlled trials, prospective and retrospective observational studies, case-control studies and case series with at least ten participants were included in this systematic review. No restriction on publication date was imposed. The studies pertained to the post-diagnosis administration of any form of vitamin D to adult (>18 years of age) patients diagnosed with COVID-19. Our studied outcomes were: duration of hospitalization, need for mechanical ventilation/intubation, ICU admission and all-cause mortality.

Studies on the chronic supplementation with vitamin D and studies focusing on paediatric populations were excluded from this systematic review. Congress abstracts, letters to the editor, case reports, case series of less than ten patients, ecological studies, reviews and meta-analyses were also excluded.

Jevalikar et al. [25] included a small number of children in their cohort. Here we only report findings based on the data relevant to vitamin D administration in a sub-population of the initial cohort, but the presence of children in this sub-group is not specified.

2.4. Data Extraction

Using a pre-determined data table, two of the authors (A.B. and K.P.) performed the data extraction. The following data were extracted: First Author's Name, Month and Year of Publication, Study Design, Vitamin D Administration Scheme, Control Method, Population Size and Number of Participants in each group, Male to Female Ratio, Mean Age, Presence Of Comorbidities (Hypertension, Cancer, Myocardial Infarction, Diabetes Mellitus, Chronic Obstructive Pulmonary Disease, Chronic Kidney Disease, Obesity), Baseline And Post-Intervention Serum Vitamin D Levels in each group, Mortality, Length Of Hospital Stay, ICU Admissions and Intubation events in each group, Mortality Time Point and Length of Follow-Up.

2.5. Quality Assesment

Quality scoring was performed using the Cochrane Risk of Bias (RoB) [26] tool for the Randomized Controlled Trials and the Methodological Index For Non-Randomized Studies (MINORS) [27] for the observational studies. The RoB tool calculates the risk of bias accounting for the randomization process, the deviations from the intended interventions, potential missing data, the outcome measuring methods and the selection of the reported result. The MINORS tool evaluates twelve factors, relevant to the aim and design of the study, patient selection and grouping, follow-up, potential size calculation and result assessment and analysis on a scale of 0–24.

3. Results

3.1. Search Results

The literature search yielded a total of 1376 articles (832 on PubMed and 544 on Scopus), among which 189 were selected to be evaluated as full texts. Finally, a total of 11 [25,28–37] articles fully met our inclusion criteria and were included in this systematic review (Figure 1).

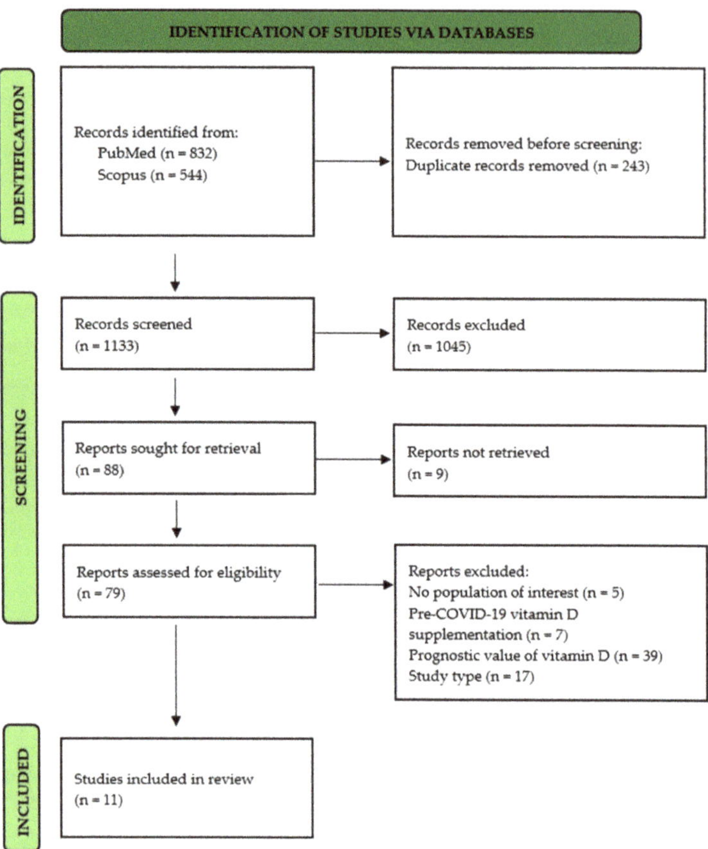

Figure 1. PRISMA flow diagram.

3.2. Study Characteristics

The studies were published from October 2020 to September 2021 and were conducted in four different continents. Three studies took place in Spain [31,33,34] and one in each of the following countries: France [28], USA [32], Brazil [35] Turkey [30], Singapore [36], Saudi Arabia [29], India [25] and Egypt [37]. The majority [25,28,30,31,33,36,37] were single-center, while in four studies patients from two [35], three [29,32] or five [34] centers were recruited. Our study collection includes four randomized controlled trials [29,32,33,35], one non-randomized controlled trial [28] and six observational cohort studies [25,30,31,34,36,37], among which two [25,31] were reported as prospective and three [34,36,37] as retrospective.

All patients examined in the aforementioned studies were hospitalized for COVID-19 infection. Vitamin D deficiency was not always a prerequisite for inclusion in the studies. A few studies focused on specific subpopulations of COVID-19 patients. More specifically, Güven et al. [30] reported only on vitamin D deficient (25(OH)D3 < 12 ng/mL) patients who had already been admitted to the ICU. In terms of age and comorbidities, Nogues et al. [31] studied high risk patients, i.e., with severe COVID-19 and/or comorbidities, Tan et al. [36] included only patients of age 50 or older, Soliman et al. [37] selected elderly (>60 years of age) vitamin D deficient (<20 ng/mL) Type II diabetics, while Annweiler et al. [28] focused on frail elderly inpatients at a geriatric acute care unit.

The studies and their characteristics are presented in Table 1.

Table 1. Study Characteristics.

Author, Date of Publication	Study Design	Treatment		Population, Male/Female Ratio, Mean Age, Baseline Vitamin D Levels (ng/mL)	
		Intervention	Control	Intervention	Control
Annweiler [28] Nov-2020	non-randomized clinical trial	80,000 IU oral vitamin D_3 plus standard care	standard care	16 11/5 85 (IQR = 84–89) NA	32 19/13 88 (IQR = 84–92) NA
Sabico [29] Jun-2021	randomized controlled trial	5000 IU oral vitamin D_3	1,000 IU oral D_3	36 21/15 46.3 ± 15.2 21.4 ± 1.2 *	33 13/20 53.5 ± 12.3 25.2 ± 1 *
Güven [30] Sep-2021	observational	300,000 IU of vitamin D_3 IM	NA	113 69/44 74 (IQR = 60–81) 6.65 (5.06–9.1)	62 36/26 74 (IQR = 60–81) 7.14 (5.17–8.21)
Nogues [31] Sep-2021	prospective	oral 25(OH)D_3 (532 µg on day one plus 266µg on day 3, 7, 15, and 30) plus standard care	standard care	447 264/183 61.81 ± 15.5 13 (IQR = 8–24)	391 231/160 62.41 ± 17.2 12 (IQR = 8–19)
Elamir [32] Sep-2021	randomized controlled trial	0.5 µg 1,25(OH)$_2$$D_3$ daily for 14 days oral plus standard care	standard care	25 12/13 69 ± 18 NA	25 13/12 64 ± 16 NA
Entrenas-Castillo [33] Oct-2020	randomized controlled trial	oral 25(OH)D_3 (0.532 mg), oral calcifediol (0.266 mg) on day 3 and 7, and then weekly plus standard care	standard care	50 27/23 53.14 ± 10.77 NA	26 18/8 52.77 ± 9.35 NA
Alcala-Diaz [34] May-2021	retrospective	oral 25(OH)D_3 (0.532 mg), then 0.266 mg on day 3 and 7, and then weekly until discharge or ICU admission plus standard care	standard care	79 42/37 69 ± 15 NA	458 275/183 67 ± 16 NA
Murai [35] Mar-2021	randomized controlled trial	single dose of 200,000 IU of oral vitamin D_3	placebo	119 70/49 56.5 ± 13.8 21.2 ± 10.1	118 63/55 56.0 ± 15.0 20.6 ± 8.1
Tan [36] Nov/Dec 2020	retrospective	1000 IU/d oral vitamin D_3 and 150 mg/d oral magnesium, and 500 mcg/d oral vitamin B_{12}	NA	17 11/6 58.4 ± 7 NA	26 15/11 64.1 ± 7.9 NA
Soliman [37] Sep-2021	prospective	vitamin D_3 as a single IM (200,000 IU) injection	placebo	40 NA 71.30 ± 4.16 10.4 ± 1.3	16 NA 70.19 ± 4.57 21.17 ± 3.96
Jevalikar [25] Mar-2021	prospective	median total dose of 60,000 IU oral vitamin D_3	NA	128 NA 45.5 ± 18.2 NA	40 NA 48.8 ± 14.7 NA

IU: International Units, IM: intramuscular, d: day, mg: milligrams, µg: micrograms, ng/mL: nanograms per milliliter, IQR: Interquartile Range, NA: not available. * Originally given at nmol/L, but converted here to ng/mL for consistency.

3.3. Interventions

The administered substance, its administration route and dosing scheme varied significantly among studies. Seven of them investigated the effect of vitamin D_3 (cholecalciferol), administered daily per os [29,36], as a high single oral dose of 60,000 IU [25], 80,000 IU [28] or 200,000 IU [35] or as an intramuscular injection of 200,000 [37] or 300,000 IU [30]. Three studies [31,33,34] applied various regimens of oral 25(OH)D3 (calcifediol) and one trial [32] used oral $1,25(OH)_2D_3$ (calcitriol) at 0.5μg/day for 14 days.

With two exceptions [29,36], the intervention and control groups did not receive any further treatments other than the appropriate standard of care of their centers or placebo. However, in a retrospective study by Tan et al. [36], the intervention group received 1,000 IU/day oral vitamin D3, 150 mg/day oral magnesium and 500 mcg/day oral vitamin B12 for a median interval of 5 days. Finally, in a randomized controlled trial by Sabico et al. [29] both groups received oral vitamin D3, but at different doses (5000 IU vs. 1000 IU).

No severe adverse effects related to this treatment were observed in any of the studies.

3.4. Length of Hospital Stay

Out of 10 studies of vitamin D-supplemented vs. vitamin D-non-supplemented patients, three reported on the length of hospitalization. Neither a single dose of 300,000 IU of intramuscular vitamin D_3 [30], a single dose of 200,000 IU of oral D3 [35] or a 14-day regimen of 0.5 μg 1,25(OH)2D3 per day [32] managed to affect the duration of hospital stay for the intervention group [9(6–16) vs. 9(5–17), p-value = 0.649, 7.0(4.0–10.0) vs. 7.0(5.0–13.0) days, p-value = 0.59, 5.5 ± 3.9 vs. 9.24 ± 9.4 days, p-value = 0.14 respectively]. Additionally, no difference in hospitalization duration was observed between the 5000 IU and the 1000 IU oral D3 group in the randomized controlled trial by Sabico et al. [29] [6(5–8) vs. 7(0–10), p-value = 0.14] (Table 2).

Table 2. Patient Outcomes.

Author	Length of Hospital Stay (Days), Mean ± SD or Median (IQR)		ICU Admission (n/N,%)		Mechanical Ventilation (n/N,%)		All-Cause Mortality (n/N,%)	
	Intervention	Control	Intervention	Control	Intervention	Control	Intervention	Control
Annweiler [28]	NA	NA	all (the study recruited patients already admitted in the ICU)		NA	NA	3/16, 19%	10/32, 31%
Sabico [29]	6 (5–8)	7 (0–10)	2/36, 5.6%	3/33, 9.1%	NA	NA	1/36, 2.8%	0/33, 0%
Güven [30]	9 (6–16)	9 (5–17)	all (the study recruited patients already admitted in the ICU)		44/113, 39%	13/62, 21%	43/113, 38%	30/62, 48%
Nogues [31]	NA	NA	20/447, 4.5%	82/39, 21%	NA	NA	21/447, 4.7%	62/391, 16%
Elamir [32]	5.5 ± 3.9	9.24 ± 9.4	5/25, 20%	8/25, 32%	0/25, 0%	2/25, 8%	0/25, 0%	3/25, 12%
Entrenas-Castillo [33]	NA	NA	1/50, 2%	13/26, 50%	NA	NA	0/50, 0%	2/26, 7.7%
Alcala-Diaz [34]	NA	NA	NA	NA	3/79, 3.8%	26/458, 5.7%	4/79, 5.1%	90/458, 20%
Murai [35]	7.0 (4.0–10.0)	7.0 (5.0–13.0)	16.0 % (9.9–22.5)	21.2% (14.2–29.7)	7.6% (3.5–13.9)	14.4% (8.6–22.1)	7.6% (3.5–13.9)	5.1% (1.9–10.7)
Tan [36]	NA	NA	1/17, 5.9%	8/26, 31%	NA	NA	0/17, 0%	0/26, 0%
Soliman [37]	NA	NA	NA	NA	14/40, 35%	7/16, 44%	7/40, 18%	3/16, 19%
Jevalikar [25]	NA	NA	16/128, 13%	13/40, 33%	NA	NA	1/128, 0.8%	3/40, 7.5%

ICU: Intensive Care Unit, IQR: Interquartile Range, NA: not available.

3.5. Need for Intubation and ICU Admission

Ten out of eleven studies provided data regarding either the need for intubation and mechanical ventilation (three studies) or intensive care admission (four studies) or both (two studies). Entrenas-Castillo et al. [33], explored the effect of a regimen comprised of 0.532 mg oral 25(OH)D3 on the day of admission followed by 0.266 mg on the 3rd and 7th day and then weekly until discharge or ICU admission in a randomized controlled trial. Of 50 patients in the intervention arm, only one required ICU admission, in contrast to the 13/26 patients from the control group (p-value < 0.001).

A similar dosing scheme (0.532 mg oral 25(OH)D3 on day 1 plus 0.266 mg on days 3, 7, 15, and 30) was later investigated by Nogues et al. [31], in a large prospective study of 838 high-risk COVID-19 patients. ICU admission was necessary for 21% of the patients in the control group, compared to 4.5% in the intervention group (OR = 0.18 (0.11–0.29), p-value < 0.001), showing an 87% risk reduction following adjustment for age, gender, baseline vitamin D levels and comorbidities [OR = 0.13, (0.07–0.23), p-value < 0.001]. A statistically significant difference in vitamin D levels between ICU and non-ICU patients was also noted [10 (7–14) ng/mL vs. 13 (8–23) ng/mL, p-value < 0.001].

Tan et al. [36], evaluated the combination of vitamin D, vitamin B12 and magnesium in a retrospective study of 43 patients over 50 years of age. The combination therapy was shown to significantly (p-value = 0.006) reduce the need for any form of oxygenation therapy. Specifically, 3/17 treated patients required oxygen therapy (including 1 in the ICU), compared to 16/26 non-treated ones (including 8 in the ICU). A subgroup analysis focusing on 30 non-diabetic patients aged 50–60 years was later performed and failed to show a statistically significant difference in oxygenation needs [25% vs. 58.3%, p-value = 0.197 and 12.5% vs. 41.7% in regard to ICU admission].

The remaining eight studies, among which the trial of 5000 IU vs. 1000 IU of oral vitamin D3 by Sabico et al. [29] did not show a statistically significant difference in ICU admission [25,29,32,35] and need for intubation [30,32,34,35,37] between study groups (Table 2).

3.6. Mortality

All eleven studies reported on the in-hospital mortality of COVID-19 patients. In a multi-center retrospective analysis of 537 patients by Alcala-Diaz et al. [34], 79 patients had received 0.532 mg of oral 25(OH)D3 on day 1 followed by 0.266 mg on day 3 and 7 and then weekly until hospital discharge or ICU admission. Mortality rates among these patients were significantly lower than those of the control group [5% versus. 20%, p-value < 0.001, OR = 0.22 (0.08–0.61), p-value < 0.01]. Given that all intervention group patients were from the same center and the patients in the control group had a greater comorbidity burden and worse clinical image upon admission, an analysis adjusted for age, center, CURB-65, ARDS at admission, neutrophil/lymphocytes ratio and comorbidities followed and still demonstrated the favorable position of the intervention group in terms of mortality [OR = 0.16 (95%CI = 0.03–0.80), p-value = 0.02]. The elderly (>65 years) subgroup with oxygen saturation <96% also greatly benefited from calcifediol administration [OR 0.06 (0.04–0.8), p-value = 0.04].

Nogues et al. [31] also attributed a reduction of death rates to 25(OH)D3 administration both in the initial [4.7% vs. 15.9%, OR: 0.26 (0.15–0.43), p-value < 0.001] and the adjusted analysis for age, gender, vitamin D levels and comorbidities [OR = 0.21; (95%CI, 0.10–0.43)], which translates into a 70% mortality risk reduction. Baseline vitamin D levels were greater in survivors compared to non-survivors [13 (8–22.7) ng/mL vs. 9 (6–13.5) ng/mL, p-value < 0.001].

In this study, 53 of 82 patients from the control group who required intensive care were started on the 25(OH)D3 regimen upon ICU admission. A sub-analysis of a total of 102 ICU COVID-19 patients was then performed. Interestingly in these patients, administration of vitamin D upon initial hospital admission was associated with lower mortality than initiation of supplementation upon ICU admission, while never receiving vitamin D at any point of the disease course had the worst prognosis. However, these differences in mortality were considered statistically insignificant (10.0% vs. 28.3% vs. 31% respectively).

No other study observed significantly different death rates among study groups (Table 2).

3.7. Quality Assessment and Risk of Bias

The bias risk for the randomized controlled trials varied significantly, as seen in Figure 2. One study [35] is marked as low-risk, one [29] as moderate risk and two [32,33] as high risk, with concerns arising mainly form the randomization process bias.

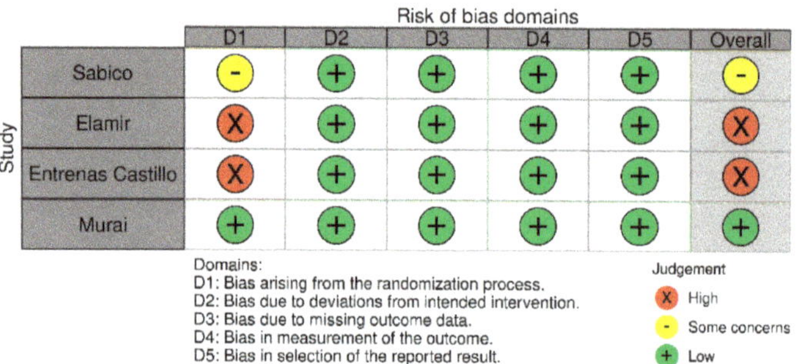

Figure 2. Risk of Bias of Randomized Controlled Trials.

The quality of the comparative observational studies ranged from 17 to 22 out of 24, based on the MINORS tool, which translates into moderate and high quality in five [28,30,34,36,37] and two [25,31] studies respectively. MINORS scores for each individual study are reported in Table 3.

Table 3. MINORS Score for non-randomized trials.

Author	MINORS Score (Out of 24)
Annweiler	18
Guven	18
Nogues	19
Alcala Diaz	17
Tan	18
Jevalikar	22
Soliman	17

4. Discussion

To our knowledge, this is the largest and most updated systematic review focusing exclusively on post-COVID-19 diagnosis administration of vitamin D, having included more recent articles compared to previous work. Thus, we have distinguished the therapeutic administration of vitamin D in hospitalized patients following COVID-19 diagnosis from chronic vitamin D supplementation for unrelated purposes.

The aim of this systematic review was to explore the impact of vitamin D administration on important parameters of COVID-19 disease course, such as length of hospital stay, ICU admissions and mortality. Of the four studies mentioning vitamin D and hospitalization duration, none managed to prove an association. Moreover, the majority of studies did not observe significant differences in the need for intubation, ICU admission or mortality, since only four out of eleven studies finally support vitamin D administration to prevent one or multiple among these unfavorable outcomes.

Evidence in favor of the use of vitamin D were identified in one randomized controlled trial of 76 patients [33], one large multi-center prospective study of 838 participants [31] and two retrospective studies [34,36] of 537 and 43 patients respectively. The observational studies, which lacked randomization, performed linear regression analyses adjusted for the confounders that were of statistical significance between the two groups and their results remained consistent with the initial findings.

It is possible that the active substance used in each study could have determined its results. Administration of vitamin D3 or 1,25$(OH)_2$D3 alone in any form or dose failed to improve any of the outcomes. On the contrary, three out of eleven studies used 25(OH)D3 and all of them reached statistical significance regarding ICU admission, mortality or both. They all took place in Spain and employed a very similar intervention scheme, comprised of an initial oral dose of 0.532 mg 25(OH)D3 followed by 0.266 mg on days 3, 7, 15 and then weekly [33,34] or on days 3, 7, 15 and 30 in the case of Nogues et al. [31]. The fourth study [36] supporting the use of vitamin D supplements to reduce oxygenation and ICU admission used a triple combination of 1000 IU/day oral vitamin D3, 150 mg/day oral magnesium and 500 mcg/day oral vitamin B12 for a median duration of 5 days.

The active vitamin D substance chosen for administration might be of special importance in the setting of renal or liver disease. As expected from the fact that the activation of vitamin D takes place in these tissues, there is a high prevalence for vitamin D deficiency among patients with renal and liver disease [38,39]. Future studies should thus consider administering the fully activated $1,25(OH)_2D3$ to these subgroups or even 25(OH)D3 in the case of liver failure, to bypass the possibly inadequate intrinsic hydroxylation stages.

A general micronutrient sufficiency was shown to reduce SARS-CoV-2 infection and severe illness in a large meta-analysis [40]. Although most heated discussions revolve around vitamin D, other dietary supplements have also been administrated by clinicians in an off-label basis, thanks to their broad role in immune system function and minimal adverse effect burden. Vitamin C [41] and zinc [42] offered no benefit regarding disease outcomes. Vitamin B12, which was co-administered with vitamin D and magnesium in one of our included studies, might facilitate symptom alleviation in COVID-19 [43]. Curcumin, on the other hand, seems to be a more promising agent, associated with faster recovery and lower mortality in a systematic review of six trials [44].

Since the beginning of the COVID-19 pandemic, the use of vitamin D as a prognostic marker and a therapeutic agent has been debatable. This hypothesis was based on pre-existing knowledge from studies on its association with other respiratory tract infections, summarized in recent systematic reviews and meta-analyses, where vitamin D deficiency was found to increase susceptibility to infection [45], while vitamin D seemed to prevent [46,47] or improve [46] the disease course. Similar to our systematic review, a major source of concern on the reliability of these conclusions is the highly variable form of vitamin D analog, its dose and route of administration employed in each of the analyzed studies.

As far as COVID-19 is concerned, vitamin D status is regularly proven to attain a prognostic value in large recent meta-analyses. Lower vitamin D levels are measured in COVID-19 patients than in healthy individuals [42,48], indicating a possible link with susceptibility to infection. Indeed, vitamin D deficiency increased the odds of contracting SARS-CoV-2 by 80% [49]. When it comes to outcomes, a lower vitamin D status was observed in severe disease cases [48], while deficient COVID-19 patients were at an increased risk for prolonged hospitalization [50], ICU admission [51] and death [50,51], although its effect on mortality is quite debatable [48,52].

In the studies presented in this systematic review, no association was observed between baseline levels of vitamin D and the benefits of vitamin D administration. More specifically, two studies [30,37] recruited vitamin D deficient patients only, but no differences were observed between the intervention and control groups. Among the studies demonstrating significant improvements following vitamin D administration, Nogues et al. [31] was the only one providing data on baseline vitamin D levels and these were similar between groups. In any case, vitamin D status should be taken into consideration in the design of future trials.

When it comes to vitamin D as a treatment option, the effect on outcomes other than length of hospital stay, intubation and mortality have also been investigated. High (60,000–80,000 IU) total doses of vitamin D3 failed to reduce the incidence of severe COVID-19, defined as Ordinal Scale for Clinical Improvement (OSCI) score equal to or greater than 5 both in frail elderly [28] and vitamin-D-deficient patients [25]. Furthermore, the effect of vitamin D on inflammatory markers varied across studies. In the aforementioned prospective study by Jevalikar et al. [25], no difference was observed in the fluctuation of any of the inflammatory markers (D-dimers, CRP, LDH, IL6, Ferritin) between the intervention and control groups. The same was reported by Sánchez-Zuno et al. [53], regarding vitamin D3 treated outpatients in regards to transferrin, ferritin and D-dimers. Among a small group of high-dose D3 supplemented and non-supplemented asymptomatic or mildly symptomatic patients the only significantly different decrease was observed in the fibrinogen levels [54]. On the contrary, a similar trial with mildly-moderately affected patients with vitamin D insufficiency reached statistical significance in all (N/L ratio, CRP, LDH, IL6, Ferritin) measured markers [55]. Vitamin D also facilitated symptom alleviation [53] and viral clearance [54] in one of two studies that reported these outcomes.

The role of vitamin D in the treatment plan against COVID-19 had been discussed in previous systematic reviews and meta-analyses. Our conclusions differ from a meta-analysis published by Pal et al. [56], who considered vitamin D supplementation to be beneficial with regards to COVID-19-related ICU admissions and mortality. This is the largest meta-analysis so far, including 13 studies, five of which are common with the ones presented in this systematic review. The difference in our conclusions may be attributed to the study selection. Pal et al. were able to include additional studies compared to our systematic review after contacting their respective authors for data which were not available in the original studies. However, studies associating COVID-19 outcomes with regular vitamin D supplementation, which were excluded in our methodology, were taken into consideration by Pal et al., who subsequently concluded that it is inferior to vitamin D administration after COVID-19 diagnosis. Finally, that meta-analysis does not take into consideration six of the eleven studies presented here, including the five most recent ones.

Previous systematic reviews and meta-analyses containing smaller subsets of articles have reached varying conclusions. Da Rocha et al. [57] were the first to publish a systematic review including three randomized controlled trials on November 2020. These three trials were also the basis for another systematic review by Stroehlein et al. [58] and a meta-analysis by Bassatne et al. [59]. The general conclusion was that vitamin D may have a therapeutic potential, but due to the insufficient, then available, evidence, the need for more, higher quality trials was highlighted.

Other systematic reviews have used subsets of the aforementioned studies and have reached conflicting conclusions supporting or disregarding the therapeutic value of vitamin D in COVID-19. An early meta-analysis by Shah et al. [60] observed the potential of vitamin D to reduce ICU admissions only. A meta-analysis of five studies [41] reported no statistically significant improvements in acute inflammatory markers, ventilation/ICU needs and mortality among patients receiving a variety of different supplementation regimens. This totally contradicts the conclusions of Dramé et al. [61] and Petrelli et al. [62], who express themselves in favor of vitamin D administration to improve all major outcomes. The co-presence of both regular supplementation regimens and post-diagnosis administration as interventions in the included studies is common among many of the systematic reviews and meta-analyses. The common denominator among all these, some of which date back to the very beginning of the pandemic, is the call for large randomized controlled trials. Indeed, the inconsistencies in population selection and more importantly in vitamin D form, dosage and route of administration among the existing studies prevents the extraction of definite conclusions, even two years into the pandemic. Therefore, as we highlight again the necessity for further research, we distinguish calcifediol from all other agents, identifying it as the most promising to be evaluated in upcoming trials.

5. Limitations

It has to be noted that, with one exception [35], the clinical trials presented in this review recruited a relatively small number of participants (<100, usually around 50) and this might be a reason for their failure to reach statistical significance.

This systematic review focuses only on the administration of vitamin D following COVID-19 diagnosis to improve important outcomes, such as length of hospital stay, intubation and ICU admission and mortality. Studies discussing the effect of vitamin D as a pre-existing regular supplementation were excluded.

It was also noticed that the included studies employed a highly variable intervention scheme, which consisted of different forms, doses and administration routes of vitamin D which, on one occasion, was co-administered with other agents. It was therefore hypothesized that it could affect the study results making data unsuitable to be pooled or processed in a meta-analysis. Indeed, the form of vitamin D analog seemed to affect outcomes, with 25(OH)D3 being associated with lower ICU admission and mortality, as opposed to vitamin D3 and 1,25$(OH)_2$D3.

As about 80% of vitamin D reserves are derived from its biosynthesis in the skin, differences in exposure to UV radiation could influence the results of the included studies. Finally, cases of liver and kidney disease in the studied cohorts might underlie the lack of response to non-activated vitamin D compounds.

6. Conclusions

In this systematic review we have summarized existing knowledge regarding the role of vitamin D on important COVID-19 outcomes indicative of disease severity (length of hospital stay, ICU admission, mortality). Despite the conflicting evidence surrounding the effect of vitamin D across the reviewed studies, we observed 25(OH)D3 (calcifediol) to be by far the most successful agent in reducing intensive care needs and mortality. Therefore, given the insufficient level of evidence of these studies, we are looking forward to larger randomized controlled trials to evaluate calcifediol's role as an adjuvant to the existing treatment regimens. Finally, given that different SARS-CoV-2 variants are currently spreading worldwide, it could be interesting and useful for further studies to include data on the effect of vitamin D on different variants as well as the patients' viral load.

Supplementary Materials: The following supporting information can be downloaded at: https://www.mdpi.com/article/10.3390/jpm12030419/s1, Document S1: Literature search algorithms.

Author Contributions: Conceptualization, A.B., G.M., D.M., V.T., K.G. and I.P.; methodology, A.B., G.M., E.T.B., A.A., D.M., V.T., K.G. and I.P.; investigation, A.B., K.P., G.M., M.M. and V.K.; data curation, A.B., K.P., G.M., M.M. and I.P.; writing—original draft preparation, A.B., K.P., G.M., M.M., E.T.B., A.A., V.K., D.M., V.T., K.G. and I.P.; writing—review and editing, A.B., K.P., G.M., M.M., E.T.B., A.A., V.K., D.M., V.T., K.G. and I.P.; visualization, A.B., K.P. and G.M.; supervision, G.M. and I.P.; project administration, I.P.; All authors have read and agreed to the published version of the manuscript.

Funding: This research received no external funding.

Institutional Review Board Statement: Not applicable.

Informed Consent Statement: Not applicable.

Data Availability Statement: Data are available upon request.

Conflicts of Interest: The authors declare no conflict of interest.

References

1. WHO Coronavirus (COVID-19) Dashboard. Available online: https://covid19.who.int (accessed on 4 December 2021).
2. COVID-19 Treatment Guidelines Panel Coronavirus Disease 2019 (COVID-19) Treatment Guidelines. Available online: https://www.covid19treatmentguidelines.nih.gov/ (accessed on 18 February 2022).
3. Holick, M.F.; MacLaughlin, J.A.; Clark, M.B.; Holick, S.A.; Potts, J.T.; Anderson, R.R.; Blank, I.H.; Parrish, J.A.; Elias, P. Photosynthesis of Previtamin D_3 in Human Skin and the Physiologic Consequences. *Science* **1980**, *210*, 203–205. [CrossRef] [PubMed]
4. Bikle, D.D. Vitamin D Metabolism, Mechanism of Action, and Clinical Applications. *Chem. Biol.* **2014**, *21*, 319–329. [CrossRef] [PubMed]
5. Nurminen, V.; Seuter, S.; Carlberg, C. Primary Vitamin D Target Genes of Human Monocytes. *Front. Physiol.* **2019**, *10*, 194. [CrossRef] [PubMed]
6. Carlberg, C. Vitamin D: A Micronutrient Regulating Genes. *Curr. Pharm. Des.* **2019**, *25*, 1740–1746. [CrossRef] [PubMed]

7. Pike, J.W.; Meyer, M.B. The Vitamin D Receptor: New Paradigms for the Regulation of Gene Expression by 1,25-Dihydroxyvitamin D3. *Endocrinol. Metab. Clin. N. Am.* **2010**, *39*, 255–269. [CrossRef] [PubMed]
8. Holick, M.F.; Binkley, N.C.; Bischoff-Ferrari, H.A.; Gordon, C.M.; Hanley, D.A.; Heaney, R.P.; Murad, M.H.; Weaver, C.M. Endocrine Society Evaluation, Treatment, and Prevention of Vitamin D Deficiency: An Endocrine Society Clinical Practice Guideline. *J. Clin. Endocrinol. Metab.* **2011**, *96*, 1911–1930. [CrossRef]
9. Marino, R.; Misra, M. Extra-Skeletal Effects of Vitamin D. *Nutrients* **2019**, *11*, 1460. [CrossRef]
10. Aygun, H. Vitamin D Can Prevent COVID-19 Infection-Induced Multiple Organ Damage. *Naunyn. Schmiedebergs Arch. Pharmacol.* **2020**, *393*, 1157–1160. [CrossRef]
11. Mercola, J.; Grant, W.B.; Wagner, C.L. Evidence Regarding Vitamin D and Risk of COVID-19 and Its Severity. *Nutrients* **2020**, *12*, 3361. [CrossRef] [PubMed]
12. Dimitrov, V.; White, J.H. Species-Specific Regulation of Innate Immunity by Vitamin D Signaling. *J. Steroid Biochem. Mol. Biol.* **2016**, *164*, 246–253. [CrossRef]
13. Peterson, C.A.; Heffernan, M.E. Serum Tumor Necrosis Factor-Alpha Concentrations Are Negatively Correlated with Serum 25(OH)D Concentrations in Healthy Women. *J. Inflamm. Lond. Engl.* **2008**, *5*, 10. [CrossRef] [PubMed]
14. Cantorna, M.T.; Snyder, L.; Lin, Y.-D.; Yang, L. Vitamin D and 1,25(OH)2D Regulation of T Cells. *Nutrients* **2015**, *7*, 3011–3021. [CrossRef] [PubMed]
15. Talmor, Y.; Bernheim, J.; Klein, O.; Green, J.; Rashid, G. Calcitriol Blunts Pro-Atherosclerotic Parameters through NFkappaB and P38 in Vitro. *Eur. J. Clin. Investig.* **2008**, *38*, 548–554. [CrossRef] [PubMed]
16. Fisher, S.A.; Rahimzadeh, M.; Brierley, C.; Gration, B.; Doree, C.; Kimber, C.E.; Plaza Cajide, A.; Lamikanra, A.A.; Roberts, D.J. The Role of Vitamin D in Increasing Circulating T Regulatory Cell Numbers and Modulating T Regulatory Cell Phenotypes in Patients with Inflammatory Disease or in Healthy Volunteers: A Systematic Review. *PLoS ONE* **2019**, *14*, e0222313. [CrossRef] [PubMed]
17. Chen, G.; Wu, D.; Guo, W.; Cao, Y.; Huang, D.; Wang, H.; Wang, T.; Zhang, X.; Chen, H.; Yu, H.; et al. Clinical and Immunological Features of Severe and Moderate Coronavirus Disease 2019. *J. Clin. Investig.* **2020**, *130*, 2620–2629. [CrossRef]
18. López-Castro, J. Coronavirus Disease-19 Pandemic and Vitamin D: So Much for so Little? *Rev. Investig. Clin. Organo Hosp. Enferm. Nutr.* **2021**, *73*, 408. [CrossRef] [PubMed]
19. Sieiro-Santos, C.; López-Castro, J. Post-Coronavirus Disease Syndrome and Disseminated Microthrombosis: The Role of the von Willebrand Factor and Antiphospholipid Antibodies. *Clinics* **2021**, *76*, e2784. [CrossRef]
20. Hoffmann, M.; Kleine-Weber, H.; Schroeder, S.; Krüger, N.; Herrler, T.; Erichsen, S.; Schiergens, T.S.; Herrler, G.; Wu, N.-H.; Nitsche, A.; et al. SARS-CoV-2 Cell Entry Depends on ACE2 and TMPRSS2 and Is Blocked by a Clinically Proven Protease Inhibitor. *Cell* **2020**, *181*, 271–280.e8. [CrossRef]
21. Imai, Y.; Kuba, K.; Rao, S.; Huan, Y.; Guo, F.; Guan, B.; Yang, P.; Sarao, R.; Wada, T.; Leong-Poi, H.; et al. Angiotensin-Converting Enzyme 2 Protects from Severe Acute Lung Failure. *Nature* **2005**, *436*, 112–116. [CrossRef]
22. Vaidya, A.; Forman, J.P.; Hopkins, P.N.; Seely, E.W.; Williams, J.S. 25-Hydroxyvitamin D Is Associated with Plasma Renin Activity and the Pressor Response to Dietary Sodium Intake in Caucasians. *J. Renin-Angiotensin-Aldosterone Syst.* **2011**, *12*, 311–319. [CrossRef] [PubMed]
23. Forman, J.P.; Williams, J.S.; Fisher, N.D.L. Plasma 25-Hydroxyvitamin D and Regulation of the Renin-Angiotensin System in Humans. *Hypertension* **2010**, *55*, 1283–1288. [CrossRef]
24. Xu, J.; Yang, J.; Chen, J.; Luo, Q.; Zhang, Q.; Zhang, H. Vitamin D Alleviates Lipopolysaccharide-induced Acute Lung Injury via Regulation of the Renin-angiotensin System. *Mol. Med. Rep.* **2017**, *16*, 7432–7438. [CrossRef] [PubMed]
25. Jevalikar, G.; Mithal, A.; Singh, A.; Sharma, R.; Farooqui, K.J.; Mahendru, S.; Dewan, A.; Budhiraja, S. Lack of Association of Baseline 25-Hydroxyvitamin D Levels with Disease Severity and Mortality in Indian Patients Hospitalized for COVID-19. *Sci. Rep.* **2021**, *11*, 6258. [CrossRef] [PubMed]
26. Sterne, J.A.C.; Savović, J.; Page, M.J.; Elbers, R.G.; Blencowe, N.S.; Boutron, I.; Cates, C.J.; Cheng, H.-Y.; Corbett, M.S.; Eldridge, S.M.; et al. RoB 2: A Revised Tool for Assessing Risk of Bias in Randomised Trials. *BMJ* **2019**, *366*, l4898. [CrossRef] [PubMed]
27. Slim, K.; Nini, E.; Forestier, D.; Kwiatkowski, F.; Panis, Y.; Chipponi, J. Methodological Index For Non-Randomized Studies (MINORS): Development And Validation of A New Instrument. *ANZ J. Surg.* **2003**, *73*, 712–716. [CrossRef]
28. Annweiler, G.; Corvaisier, M.; Gautier, J.; Dubée, V.; Legrand, E.; Sacco, G.; Annweiler, C. Vitamin D Supplementation Associated to Better Survival in Hospitalized Frail Elderly COVID-19 Patients: The GERIA-COVID Quasi-Experimental Study. *Nutrients* **2020**, *12*, 3377. [CrossRef] [PubMed]
29. Sabico, S.; Enani, M.A.; Sheshah, E.; Aljohani, N.J.; Aldisi, D.A.; Alotaibi, N.H.; Alshingetti, N.; Alomar, S.Y.; Alnaami, A.M.; Amer, O.E.; et al. Effects of a 2-Week 5000 IU vs. 1000 IU Vitamin D3 Supplementation on Recovery of Symptoms in Patients with Mild to Moderate Covid-19: A Randomized Clinical Trial. *Nutrients* **2021**, *13*, 2170. [CrossRef]
30. Güven, M.; Gültekin, H. The Effect of High-Dose Parenteral Vitamin D3 on COVID-19-Related Inhospital Mortality in Critical COVID-19 Patients during Intensive Care Unit Admission: An Observational Cohort Study. *Eur. J. Clin. Nutr.* **2021**, *75*, 1383–1388. [CrossRef]
31. Nogues, X.; Ovejero, D.; Pineda-Moncusí, M.; Bouillon, R.; Arenas, D.; Pascual, J.; Ribes, A.; Guerri-Fernandez, R.; Villar-Garcia, J.; Rial, A.; et al. Calcifediol Treatment and COVID-19-Related Outcomes. *J. Clin. Endocrinol. Metab.* **2021**, *106*, e4017–e4027. [CrossRef]

32. Elamir, Y.M.; Amir, H.; Lim, S.; Rana, Y.P.; Lopez, C.G.; Feliciano, N.V.; Omar, A.; Grist, W.P.; Via, M.A. A Randomized Pilot Study Using Calcitriol in Hospitalized COVID-19 Patients. *Bone* **2022**, *154*, 116175. [CrossRef]
33. Entrenas Castillo, M.; Entrenas Costa, L.M.; Vaquero Barrios, J.M.; Alcalá Díaz, J.F.; López Miranda, J.; Bouillon, R.; Quesada Gomez, J.M. Effect of Calcifediol Treatment and Best Available Therapy vs. Best Available Therapy on Intensive Care Unit Admission and Mortality among Patients Hospitalized for COVID-19: A Pilot Randomized Clinical Study. *J. Steroid Biochem. Mol. Biol.* **2020**, *203*, 105751. [CrossRef] [PubMed]
34. Alcala-Diaz, J.F.; Limia-Perez, L.; Gomez-Huelgas, R.; Martin-Escalante, M.D.; Cortes-Rodriguez, B.; Zambrana-Garcia, J.L.; Entrenas-Castillo, M.; Perez-Caballero, A.I.; López-Carmona, M.D.; Garcia-Alegria, J.; et al. Calcifediol Treatment and Hospital Mortality Due to COVID-19: A Cohort Study. *Nutrients* **2021**, *13*, 1760. [CrossRef] [PubMed]
35. Murai, I.H.; Fernandes, A.L.; Sales, L.P.; Pinto, A.J.; Goessler, K.F.; Duran, C.S.C.; Silva, C.B.R.; Franco, A.S.; Macedo, M.B.; Dalmolin, H.H.H.; et al. Effect of a Single High Dose of Vitamin D3 on Hospital Length of Stay in Patients With Moderate to Severe COVID-19. *JAMA* **2021**, *325*, 1053–1060. [CrossRef] [PubMed]
36. Tan, C.W.; Ho, L.P.; Kalimuddin, S.; Cherng, B.P.Z.; Teh, Y.E.; Thien, S.Y.; Wong, H.M.; Tern, P.J.W.; Chandran, M.; Chay, J.W.M.; et al. Cohort Study to Evaluate the Effect of Vitamin D, Magnesium, and Vitamin B12 in Combination on Progression to Severe Outcomes in Older Patients with Coronavirus (COVID-19). *Nutrition* **2020**, *79–80*, 111017. [CrossRef] [PubMed]
37. Soliman, A.R.; Abdelaziz, T.S.; Fathy, A. Impact of Vitamin D Therapy on the Progress COVID-19: Six Weeks Follow-Up Study of Vitamin D Deficient Elderly Diabetes Patients. *Proc. Singap. Healthc.* **2021**, 201010582110414. [CrossRef]
38. Arteh, J.; Narra, S.; Nair, S. Prevalence of Vitamin D Deficiency in Chronic Liver Disease. *Dig. Dis. Sci.* **2010**, *55*, 2624–2628. [CrossRef]
39. Kim, S.M.; Choi, H.J.; Lee, J.P.; Kim, D.K.; Oh, Y.K.; Kim, Y.S.; Lim, C.S. Prevalence of Vitamin D Deficiency and Effects of Supplementation with Cholecalciferol in Patients with Chronic Kidney Disease. *J. Ren. Nutr. Off. J. Counc. Ren. Nutr. Natl. Kidney Found.* **2014**, *24*, 20–25. [CrossRef]
40. Wang, M.X.; Gwee, S.X.W.; Pang, J. Micronutrients Deficiency, Supplementation and Novel Coronavirus Infections-A Systematic Review and Meta-Analysis. *Nutrients* **2021**, *13*, 1589. [CrossRef]
41. Rawat, D.; Roy, A.; Maitra, S.; Shankar, V.; Khanna, P.; Baidya, D.K. Vitamin D Supplementation and COVID-19 Treatment: A Systematic Review and Meta-Analysis. *Diabetes Metab. Syndr.* **2021**, *15*, 102189. [CrossRef]
42. Szarpak, L.; Rafique, Z.; Gasecka, A.; Chirico, F.; Gawel, W.; Hernik, J.; Kaminska, H.; Filipiak, K.J.; Jaguszewski, M.J.; Szarpak, L. A Systematic Review and Meta-Analysis of Effect of Vitamin D Levels on the Incidence of COVID-19. *Cardiol. J.* **2021**, *28*, 647–654. [CrossRef]
43. Batista, K.S.; Cintra, V.M.; Lucena, P.A.F.; Manhães-de-Castro, R.; Toscano, A.E.; Costa, L.P.; Queiroz, M.E.B.S.; de Andrade, S.M.; Guzman-Quevedo, O.; de S Aquino, J. The Role of Vitamin B12 in Viral Infections: A Comprehensive Review of Its Relationship with the Muscle-Gut-Brain Axis and Implications for SARS-CoV-2 Infection. *Nutr. Rev.* **2022**, *80*, 561–578. [CrossRef] [PubMed]
44. Vahedian-Azimi, A.; Abbasifard, M.; Rahimi-Bashar, F.; Guest, P.C.; Majeed, M.; Mohammadi, A.; Banach, M.; Jamialahmadi, T.; Sahebkar, A. Effectiveness of Curcumin on Outcomes of Hospitalized COVID-19 Patients: A Systematic Review of Clinical Trials. *Nutrients* **2022**, *14*, 256. [CrossRef] [PubMed]
45. Shokri-Mashhadi, N.; Kazemi, M.; Saadat, S.; Moradi, S. Effects of Select Dietary Supplements on the Prevention and Treatment of Viral Respiratory Tract Infections: A Systematic Review of Randomized Controlled Trials. *Expert Rev. Respir. Med.* **2021**, *15*, 805–821. [CrossRef]
46. Abioye, A.I.; Bromage, S.; Fawzi, W. Effect of Micronutrient Supplements on Influenza and Other Respiratory Tract Infections among Adults: A Systematic Review and Meta-Analysis. *BMJ Glob. Health* **2021**, *6*, e003176. [CrossRef]
47. Jolliffe, D.A.; Camargo, C.A.; Sluyter, J.D.; Aglipay, M.; Aloia, J.F.; Ganmaa, D.; Bergman, P.; Borzutzky, A.; Damsgaard, C.T.; Dubnov-Raz, G.; et al. Vitamin D Supplementation to Prevent Acute Respiratory Infections: Systematic Review and Meta-Analysis of Aggregate Data from Randomised Controlled Trials. *medRxiv* **2020**. [CrossRef]
48. Crafa, A.; Cannarella, R.; Condorelli, R.A.; Mongioì, L.M.; Barbagallo, F.; Aversa, A.; La Vignera, S.; Calogero, A.E. Influence of 25-Hydroxy-Cholecalciferol Levels on SARS-CoV-2 Infection and COVID-19 Severity: A Systematic Review and Meta-Analysis. *EClinicalMedicine* **2021**, *37*, 100967. [CrossRef] [PubMed]
49. Teshome, A.; Adane, A.; Girma, B.; Mekonnen, Z.A. The Impact of Vitamin D Level on COVID-19 Infection: Systematic Review and Meta-Analysis. *Front. Public Health* **2021**, *9*, 624559. [CrossRef]
50. Wang, Z.; Joshi, A.; Leopold, K.; Jackson, S.; Christensen, S.; Nayfeh, T.; Mohammed, K.; Creo, A.; Tebben, P.; Kumar, S. Association of Vitamin D Deficiency with COVID-19 Infection Severity: Systematic Review and Meta-Analysis. *Clin. Endocrinol.* **2021**, *93*, 281–287. [CrossRef]
51. Ben-Eltriki, M.; Hopefl, R.; Wright, J.M.; Deb, S. Association between Vitamin D Status and Risk of Developing Severe COVID-19 Infection: A Meta-Analysis of Observational Studies. *J. Am. Coll. Nutr.* **2021**, 1–11, Ahead of print. [CrossRef]
52. Ghasemian, R.; Shamshirian, A.; Heydari, K.; Malekan, M.; Alizadeh-Navaei, R.; Ebrahimzadeh, M.A.; Ebrahimi Warkiani, M.; Jafarpour, H.; Razavi Bazaz, S.; Rezaei Shahmirzadi, A.; et al. The Role of Vitamin D in the Age of COVID-19: A Systematic Review and Meta-analysis. *Int. J. Clin. Pract.* **2021**, *75*, e14675. [CrossRef]

53. Sánchez-Zuno, G.A.; González-Estevez, G.; Matuz-Flores, M.G.; Macedo-Ojeda, G.; Hernández-Bello, J.; Mora-Mora, J.C.; Pérez-Guerrero, E.E.; García-Chagollán, M.; Vega-Magaña, N.; Turrubiates-Hernández, F.J.; et al. Vitamin D Levels in COVID-19 Outpatients from Western Mexico: Clinical Correlation and Effect of Its Supplementation. *J. Clin. Med.* **2021**, *10*, 2378. [CrossRef] [PubMed]
54. Rastogi, A.; Bhansali, A.; Khare, N.; Suri, V.; Yaddanapudi, N.; Sachdeva, N.; Puri, G.D.; Malhotra, P. Short Term, High-Dose Vitamin D Supplementation for COVID-19 Disease: A Randomised, Placebo-Controlled, Study (SHADE Study). *Postgrad. Med. J.* **2020**, *98*, 87–90. [CrossRef] [PubMed]
55. Lakkireddy, M.; Gadiga, S.G.; Malathi, R.D.; Karra, M.L.; Raju, I.S.S.V.P.M.; Ragini; Chinapaka, S.; Baba, K.S.S.S.; Kandakatla, M. Impact of Daily High Dose Oral Vitamin D Therapy on the Inflammatory Markers in Patients with COVID 19 Disease. *Sci. Rep.* **2021**, *11*, 10641. [CrossRef]
56. Pal, R.; Banerjee, M.; Bhadada, S.K.; Shetty, A.J.; Singh, B.; Vyas, A. Vitamin D Supplementation and Clinical Outcomes in COVID-19: A Systematic Review and Meta-Analysis. *J. Endocrinol. Investig.* **2021**, *45*, 53–68. [CrossRef]
57. da Rocha, A.P.; Atallah, A.N.; Aldrighi, J.M.; Pires, A.L.R.; dos Santos Puga, M.E.; Pinto, A.C.P.N. Insufficient Evidence for Vitamin D Use in COVID-19: A Rapid Systematic Review. *Int. J. Clin. Pract.* **2021**, *75*, e14649. [CrossRef] [PubMed]
58. Stroehlein, J.K.; Wallqvist, J.; Iannizzi, C.; Mikolajewska, A.; Metzendorf, M.-I.; Benstoem, C.; Meybohm, P.; Becker, M.; Skoetz, N.; Stegemann, M.; et al. Vitamin D Supplementation for the Treatment of COVID-19: A Living Systematic Review. *Cochrane Database Syst. Rev.* **2021**, *5*, CD015043. [CrossRef] [PubMed]
59. Bassatne, A.; Basbous, M.; Chakhtoura, M.; El Zein, O.; Rahme, M.; El-Hajj Fuleihan, G. The Link between COVID-19 and VItamin D (VIVID): A Systematic Review and Meta-Analysis. *Metabolism* **2021**, *119*, 154753. [CrossRef]
60. Shah, K.; Saxena, D.; Mavalankar, D. Vitamin D Supplementation, COVID-19 and Disease Severity: A Meta-Analysis. *QJM Int. J. Med.* **2021**, *114*, 175–181. [CrossRef]
61. Dramé, M.; Cofais, C.; Hentzien, M.; Proye, E.; Coulibaly, P.S.; Demoustier-Tampère, D.; Destailleur, M.-H.; Lotin, M.; Cantegrit, E.; Cebille, A.; et al. Relation between Vitamin D and COVID-19 in Aged People: A Systematic Review. *Nutrients* **2021**, *13*, 1339. [CrossRef]
62. Petrelli, F.; Luciani, A.; Perego, G.; Dognini, G.; Colombelli, P.L.; Ghidini, A. Therapeutic and Prognostic Role of Vitamin D for COVID-19 Infection: A Systematic Review and Meta-Analysis of 43 Observational Studies. *J. Steroid Biochem. Mol. Biol.* **2021**, *211*, 105883. [CrossRef] [PubMed]

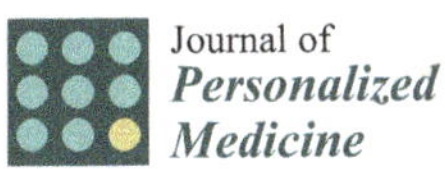

Journal of *Personalized Medicine*

MDPI

Article

Prevalence of Hemorrhagic Complications in Hospitalized Patients with Pulmonary Embolism

Nikolaos Pagkratis [1], Miltiadis Matsagas [2], Foteini Malli [3], Konstantinos I. Gourgoulianis [4] and Ourania S. Kotsiou [3,*]

1 Psychiatric Clinic, General Hospital of Corfu, 49100 Corfu, Greece; nikos.pag@hotmail.com
2 Department of Respiratory Medicine, Faculty of Medicine, University of Thessaly, 41110 Larissa, Greece; mimats@med.uth.gr
3 Vascular Surgery Department, Faculty of Medicine, University of Thessaly, 41110 Larissa, Greece; mallifoteini@yahoo.gr
4 Faculty of Nursing, University of Thessaly, 41110 Larissa, Greece; kgourg@med.uth.gr
* Correspondence: raniakotsiou@gmail.com

Abstract: Background: The prevalence of anticoagulant therapy-associated hemorrhagic complications in hospitalized patients with pulmonary embolism (PE) has been scarcely investigated. Aim: To evaluate the prevalence of hemorrhages in hospitalized PE patients. Methods: The Information System "ASKLIPIOS™ HOSPITAL" implemented in the Respiratory Medicine Department, University of Thessaly, was used to collect demographic, clinical and outcome data from January 2013 to April 2021. Results: 326 patients were included. Males outnumbered females. The population's mean age was 68.7 ± 17.0 years. The majority received low molecular weight heparin (LMWH). Only 5% received direct oral anticoagulants. 15% of the population were complicated with hemorrhage, of whom 18.4% experienced a major event. Major hemorrhages were fewer than minor (29.8% vs. 70.2%, $p = 0.001$). Nadroparin related to 83.3% of the major events. Hematuria was the most common hemorrhagic event. 22% of patients with major events received a transfusion, and 11% were admitted to intensive care unit (ICU). The events lasted for 3 ± 2 days. No death was recorded. Conclusions: 1/5 of the patients hospitalized for PE complicated with hemorrhage without a fatal outcome. The hemorrhages were mainly minor and lasted for 3 ± 2 days. Among LMWHs, nadroparin was related to a higher percentage of hemorrhages.

Keywords: pulmonary embolism; venous thromboembolism; bleeding complications; anticoagulant treatment; prediction of bleeding; in-hospital bleeding

Citation: Pagkratis, N.; Matsagas, M.; Malli, F.; Gourgoulianis, K.I.; Kotsiou, O.S. Prevalence of Hemorrhagic Complications in Hospitalized Patients with Pulmonary Embolism. *J. Pers. Med.* **2022**, *12*, 1133. https://doi.org/10.3390/jpm12071133

Academic Editor: Giovanni Squadrito

Received: 11 June 2022
Accepted: 12 July 2022
Published: 13 July 2022

1. Introduction

Pulmonary embolism (PE) is defined as a blockage in the pulmonary artery and its branches. It is caused by detached blood clots that move through the large veins to the pulmonary arteries. Embolism is usually caused by blood clots in the deep network of veins of the lower limbs—mainly in their proximal parts—such as by blood clots in the pelvic network, the upper limbs, and the right part of the heart. Rarely PE is caused by nonthrombotic sources, such as amniotic fluid, tumors, fat, large amounts of air and foreign bodies. In every patient suffering from PE, there is a degree of pulmonary obstruction. The effects of the mechanical obstruction depend on the percentage of the pulmonary circulation that is obstructed, the existence or non-existence of a cardio-respiratory disease and on time taken for the obstruction to occur [1]. If the amount of obstruction is higher than 30%, then the pressure in the pulmonary artery is increased well beyond normal, and consequently, the right part of the heart is beaten. A serious obstruction cannot be compensated by pulmonary capillaries, thus leading to increased pulmonary vascular resistance. This, in turn, provokes an increase in the right ventricular afterload, which results in increased parietal tension and finally, ischemia. Respiratory effects include tachypnea in 92% of patients and serious hypoxemia (PaO_2 < 70%) in a 63% [2].

PE presents a wide range of hemodynamic effects, from asymptomatic and undiagnosed disease to life-threatening emergencies. It is the third most frequent cause of death in hospitalized patients and a major cause of morbidity and mortality, with a total annual effect of 62 to 112 cases per 100,000 inhabitants [3]. Prognosis may worsen in PE patients, during intrahospital treatment, by experiencing hemorrhagic complications, which are mainly attributed to anticoagulant therapy [4].

Even with the best-coordinated care, hemorrhagic complications may occur. A minor hemorrhage could predict a major one and lead to modification of the anticoagulant therapy, underlying its importance for the prognosis and the efficient management of the major hemorrhagic episodes [1]. Hemorrhage is the most frequent complication caused by any anticoagulant [5].

Only a few studies investigated the in-hospital hemorrhage cases in patients with PE. Data regarding the in-hospital hemorrhagic complications in patients with PE presented with hemodynamic instability have also been scarcely noted, while the percentage of hemorrhagic complications has not been clarified in those receiving thrombolytic therapy. It is also important that there are no references regarding minor hemorrhages in patients hospitalized for PE.

In that context, this study aimed to evaluate the prevalence of hemorrhagic events in hospitalized PE patients and investigate the correlation of hemorrhagic events with the type of anticoagulant treatment, patients' demographic and clinical parameters, clinical burden, and outcome.

2. Materials and Methods

2.1. Study Participants

This was a retrospective study recording the hemorrhagic complications of patients with confirmed PE who were hospitalized in the Department of Respiratory Medicine of the University of Thessaly from January 2013 to April 2021. This research included all hospitalized patients in the Department of Respiratory Medicine, University of Thessaly with a discharge diagnosis I-26 Pulmonary Embolism (coding in ICD-10).

2.2. Data Collection

Demographic, clinical data, the type of anticoagulant treatment, the burden of disease, hemorrhagic events and outcomes were recorded by the Health Information System "ASKLIPIOS™ HOSPITAL" of the University Hospital of Larissa. Overview of all parameters extracted from the recordings are presented in Table 1.

Table 1. The parameters were extracted from the e-recordings of the patients hospitalized with PE.

Demographic Data	**Medical History**	**Symptomatology, Clinical Picture, Estimation of Clinical Probability**
Laboratory testing on admission and variation of laboratory parameters	The size of pulmonary emboli	Initial therapy
The burden of hemorrhagic episode	Anticoagulant therapy	Intensive care unit entrance, hospitalization length

2.3. Statistical Analysis

The chi-square test was used to make comparisons between frequencies. Unpaired t-tes was used for comparing parametric data between two groups, while non-parametric data were analyzed with the Mann–Whitney U test. Parametric data comparing three or more groups were analyzed with one-way ANOVA and Tukey's multiple comparisons test, while non-parametric were analyzed with the Kruskal–Wallis test and Dunn's multiple comparison test. Spearman's correlation was used for correlation analysis. Multiple logistic regression was used to examine a series of predictor variables to determine those that best predict a hemorrhagic event. Statistical analyses were performed with IBM SPSS Statistics for Windows, version 23.0, IBM Corp., Armonk, NY, USA.

3. Results

The study included 326 patients with a mean age of 68.7 ± 17.0 years. 57.7% (188) of them were men and much younger than the women. 97.5% of patients were Greek, 1.2% were refugees, and the rest 1.3% were of other nationalities. 86.2% of the population had at least one comorbidity, with arterial hypertension being the most frequent one (52.5% of the patients).

Demographics and comorbidities are presented in Table 2. 8.9% of the total population had no prior medical history. 61.1% of men had had recent surgery in the last three months. Three of these operations had been performed on the vertebral column. In females, three cases of PE were noted in the postnatal period, three cases noted after a recent fracture and immobilization, and two cases after a recent fracture.

Table 2. Demographics and comorbidities of the sample, n = 326.

Characteristics	Total n = 326	Males n = 188 (57.7)	Females n = 138 (42.3)
Age (years)	68.7 ± 17.0	64.9 ± 17.5	74.0 ± 15
Any comorbidity	281 (86.2)	162 (57.7)	119 (42.3)
No comorbidity	29 (8.9)	17 (58.7)	12 (41.3)
Malignancy	56 (17.1)	35 (62.5)	21 (37.5)
Lung cancer	12 (3.7)	12 (100)	0
First diagnosis of malignancy	9 (2.8)	6 (66.7)	3 (33.3)
History of thrombosis	82 (25.1)	52 (63.4)	30 (36.6)
Antiplatelet treatment	56 (17.1)	32 (57.1)	24 (42.9)
Previous hemorrhage	19 (5.8)	11 (57.9)	8 (42.1)
Thrombophilia	30 (9.2)	21 (70)	9 (30)

Note: Data are expressed as mean ± SD or as frequencies (percentages).

17.1% had a history of malignancy and 7.3% of them had a gender-related active disease. An absolute predominance of men (3.7% of the total population) was observed in the most frequent malignancy which is lung cancer. Surprisingly, in the present study, cancer was firstly diagnosed in 2.8% of patients, and more specifically, PE was the first sign of malignancy. 25.2% of the patients (82 people) had a history of thrombosis. 17.2% of the population received antiplatelet agents without any difference in the gender noticed. 5.8% (19) of the patients mentioned a previous episode of hemorrhage, and 21.1% presented a new hemorrhage during the hospitalization because of the PE. 9.2% of the population had a history of thrombophilia.

During the hospital admission, 44.2% presented dyspnea, 32% presented thoracic pain, 26.7% presented fever, and 7.7% had bloody sputum, while 4% of the population was asymptomatic. 18% presented tachycardia in the electrocardiogram (ECG).

Wells scores and Geneva scores, as well as the rates of the laboratory on patients' admission are presented in Table 3. 26% of the population had respiratory failure and 54% had hypocapnia on admission.

3.3% of the population presented with thrombocytopenia on admission. 10% were complicated by a fall in the number of platelets and thrombocytopenia during the hospitalization. 3.3% had an abnormal international normalized ratio (INR) >1.50, and 19.9% presented uremia on admission. 50% of the patients had a proximal deep vein thrombosis (DVT). 1.8% of the population had a paradox embolism.

Table 3. Wells scores, Geneva scores, clinical and laboratory data on patients' admission, $n = 326$.

Parameter	Total ($n = 326$)	Men ($n = 188$)	Women ($n = 138$)	p-Value
Wells score	5 ± 4	5 ± 4	5 ± 4	0.849
Geneva score	3 ± 4	3 ± 4	3 ± 4	0.955
PO2	70 ± 17	70 ± 19	69 ± 18	0.734
PCO2	34 ± 8	34 ± 9	34 ± 6	0.612
Platelets	257 ± 104	264 ± 111	248 ± 93	0.258
Urea	41 ± 20	42 ± 22	39 ± 16	0.161
Creatinine	1.17 ± 0.07	1.32 ± 2.3	0.9 ± 0.3	0.132
CRP	6.5 ± 6.4	6.3 ± 6.2	6.7 ± 6.1	0.641
D-dimer	2121 ± 1813	2083 ± 1722	2167 ± 1928	0.748
BNP	4283 ± 4442	3995 ± 4414	4860 ± 5122	0.767
AST	37 ± 30	34 ± 21	40 ± 12	0.636
ALT	33 ± 20	32 ± 23	34 ± 22	0.814
HCT	39 ± 6	39.4 ± 5.4	39.2 ± 6.8	0.839

Note: Data are expressed as mean ± SD; Abbreviations: ALT, Alanine Aminotransferase; AST, Aspartate Aminotransferase; BNP, Brain; Natriuretic Peptide; CRP, C-reactive protein; HCT, hematocrit; PO2, partial pressure of oxygen; PCO2, partial pressure of carbon dioxide.

Most of the patients admitted (92.4%) received LMWH, as shown in Table 3. 74.7% of them received 12-h action LMWH, and the rest received one subcutaneous dosage daily.

The anticoagulant therapy administered during patients' hospitalization is presented in Table 4. In 57.3% of the population, the treatment was modified during hospitalization. Specifically, 51.8% shifted to direct oral anticoagulants (DOACs), with which they were discharged. In 9.2% of the population, there had been a shift from 12-h to 24-h action Low-Molecular-Weight Heparin (LMWH), while in 0.9%, there had been a shift from 24-h to 12-h action LMWH. There was only one case of switching from DOAC to LMWH after an episode of gastric bleeding. The patients more frequently received rivaroxaban (75%) and less frequently dabigatran (12.5%) and apixaban (12.5%).

Table 4. Anticoagulant therapy administered during patients' hospitalization, $n = 326$.

Preparation	Frequency n, (%)
Low-Molecular-Weight Heparin (not specified)	132 (40.4)
Fondaparinux	73 (22.3)
Nadroparin	47 (14.4)
Enoxaparin	26 (8)
Tinzaparin	23 (7.1)
Classic heparin	1 (0.3)
Rivaroxaban	13 (4)
Apixaban	1 (0.3)
Dabigatran	2 (0.6)
Acenocoumarol	8 (2.4)
Total	326

Data are expressed as frequencies (percentages).

15% of the hospitalized patients (49 people) experienced an episode of hemorrhage without any gender difference (12.2% of men vs. 17.4% of women, $p = 0.240$). 18.4% of them experienced a major hemorrhage, without any difference regarding the gender noticed. Major hemorrhages were much fewer than the minor ones (18.4% vs. 81.6%, $p = 0.001$), while the average duration of hemorrhage was 3 ± 2 days. The sites of the hemorrhage are presented in Table 5.

Table 5. The hemorrhagic sites of patients hospitalized due to PE, $n = 326$.

		Site of Hemorrhage						Total
		Gastric Bleeding	Hemoptysis	Bloody Sputum	Hematoma	Hematuria	Metrorrhagia	
Gender	Males	4 (18.1)	1 (4.5)	1 (4.5)	0	16 (72.7)	0	22
	Females	1 (3.7)	4 (14.8)	3 (11.1)	6 (22.2)	13 (48.1)	1 (3.7)	27
Total		5 (10.2)	5 (10.2)	4 (8.1)	6 (12.2)	29 (59.1)	1 (2)	49

Data are expressed as frequencies (percentages).

16% of the patients with hemorrhagic complications (2.1% of the sum) needed a transfusion. The patients who had been transfused were the ones that presented major hemorrhages. 2.1% of the patients with hemorrhagic complications (0.3% of the total population) needed to be transferred to an ICU because of the bleeding.

4.2% of patients with hemorrhagic complications had to interrupt the anticoagulant therapy by missing doses, and 19.1% had to shift to 12-h action LMWH, especially enoxaparin. One out of the 49 patients with hemorrhagic complications who interrupted the therapy experienced a thrombotic event (2.1%). The average duration of hospitalization was 8 ± 5 days. 5.2% of the patients died. No death due to hemorrhagic complications was recorded.

The highest Wells score and the highest rate of creatinine (1.3 vs. 12 + 0.2, $p = 0.029$) were positively correlated with the risk of hospital bleeding. An accounting regression model was used to search for dependent variables (age, gender, comorbidities, the presence of cancer, Wells score, INR on admission, uremia on admission, location of PE, PESI score, ICU, platelet count on admission, right heart failure, instability, antithrombotics) to identify the parameters that could predict hospital bleeding, but no clinical or laboratory predictors were identified.

4. Discussion

The frequency of hemorrhagic complications during the hospitalization of patients with PE has not been previously determined in Greece. The present study was the first to investigate this issue. We found that 15% of the population hospitalized due to PE were complicated with hemorrhage, of whom 18.4% experienced a major event. Major hemorrhages were fewer than minor. Nadroparin related to 83.3% of the major events. Hematuria was the most common hemorrhagic event. 22% of patients with major events received a transfusion, and 11% were admitted to ICU. The events lasted for 3 ± 2 days. No death was recorded.

We found that among the hospitalized patients due to PE, males outnumbered females, a finding following the literature supporting that the risk of PE is higher in men than in women [6]. In some studies, the frequency of unprovoked PE varies between 16.5% and 51%, up to 69–76% [7–9]. We considered that unprovoked PE should be accepted when there are no comorbidities or provocations with proven PE hazards. Based on this definition, it was found that the frequency of unprovoked PE was 8.9% in our study. However, major predisposing factors were detected in the majority population, such as major surgery, fractures, and postnatal period [10].

The delayed diagnosis of PE was a finding of great interest that accords with previous reports commenting that PE has no typical symptomatology, thus, confirming the difficulty in PE diagnosis [11]. Patient delay of an average of 4.2 days and delay in primary care of an average of 3.9 days were the major contributors to this delay [12]. However, diagnostic delay of PE of more than seven days is common in primary care, especially in the elderly, and if chest symptoms, like pain on inspiration, are absent [13,14].

Surprisingly, in the present study, cancer was firstly diagnosed in 2.8% of patients, and more specifically, PE was the first sign of malignancy. In the case of cancer, the venous thromboembolism (VTE) risk is increased from 7 up to 28 times [15]. Neoplasia is caused when the tumor secretes substances with a prothrombotic effect, such as adhesion molecules that activate the macrophages and the platelets [16]. It has been reported that cancer is usually diagnosed within the first months after a VTE episode, with an overall incident rate of 4.1% in 1 month and 6.3% in 1 year [17].

25.2% of the patients had a previous history of thrombosis. The location and manifestation of thrombosis are of great predictive value for the risk of re-thrombosis. In a meta-analysis of patients with PE or/and DVT, the re-thrombosis percentages were 22% for PE and 26.4% for DVT [18]. The risk for a new PE was 3.1 times higher in patients with symptomatic PE than in those with proximal DVT. The patients with proximal DVT had a 4.8 times higher percentage of relapse than those with peripheral DVT [19].

In the present study, 3.1% of the patients were suffering from chronic renal failure (CRF), a disease associated with an increased risk for hemorrhage, because of the platelet dysfunction and uremic toxins in the blood, which harms the primary hemostasis [20]. Also, patients with moderate or severe CRF present higher rates of major hemorrhage than those with mild to non-CRF during the next 12 days after VTE diagnosis, despite the administration of anticoagulant therapy [20,21].

Moreover, 1.5% of the patients had asthma, and 4.3% had chronic obstructive pulmonary disease (COPD). It has been shown that asthma increases the risk for PE. In comparison with the non-asthmatic people, asthmatic patients of all age groups run an increased risk for PE, which is even more increased depending on the age and the severity of the respiratory disease [22]. Even in a stable phase, COPD is considered an independent risk factor for PE. At the same time, a meta-analysis suggests that one out of four patients with a COPD exacerbation who need hospitalization may suffer from PE [18,22].

Diabetes mellitus (DM) appeared in 12.2% of the patients. Clinically, patients with PE who suffer from DM have a higher risk of mortality than those who do not suffer from DM, while it seems that elevated glucose rates increase the risk of VTE [23]. Also, a study on the Asian population considers insulin-independent diabetes as an independent risk factor for the development of DVT and PE [24].

15% of the hospitalized population were complicated with hemorrhage, of whom 18.4% experienced a major event. Major hemorrhages were fewer than minor (29.8% vs. 70.2%, p = 0.001). Hematuria was the most common hemorrhagic event. The overall prevalence of bleeding in acute PE cohorts is approximately 10/100 patient-years [25–28].

Specifically, in the MAPPET registry, among 1001 cases of PE, 92 (9.2%) presented a major hemorrhage required a transfusion of blood units or discontinuation of the anticoagulant therapy [29]. In the EMPEROR registry, 10.3% of the patients with massive pulmonary embolism (MPE) and 3.5% of those without MPE had hemorrhagic complications. 3 out of the 63 patients in the second group died because of the hemorrhage [7].

In the IPER registry, among 1716 patients with PE, a loss of hemoglobin > 4 g/dL was reported in 53 patients (3.1%), while 6 out of 10 patients with intracranial hemorrhage died [30]. In the ZATPOL registry, hemorrhagic complications were reported in 6% (67 out of 1112) of the patients with PE. Major hemorrhage was reported in 3.6% of the patients, while 0.5% had a fatal hemorrhage. Among the patients receiving anticoagulant therapy, 24% (29 patients) presented hemorrhagic complications. Specifically, 19% (23 cases) of the hemorrhages were major and 5% were (6 cases) minor. 38 hemorrhagic cases were reported in patients who had not received thrombolysis. 17 of them were major and 21 were minor. Among the 67 cases that presented hemorrhagic complications, 17 were presented after oral anticoagulant therapy was initiated [31].

Recently, a higher risk of bleeding (RR: 2.53, 95% CI: 1.60–4.00; I 2: 65%) has been reported in ICU patients receiving an anticoagulant therapeutic regimen [26,27]. In the elderly population, in which the risk of acute PE is increased due to advanced age, bleeding is even more pronounced, with the risk of major bleeding including intracerebral bleeding doubling in patients aged above 80 years and the risk of hemorrhagic complications is highest in the early days of treatment [32–35]. Interestingly, the risk of bleeding resulting in hospitalization or death within 3 and 12 months after the index PE admission increased over the last years [36].

Several bleeding risk prediction scores have been proposed, including the VTE-BLEED, RIETE, HASBLED, and HEMORR2HAGES scores [31–35], that have several limitations as most are retrospective, few focus on real-life cohorts, and patients in the stable (not acute) phase of anticoagulation are mainly included [37].

Most patients hospitalized due to PE received LMWH related to 6 major and 39 minor hemorrhagic episodes. Fondaparinux was only related to minor episodes of hemorrhage. According to studies that have compared it with enoxaparin, the percentage of major hemorrhage in 9 days is much lower when fondaparinux is used rather than enoxaparin [38]. On the other hand, we found that nadroparin related to 83.3% of the major events. Generally, it has been reported that absolute major bleeding rates are low for all LMWH agents [38]. Nevertheless, twice-daily dosing with nadroparin appeared to be associated with a 1.77 times greater bleeding risk as compared with once-daily dosing, as also suggested in a meta-analysis of controlled clinical trials [38,39].

As initial therapy, low-risk patients can receive DOACs, specifically rivaroxaban or apixaban [29]. Rivaroxaban and apixaban can be given in a higher initial dose without previous heparin therapy [29]. In the present study, 4.1% were receiving DOACs, and they underwent one major and one minor hemorrhagic episode. Multiple clinical studies support the safer bleeding profile of DOACs over Vitamin K antagonists [38]. However, it has been supported that DOACs at standard dose, except apixaban, had a higher risk of major gastrointestinal bleeding compared to warfarin. Apixaban had a lower rate of major gastrointestinal bleeding compared to dabigatran and rivaroxaban [40].

2% of patients with major events received a transfusion, and 11% were admitted to ICU. The bleeding events lasted for 3 ± 2 days. No death was recorded. Hemorrhagic complications were associated with an average hospitalization of 10.7 days, with higher risk of hospital-acquired infection and higher healthcare cost, compared to 7.4 days of hospitalization for those without bleeding, In-hospital major bleeding has been identified as strong predictor of in-hospital (OR 7.7, 95% CI 2.3–25.8) and 1-year mortality (HR 3.6, 95% CI 2.0–6.6), especially in normotensive patients [41]. Generally, an improvement in mortality has been reported over years attributed to both a real improvement in patient care and "over-diagnosis" of incidental and sub-segmental PE [36].

According to a recent meta-analysis of 14 randomized controlled trials and 13 cohort studies, including 9982 patients who received a vitamin K antagonist and 7220 received a DOAC, it has been supported that the incidence of major bleeding was statistically significantly higher among those who had creatinine clearance less than 50 mL/min [42]. Accordingly, in the present study, we found a correlation between high serum creatinine levels and hemorrhagic complications, but the regression model did not prove that this variable was an independent predictor of hemorrhage. A few limitations need to be noted regarding the present study. A major limitation of this study was its retrospective design that it might generate a great deal of missed data. There was also absence of data on potential confounding factors.

5. Conclusions

15% of the hospitalized patients of the study (49 patients) presented an episode of hemorrhage, while 18.4% of them presented an episode of major hemorrhage. Hemorrhages were mainly minor and there was no hemorrhage leading to death. 16.2% of the patients with hemorrhagic complication (2.1% of the total population) needed transfusion. The average duration of hemorrhage was 3 ± 2 days. 2.1% of the patients with major hemorrhage (0.3% of the total population) needed to be transferred to an ICU, because of the hemorrhagic complication. 83.3% of the cases that presented major hemorrhage and received LMWH were given nadroparin. There was not any independent predictor of hemorrhage, but there was a correlation between high Wells score or high levels of serum creatinine and hemorrhagic complication.

Only a few studies investigated the in-hospital hemorrhage cases in patients with PE, as detecting these rare events in large datasets remains difficult. The present study evaluating data throughout an 8-year period highlights a significant likelihood of bleeding and a small, but not negligible, possibility of major hemorrhage in patients hospitalized for PE. We found that nadroparin administration was associated with major hemorrhagic events; thus, it should probably not be the first therapeutic choice among other LMWH during the in-hospital treatment of patients with PE. Until now, there are no clear guidelines and scientific evidence available for physicians in this field for early diagnosis and tools to avoid hemorrhagic complications in patients hospitalized for PE. The optimal management of bleeding involves the application of predictive scores in combination with anticoagulant reversal strategies. However, risk assessment tools are relevant in managing patients with atrial fibrillation but are not widely validated in PE patients. Hence, the performance of existing prediction models in patients with PE should be further assessed. More comprehensively, the combination of clinical, biological, and genetic markers should be incorporated to build predictive scores to estimate the risk of bleeding and help the decision process about the proper type of anticoagulant treatment.

Author Contributions: Conceptualization, O.S.K., M.M., K.I.G. and N.P.; methodology, O.S.K. and N.P.; validation, M.M., K.I.G., F.M. and O.S.K.; formal analysis, O.S.K.; investigation, N.P.; data curation, N.P.; writing—original draft preparation, N.P. and O.S.K.; writing—review and editing, N.P., O.S.K. and M.M.; supervision, O.S.K.; project administration, O.S.K. All authors have read and agreed to the published version of the manuscript.

Funding: This research received no external funding.

Institutional Review Board Statement: The study was conducted in accordance with the Declaration of Helsinki and approved by the Ethics Committee of the University of Thessaly (No. 2800-01/11/2020; approved on 1 November 2020).

Informed Consent Statement: Patient consent was waived due to the retrospective nature of this study and the analysis used anonymous clinical data.

Data Availability Statement: The data that support the findings of this study are available on request from the corresponding author, O.S.K.

Conflicts of Interest: The authors declare no conflict of interest.

References

1. Limbrey, R.; Howard, L. Developments in the management and treatment of pulmonary embolism. *Eur. Respir. Rev.* **2015**, *24*, 484–497. [CrossRef]
2. Kotsiou, O.S.; Karadontas, V.; Daniil, Z.; Zakynthinos, E.; Gourgoulianis, K. Transcutaneous carbon dioxide monitoring as a predictive tool for all-cause 6-month mortality after acute pulmonary embolism. *Eur. J. Intern. Med.* **2019**, *68*, 44–50. [CrossRef]
3. Cohen, A.T.; Agnelli, G.; Anderson, F.A.; Arcelus, J.I.; Bergqvist, D.; Brecht, J.G.; Greer, I.A.; Heit, J.A.; Hutchinson, J.L.; Kakkar, A.K.; et al. Venous thromboembolism (VTE) in Europe. The number of VTE events and associated morbidity and mortality. *Thromb. Haemost.* **2007**, *98*, 756–764.
4. Kucher, N.; Tapson, V.F.; Goldhaber, S.Z.; DVT FREE Steering Committee. Risk factors associated with symptomatic pulmonary embolism in a large cohort of deep vein thrombosis patients. *Thromb. Haemost.* **2005**, *93*, 494–498.
5. Proietti, M.; Rivera-Caravaca, J.M.; Esteve-Pastor, M.A.; Romiti, G.F.; Marin, F.; Lip, G.Y.H. Predicting Bleeding Events in Anticoagulated Patients With Atrial Fibrillation: A Comparison Between the HAS-BLED and GARFIELD-AF Bleeding Scores. *J. Am. Heart Assoc.* **2018**, *7*, e009766. [CrossRef]
6. Ageno, W.; Pomero, F.; Fenoglio, L.; Squizzato, A.; Bonzini, M.; Dentali, F. Time trends and case fatality rate of in-hospital treated pulmonary embolism during 11 years of observation in Northwestern Italy. *Thromb. Haemost.* **2016**, *115*, 399–405.
7. Pollack, C.V.; Schreiber, D.; Goldhaber, S.Z.; Slattery, D.; Fanikos, J.; O'Neil, B.J.; Thompson, J.R.; Hiestand, B.; Briese, B.A.; Pendleton, R.C.; et al. Clinical characteristics, management, and outcomes of patients diagnosed with acute pulmonary embolism in the emergency department: Initial report of EMPEROR (Multicenter Emergency Medicine Pulmonary Embolism in the Real World Registry). *J. Am. Coll. Cardiol.* **2011**, *57*, 700–706.
8. Miniati, M.; Cenci, C.; Monti, S.; Poli, D. Clinical presentation of acute pulmonary embolism: Survey of 800 cases. *PLoS ONE* **2012**, *7*, e30891.
9. Gjonbrataj, E.; Kim, J.N.; Gjonbrataj, J.; Jung, H.I.; Kim, H.J.; Choi, W.I. Risk factors associated with provoked pulmonary embolism. *Korean J. Intern. Med.* **2017**, *32*, 95–101.
10. Anderson, F.A., Jr.; Spencer, F.A. Risk factors for venous thromboembolism. *Circulation* **2003**, *107* (Suppl. S1), I9–I16. [CrossRef]

11. Huisman, M.V.; Barco, S.; Cannegieter, S.C.; Le Gal, G.; Konstantinides, S.V.; Reitsma, P.H.; Rodger, M.; Vonk Noordegraaf, A.; Klok, F.A. Pulmonary embolism. *Nat. Rev. Dis. Prim.* **2018**, *4*, 18028. [CrossRef]
12. Walen, S.; Damoiseaux, R.A.; Uil, S.M.; van den Berg, J.W. Diagnostic delay of pulmonary embolism in primary and secondary care: A retrospective cohort study. *Br. J. Gen. Pract.* **2016**, *66*, e444–e450.
13. Hendriksen, J.M.; Koster-van Ree, M.; Morgenstern, M.J.; Oudega, R.; Schutgens, R.E.; Moons, K.G.; Geersing, G.J. Clinical characteristics associated with diagnostic delay of pulmonary embolism in primary care: A retrospective observational study. *BMJ Open.* **2017**, *7*, e012789.
14. Vinson, D.R.; Hofmann, E.R.; Johnson, E.J.; Rangarajan, S.; Huang, J.; Isaacs, D.J.; Shan, J.; Wallace, K.L., Rauchwerger, A.S.; Reed, M.E.; et al. PEPC Investigators of the KP CREST Network. Management and Outcomes of Adults Diagnosed with Acute Pulmonary Embolism in Primary Care: Community-Based Retrospective Cohort Study. *J. Gen. Intern. Med* **2022**. [CrossRef]
15. Noble, S.; Pasi, J. Epidemiology and pathophysiology of cancer-associated thrombosis. *Br. J. Cancer* **2010**, *102* (Suppl. S1), S2–S9. [CrossRef]
16. Lyman, G.H. Venous thromboembolism in the patient with cancer: Focus on burden of disease and benefits of thromboprophylaxis. *Cancer* **2011**, *117*, 1334–1349.
17. Sorensen, H.T.; Svaerke, C.; Farkas, D.K.; Christiansen, C.F.; Pedersen, L.; Lash, T.L.; Prandoni, P.; Baron, J.A. Superficial and deep venous thrombosis, pulmonary embolism and subsequent risk of cancer. *Eur. J. Cancer* **2012**, *48*, 586–593.
18. Rizkallah, J.; Man, S.F.P.; Sin, D.D. Prevalence of pulmonary embolism in acute exacerbations of COPD: A systematic review and metaanalysis. *Chest* **2009**, *135*, 786–793.
19. Baglin, T.; Douketis, J.; Tosetto, A.; Marcucci, M.; Cushman, M.; Kyrle, P.; Palareti, G.; Poli, D.; Tait, R.; Iorio, A. Does the clinical presentation and extent of venous thrombosis predict likelihood and type of recurrence? A patient-level meta-analysis. *J. Thromb. Haemost.* **2010**, *8*, 2436–2442.
20. Bhatia, H.S.; Hsu, J.C.; Kim, R.J. Atrial fibrillation and chronic kidney disease: A review of options for therapeutic anticoagulation to reduce thromboembolism risk. *Clin. Cardiol.* **2018**, *41*, 1395–1402.
21. Goto, S.; Haas, S.; Ageno, W.; Goldhaber, S.Z.; Turpie, A.G.G.; Weitz, J.I.; Angchaisuksiri, P.; Nielsen, J.D.; Kayani, G.; Farjat, A.; et al. Assessment of outcomes among patients with venous thromboembolism with and without chronic kidney disease. *JAMA Netw. Open* **2020**, *3*, e2022886.
22. Keramidas, G.; Gourgoulianis, K.I.; Kotsiou, O.S. Venous Thromboembolic Disease in Chronic Inflammatory Lung Diseases: Knowns and Unknowns. *J. Clin. Med.* **2021**, *10*, 2061. [CrossRef]
23. Bell, E.J.; Selvin, E.; Lutsey, P.L.; Nambi, V.; Cushman, M.; Folsom, A.R. Glycemia (hemoglobin A_{1c}) and incident venous thromboembolism in the atherosclerosis risk in communities cohort study. *Vasc. Med.* **2013**, *18*, 245.
24. Chung, W.-S.; Lin, C.-L.; Kao, C.-H. Diabetes increases the risk of deep-vein thrombosis and pulmonary embolism. *Thromb. Haemost.* **2015**, *114*, 812–818.
25. Kruger, P.C.; Eikelboom, J.W.; Douketis, J.D.; Hankey, G.J. Pulmonary embolism: Update on diagnosis and management. *Med. J. Aust.* **2019**, *211*, 82–87. [CrossRef]
26. Parisi, R.; Costanzo, S.; Di Castelnuovo, A.; de Gaetano, G.; Donati, M.B.; Iacoviello, L. Different Anticoagulant Regimens, Mortality, and Bleeding in Hospitalized Patients with COVID-19: A Systematic Review and an Updated Meta-Analysis. *Semin. Thromb. Hemost.* **2021**, *47*, 372–391.
27. Dreijer, A.R.; Diepstraten, J.; Brouwer, R.; Croles, F.N.; Kragten, E.; Leebeek, F.W.G.; Kruip, M.J.H.A.; van den Bemt, P.M.L.A. Risk of bleeding in hospitalized patients on anticoagulant therapy: Prevalence and potential risk factors. *Eur. J. Intern. Med.* **2019**, *62*, 17–23.
28. Piovella, C.; Dalla Valle, F.; Trujillo-Santos, J.; Pesavento, R.; Lopez, L.; Font, L.; Valle, R.; Nauffal, D.; Monreal, M.; Prandoni, P.; et al. Comparison of four scores to predict major bleeding in patients receiving anticoagulation for venous thromboembolism: Findings from the RIETE registry. *Intern. Emerg. Med.* **2014**, *9*, 847–852. [CrossRef]
29. Kasper, W.; Konstantinides, S.; Geibel, A.; Olschewski, M.; Heinrich, F.; Grosser, K.D.; Rauber, K.; Iversen, S.; Redecker, M.; Kienast, J. Management strategies and determinants of outcome in acute major pulmonary embolism: Results of a multicenter registry. *J. Am. Coll. Cardiol.* **1997**, *30*, 1165–1171. [CrossRef]
30. Casazza, F.; Becattini, C.; Bongarzoni, A.; Cuccia, C.; Roncon, L.; Favretto, G.; Zonzin, P.; Pignataro, L.; Agnelli, G. Clinical features and short term outcomes of patients with acute pulmonary embolism. The Italian Pulmonary Embolism Registry (IPER). *Thromb. Res.* **2012**, *130*, 847–852. [CrossRef]
31. Budaj-Fidecka, A.; Kurzyna, M.; Fijałkowska, A.; Żyłkowska, J.; Wieteska, M.; Florczyk, M.; Szewczyk, G.; Torbicki, A.; Filipiak, K.J.; Opolski, G. In-hospital major bleeding predicts mortality in patients with pulmonary embolism: An analysis of ZATPOL Registry data. *Int. J. Cardiol.* **2013**, *1013*, 3543–3549.
32. Spencer, F.A.; Emery, C.; Joffe, S.W.; Pacifico, L.; Lessard, D.; Reed, G.; Gore, J.M.; Goldberg, R.J. Incidence rates, clinical profile, and outcomes of patients with venous thromboembolism. The Worcester VTE study. *J. Thromb. Thrombolysis* **2009**, *28*, 401–409. [CrossRef]
33. Konstantinides, S.V.; Barco, S.; Lankeit, M.; Meyer, G. Management of Pulmonary Embolism: An update. *J. Am. Coll. Cardiol.* **2016**, *67*, 976–990. [CrossRef]

34. Faller, N.; Limacher, A.; Mean, M.; Righini, M.; Aschwanden, M.; Beer, J.H.; Frauchiger, B.; Osterwalder, J.; Kucher, N.; Lämmle, B.; et al. Predictors and causes of long-term mortality in elderly patients with acute venous thromboembolism: A Prospective cohort study. *Am. J. Med.* **2017**, *130*, 198–206.
35. Riva, N.; Bellesini, M.; Di Minno, M.N.; Mumoli, N.; Pomero, F.; Franchini, M.; Fantoni, C.; Lupoli, R.; Brondi, B.; Borretta, V.; et al. Poor predictive value of contemporary bleeding risk scores during long-term treatment of venous thromboembolism. A multicentre retrospective cohort study. *Thromb. Haemost.* **2014**, *112*, 511–521.
36. Kempny, A.; McCabe, C.; Dimopoulos, K.; Price, L.C.; Wilde, M.; Limbrey, R.; Gatzoulis, M.A.; Wort, S.J. Incidence, mortality and bleeding rates associated with pulmonary embolism in England between 1997 and 2015. *Int. J. Cardiol.* **2019**, *277*, 229–234.
37. Skowrońska, M.; Furdyna, A.; Ciurzyński, M.; Pacho, S.; Bienias, P.; Palczewski, P.; Kurnicka, K.; Jankowski, K.; Lipińska, A.; Uchacz, K.; et al. D-dimer levels enhance the discriminatory capacity of bleeding risk scores for predicting in-hospital bleeding events in acute pulmonary embolism. *Eur. J. Intern. Med.* **2019**, *69*, 8–13.
38. van Rein, N.; Biedermann, J.S.; van der Meer, F.J.M.; Cannegieter, S.C.; Wiersma, N.; Vermaas, H.W.; Reitsma, P.H.; Kruip, M.J.H.A.; Lijfering, W.M. Major bleeding risks of different low-molecular-weight heparin agents: A cohort study in 12,934 patients treated for acute venous thrombosis. *J. Thromb. Haemost.* **2017**, *15*, 1386–1391.
39. Zhang, Y.; Zhang, M.; Tan, L.; Pan, N.; Zhang, L. The clinical use of Fondaparinux: A synthetic heparin pentasaccharide. *Prog. Mol. Biol. Transl. Sci.* **2019**, *163*, 41–53. [CrossRef]
40. Radadiya, D.; Devani, K.; Brahmbhatt, B.; Reddy, C. Major gastrointestinal bleeding risk with direct oral anticoagulants: Does type and dose matter?—A systematic review and network meta-analysis. *Eur. J. Gastroenterol. Hepatol.* **2021**, *33* (Suppl. S1), e50–e58.
41. Kresoja, K.P.; Ebner, M.; Rogge, N.I.J.; Sentler, C.; Keller, K.; Hobohm, L.; Hasenfuß, G.; Konstantinides, S.V.; Pieske, B.; Lankeit, M. Prediction and prognostic importance of in-hospital major bleeding in a real-world cohort of patients with pulmonary embolism. *Int. J. Cardiol.* **2019**, *290*, 144–149.
42. Khan, F.; Tritschler, T.; Kimpton, M.; Wells, P.S.; Kearon, C.; Weitz, J.I.; Büller, H.R.; Raskob, G.E.; Ageno, W.; Couturaud, F.; et al. Long-Term Risk for Major Bleeding During Extended Oral Anticoagulant Therapy for First Unprovoked Venous Thromboembolism: A Systematic Review and Meta-analysis. *Ann. Intern. Med.* **2021**, *174*, 1420–1429.

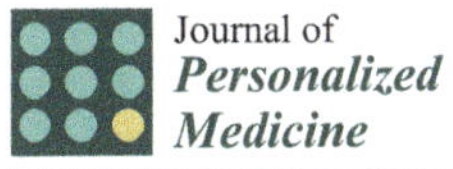

Article

Exercise Preferences and Benefits in Patients Hospitalized with COVID-19

Sevasti Kontopoulou [1], Zoe Daniil [1], Konstantinos I. Gourgoulianis [1] and Ourania S. Kotsiou [2,*]

[1] Department of Respiratory Medicine, University of Thessaly, 41110 Larissa, Greece; sevi_kon@hotmail.com (S.K.); zdaniil@uth.gr (Z.D.); kgourg@med.uth.gr (K.I.G.)
[2] Faculty of Nursing, University of Thessaly, 41110 Larissa, Greece
* Correspondence: raniakotsiou@gmail.com

Abstract: Background: Obese people are at risk of becoming severely ill due to SARS-CoV-2. The exercise benefits on health have been emphasized. Aim: To investigate the correlation of obesity with the length of hospitalization, the pre- and post-hospitalization exercise preferences of COVID-19 patients, and the impact of pre-admission or post-hospitalization physical activity on dyspnea one month after hospitalization and recovery time. Methods: A telephone survey was conducted in patients hospitalized at the Respiratory Medicine Department, University of Thessaly, Greece, from November to December 2020. Results: Two-thirds of the patients were obese. Obesity was not associated with the hospitalization time. Two-thirds of the patients used to engage in physical activity before hospitalization. Males exercised in a higher percentage and more frequently than women before and after hospitalization. The methodical pre-hospitalization exercise was associated with lower levels of dyspnea one month after hospitalization. In-hospital weight loss, comorbidities, and dyspnea on admission independently predicted longer recovery time. Lockdown had boosted men's desire to exercise than females who were negatively affected. Conclusions: Obesity is common in COVID-19 hospitalized patients. In-hospital weight loss, comorbidities, and dyspnea on admission predicted a longer post-hospitalization recovery time. The pre-hospitalization exercise was associated with less post-hospitalization dyspnea and recovery time.

Keywords: dyspnea; exercise; hospitalization; recovery

Citation: Kontopoulou, S.; Daniil, Z.; Gourgoulianis, K.I.; Kotsiou, O.S. Exercise Preferences and Benefits in Patients Hospitalized with COVID-19. *J. Pers. Med.* **2022**, *12*, 645. https://doi.org/10.3390/jpm12040645

Academic Editor: Bruno Mégarbané

Received: 13 February 2022
Accepted: 14 April 2022
Published: 17 April 2022

1. Introduction

COVID-19 is a multisystemic and multivessel disease that involves the respiratory, cardiovascular, renal, gastrointestinal, and central nervous systems. The presence of comorbidities increases the risk for severe illness due to SARS-CoV-2. More often, people with underlying medical conditions display respiratory failure that requires admission to the ICU, multiorgan failure, or even loss of their lives [1].

Obesity exposes infected individuals to peril, increasing the required days of hospitalization and recovery. This connection occurs because the chronic storage of body fat is directly associated with a chronic pro-inflammatory state, weakening the immune system and creating an ideal environment for the virus to grow inside the fat cells. Obesity, combined with comorbidities, aggravates the symptoms of the COVID-19 disease by extending the time of needed hospitalization and eventually raising the mortality rate. Regular body fat storage and a sedentary lifestyle adopted due to the mandatory quarantine can create the perfect conditions for infection and growth of contagious pathogens, such as the SARS-CoV-2 virus among the more vulnerable population [2].

Consequently, a risk factor for severe illness and needed admission to the Intensive Care Unit (ICU) is the increased body mass index (BMI), namely the increased storage of body fat [3]. A recently conducted study pointed out that the need for intensive mechanical ventilation for COVID-19 patients under 60 was seven times higher for those with a BMI over 35 kg/m^2 compared to those with a BMI under or equal to 25 kg/m^2 [4].

Starting on 4 May 2020, a 42-day strict lockdown was implemented in Greece. Movements of individuals to serve their needs outside the house were permitted only for seven categories of reasons: (i) transition to the workplace during work hours; (ii) going to the pharmacy or visiting a doctor; (iii) going to a food store; (iv) going to the bank for services not possible online; (v) helping a person; (vi) going to a significant ritual (funeral, marriage, baptism) or movement, for divorced parents, which was essential for contact with their children; and (vii) moving outdoors for exercising or taking one's pet out, individually or in pairs. Again, from 7 November 2020, Greece implemented new measures and restrictions on movement and business activity. Kindergartens, primary and special schools initially remained open, and from 18 November 2020, they switched to distance learning. On 14 December 2020, shops, hairdressers, and other facilities were allowed to open, while schools and restaurants remained closed [5].

At the beginning of the quarantine, people generally adopted a sedentary lifestyle with decreased physical activity, ultimately harming their physical and psychological health and their quality and quantity of sleep [6]. Multiple vulnerabilities and an interplay leading from simple anxiety to clinical depression and suicidality through distress were revealed among the Greek population [7].

Moderate to intense exercise entrains important positive adjustments to the cardiorespiratory ability, reduces the levels of chronic inflammation that may have preexisted due to related diseases, and improves the immune system's function for a faster reaction against viral infection such as COVID-19 [8], improves lipid profile, reduces the BMI, and can have a positive effect on our psychological health [9]. Moreover, physical exercise can help individuals maintain their muscle mass, good respiratory function, and boost the immune system to keep respiratory function levels high [10].

An international online survey including 41 research institutions from Europe, Western-Asia, North-Africa, and the Americas, documented that COVID-19 lockdown deleteriously affected physical activity and sleep patterns [11]. A recently conducted Greek study supported that during a pandemic, compared with a typical week, physical activity of a high and moderate intensity decreased for 43.0% and 37.0% of participants, did not change in 32.9% and 36.1% of participants, and increased only in 24.1% and 26.9%, respectively, whereas walking time decreased in 31.3%, did not change in 27.3%, and increased in 41.5% of participants [12]. In fact, after consecutive lockdown periods were examined, a decline in overall physical activity was evident in all age and gender groups during each lockdown phase [13].

During the pandemic, health regulators constantly point out, mainly to the elderly confined by the quarantine, to avoid a sedentary way of life and engage in any form of physical activity [8]. Furthermore, recent studies mention that exercise reduces hospitalizations due to the COVID-19 disease [14].

This study aimed to investigate the correlation of obesity with the duration of hospitalization, the pre–and post-hospitalization exercise preferences of COVID-19 patients, and the impact of pre-admission or post-hospitalization physical activity on dyspnea one month after hospitalization.

2. Materials and Methods

2.1. Procedure

This retrospective study was conducted via a telephone survey from February 2021 to March 2021. One specialized trainer was the researcher of this study and contacted previously hospitalized patients via telephone to interview by asking them a list of predetermined questions.

2.2. Participants

In the study were included all patients regardless of their age who were infected by the SARS-CoV-2 virus and were hospitalized at the Infection Diseases Unit (COVID-19) of the Department of Respiratory Medicine of the University of Thessaly from November to

December 2020. An exclusion criterion was the inability to acquire information due to their non-consent or lack of good cooperation.

2.3. Study Tools

In this study, we used an original self-reported questionnaire with 26 questions regarding:

(i) Demographics and the body metrics data of every patient before and after hospitalization (age, weight, height, body mass index were recorded);
(ii) The presence and types of comorbidities;
(iii) The dyspnea levels according to the Modified Medical Research Council (mMRC) dyspnea scale before and one month after hospitalization. Modified Medical Research Council (mMRC) Dyspnea Scale. Dyspnea is defined as the feeling of difficult and labored breathing that results from insufficient aeration. The mMRC scale used by the Medical Research Council classifies dyspnea from level 0 (dyspnea only during intense exercise) to level 4 (severe dyspnea that prevents individuals from leaving their home or even getting dressed) [8].
(iv) The length of hospitalization, (v) the physical state before and after hospitalization. As parameters of physical activity in our study, resistance training, either using the bodyweight (Pilates, yoga) or with the assistance of additional equipment (weights, resistance equipment, TRX), aerobics (running, walking, cycling, swimming), as well as work-related physical activity were included, (vi) the number of days per week spent on exercising before and after hospitalization, (vii) the different kinds of exercise before and after hospitalization, and (viii) whether the enforcement of restrictive measures negatively affected the frequency or the desire to exercise.

2.4. Statistical Analysis

The statistical analysis was conducted with the IBM SPSS v23. The quantitative variables were presented as mean value ± standard deviation (SD), and the qualitative variables were presented as an absolute value (frequency). The frequencies were compared with the chi-square statistical test. The *t*-test was used to test the difference between two mean values from independent samples. The nonparametric data were analyzed with the Mann–Whitney U test. The parametric data that compare three or more groups were analyzed with the ANOVA unidirectional Variance Analysis and the post hoc Bonferroni multiple comparison test. In contrast, the nonparametric data were analyzed with the Kruskal–Wallis test and the Dunn multiple comparison test. Spearman's correlation was used for the correlation analysis. A multiple linear regression model was utilized to examine a series of prediction variables to find those that can better predict faster recovery time in days.

3. Results

3.1. Demographics, Clinical Parameters, and Symptomatology of the Hospitalized COVID-19 Population

In total, 42 men (66%) and 22 women (34%) were included in the study, with a mean age of 62.2 ± 13.2 years old (min = 21 years, max = 91 years). The demographic and clinical parameters of the study's population and comparisons according to sex are presented in Table 1.

The men were significantly taller and heavier than the women, as expected (Table 1). The study's patients were overweight on average with no BMI difference between the genders. A total of 45.3% of the patients (29 patients) were overweight, while 23.4% (15 patients) were obese. Only 31% of the patients had normal weight. The comorbidities of the sample hospitalized due to COVID-19 and their comparison based on sex can be found in Table 2.

Table 1. Demographic and clinical data of the study's population and their comparison according to sex.

Parameters	Sum n = 64	Men n = 42	Women n = 22	p-Value
Age	62.2 ± 13.2	61.1 ± 11.9	64.2 ± 15.5	0.385 *
Height (cm)	171.0 ± 10.3	176.2 ± 7.5	161.0 ± 7.1	<0.001 *
Weight	81.6 ± 14.2	84.9 ± 13.2	75.2 ± 13.4	0.010 *
BMI	28 ± 4	27 ± 3	29 ± 5	0.113 *
mMRC before hospitalization	1 ± 1	1 ± 1	1 ± 1	0.724 *
mMRC after hospitalization	2 ± 1	2 ± 1	2 ± 1	0.068 *

Note: The data are presented as mean value ± SD; * Student's *t*-test.

Table 2. Comorbidities of the study's population and their comparison based on sex, n = 64.

Parameters	Sum n = 64	Men n = 42	Women n = 22	p-Value
At least one comorbidity	42 (65.5)	26 (61.9)	16 (72.7)	0.280 *
Number of comorbidities	2 ± 1	2 ± 1	2 ± 1	0.258 *
Hypertension	19 (29.7)	10 (23.8)	9 (40.9)	0.129 *
Cardiovascular diseases (CD, CVA)	12 (18.7)	7 (16.7)	5 (22.7)	0.392 *
DM	14 (21.9)	6 (14.3)	8 (36.4)	0.046 *
HDL	10 (15.6)	5 (11.9)	5 (22.7)	0.218 *
Malignancy	6 (9.3)	3 (7.1)	3 (13.6)	0.336 *
Autoimmune diseases	3 (4.7)	1 (2.4)	2 (9.1)	0.270 *
COPD	3 (4.7)	3 (7.1)	0	0.270 *
Asthma	2 (3.1)	1 (2.4)	1 (4.5)	0.573 *
Chronic Hepatitis	2 (3.1)	0	2 (9.1)	0.427 *
Thyroid Disease	2 (3.1)	2 (4.8)	0	0.427 *

Note: The data are presented as frequencies (percentages) or mean values ± SD; * Chi-square Test of independence; Abbreviations: CD, coronary disease; CVA, cardiovascular accidents; DM, diabetes mellitus; COPD, chronic obstructive pulmonary disease; HLD, hyperlipidaemia.

The most common comorbidity of the sample was hypertension. The women suffered from DM in a greater frequency than men. The patients with comorbidities were significantly older than those without (65 ± 12 vs. 57 ± 13 years old, $p = 0.019$), as expected.

Older age was positively associated with the level of mMRC dyspnea on admission ($r = 0.402$, $p = 0.001$) and after hospitalization ($r = 0.280$, $p = 0.025$). The number of comorbidities was positively associated with the level of mMRC dyspnea before ($r = 0.499$, $p = 0.001$) and after ($r = 0.298$, $p = 0.050$) hospitalization. Patients hospitalized due to COVID-19 with high blood pressure, or another cardiovascular disease displayed higher levels of mMRC dyspnea at the time before their admission to the hospital by comparison with those who did not have any comorbidities (2 ± 1 vs. 1 ± 1, $p < 0.001$). Patients with COPD hospitalized due to COVID-19 also displayed higher levels of mMRC dyspnea before their hospital admission than those who had no comorbidities (4 ± 1 vs. 1 ± 1, $p < 0.001$).

The symptomatology of the study's population on admission and the comparisons based on the presence or absence of comorbidities are presented in Table 3.

The most frequently displayed symptom during hospital admissions among the study's population was fever. There was no differentiation on the symptoms during admission between genders. Patients with at least one comorbidity more often had dyspnea and fever than the healthy patients prior to infection (Table 3). There was no significant difference in length of stay between patients with and without comorbidities.

Table 3. Population's symptomatology during admission and their comparison based on the presence or absence of comorbidities n = 64.

Symptomatology	Sum n = 64	Presence of Comorbidities (n = 42)	Absence of Comorbidities (n = 22)	*p*-Value
Number of symptoms	2 ± 1	2 ± 1	2 ± 1	0.648
Fever	54 (84%)	32 (76.2%)	22 (100%)	0.010 *
Dyspnea	29 (45%)	24 (57.1%)	5 (22.7%)	0.008 *
Cough	22 (34%)	14 (33.3%)	8 (36.4%)	0.510
Sore throat	7 (11%)	5 (11.9%)	2 (9.1%)	0.546 *
Abdominal pain	4 (6%)	3 (7.1%)	1 (4.5%)	0.574 *
Joint pain	4 (6%)	1 (2.3%)	3 (13.6%)	0.113 *
Myalgia	4 (6%)	3 (7.1%)	1 (4.5%)	0.574 *
Loss of taste	3 (5%)	1 (2.4%)	2 (9.1%)	0.730 *
Expectoration	2 (3%)	1 (2.4%)	1 (4.5%)	0.427 *
Loss of smell	0	0	0	-
Nasal discharge	0	0	0	-
Days of hospitalization	15 ± 12	16 ± 13	12 ± 7	0.129 *

Note: The data are presented as frequencies (percentages) or on average ± SD; * Chi-square Test of independence.

3.2. Physical Activity Preferences of the Population before Hospitalization

The physical activity of the study's population before hospitalization and their comparison based on sex can be found in Table 4.

Table 4. Physical activity of the study's population before hospitalization and comparisons based on sex, n = 64.

Parameters	Sum n = 64	Men n = 42	Women n = 22	*p*-Value
Physical exercise before hospitalization	42 (65%)	32 (76.2%)	10 (45.5%)	0.015 *
Days of exercising per week	5 ± 1	5 ± 1	4 ± 1	0.023
Walking	33 (51.6%)	24 (57.1%)	9 (40.9%)	0.166 *
Activity at work	18 (28.1%)	13 (31.1%)	5 (22.7%)	0.348 *
Resistance training	4 (6.2%)	4 (9.5%)	0	0.176 *
Aerobic exercise	5 (7.8%)	5 (11.9%)	0	0.112 *
TRX	2 (3.1%)	2 (4.8%)	0	0.427 *
Cycling	0	0	0	-

Note: The data are presented as frequencies (percentages) or mean values ± SD; * Chi-square Test of independence.

In total, 65% of the sample mentioned their engagement with at least one form of physical activity before being hospitalized. The men were exercising at a higher percentage than the women before their hospitalization and with greater frequency (Table 4). Overall, 51.6% of the study's population engaged in physical activity mentions walking as their primary exercise before hospitalization despite gender (Table 4).

The patients with at least one chronic disease were used to engage less in aerobic exercise (!8.2% vs. 2.4%, $p = 0.044$) and resistance training (18.2% vs. 0%, $p = 0.010$) compared to individuals without comorbidities.

3.3. Physical Activity Preferences of the Population after Hospitalization

The post-hospitalization physical activity of the study's population and their comparison based on sex is presented in Table 5.

Table 5. Post-hospitalization physical activity of the study's population and their comparison based on sex n = 64.

Parameters	Sum n = 64	Men n = 42	Women n = 22	p-Value
Physical activity	44 (68.8%)	34 (81%)	10 (45.5%)	0.005 *
Days of exercise per week	5 ± 2	5 ± 2	4 ± 2	0.033 *
Walking	37 (57.8%)	28 (66.7%)	9 (40.9%)	0.043 *
Activity at work	13 (20.3%)	10 (23.8%)	3 (13.6%)	0.268 *
Resistance training	6 (9.3%)	5 (11.9%)	1 (4.5%)	0.320 *
Aerobic exercise	4 (6.2%)	4 (9.5%)	0	0.176 *
Cycling	0	0	0	-
TRX	0	0	0	-

Note: The data are presented as frequencies (percentages); * Chi-square Test of independence.

Overall, 68.8% of the study's population started or continued to exercise after their hospitalization. Men continued to exercise on a larger scale and at a greater frequency than women after their hospitalization (Table 5). In 57.8% of the abovementioned population engaged in any form of physical activity after their hospitalization mentioned walking as their primary physical activity, with the male percentages being significantly higher compared to those of females (Table 5). In 36 out of the 42 individuals (85.7%) exercising before their hospitalization continued to exercise after it. In 8 out of the 44 individuals (18.2%) exercising after their hospitalization had just started, and they were not before.

3.4. Changes of Body Weight before and after Hospitalization, and Views about the Effects of Hospitalization or Lockdown on the Frequency and the Desire of Exercise after Discharge

The change of body weight before and after hospitalization, the various views about the effects of hospitalization or lockdown on the frequency and the desire of exercise after discharge and comparisons based on sex are shown on Table 6.

The BMI was not associated with the duration of hospitalization. However, the days of hospitalization were positively associated with more extensive changes in the patients' weight ($r = 0.809$, $p < 0.001$). Patients who experienced in-hospital weight loss were hospitalized more days than those who had gained weight (19 ± 14 vs. 9 ± 4, $p < 0.001$).

At a significantly higher percentage than the women, the men stated that their hospitalization or lockdown measures did not affect their exercise frequency after discharge from the hospital. In total, 50% of the men (a more considerable percentage than the women at 9%) supported that the restrictive measures did not affect the frequency of their desire to exercise. Actually, among men, 38.1% that were not previously exercising mentioned that the lockdown increased their desire to begin. Approximately half of women (45.5%) were negatively affected by the lockdown regarding their frequency and desire to exercise, a significantly higher percentage compared to the men.

Both the men and the women that did not exercise (before or after hospitalization) were those individuals who supported the harmful effects of the lockdown to their desire for exercise in comparison to those physically active before their hospitalization. The men and the women that believed in the positive effects of their hospitalization to their desire for exercise were also those who supported the positive effects of the restrictive measures to that desire.

The frequency of exercise before hospitalization was positively associated with the frequency of exercise after hospitalization ($r = 0.645$, $p < 0.001$). The patients previously engaged in physical activity needed significantly lesser time to recover (22 ± 14 vs. 65 ± 32 days, $p < 0.001$) and displayed significantly lower levels of dyspnea on the mMRC scale (1 ± 1 vs. 3 ± 1, $p < 0.001$) after their hospitalization compared to the patients with no history of physical activity. In fact, the frequency of exercise (days per week) was negatively associated with the levels of mMRC dyspnea after hospitalization ($r = -0.342$, $p = 0.026$). On the contrary, the recovery time in days was positively associated with the time of hospitalization (r = 0.408, $p = 0.001$). Of all forms of exercise, walking was associated with a shorter recovery time (23 ± 15 vs. 55 ± 34, $p < 0.001$) and a lower score on the mMRC dyspnea scale (1 ± 1 vs. 2 ± 1, $p = 0.04$) in comparison to the absence of any previous physical activity.

Table 6. Changes in body weight before and after hospitalization, views about the effects of hospitalization on the frequency of exercise after discharge and during recovery, effects of the lockdown to the frequency and the desire of the study's population to exercise and their comparison based on sex, n = 64.

Parameters	Sum n = 64	Men n = 42	Women n = 22	*p*-Value
Changes in body weight after hospitalization				
Weight loss	36 (56.3%)	26 (61.9%)	10 (45.5%)	0.459 *
Weight increase	12 (18.7%)	7 (16.7%)	5 (22.7%)	
Consistent weight	16 (25%)	9 (21.4%)	7 (31.8%)	
Weight change in Kg #	8 ± 6	8 ± 6	7 ± 5	0.388 *
Return to the pre-infection physical condition	56 (87.5%)	39 (92.9%)	17 (77.3%)	0.085 *
Recovery time after hospitalization (days)	35 ± 29	31 ± 28	45 ± 29	0.070 *
Hospitalization effects on the frequency of exercise				
Frequency increase	17 (26.6%)	11 (26.2%)	6 (27.3%)	0.396 *
Frequency decrease	9 (14%)	5 (11.9%)	4 (18.2%)	0.396 *
Consistent frequency	23 (35.9%)	21 (50%)	2 (9%)	0.002 **
No exercise	15 (23.4%)	5 (11.9%)	10 (45.5%)	0.002 **
Effects of exercise on the recovery time				
Negative	2 (3.1%)	1 (2.4%)	1 (4.5%)	0.876 *
Positive	54 (84.4%)	36 (66.7%)	18 (33.3%)	0.703 *
Do Not Know	8 (12.5%)	5 (11.9%)	3 (13.6%)	0.876 *
Lockdown effects on the frequency of exercise				
Frequency increase	17 (26.6%)	11 (26.2%)	6 (27.3%)	0.066 *
Frequency decrease	9 (14%)	5 (11.9%)	4 (18.2%)	0.066 *
Consistent frequency	23 (35.9%)	21 (50%)	2 (%)	0.002 **
No exercise	15 (23.4%)	5 (11.9%)	10 (45.5%)	0.002 **
Lockdown effects on the desire for exercise				
Negative	23 (35.9%)	10 (23.8%)	13 (59%)	<0.001 **
Positive	25 (39%)	16 (38.1%)	9 (40.9%)	0.650 *
Do Not Know	26 (25%)	16 (38.1%)	0	<0.001 **

Note: The data are presented as frequencies (percentages) or mean values ± SD; * Chi-square Test of independence; ** Bonferonni method; # Weight change refers to weight gain or loss.

The patients engaged in physical activity after their hospitalization displayed significantly lower levels of dyspnea on the mMRC scale (1 ± 1 vs. 3 ± 1, $p = 0.001$) compared to those who did not engage in any physical activity after their hospitalization. Of all the different kinds of post-hospitalization exercise, walking was positively associated with the most remarkable improvement of dyspnea after hospitalization (1 ± 1 vs. 2 ± 1, $p = 0.004$).

A multiple linear regression model was used to research those parameters that can independently predict a quicker recovery. The weight loss in Kg, the presence of chronic disease, and dyspnea on admission, were found to be independent predictors of a faster recovery time (in days) of patients hospitalized due to COVID-19 (R^2 = 92.0, adjusted R^2: 89.4) (Table 7).

Table 7. Multiple linear regression model to predict a faster recovery time (a).

Model	Unstandardized Coefficients		Standardized Coefficients	t	Sig.	95.0% Confidence Interval for B	
	B	Std. Error	Beta			Lower Bound	Upper Bound
(Constant)	35.021	10.073		3.477	0.007	12,233	57,808
b. Weight loss	2.906	0.225	1.002	9.322	<0.001	1587	2604
b. Chronic Disease	−24.648	5.002	−0.479	−4.927	<0.001	−35,964	−13,331
b. Dyspnea	13.669 Adjusted	3.112	0.485	4.392	0.002	6628	20,710

a. Dependent Variable: recovery time in days; b. Predictors: (Constant), weight loss, chronic disease, dyspnea.

4. Discussion

In this study, we investigated the correlation of obesity with the duration of hospitalization, the pre- and post-hospitalization exercise preferences of COVID-19 patients, and the impact of pre-admission or post-hospitalization physical activity on dyspnea one month after hospitalization or recovery time after discharge. We found that two-thirds of the patients were obese; however, obesity was not associated with the hospitalization time. Two-thirds of the patients used to engage in physical activity before hospitalization. The men exercised in a higher percentage and more frequently than women before and after hospitalization. The methodical pre-hospitalization exercise was associated with lower levels of dyspnea one month after hospitalization and less recovery time in days. Weight loss in Kg, preexisting comorbidity, and dyspnea on admission were independent predictors for faster recovery time in days. Most males used to exercise before infection supported that the lockdown had boosted their desire to exercise, compared to females who were negatively affected.

In our study, the average age of the sample of hospitalized patients in November and December 2020 was 62.2 ± 13.2 years old. It is distinctively mentioned that the frequency of infection is increased for men over 60 years old, who also display higher mortality rates than the women of the study up to 50%. According to the World Health Organization, there were expected differences between the two genders regarding the body metric data, while the population studied was overweight on average, without any statistically significant difference among genders.

Comorbidities were positively associated with age, as expected. It has been reported that 60 to 90% of patients who need hospitalization due to COVID-19, display at least one comorbidity [15,16]. The most common comorbidities mentioned in the literature are hypertension (57% of the patients), respiratory diseases (10% of the patients), and malignancy (8% of the patients) [15,16]. In a recent meta-analysis of 10 studies that included 76,993 patients, the prevalence of high blood pressure was 17.37% (95%CI, 10.15–23.65%), of cardiovascular disease 12.11% (95%CI 4.40–22.75%) and of DM 7.87% (95%CI 6.57–9.28%) [17]. Accordingly, the present study revealed that two-thirds of the population had at least one of the following comorbidities in descending order, high blood pressure (29.7%), DM (21.9%), cardiovascular diseases (CD, CVA) (18.7%), hypercholesterolemia/dyslipidemia (15.6%), malignancy (9.3%), coexistent autoimmune disease (4.7%), COPD (4.7%), asthma (3.1%), chronic hepatitis (3.1%), and thyroid disease (3.1%).

It has been reported that patients with more than one comorbidity experience more dyspnea [18]. In the present study, there was a positive association of dyspnea before and after hospitalization with the presence of comorbidities. Furthermore, advanced age was positively associated with the level of mMRC dyspnea on admission and after discharge. It has been reported that at least 87% of the infected by the virus still displayed at least one of the common symptoms after their recovery, more often dyspnea and fatigue, while 15% of the examined patients displayed increased breathing difficulty as a complication of the virus [19].

Patients with increased BMI are more likely to be severely infected by the new coronavirus. A large percentage of patients that need intensive care are overweight or obese [20].

We found that increased BMI was not associated with hospitalization time. However, it is essential to point out that the patients with more weight included in this study were exercising more often before their hospitalization, and the benefits of their exercise could possibly counterbalance their increased BMI. Physical activity is an important means of promoting health. In addition to improving functions related to cardiovascular and respiratory function, as well as avoiding the deposition of body fat, physical activity has many benefits for avoiding infectious diseases, or in the case of hospitalization, for faster recovery [10,21].

More specifically, physical activity improves inflammation associated with COVID-19 independent of body fat, explaining why bodyweight was not an independent contributor to hospitalization. There are data demonstrating that regular bouts of short-lasting (i.e., 45–60 min), moderate-intensity exercise (50–70% VO2max), performed at least three times per week is beneficial for the host immune defense, particularly in older adults and people with comorbidities [22,23], compared to prolonged and/or intense bout of endurance exercise that makes humans more susceptible to infection. Moderate-intensity exercise has been linked to increased leukocyte function in humans [24]. It has been found to enhance chemotaxis, degranulation, phagocytosis, cytotoxic activity, and the oxidative activity of macrophages and neutrophils in rats [25]. Increased cytolytic activity of NK cells and NK cell-activating lymphokine during 60 min of moderate-intensity exercise by healthy cyclists was also reported [11]. On the contrary, the long-duration/intense exercise-induced immunomodulation is associated with markers of immunosuppression, such as increased production of proinflammatory cytokines [26] reduced activity of NK cells, T and B lymphocytes, and neutrophils; reduced production of salivary IgA and plasma IgM and IgG; and a low expression of major histocompatibility complex II in macrophages [27,28]. These changes can be detected hours to days after the end of a prolonged and/or intense endurance exercise. Physical activity controls the viral gateway, modulates inflammation, stimulates NO production pathways, and establishes control over oxidative stress. Adaptation to usual exercise appears to affect immune function, particularly innate and adaptive immunity, and improve humoral immunity with increased vaccination responses. Exercise may at least partially counteract the detrimental effect of SARS-CoV-2 binding to the angiotensin-converting enzyme receptor [22]. Physical can activate anti-inflammatory signaling pathways. In this regard, the release of anti-inflammatory cytokines from skeletal muscle contraction, cortisol elevations, prostaglandin E2, and soluble receptors against tumor necrosis factor and interleukin 2, and increased mobilization of immunoregulatory leukocyte subtypes may be relevant in attenuating the cytokine release in COVID-19. Exercise may enhance alternative routes of NO production, stimulating eNO with antiviral effects and post-infection lung recovery of COVID-19. The control of oxidative stress, which produce cell damage, is modulated by the practice of physical activity by two mechanisms, the inhibition of NF-κB, and the stimulation of Nrf2 pathways [22].

A total of 65% of the studied sample mentioned that they engaged at least in one form of physical activity before their hospitalization, with walking being the most common. The men, compared to the women, were exercising more frequently both before and after their hospitalization. Our results are in agreement with previous studies documenting that woman were less active than men [29] and that levels of physical activity decreased progressively with age especially among women [30]. Another study reported that women were less likely than men to prefer activities that require skill and practice or done outdoors [31].

Conversely, a recent Italian study reported that women, who previously had a lower level of physical activity than men, showed a lower tendency to reduce it during lockdown, revealing greater resilience than men. During that period, women were motivated by weight loss and toning more than men [32,33], being concerned with controlling their weight, improving their physical appearance, or counteracting the effects of aging. In the present study, the factor that affected their pursuit of physical activity differs between the two sexes, and the leading cause of this phenomenon may be that Greek women tend to spend more time handling family matters and everyday family needs [34], despite the fact that females reported higher motivation for appearance and physical condition than males [33]. A study that was conducted before the COVID-19 pandemic documented that half of the studied population were physically inactive, indicating that sedentary lifestyles have become a serious epidemic in Greece [35].

An interesting finding of this study was that the patients methodically exercising had lower levels of dyspnea one month after hospitalization, needed less time to recover from the infection and return to their previous physical condition. Out of all kinds of exercise we included, walking was positively associated with a faster recovery time of the hospitalized patients. Given that in the present study the age group is over 60, we assume that it is not the walking itself in regard to intensity and how it affects the body but the fact that we had a high number of individuals in that category. Walking is a type of physical activity that is relevant to older adults as the walking ability is of primary importance for older adults [36]. On the other hand, there are data demonstrating that regular bouts of moderate-intensity exercise performed at least three times per week is more beneficial in immunomodulation compared to high intensity exercise, as mentioned above.

Exercise positively affects the immune system contributing considerably to its improvement, bearing in mind the kind, the intensity, and the duration of exercise [37]. Overall, it is a fact that mild exercises stimulate cellular immunity, increase the anti-infective activity of the macrophages and the effect of the inflammatory cytokines, contributing to the faster cure from the infection [37]. There are no data regarding the improvement of the immune response to COVID-19 infection through exercise; however, there are indications, from past viral infections of the respiratory system, of physical activity decreasing the duration and the severity of the symptoms, as well as the mortality rates of the viral disease. Physical activity of mild intensity could be considered nonmedicinal means to the fight against respiratory infections [37].

Regarding the physical activity after hospitalization, walking was again the main preferable exercise by 57.8%. It is essential to mention that this percent value increased (up to 68.8%) because most patients continued to exercise, and at the same time, some patients had begun to exercise after their recovery. Similarly, in that situation, there were more men who continued to exercise than women. In addition, the men stated that the hospitalization and restrictive measures did not affect their frequency or desire to exercise and they continued to work out the same after being cured, some even more, however, the women were affected negatively and reduced their exercise frequency.

A percentage of men and women believed that their hospitalization and the restrictive measures increased their desire to exercise. Mainly, the patients who exercised before infection claimed that their desire decreased, and their exercise after hospitalization became even more intense. On the other hand, the patients that were not exercising at all continued to keep their distance from physical activity and demonstrated that the confinement and the hospitalization affected their desire to exercise negatively. A large proportion of patients (20%) with COVID-19 will continue to have clinical manifestations of the disease, such as fatigue, weakness, severe dyspnea, and headaches for a period that may exceed one month. There is considerable evidence that physical activity has long-term health benefits that mitigate or even prevent the development of chronic non-communicable diseases (lung disease, heart disease, neurocognitive problems, musculoskeletal problems). On the other hand, physical inactivity has been associated with serious COVID-19 problems, including dyspnea [38]. Accordingly, the Centers for Disease Control and Prevention (CDC) advise not only to engage the inactive population in physical activity, but also to establish it as a tool in the management of patients with post-COVID-19 syndrome. Since exercise has been shown to be beneficial for many viral infections such as COVID-19, it is worth highlighting and further examining the extent of the favorable impacts of exercise [38]. It is also important to mention that moderate physical activity significantly increases the anti-pathogenic activity of macrophages, increases the circulation of immune cells, immunoglobulins, and anti-inflammatory cytokines while reducing the possibility of organ damage (such as the lung) due to COVID-induced inflammation [38]. Therefore, physical exercise is shown to be a non-pharmacological intervention that achieves immune enhancement and reduces the negative effects of the disease [36].

Nevertheless, it is crucial to direct our attention to that significant part of the examined sample (36.4%) that did not exercise before the lockdown and started to, not so much, of course, as those who were already used to exercise regularly. A lower frequency of exercise is imperative to eventually adopt a healthier way of life in general than no physical activity at all. This mainly happened due to the shutdown of almost all businesses which left more free time for people. At the same time, while physical activity is the only way of transportation outside the house, even for an hour, a motive has been provided to a vast part of the population to engage in physical activities and follow a healthier way of living [38].

The recovery time was positively associated with the days of hospitalization, as the more days a patient was hospitalized, the more time they needed to return to their physical condition before infection. The data of many studies support that those patients hospitalized for a long time or subjected to invasive ventilation for a prolonged period displayed respiratory and muscle difficulties, a key factor for their recovery time and the restoration of their previous physical condition to how it was before hospitalization [39].

Together, in the present study we found that preexisting comorbidities, dyspnea on admission, and weight loss in Kg during hospitalization were independent predictors for a longer recovery time after the hospitalization. The days of hospitalization were associated with more significant weight fluctuations, either weight gain or weight loss. In total, 56.3% of the patients displayed weight loss. This study showed that weight loss in Kg is an independent indicating factor for greater needed time for recovery. The severe inflammation caused by the virus and results in the release of much more acute phase proteins disorganizes the metabolism and causes weight loss. Additionally, the decreased food intake mostly connected with loss of appetite due to the disease's symptoms is one more main factor. Another important cause of weight loss is the anxiety brought on the surface due to the disease and bad sleep quality during hospitalization. In addition, immobility due to hospitalization undoubtedly contributes to muscle atrophy, a decrease in adipose tissue, sarcopenia, and, eventually, weight loss. The decreased weight and cachexia due to hospitalization increase the time patients need to return to their state prior to infection [39].

Several limitations need to be noted regarding the present study. A main limitation is that the data-stream provided by self-reporting is not shielded from potential acquiescence response bias. For this reason, the self-reported administered questionnaires were used, measured physical activities that were relevant to older adults over a relatively short period of time before and after hospitalization to minimize reporting errors [40]. In addition, reliability measures were not used in the study, but only self-report questionnaires were used to collect data. Moreover, the physical activity is not the only predictor for obesity but there are other factors as well that should be evaluated in future studies. Furthermore, we do recognize that our study was obviously limited by the small sample size. Even though we aimed to have a larger sample size, the actual response rate was much lower. Nevertheless, this study for the first time evaluated the frequency and type of physical activity among adults previously hospitalized due to COVID-19 in Greece.

5. Conclusions

We found that two-thirds of the hospitalized patients were overweight or obese. The increased BMI was not associated with the hospitalization time. This study also showed that weight loss in Kg, a pre-existing chronic disease, and dyspnea as a symptom during hospital admission could independently predict a longer recovery time. Two-thirds of the patients used to engage in some form of physical activity before infection. The men were exercising in a higher percentage and more frequently than the women before their hospitalization. Most of the patients that used to exercise before infection supported that the lockdown had boosted their desire to exercise. At a significantly higher percentage than women, men supported that their hospitalization and the restrictive measures did not affect their frequency or desire to exercise after discharge from the hospital. Women in their majority were negatively affected by the lockdown, at a higher percentage than men, regarding their frequency and desire to exercise.

Hence, obesity is a common comorbidity in patients with COVID-19 that was not proven to be associated with recovery time. Physical activity has long-term health benefits in COVID-19 patients given that those with methodical contact with exercise before infection had low levels of dyspnea after their hospitalization and less recovery time. Avoiding a sedentary life and adopting a healthier way of living by engaging in any form of physical activity are proven to positively affect the rehabilitation from the immensely severe COVID-19 disease that requires hospitalization.

Author Contributions: Conceptualization, K.I.G., Z.D. and O.S.K.; methodology, K.I.G., O.S.K. and S.K.; formal analysis, S.K.; investigation, S.K. and O.S.K.; writing—original draft preparation, O.S.K.; writing—review and editing, O.S.K.; supervision, K.I.G., Z.D. and O.S.K. All authors have read and agreed to the published version of the manuscript.

Funding: This research received no external funding.

Institutional Review Board Statement: The study was conducted in accordance with the Declaration of Helsinki and approved by the Institutional Review Board (or Ethics Committee) of University of Thessaly (No. 2800-01/11/2020; approved on 1 November 2020).

Informed Consent Statement: Informed consent was obtained from all subjects involved in the study.

Data Availability Statement: The data that support the findings of this study are available on request from the corresponding author, OSK.

Conflicts of Interest: The authors declare no conflict of interest.

References

1. Wynants, L.; Van Calster, B.; Collins, G.S.; Riley, R.D.; Heinze, G.; Schuit, E.; Bonten, M.M.J.; Dahly, D.L.; Damen, J.A.A.; Debray, T.P.A.; et al. Prediction models for diagnosis and prognosis of covid-19: Systematic review and critical appraisal. *BMJ* **2020**, *369*, m1328. [CrossRef] [PubMed]
2. Blüher, M. Obesity: Global epidemiology and pathogenesis. *Nat. Rev. Endocrinol.* **2019**, *15*, 288–298. [CrossRef] [PubMed]
3. Sattar, N.; McInnes, I.B.; McMurray, J.J.V. Obesity Is a Risk Factor for Severe COVID-19 Infection: Multiple Potential Mechanisms. *Circulation* **2020**, *142*, 4–6. [CrossRef] [PubMed]
4. Petrilli, C.M.; Jones, S.A.; Yang, J.; Rajagopalan, H.; O'Donnell, L.; Chernyak, Y.; Tobin, K.A.; Cerfolio, R.J.; Francois, F.; Horwitz, L.I. Factors associated with hospital admission and critical illness among 5279 people with coronavirus disease 2019 in New York City: Prospective cohort study. *BMJ* **2020**, *369*, m1966. [CrossRef]
5. COVID-19 Pandemic in Greece. Available online: https://en.wikipedia.org/wiki/COVID-19_pandemic_in_Greece (accessed on 4 April 2022).
6. Janssen, X.; Fleming, L.; Kirk, A.; Rollins, L.; Young, D.; Grealy, M.; MacDonald, B.; Flowers, P.; Williams, L. Changes in physical activity, sitting and sleep across the COVID-19 national lockdown period in Scotland. *Int. J. Environ. Res. Public Health* **2020**, *17*, 9362. [CrossRef]
7. Fountoulakis, K.N.; Apostolidou, M.K.; Atsiova, M.B.; Filippidou, A.K.; Florou, A.K.; Gousiou, D.S.; Katsara, A.R.; Mantzari, S.N.; Padouva-Markoulaki, M.; Papatriantafyllou, E.I.; et al. Self-reported changes in anxiety, depression and suicidality during the COVID-19 lockdown in Greece. *J. Affect Disord.* **2021**, *279*, 624–629. [CrossRef]
8. Cunningham, C.; O'Sullivan, R. Why physical activity matters for older adults in a time of pandemic. *Eur. Rev. Aging Phys. Act.* **2020**, *17*, 16. [CrossRef]
9. Baena Morales, S.; Tauler Riera, P.; Aguiló Pons, A.; García Taibo, O. Physical activity recommendations during the COVID-19 pandemic: A practical approach for different target groups. *Nutr. Hosp.* **2021**, *38*, 194–200.
10. Lavie, C.J.; Ozemek, C.; Carbone, S.; Katzmarzyk, P.T.; Blair, S.N. Sedentary Behavior, Exercise, and Cardiovascular Health. *Circ. Res.* **2019**, *124*, 799–815. [CrossRef]
11. Trabelsi, K.; Ammar, A.; Masmoudi, L.; Boukhris, O.; Chtourou, H.; Bouaziz, B.; Brach, M.; Bentlage, E.; How, D.; Ahmed, M.; et al. Sleep Quality and Physical Activity as Predictors of Mental Wellbeing Variance in Older Adults during COVID-19 Lockdown: ECLB COVID-19 International Online Survey. *Int. J. Environ. Res. Public Health* **2021**, *18*, 4329. [CrossRef]
12. Papazisis, Z.; Nikolaidis, P.T.; Trakada, G. Sleep, Physical Activity, and Diet of Adults during the Second Lockdown of the COVID-19 Pandemic in Greece. *Int. J. Environ. Res. Public Health* **2021**, *18*, 7292. [CrossRef] [PubMed]

13. Bourdas, D.I.; Zacharakis, E.D. Evolution of changes in physical activity over lockdown time: Physical activity datasets of four independent adult sample groups corresponding to each of the last four of the six COVID-19 lockdown weeks in Greece. *Data Brief* **2020**, *32*, 106301. [CrossRef] [PubMed]
14. Scartoni, F.R.; Sant'Ana, L.O.; Murillo-Rodriguez, E.; Yamamoto, T.; Imperatori, C.; Budde, H.; Vianna, J.M.; Machado, S. Physical Exercise and Immune System in the Elderly: Implications and Importance in COVID-19 Pandemic Period. *Front. Psychol.* **2020**, *11*, 593903. [CrossRef] [PubMed]
15. Wiersinga, W.J.; Rhodes, A.; Cheng, A.C.; Peacock, S.J.; Prescott, H.C. Pathophysiology, Transmission, Diagnosis, and Treatment of Coronavirus Disease 2019 (COVID-19): A Review. *JAMA* **2020**, *324*, 782–793. [CrossRef] [PubMed]
16. Gao, Y.D.; Ding, M.; Dong, X.; Zhang, J.J.; Kursat Azkur, A.; Azkur, D.; Gan, H.; Sun, Y.L.; Fu, W.; Li, W.; et al. Risk factors for severe and critically ill COVID-19 patients: A review. *Allergy* **2021**, *76*, 428–455. [CrossRef] [PubMed]
17. Emami, A.; Javanmardi, F.; Pirbonyeh, N.; Akbari, A. Prevalence of Underlying Diseases in Hospitalized Patients with COVID-19: A Systematic Review and Meta-Analysis. *Arch. Acad. Emerg. Med.* **2020**, *8*, e35.
18. Berliner, D.; Schneider, N.; Welte, T.; Bauersachs, J. The Differential Diagnosis of Dyspnea. *Dtsch. Arztebl. Int.* **2016**, *113*, 834–845. [CrossRef]
19. Carfi, A.; Bernabei, R.; Landi, F. Gemelli Against COVID-19 Post-Acute Care Study Group. Persistent Symptoms in Patients After Acute COVID-19. *JAMA* **2020**, *324*, 603–605. [CrossRef]
20. Albashir, A.A.D. The potential impacts of obesity on COVID-19. *Clin. Med.* **2020**, *20*, e109–e113. [CrossRef]
21. Katzmarzyk, P.T.; Powell, K.E.; Jakicic, J.M.; Troiano, R.P.; Piercy, K.; Tennant, B. 2018 PHYSICAL ACTIVITY GUIDELINES ADVISORY COMMITTEE. Sedentary Behavior and Health: Update from the 2018 Physical Activity Guidelines Advisory Committee. *Med. Sci. Sports Exerc.* **2019**, *51*, 1227–1241. [CrossRef]
22. Leandro, C.G.; Ferreira, E.; Silva, W.T.; Lima-Silva, A.E. Covid-19 and Exercise-Induced Immunomodulation. *Neuroimmunomodulation* **2020**, *27*, 75–78. [CrossRef] [PubMed]
23. Simpson, R.J.; Campbell, J.P.; Gleeson, M.; Krüger, K.; Nieman, D.C.; Pyne, D.B.; Turner, J.E.; Walsh, N.P. Can exercise affect immune function to increase susceptibility to infection? *Exerc. Immunol. Rev.* **2020**, *26*, 8–22. [PubMed]
24. Bigley, A.B.; Rezvani, K.; Pistillo, M.; Reed, J.; Agha, N.; Kunz, H.; O'Connor, D.P.; Sekine, T.; Bollard, C.M.; Simpson, R. Acute exercise preferentially redeploys NK-cells with a highly-differentiated phenotype and augments cytotoxicity against lymphoma and multiple myeloma target cells. Part II: Impact of latent cytomegalovirus infection and catecholamine sensitivity. *Brain Behav. Immun.* **2015**, *49*, 59–65. [CrossRef] [PubMed]
25. Senna, S.M.; Torres, M.K.; Lopes, D.A.; Alheiros-Lira, M.C.; de Moura, D.B.; Pereira, V.R.; de Aguiar, F.C., Jr.; Ferraz, J.C.; Leandro, C.G. Moderate physical training attenuates perinatal low-protein-induced spleen lymphocyte apoptosis in endotoxemic adult offspring rats. *Eur. J. Nutr.* **2016**, *55*, 1113–1122. [CrossRef]
26. Ferreira, G.A.; Felippe, L.C.; Bertuzzi, R.; Bishop, D.J.; Barreto, E.; De-Oliveira, F.R.; Lima-Silva, A.E. The Effects of Acute and Chronic Sprint-Interval Training on Cytokine Responses Are Independent of Prior Caffeine Intake. *Front. Physiol.* **2018**, *9*, 671. [CrossRef]
27. Leandro, C.G.; Martins de Lima, T.; Folador, A.; Alba-Loreiro, T.; do Nascimento, E.; Manhães de Castro, R.; de Castro, C.M.; Pithon-Curi, T.; Curi, R. Physical training attenuates the stress-induced changes in rat T-lymphocyte function. *Neuroimmunomodulation* **2006**, *13*, 105–113. [CrossRef]
28. Leandro, C.G.; de Lima, T.M.; Alba-Loureiro, T.C.; do Nascimento, E.; Manhães de Castro, R.; de Castro, C.M.; Pithon-Curi, T.C.; Curi, R. Stress-induced downregulation of macrophage phagocytic function is attenuated by exercise training in rats. *Neuroimmunomodulation* **2007**, *14*, 4–7. [CrossRef]
29. Gretebeck, K.A.; Sabatini, L.M.; Black, D.R.; Gretebeck, R.J. Physical Activity, Functional Ability, and Obesity in Older Adults: A Gender Difference. *J. Gerontol. Nurs.* **2017**, *43*, 38–46. [CrossRef]
30. Li, W.; Procter-Gray, E.; Churchill, L.; Crouter, S.E.; Kane, K.; Tian, J.; Franklin, P.D.; Ockene, J.K.; Gurwitz, J. Gender and Age Differences in Levels, Types and Locations of Physical Activity among Older Adults Living in Car-Dependent Neighborhoods. *J. Frailty Aging* **2017**, *6*, 129–135. [CrossRef]
31. van Uffelen, J.G.Z.; Khan, A.; Burton, N.W. Gender differences in physical activity motivators and context preferences: A population-based study in people in their sixties. *BMC Public Health* **2017**, *17*, 624. [CrossRef]
32. Molanorouzi, K.; Khoo, S.; Morris, T. Motives for adult participation in physical activity: Type of activity, age, and gender. *BMC Public Health* **2015**, *15*, 66. [CrossRef] [PubMed]
33. Orlandi, M.; Rosselli, M.; Pellegrino, A.; Boddi, M.; Stefani, L.; Toncelli, L.; Modesti, P.A. Gender differences in the impact on physical activity and lifestyle in Italy during the lockdown, due to the COVID-19 pandemic. *Nutr. Metab. Cardiovasc. Dis.* **2021**, *31*, 2173–2180. [CrossRef] [PubMed]
34. Sallis, J.F.; Hovell, M.F.; Hofstetter, C.R. Predictors of adoption and maintenance of vigorous physical activity in men and women. *Prev. Med.* **1992**, *21*, 237–251. [CrossRef]
35. Pitsavos, C.; Panagiotakos, D.B.; Lentzas, Y.; Stefanadis, C. Epidemiology of leisure-time physical activity in socio-demographic, lifestyle and psychological characteristics of men and women in Greece: The ATTICA Study. *BMC Public Health* **2005**, *5*, 37. [CrossRef] [PubMed]
36. Kimura, T.; Kobayashi, H.; Nakayama, E.; Kakihana, W. Seasonality in physical activity and walking of healthy older adults. *J. Physiol. Anthropol.* **2015**, *34*, 33. [CrossRef] [PubMed]

37. da Silveira, M.P.; da Silva Fagundes, K.K.; Bizuti, M.R.; Starck, É.; Rossi, R.C.; de Resende, E.; Silva, D.T. Physical exercise as a tool to help the immune system against COVID-19: An integrative review of the current literature. *Clin. Exp. Med.* **2021**, *21*, 15–28. [CrossRef] [PubMed]
38. Jimeno-Almazán, A.; Pallarés, J.G.; Buendía-Romero, Á.; Martínez-Cava, A.; Franco-López, F.; Sánchez-Alcaraz Martínez, B.J.; Bernal-Morel, E.; Courel-Ibáñez, J. Post-COVID-19 Syndrome and the Potential Benefits of Exercise. *Int. J. Environ. Res. Public Health* **2021**, *18*, 5329. [CrossRef]
39. Morley, J.E.; Kalantar-Zadeh, K.; Anker, S.D. COVID-19: A major cause of cachexia and sarcopenia? *J. Cachexia Sarcopenia Muscle* **2020**, *11*, 863–865. [CrossRef]
40. Nigg, C.R.; Fuchs, R.; Gerber, M.; Jekauc, D.; Koch, T.; Krell-Roesch, J.; Lippke, S.; Mnich, C.; Novak, B.; Ju, Q.; et al. Assessing physical activity through questionnaires—A consensus of best practices and future directions. *Psychol. Sport Exerc.* **2020**, *50*, 101715. [CrossRef]

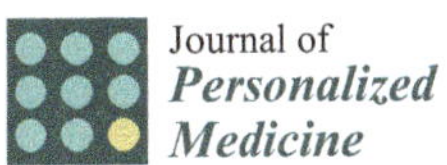

Journal of *Personalized Medicine*

MDPI

Review

Bronchial Asthma and Sarcopenia: An Upcoming Potential Interaction

Nikolaos D. Karakousis [1], Ourania S. Kotsiou [2,3,*] and Konstantinos I. Gourgoulianis [3]

1 Primary Healthcare, Internal Medicine Department, Amarousion, 15125 Athens, Greece
2 Faculty of Nursing, University of Thessaly, 41500 Larissa, Greece
3 Department of Respiratory Medicine, Faculty of Medicine, University of Thessaly, 41110 Larissa, Greece
* Correspondence: raniakotsiou@gmail.com or okotsiou@uth.gr

Abstract: Background: Sarcopenia seems to be an emerging health issue worldwide, concerning the progressive loss of skeletal muscle mass, accompanied by adverse outcomes. Asthma is a chronic inflammatory respiratory condition that is widespread in the world, affecting approximately 8% of adults. Although data are scarce, we aim to shed light on the potential association between low muscle mass and asthma and point out any probable negative feedback on each other. Methods: We searched within the PubMed, Scopus, MEDLINE, and Google Scholar databases. Study selections: Three studies were included in our analysis. Only original studies written in English were included, while the references of the research articles were thoroughly examined for more relevant studies. Moreover, animal model studies were excluded. Results: 2% to 17% of asthmatics had sarcopenia according to the existent literature. Sarcopenic asthmatic patients seem to have reduced lung function, while their mortality risk may be increased. Furthermore, patients with asthma- chronic obstructive pulmonary disease (COPD) overlap syndrome phenotype and sarcopenia might have a higher risk of osteopenia and osteoporosis progression, leading consequently to an increased risk of fractures and disability. Conclusions: Emerging data support that pulmonologists should be aware of the sarcopenia concept and be prepared to evaluate the existence of low muscle mass in their asthmatic patients.

Keywords: asthma; sarcopenia; low muscle mass; inflammation; respiratory disease

Citation: Karakousis, N.D.; Kotsiou, O.S.; Gourgoulianis, K.I. Bronchial Asthma and Sarcopenia: An Upcoming Potential Interaction. *J. Pers. Med.* **2022**, *12*, 1556. https://doi.org/10.3390/jpm12101556

Academic Editor: Bruno Mégarbané

Received: 23 August 2022
Accepted: 16 September 2022
Published: 21 September 2022

1. Introduction

Worldwide, it there is an emerging interest concerning the progressive loss of skeletal muscle mass and loss of muscle function, broadly known as sarcopenia [1]. Sarcopenia prevalence in the elderly is considered quite variable, ranging from 5% to 50%, depending on different factors such as age, gender, pathological conditions, and last but not least, criteria concerning diagnosis [1]. Moreover, it is closely related to frailty syndrome, which is related to increased vulnerability [2]. Besides the aging process, low muscle mass can also be associated with pathological conditions. Among these conditions are chronic liver and kidney disease, inflammatory bowel disease, diabetic foot, and many others [2–5].

Asthma is a chronic inflammatory disorder concerning the airways [6]. It is characterized by chronic airway inflammation, which is manifested as variable airway narrowing leading to wheezes, dyspnea, and cough [7]. Asthma affected an estimated 262 million people in 2019 [1] and caused 455,000 deaths [8]. It seriously affects people's physical along with their mental health, resulting in limited physical activity and decreased quality of life (QoL) [8].

In this non-systematic review, we aim to investigate the potential interplay between these two clinical entities, even though data are limited and further studies are needed to validate this interaction.

1.1. The Concept of Sarcopenia: Where We Stand?

The combination of low muscle mass and low muscle function is characterized as sarcopenia [9,10]. Even though this term was used to describe the loss of muscle mass and physical performance associated with aging, nowadays, factors harming sarcopenia progression may concern chronic diseases, an idle lifestyle, disability, and malnutrition [9,11]. It is already established that alterations in mitochondrial function, muscle fiber types, myokines, nicotinamide adenine dinucleotide (NAD+) metabolism, and gut microbiota are present in aged muscle compared to young muscle or healthy aged muscle [12]. Several age-related factors, such as neuromuscular degeneration, changes in hormone levels, chronic inflammation, and oxidative stress, are related to the development of low muscle mass [13]. On the other hand, low muscle mass might be related to pathological clinical conditions such as chronic kidney disease (CKD), chronic liver disease, respiratory disease, endocrine disorders, and others [4,14–16].

Sarcopenia is an important component of the syndrome of frailty, which is associated with increased vulnerability, a decline in the physiological reserves of several systems of the human body and augmented susceptibility to both endogenous and exogenous stressors [17,18]. Frailty syndrome has also been associated and linked to the aging population, and other pathological conditions such as postoperative complications, metabolic syndrome, cardiovascular disease, inflammation and many others [17,19,20].

In 2010, the European Working Group on Sarcopenia in Older People (EWGSOP) published a sarcopenia definition. Still, in early 2018, the Working Group carried out a new meeting (EWGSOP2) to determine an update concerning the description of this condition. In its 2018 definition, EWGSOP2 uses low muscle strength as the basic parameter of sarcopenia [21]. The updated consensus on sarcopenia uses detection of low muscle quantity and quality to confirm the sarcopenia diagnosis while it identifies poor physical performance as indicative of severe sarcopenia. Moreover, it updates the clinical algorithm used for sarcopenia case-finding, diagnosis and confirmation, and severity determination and provides clear cut-off points for measurements of variables that identify and characterize sarcopenia [21].

To monitor sarcopenia among individuals, there are specific tools. One screening tool for sarcopenia is SARC-F, which is a questionnaire consisting of five questions: Strength (S), Assistance walking (A), Rising from a chair (R), Climbing stairs (C), and Falls (F) on a scale of 0 to 2. The cutoff value recommended is ≥4 points [22,23]. In addition, tools such as grip strength and chair stand test (chair rise test), gait speed, timed-up-and-go test (TUG), 400-m walk or long-distance corridor walk (400-m walk) and short physical performance battery (SPPB) may also be of great importance to assess skeletal muscle strength and physical performance [21].

The laboratory evaluation of skeletal muscle mass, or skeletal muscle quality, can be carried out by appendicular skeletal muscle mass (ASMM) by Dual-energy X-ray absorptiometry (DXA), muscle ultrasonography, neutron activation (NAA), electrical impedance myography (EIM), whole-body skeletal muscle mass (SMM) or ASMM predicted by Bioelectrical impedance analysis (BIA) and lumbar muscle cross-sectional area by CT or MRI [21,24,25].

Interventions concerning sarcopenia are also critical to prevent its progression and adverse outcomes. Among these interventions are dietary supplementation, exercise interventions, and combined diet and exercise interventions or lifestyle interventions [26].

Both aerobic and resistance training seem to increase muscle strength and improve physical function in general [13]. Specifically, in the early 1990s, a series of studies established the role of Progressive Resistance Exercise Training (PRT) in increasing muscle size, muscle strength, and functional capacity in the elderly. At the same time, in 2009, a Cochrane review on 121 trials concluded that PRT could be imperative to improve physical performance along with muscle strength, including gait speed and getting up from a chair. PRT should be considered a first-line treatment strategy for managing and preventing sarcopenia and its adverse outcomes, but trained therapists and special equipment are required for its implementation [13].

It is already well-established that malnutrition is related to the pathogenesis of low muscle mass, specifically in frail and vulnerable elderly patients [13,18,27,28]. Interventions concerning nutrition may include increased protein, vitamin D supplementation, creatine monohydrate, antioxidants, omega-3 fatty acids, and other nutritional strategies, but all these are under consideration [13,18,29].

1.2. Bronchial Asthma: A Respiratory Key Competitor

Bronchial asthma is a medical condition that may have detrimental effects, while its prevalence globally has demonstrated a rapid increase during the last century [30,31]. It is a common clinical condition due to chronic inflammation of the lower respiratory tract, whilst due to the fact that it is a quite heterogenic clinical condition, it is often underdiagnosed, despite the fact that its clinical manifestation is already well-established and there are already valid and quite effective treatment strategies in order to confront this medical issue [32].

The risk factors concerning the bronchial asthma are already validated and it seems that gene-environment interactions have a pivotal role [32,33]. As has already been proven, genetics and heritability have an important role in bronchial asthma development along with epigenetic variation, whilst respiratory infections, particularly viral, are associated with environmental exposures, tobacco smoke, pollutants, ozone, atopic conditions, chemical exposures and effects of the microbiome, stress and metabolites [32–35].

The pathophysiology of this clinical issue is closely linked to the inflammation of the lower airway. This is most likely to derive from the combination of environmental exposures, genetic profile of its individual and probably alterations in the microbiome and metabolites [32,36]. It is well-established that the most frequent type of inflammation in asthmatic patients is the type 2 inflammation which can be associated with eosinophilic disorders, allergic diseases and parasite infections [32,37]. In addition, type 2 inflammation in asthmatic individuals can be characterized by increased IL-33 and thymic stromal lymphopoietin, increased OX40L expression and lymph node migration affecting lymphocyte maturation, metaplasia and increased mucin stores, increased TH2 bias with downregulation of Treg cells, along with increased IL-4, IL-5 and IL-13, increased IgE-producing plasma cells, IL-5–mediated accumulation and increased IgE binding and mediator storage [32,37]. All these alterations, which happen in the lower airways may lead to a remodeling status of the lung tissue in asthmatic subjects, in the mucosa and submucosa, including epithelial hyperplasia and metaplasia of goblet cells along with increased mucus production, smooth muscle hypertrophy, collagen deposition and larger mucous glands leading to airways remodeling and narrowing and increased mucous production [32,38,39]. Moreover, it is of great importance to point out, that in individuals with asthma, chest wall geometry is modified, shortening the inspiratory muscles and as a result the ability of these muscles to generate tension is quite reduced [40].

There are four essential symptoms concerning individuals living with bronchial asthma. Among these symptoms are: wheezing, coughing, shortness of breath / dyspnea and chest tightness [32,41], whilst the differential diagnosis includes medical conditions such as reactive airway disease, bronchopulmonary dysplasia, bronchiolitis and chronic obstructive pulmonary disease (COPD) [32,42].

Bronchial asthma classification concerns intermittent or persistent asthma, ranging from mild to severe, while certain asthmatic patients may have intermittent to persistent asthma [6]. Moreover, another classification concerning specific types of asthma causes and manifestations such as non-allergic, allergic, aspirin-exacerbated respiratory disease, occupational, potentially fatal, exercise-induced, and cough variant asthma [6].

Asthma management remains still quite intriguing, with acute asthma being a medical emergency that could be fatal [43]. In addition, it is well-known that asthma severity is characterized by the presence of exacerbations [43]. The four fundamental components of asthma management include patient education, monitoring and recording of symptoms and lung function, control of triggering factors and conditions that fuel comorbidity, requiring pharmacologic treatment administration [44–46].

Asthma treatment strategy is associated with the administration of inhaled corticosteroids (ICS), which have the ability to reduce asthma exacerbations and generally ameliorate the disease control [46]. In addition, in individuals living with this chronic respiratory disease, poorly controlled asthma and a history of prior asthma exacerbations, the combined administration of ICS and long-acting β-agonists (LABA), such as budesonide and formoterol, can lead to a significant reduction of asthma exacerbations compared to ICS administration alone, whilst the prescription of ICS/LABA combinations, both for maintenance and symptom relief, has demonstrated reduction concerning asthma exacerbations [46,47]. Regarding other treatment strategies, leukotriene antagonists seem to reduce exacerbations both in children and adults, while montelukast reduced asthma exacerbations to RV infections among children, even if adding montelukast to inhaled budesonide was as effective as doubling the dose of inhaled budesonide [46]. Last but not least, the administration of anticholinergic drugs, such as tiotropium, reduces the frequency of asthma exacerbations and is approved by Food and Drug Administration (FDA) for long-term, maintenance treatment for individuals 6 years of age and older with persistent asthma, uncontrolled with ICS along with the use of one or more drugs against bronchial asthma [46,48].

It is important to underline that, in severe conditions of bronchial asthma, there is availability of biologic therapies in the form of anti-IgE (omalizumab) and anti-IL5 therapies (mepolizumab and reslizumab) [49].

Asthma and obesity, both of which are considered global health issues, tend to increase in parallel indicating a potential link between these two conditions [50,51]. There is a debate whether body mass index (BMI) status is associated with asthma control, i.e., the persistence and intensity of symptoms of asthma. [50,51].

1.3. Literature Review Organization

In this non-systematic review article, the current literature was retrieved using the PubMed, Scopus, MEDLINE, and Google Scholar databases from the date of the idea's inception concerning this review from July 1975 until August 2022. We have searched for the following terms: "sarcopenia and asthma" OR "sarcopenia and bronchial asthma" OR "low muscle mass and asthma" OR "low muscle mass and bronchial asthma". Only original studies written in English were included, while the references of the research articles were thoroughly examined for relevant studies. Animal model studies were excluded. In this study, we tried to highlight the existing literature concerning the interaction between these two entities (Table 1).

Table 1. The interplay between sarcopenia and bronchial asthma.

Authors [Ref]/Year	Study Design	Study Population	Findings	% of Sarcopenia in Asthmatics	Low Muscle Mass Evaluation
Won et al. [50]/2022	Cross-sectional	320 elderly asthmatics	Decreased muscle mass and physical activity levels may contribute to reduced lung function concerning elderly asthmatics. Sarcopenic asthma was associated with low BMI, aging, reduced lung function.	15% asthmatics has sarcopenia	Appendicular skeletal muscle was calculated as the sum of the skeletal muscle mass.
Benz et al. [51]/2022	Population-based study	4482 participants (aged > 55 years; 57.3% female) from the population-based Rotterdam Study	Middle-aged and older people with COPD, higher SII levels or sarcopenia had an independently increased mortality risk, whilst routinely evaluating sarcopenia and SII in older people with COPD or asthma is recommended	1.4% asthmatics with sarcopenia, 2.1% COPD patients with sarcopenia	Handgrip strength evaluated by hydraulic dynamometer and appendicular lean mass measured by DXA
Lee et al. [52]/2017	Comparative study	947 subjects were included in the study: 89 had asthma, 748 COPD, and 110 ACOS	In the ACO phenotype, sarcopenic individuals had a higher prevalence rate and risks of osteopenia and osteoporosis than those non-sarcopenic	17.1% asthmatics with sarcopenia, 50.5% COPD patients with sarcopenia	Assessment by DXA

Abbreviations: ACO, Asthma—COPD overlap, COPD, chronic obstructive pulmonary disease; DXA, Dual-energy X-ray overlap.

1.4. Sarcopenia and Bronchial Asthma: The Intriguing Interplay

The association between sarcopenia and bronchial asthma seems to have been under medical investigation in recent years. Researchers worldwide tried to investigate the potential impact of these two entities on each other. Still, there is enough scientific space for a further and more thorough investigation.

Won et al. tried to investigate the association between sarcopenia and asthma in the elderly, mainly concerning asthma control and lung function [52]. The groups under investigation were divided and analyzed related to muscle mass, asthma, and physical activity. They have demonstrated that sarcopenic asthma had a younger onset and reduced physical activity than non-sarcopenic asthma, whilst asthma control was not associated with physical activity and low muscles mass [52]. Moreover, using multivariate logistic regression analyses, they further pointed out that sarcopenic asthma was associated with airway obstruction (FEV1 < 60%), older age, male gender, and lower body mass index (BMI), compared with non-sarcopenic asthma [52]. Their conclusions highlighted that intense physical activity and sarcopenia might contribute to reduced lung function in elderly asthmatics [52].

Benz et al. focused on investigating the association between sarcopenia, higher systemic immune-inflammation index (SII), COPD or asthma, and all-cause mortality in a large-scale population-based setting, taking under serious consideration that SII and sarcopenia are associated with higher morbidity in patients with COPD or asthma [53]. 4482 participants, aged > 55 years, with 57.3% being female, from the population-based Rotterdam Study were included. Asthma and COPD patients were diagnosed based on spirometry and clinical examination [53]. They defined sarcopenia according to the updated EWGSOP2 criteria while handgrip strength was obtained from the non-dominant hand using a hydraulic dynamometer, and appendicular lean mass was measured by DXA [53]. Independent of the presence of sarcopenia, COPD or asthma participants had a higher risk of all-cause mortality (HR: 2.13, 95% CI 1.46–3.12 and HR: 1.70, 95% CI 1.32–2.18 for those with and without sarcopenia, respectively, while higher SII levels increased mortality risk even in people without sarcopenia, COPD or asthma [53]. In conclusion, they pointed out that middle-aged and older people with COPD, higher SII levels, or sarcopenia had an independently increased mortality risk. At the same time, they recommended that sarcopenia and SII assessment in everyday medical practice could be predictors of worse progress in the elderly with COPD or asthma [53].

Lee et al. investigated the association between sarcopenia and bone mineral density (BMD) (which is related to osteopenia and osteoporosis) in asthma-COPD overlap (ACO), based on the existing hypothesis that sarcopenia and decreased BMD are common in the elderly and are significant comorbidities concerning obstructive airway disease (OAD) [54]. A total of 947 subjects were included in the study: 89 had asthma, 748 had COPD, and 110 ACO underwent qualified spirometry and DXA. This comparative study demonstrated that the sarcopenia group had higher risks of developing osteopenia, osteoporosis, and low BMD than the non-sarcopenia group in the ACO phenotype (OR: 6.620, 95% CI 1.129–38.828; OR: 9.611, 95% CI 1.133–81.544; and OR: 6.935, 95% CI 1.194–40.272, respectively), while in the asthma phenotype, the sarcopenia group showed no increased risk in comparison with the non-sarcopenia group [54]. They have concluded that in the ACO phenotype, individuals with sarcopenia had a higher prevalence rate and higher risks of osteopenia and osteoporosis than those without sarcopenia among all OAD phenotypes [54]. Osteoporosis is a significant factor in fractures and, as a result, disability, mortality, and morbidity [55,56]. It is already well established that the cost of osteoporosis adverse outcomes carries a significant economic burden concerning all countries, globally [57].

Figure 1 summarizes the explain the relationship between bronchial asthma and sarcopenia.

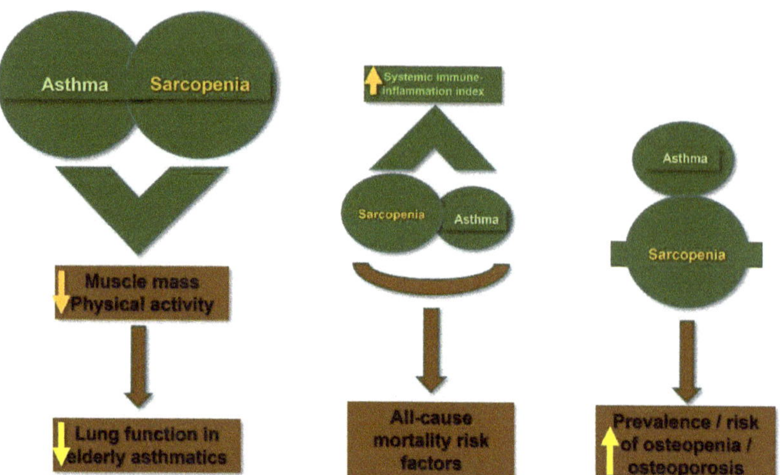

Figure 1. The relationship between bronchial asthma and sarcopenia.

2. Discussion

This non-systematic review aims to demonstrate and highlight the potential interplay between bronchial asthma and low muscle mass, known as sarcopenia. These two entities play a pivotal role in respiratory and muscle health, respectively, while they are already linked to many other pathological conditions and adverse outcomes that could deteriorate the QoL among individuals. However, the existing literature is still scarce but quite promising.

Certain limitations are related to this medical issue. These limitations are associated with the currently small number of studies investigating this intriguing interplay, while the number of patients participating in them is relatively limited.

Nevertheless, it seems that it would be intriguing if further studies could include and investigate a more significant number of patients living with bronchial asthma, not only older but also of younger age, and evaluate the existence or not of a low muscle state by muscle mass assessment. In addition, it is important to study the effect of currently used treatment against asthma in sarcopenic individuals living with asthma and whether these agents could positively impact muscle mass, apart from their chronic respiratory disease.

Another interesting approach concerning this medical topic and the potential interplay between these entities could be the development of specific indexes that could evaluate the prognosis of bronchial asthma among asthmatic sarcopenic patients, probably relying on their clinical image, along with laboratory parameters concerning both muscle mass and respiratory activity.

In addition, using specific biomarkers that could assess sarcopenia phenotype in asthmatic subjects might be of great importance. It has already been analyzed the association with plasma biomarkers such as glycoprotein Dickkopf-3 (Dkk-3), c-terminal agrin fragment-22 (CAF22), and microRNAs miR-21, miR-134a, miR-133 and miR-206 with handgrip strength (HGS) and appendicular skeletal mass index (ASMI) in male, 54–73-year-old individuals with COPD, bronchial asthma or pulmonary tuberculosis and it has been demonstrated a modest-to-significant increase in the plasma markers of oxidative stress, inflammation and muscle damage, which had varying degrees of correlations with Dkk-3, CAF22 and selected micro RNAs (miRs) in these respiratory diseases [58]. This could imply that these biomarkers could be significant and valuable tools to evaluate the phenotype of sarcopenia among older patients with diseases concerning their respiratory system [58].

Last but not least, it would be appealing if an interventional protocol could be established for sarcopenic individuals with bronchial asthma. This specific protocol could include a multimodal approach in which nutrition, exercise, and respiratory rehabilitation programs could beneficially coexist and positively affect the muscle mass, along with the asthmatic exacerbations. Ameliorating these conditions could have an upside effect on these individuals and improve their QoL.

3. Conclusions and Future Perspectives

Sarcopenic patients living with a chronic respiratory disease, such as bronchial asthma, may have reduced lung function, while their mortality risk may increase. In addition, individuals with asthma-COPD overlap syndrome phenotype and low muscle mass may have a higher risk of osteopenia and osteoporosis progression, leading consequently to an increased risk of fractures, immobilization, and disability. Pulmonologists should be aware of the sarcopenia clinical condition and be prepared to evaluate low muscle mass in bronchial asthma patients using the existing screening tools for sarcopenia. Moreover, physicians who examine sarcopenic patients with bronchial asthma should be able to appropriately collaborate with specialists who deal with nutrition and exercise, giving their patients a multimodal approach concerning these entities' interplay and the optimum treatment.

Author Contributions: Conceptualization, N.D.K. and O.S.K.; investigation, N.D.K. and O.S.K.; writing—original draft preparation, N.D.K.; writing—review and editing, N.D.K. and O.S.K.; visualization, N.D.K.; supervision, O.S.K. and K.I.G. All authors have read and agreed to the published version of the manuscript.

Funding: This research received no external funding.

Informed Consent Statement: Not applicable.

Conflicts of Interest: The authors declare no conflict of interest.

References

1. Papadopoulou, S.K. Sarcopenia: A Contemporary Health Problem among Older Adult Populations. *Nutrients* **2020**, *12*, 1293. [CrossRef]
2. Karakousis, N.D.; Pyrgioti, E.E.; Georgakopoulos, P.N.; Papanas, N. Sarcopenia, Frailty and Diabetic Foot: A Mini Narrative Review. *Int. J. Low. Extrem. Wounds* **2022**. [CrossRef]
3. Ryan, E.; McNicholas, D.; Creavin, B.; Kelly, M.E.; Walsh, T.; Beddy, D. Sarcopenia and Inflammatory Bowel Disease: A Systematic Review. *Inflamm. Bowel Dis.* **2019**, *25*, 67–73. [CrossRef]
4. Allen, S.L.; Quinlan, J.I.; Dhaliwal, A.; Armstrong, M.J.; Elsharkawy, A.M.; Greig, C.A.; Lord, J.M.; Lavery, G.G.; Breen, L. Sarcopenia in chronic liver disease: Mechanisms and countermeasures. *Am. J. Physiol. Gastrointest. Liver Physiol.* **2021**, *320*, G241–G257. [CrossRef]
5. Sabatino, A.; Cuppari, L.; Stenvinkel, P.; Lindholm, B.; Avesani, C.M. Sarcopenia in chronic kidney disease: What have we learned so far? *J. Nephrol.* **2021**, *34*, 1347–1372. [CrossRef]
6. Padem, N.; Saltoun, C. Classification of asthma. *Allergy Asthma Proc.* **2019**, *40*, 385–388. [CrossRef]
7. Nakamura, Y.; Tamaoki, J.; Nagase, H.; Yamaguchi, M.; Horiguchi, T.; Hozawa, S.; Ichinose, M.; Iwanaga, T.; Kondo, R.; Nagata, M.; et al. Japanese guidelines for adult asthma 2020. *Allergol. Int.* **2020**, *69*, 519–548. [CrossRef]
8. World Health Organization. Asthma. Available online: https://www.who.int/news-room/fact-sheets/detail/asthma (accessed on 10 September 2022).
9. Tournadre, A.; Vial, G.; Capel, F.; Soubrier, M.; Boirie, Y. Sarcopenia. *Jt. Bone Spine* **2019**, *86*, 309–314. [CrossRef]
10. Dhillon, R.J.; Hasni, S. Pathogenesis and Management of Sarcopenia. *Clin. Geriatr. Med.* **2017**, *33*, 17–26. [CrossRef]
11. Sieber, C.C. Malnutrition and sarcopenia. *Aging Clin. Exp. Res.* **2019**, *31*, 793–798. [CrossRef]
12. Dao, T.; Green, A.E.; Kim, Y.A.; Bae, S.-J.; Ha, K.-T.; Gariani, K.; Lee, M.-R.; Menzies, K.J.; Ryu, D. Sarcopenia and Muscle Aging: A Brief Overview. *Endocrinol. Metab.* **2020**, *35*, 716–732. [CrossRef] [PubMed]
13. Liguori, I.; Russo, G.; Aran, L.; Bulli, G.; Curcio, F.; Della-Morte, D.; Gargiulo, G.; Testa, G.; Cacciatore, F.; Bonaduce, D.; et al. Sarcopenia: Assessment of disease burden and strategies to improve outcomes. *Clin. Interv. Aging* **2018**, *13*, 913–927. [CrossRef] [PubMed]
14. Moorthi, R.N.; Avin, K.G. Clinical relevance of sarcopenia in chronic kidney disease. *Curr. Opin. Nephrol. Hypertens.* **2017**, *26*, 219–228. [CrossRef]
15. van Bakel, S.I.J.; Gosker, H.R.; Langen, R.C.; Schols, A.M.W.J. Towards Personalized Management of Sarcopenia in COPD. *Int. J. Chronic Obstr. Pulm. Dis.* **2021**, *16*, 25–40. [CrossRef]
16. Borba, V.Z.C.; Costa, T.L.; Moreira, C.A.; Boguszewski, C.L. MECHANISMS OF ENDOCRINE DISEASE: Sarcopenia in endocrine and non-endocrine disorders. *Eur. J. Endocrinol.* **2019**, *180*, R185–R199. [CrossRef]

17. Karakousis, N.D.; Chrysavgis, L.; Chatzigeorgiou, A.; Papatheodoridis, G.; Cholongitas, E. Frailty in metabolic syndrome, focusing on nonalcoholic fatty liver disease. *Ann. Gastroenterol.* **2022**, *35*, 234–242. [CrossRef]
18. Cruz-Jentoft, A.J.; Kiesswetter, E.; Drey, M.; Sieber, C.C. Nutrition, frailty, and sarcopenia. *Aging Clin. Exp. Res.* **2017**, *29*, 43–48. [CrossRef]
19. Soysal, P.; Arik, F.; Smith, L.; Jackson, S.E.; Isik, A.T. Inflammation, Frailty and Cardiovascular Disease. *Adv. Exp. Med. Biol.* **2020**, *1216*, 55–64.
20. Kostakopoulos, N.A.; Karakousis, N.D. Frailty assessment and postoperative complications in urologic oncology operations. *J. Frailty Sarcopenia Falls* **2020**, *5*, 57–61. [CrossRef]
21. Cruz-Jentoft, A.J.; Bahat, G.; Bauer, J.; Boirie, Y.; Bruyere, O.; Cederholm, T.; Cooper, C.; Landi, F.; Rolland, Y.; Sayer, A.A.; et al. Sarcopenia: Revised European consensus on definition and diagnosis. *Age Aging* **2019**, *48*, 601. [CrossRef]
22. Nishikawa, H.; Asai, A.; Fukunishi, S.; Takeuchi, T.; Goto, M.; Ogura, T.; Nakamura, S.; Kakimoto, K.; Miyazaki, T.; Nishiguchi, S.; et al. Screening Tools for Sarcopenia. *In Vivo* **2021**, *35*, 3001–3009. [CrossRef]
23. Beaudart, C.; McCloskey, E.; Bruyère, O.; Cesari, M.; Rolland, Y.; Rizzoli, R.; Araujo De Carvalho, I.; Amuthavalli Thiyagarajan, J.; Bautmans, I.; Bertière, M.-C.; et al. Sarcopenia in daily practice: Assessment and management. *BMC Geriatr.* **2016**, *16*, 170. [CrossRef]
24. Guglielmi, G.; Ponti, F.; Agostini, M.; Amadori, M.; Battista, G.; Bazzocchi, A. The role of DXA in sarcopenia. *Aging Clin. Exp. Res.* **2016**, *28*, 1047–1060. [CrossRef] [PubMed]
25. Tosato, M.; Marzetti, E.; Cesari, M.; Savera, G.; Miller, R.R.; Bernabei, R.; Landi, F.; Calvani, R. Measurement of muscle mass in sarcopenia: From imaging to biochemical markers. *Aging Clin. Exp. Res.* **2017**, *29*, 19–27. [CrossRef]
26. Anton, S.D.; Hida, A.; Mankowski, R.; Layne, A.; Solberg, L.M.; Mainous, A.G.; Buford, T. Nutrition and Exercise in Sarcopenia. *Curr. Protein Pept. Sci.* **2018**, *19*, 649–667. [CrossRef]
27. Cannataro, R.; Carbone, L.; Petro, J.L.; Cione, E.; Vargas, S.; Angulo, H.; Forero, D.A.; Odriozola-Martínez, A.; Kreider, R.B.; Bonilla, D.A. Sarcopenia: Etiology, Nutritional Approaches, and miRNAs. *Int. J. Mol. Sci.* **2021**, *22*, 9724. [CrossRef]
28. Ligthart-Melis, G.C.; Luiking, Y.C.; Kakourou, A.; Cederholm, T.; Maier, A.B.; de van der Schueren, M.A.E. Frailty, Sarcopenia, and Malnutrition Frequently (Co-)occur in Hospitalized Older Adults: A Systematic Review and Meta-analysis. *J. Am. Med. Dir. Assoc.* **2020**, *21*, 1216–1228. [CrossRef] [PubMed]
29. Laviano, A.; Gori, C.; Rianda, S. Sarcopenia and nutrition. *Adv. Food Nutr. Res.* **2014**, *71*, 101–136. [PubMed]
30. Stern, J.; Pier, J.; Litonjua, A.A. Asthma epidemiology and risk factors. *Semin. Immunopathol.* **2020**, *42*, 5–15. [CrossRef] [PubMed]
31. Jones, T.L.; Neville, D.M.; Chauhan, A.J. Diagnosis and treatment of severe asthma: A phenotype-based approach. *Clin. Med.* **2018**, *18* (Suppl. S2), s36–s40. [CrossRef] [PubMed]
32. Mims, J.W. Asthma: Definitions and pathophysiology. *Int. Forum Allergy Rhinol.* **2015**, *5* (Suppl. S1), S2–S6. [CrossRef]
33. Toskala, E.; Kennedy, D.W. Asthma risk factors. *Int. Forum Allergy Rhinol.* **2015**, *5* (Suppl. S1), S11–S16. [CrossRef]
34. Ntontsi, P.; Photiades, A.; Zervas, E.; Xanthou, G.; Samitas, K. Genetics and Epigenetics in Asthma. *Int. J. Mol. Sci.* **2021**, *22*, 2412. [CrossRef]
35. Guryanova, S.V.; Gigani, O.B.; Gudima, G.O.; Kataeva, A.M.; Kolesnikova, N.V. Dual Effect of Low-Molecular-Weight Bioregulators of Bacterial Origin in Experimental Model of Asthma. *Life* **2022**, *12*, 192. [CrossRef]
36. Gans, M.D.; Gavrilova, T. Understanding the immunology of asthma: Pathophysiology, biomarkers, and treatments for asthma endotypes. *Paediatr. Respir. Rev.* **2020**, *36*, 118–127. [CrossRef]
37. Fahy, J.V. Type 2 inflammation in asthma–present in most, absent in many. *Nat. Rev. Immunol.* **2015**, *15*, 57–65. [CrossRef]
38. Camoretti-Mercado, B.; Lockey, R.F. Airway smooth muscle pathophysiology in asthma. *J. Allergy Clin. Immunol.* **2021**, *147*, 1983–1995. [CrossRef]
39. Pascoe, C.D.; Green, F.H.Y.; Elliot, J.G.; James, A.L.; Noble, P.B.; Donovan, G.M. Airway remodelling with spatial correlations: Implications for asthma pathogenesis. *Respir. Physiol. Neurobiol.* **2020**, *279*, 103469. [CrossRef]
40. Silva, I.S.; Fregonezi, G.A.F.; Dias, F.A.L.; Ribeiro, C.T.D.; Guerra, R.O.; Ferreira, G.M.H. Inspiratory muscle training for asthma. *Cochrane Database Syst. Rev.* **2013**, *2013*, CD003792. [CrossRef]
41. Aaron, S.D.; Boulet, L.P.; Reddel, H.K.; Gershon, A.S. Underdiagnosis and Overdiagnosis of Asthma. *Am. J. Respir. Crit. Care Med.* **2018**, *198*, 1012–1020. [CrossRef]
42. Ramamurthy, M.B. Asthma Mimickers: Approach to Differential Diagnosis. *Indian J. Pediatr.* **2018**, *85*, 667–672. [CrossRef]
43. Ramsahai, J.M.; Hansbro, P.M.; Wark, P.A.B. Mechanisms and Management of Asthma Exacerbations. *Am. J. Respir. Crit. Care Med.* **2019**, *199*, 423–432. [CrossRef]
44. Rehman, A.; Amin, F.; Sadeeqa, S. Prevalence of asthma and its management: A review. *J. Pak. Med. Assoc.* **2018**, *68*, 1823–1827.
45. de Albornoz, S.C.; Chen, G. Relationship between health-related quality of life and subjective wellbeing in asthma. *J. Psychosom. Res.* **2021**, *142*, 110356. [CrossRef]
46. Castillo, J.R.; Peters, S.P.; Busse, W.W. Asthma Exacerbations: Pathogenesis, Prevention, and Treatment. *J. Allergy Clin. Immunol. Pract.* **2017**, *5*, 918–927. [CrossRef]
47. Olin, J.T.; Wechsler, M.E. Asthma: Pathogenesis and novel drugs for treatment. *BMJ* **2014**, *349*, g5517. [CrossRef] [PubMed]
48. Lommatzsch, M.; Virchow, J.C. Severe asthma: Definition, diagnosis and treatment. *Dtsch. Arztebl. Int.* **2014**, *111*, 847–855.
49. Chung, K.F. Precision medicine in asthma: Linking phenotypes to targeted treatments. *Curr. Opin. Pulm. Med.* **2018**, *24*, 4–10. [CrossRef] [PubMed]

50. Noal, R.B.; Menezes, A.M.B.; Macedo, S.E.C.; Dumith, S.C. Childhood body mass index and risk of asthma in adolescence: A systematic review. *Obes. Rev.* **2011**, *12*, 93–104. [CrossRef]
51. Lee, H.; Choi, H.; Nam, H.; Yang, B.; Hwangbo, B.; Kong, S.-Y.; Chung, S.J.; Yeo, Y.; Park, T.S.; Park, D.W.; et al. Body mass index change and incident asthma in adults: A nationwide cohort study. *Allergy* **2021**, *76*, 1896–1899. [CrossRef]
52. Won, H.-K.; Kang, Y.; An, J.; Lee, J.-H.; Song, W.-J.; Kwon, H.-S.; Cho, Y.S.; Moon, H.-B.; Jang, I.-Y.; Kim, T.-B. Relationship between asthma and sarcopenia in the elderly: A nationwide study from the KNHANES. *J. Asthma Off. J. Assoc. Care Asthma* **2022**, 1–10. [CrossRef] [PubMed]
53. Benz, E.; Wijnant, S.R.A.; Trajanoska, K.; Arinze, J.T.; de Roos, E.W.; de Ridder, M.; Williams, R.; van Rooji, F.; Verhamme, K.M.C.; Ikram, A.; et al. Sarcopenia, systemic immune-inflammation index and all-cause mortality in middle-aged and older people with COPD and asthma: A population-based study. *ERJ Open Res.* **2022**, *8*, 00628–2021. [CrossRef] [PubMed]
54. Lee, D.W.; Jin, H.J.; Shin, K.C.; Chung, J.H.; Lee, H.W.; Lee, K.H. Presence of sarcopenia in asthma-COPD overlap syndrome may be a risk factor for decreased bone-mineral density, unlike asthma: Korean National Health and Nutrition Examination Survey (KNHANES) IV and V (2008–2011). *Int. J. Chronic Obstr. Pulm. Dis.* **2017**, *12*, 2355–2362. [CrossRef]
55. Srivastava, M.; Deal, C. Osteoporosis in elderly: Prevention and treatment. *Clin. Geriatr. Med.* **2002**, *18*, 529–555. [CrossRef]
56. Johnston, C.B.; Dagar, M. Osteoporosis in Older Adults. *Med. Clin. North Am.* **2020**, *104*, 873–884. [CrossRef] [PubMed]
57. Rashki Kemmak, A.; Rezapour, A.; Jahangiri, R.; Nikjoo, S.; Farabi, H.; Soleimanpour, S. Economic burden of osteoporosis in the world: A systematic review. *Med. J. Islamic Repub. Iran* **2020**, *34*, 154. [CrossRef]
58. Qaisar, R.; Karim, A.; Muhammad, T.; Shah, I. Circulating Biomarkers of Accelerated Sarcopenia in Respiratory Diseases. *Biology* **2020**, *9*, 332. [CrossRef]

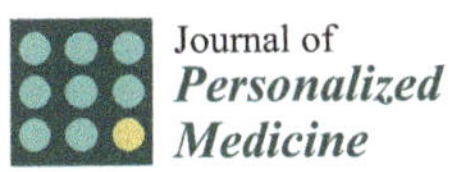
Journal of *Personalized Medicine*

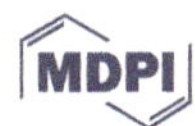

Article

Evaluating Virtual and Inpatient Pulmonary Rehabilitation Programs for Patients with COPD

Paula Irina Barata [1], Alexandru Florian Crisan [1], Adelina Maritescu [1], Rodica Anamaria Negrean [2,*], Ovidiu Rosca [3,4], Felix Bratosin [4], Cosmin Citu [5] and Cristian Oancea [1]

1 Center for Research and Innovation in Precision Medicine of Respiratory Diseases, "Victor Babes" University of Medicine and Pharmacy Timisoara, Eftimie Murgu Square 2, 300041 Timisoara, Romania
2 Faculty of Medicine and Pharmacy, University of Oradea, 410073 Oradea, Romania
3 Department XIII, Discipline of Infectious Diseases, "Victor Babes" University of Medicine and Pharmacy Timisoara, Eftimie Murgu Square 2, 300041 Timisoara, Romania
4 Methodological and Infectious Diseases Research Center, Department of Infectious Diseases, "Victor Babes" University of Medicine and Pharmacy Timisoara, Eftimie Murgu Square 2, 300041 Timisoara, Romania
5 Department of Obstetrics and Gynecology, "Victor Babes" University of Medicine and Pharmacy Timisoara, Eftimie Murgu Square 2, 300041 Timisoara, Romania
* Correspondence: rodicanegrean@yahoo.com

Abstract: Chronic obstructive pulmonary disease (COPD) is an increasingly frequent disorder that is likely to become the third leading cause of morbidity worldwide. It significantly degrades the quality of life of patients affected and poses a significant financial burden to the healthcare systems providing treatment and rehabilitation. Consequently, our study's purpose was to compare conventional inpatient pulmonary rehabilitation (PR) with virtual (online) PR using a mobile phone application. During a three-month period, two groups of patients followed the research protocol by participating in a pulmonary rehabilitation program administered and supervised by a physical therapist five times per week. A number of respiratory variables were examined before and after the test. At the end of the study period, a total of 72 patients completed the rehabilitation in the inpatient group, respectively 58 in the online group. It was observed that post-test comparison between patients undergoing the traditional and online rehabilitation methods did not show any significant differences. However, the calculated mean differences between pre-test and post-test results were significantly higher in favor of the virtual method. The most significant variations were encountered in maximal inspiratory pressure (MIP) (6.6% vs. 8.5%, p-value < 0.001), 6-min walking test (6MWT) (6.7% vs. 9.4%, p-value < 0.001), and COPD assessment test (CAT) values (4.8 vs. 6.2, p-value < 0.001), respectively. However, the maximal expiratory pressure (MEP) variation was significantly higher in patients undergoing the traditional rehabilitation method, from an average of 4.1% to 3.2% (p-value < 0.001). In this preliminary study, the online pulmonary rehabilitation program proved non-inferiority to the traditional method, with significantly better results in several measurements. Additional studies using larger cohorts of patients and longer exposure to the online rehabilitation program are required to validate these findings.

Keywords: COPD; pulmonary rehabilitation; digitalization of healthcare; respiratory disease

Citation: Barata, P.I.; Crisan, A.F.; Maritescu, A.; Negrean, R.A.; Rosca, O.; Bratosin, F.; Citu, C.; Oancea, C. Evaluating Virtual and Inpatient Pulmonary Rehabilitation Programs for Patients with COPD. *J. Pers. Med.* **2022**, *12*, 1764. https://doi.org/10.3390/jpm12111764

Academic Editors: Ioannis Pantazopoulos and Ourania S. Kotsiou

Received: 10 October 2022
Accepted: 24 October 2022
Published: 25 October 2022

1. Introduction

Chronic obstructive pulmonary disease (COPD) is a major cause of chronic morbidity and mortality in the world and is the third leading cause of global disability-adjusted life-years (DALY) [1]. COPD is a progressive respiratory disease that leads to physical inactivity, worsening dyspnoea, muscle deconditioning, and reduced quality of life [2,3].

Although there have been remarkable advances in pharmacological treatments, a large proportion of patients remain symptomatic. Pulmonary rehabilitation (PR) has been recognized as an important, standard treatment for people with COPD aimed at reducing the burden of symptoms by increasing exercise tolerance and improving self-management. The provision of PR is mandated by the National Institute for Health and Care Excellence (NICE) as a key pillar of integrated care [3].

There is level 1 evidence that PR improves dyspnoea, exercise capacity, and quality of life, regardless of disease severity [4]. Despite these findings, 5% of people who would benefit from PR undertake it [5] with a low referral (<15%) [6], high non-attendance (up to 50%), and poor completion rates (up to 30%) [7].

Moreover, approximately 50% of patients with severe and very severe COPD declined to participate in these programs, and between 30–50% dropped out before completion [8]. The barriers to the uptake of a PR program include lack of transportation, perceived benefits of PR, disruption of the usual routine, the timing of programs, lack of rehabilitation centers, and shortage of qualified health professionals [7].

Since 2015, the American Thoracic Society (ATS) and European Respiratory Society (ERS) have recommended investigating alternative approaches to PR in an attempt to increase uptake and make PR available to more patients [9]. Home-based models of PR have been proposed to increase the availability and accessibility of PR programs to patients [10], moreover during the COVID-19 pandemic to facilitate social distancing. Although telerehabilitation has existed for many years, this model's clinical efficacy is still unclear. Therefore, the objective of our study was to compare traditional inpatient PR with online PR through a mobile phone application.

2. Materials and Methods

2.1. Study Design

The patients were recruited from the Pneumocontrol application database. These were the patients who, during the SARS-CoV-2 pandemic, accessed the application for pulmonary rehabilitation information. The patients were randomly selected, and two groups were formed. The first group was the inpatient group that received a conventional pulmonary rehabilitation program, and the second group was the online group that performed PR through the application. The study was conducted over a period of three months, from January 2022 to April 2022.

All the patients were informed of the research, and informed consent was obtained before the beginning of the study. The research respected the Declaration of Helsinki regarding ethical principles for research regarding the safety of human subjects. The study design and contract forms were approved by the Ethics Committee of the "Victor Babes" Hospital (nr.3209 5 April 2022).

Both groups had to perform one pulmonary rehabilitation program conducted and supervised by a physical therapist five times a week. The duration of the program was 21 days. At the beginning and at the end of the program, all patients performed: lung volumes, maximal inspiratory and expiratory pressure (MIP/MEP), 6-min walking test, COPD assessment test (CAT), Borg scale, and modified Medical Research Council test (mMRC).

Patients in the online group were explained how to use the application, exercise with the POWERbreathe device, and how to increase weight through the sessions.

2.2. Patients

Over a period of three months, we included patients with stable COPD that were classified according to the ATS/ERS criteria for the severity of airway obstruction [11]. Inclusion criteria: age > 45 years, will participate, no exacerbation in the last three months, no prior rehabilitation in the last three months, former smoking history, non-smoking status, owning a mobile smartphone, able to use a smartphone, stationary bicycle at home (for the online group), owning a pulse oximeter.

Exclusion criteria: exacerbation in the last three months, other comorbidities that could interfere with their current health status, use of medication that could affect exercise response, active smoking status, musculoskeletal conditions that could impair exercise, an impaired vision that could affect the use of the mobile application, not having a stationary bicycle at home, a cognitive impairment that could affect the understanding of the exercises. After applying the inclusion and exclusion criteria, there were 72 patients in the inpatient group and 58 patients in the online group.

2.3. Lung Volumes and Respiratory Strength

The lung volumes and respiratory muscle strength were determined using the Smart PFY UI device (medical equipment Europe GmbH). The patients were seated in an upright position with the feet flat on the ground and performed three maximal expirations. The best value was recorded. The inclusion criteria for the patients were according to the ATS/ERS guideline using the refined ABCD assessment tool [11,12]. To determine respiratory muscle strength, three assessments were recorded, and the best value was used. All the maneuvers were performed according to standard procedures [13].

We used the same device as for spirometry but adapted with a shutter module. To determine maximal inspiratory pressure, the patients were instructed to expire to residual volume followed by a maximum inspiration against a resistance applied by the module. Three expirations were performed, and the best values was recorded. Maximal expiratory pressure was assessed by instructing the patient to breathe into total lung capacity, followed by a forced expiration against the module.

2.4. Physical Capacity, Disease Impact, and Dyspnea

Physical capacity was assessed using the 6-min walking distance test (6MWD), in which the patient had to cover as much distance as possible in the predicted time. To perform the 6MWD we used the ERS/ATS recording form, the BORG scale, pulse-oximeter and a stopwatch. The test was performed on a 30 m long corridor according to the ATS guidelines [14].

The global impact of COPD on the patient was evaluated using the COPD assessment test (CAT questionnaire). The questionnaire consists of 8 questions on a numerical scale from 0 to 5 for each question. Higher scores denote a more severe impact of COPD on a patient's life [15].

We assessed dyspnoea with the Borg breathlessness scale, which rates the difficulty of breathing. It rates the breathing on a scale from 0 to 10, where 0 means "breathing causes no difficulty" and 10, where "breathing is maximal". We also used this scale to determine the effort level during training sessions [16].

Dyspnoea was also evaluated using the modified Medical Research Council scale (mMRC), which assesses the degree of baseline functional disability due to dyspnoea. It rates dyspnoea on a scale from 0-"dyspnoea only with strenuous exercise" to 4-"too dyspneic to leave the house or breathless when dressing" [17].

2.5. Intervention

Inpatient pulmonary rehabilitation was performed with a physical therapist in the hospital. Home monitoring and training exercises were performed online through the Pneumocontrol application. The feasibility of the application was demonstrated in previous studies [18,19]. Patients were given basic instructions on how to use the online application after making sure the internet connection was working, and a brief test was performed before first use in live session with one of the researchers involved in the study. The training sessions lasted 45–60 min and included diaphragmatic breathing, pursed lips breathing, and strength and endurance training for both upper and lower extremities, according to the recommendation of the American Thoracic Society [20].

Each training session was composed of: (a) warm-up: duration 5–10 min—sitting, standing warm-up exercises, different breathing techniques; (b) endurance training: duration 20–30 min—stationary bicycle, Borg between 5–7, exercise performed continuous or intervals; strength/resistance training: duration 20–30 min—50–80% of 1 RM, 10–15 repetitions, three sets; cool-down: duration 5–10 min—stretching, different breathing techniques.

Respiratory muscle training was performed once per day before the training session with the POWERbreathe MEDIC device. Patients had to inhale through a variable-diameter orifice. The smaller the orifice, the greater the load achieved. Thirty breaths had to be performed per session at a level that was determined for each patient.

All the exercises were performed respecting basic physical education principles. Patients started with light and simple exercises, and as they progressed, the exercises became more complex. All training sessions were individualized according to the patients' possibilities, scores, and symptoms obtained from the questionnaire in the application.

2.6. Statistical Analysis

Microsoft Excel and IBM SPSS (Armonk, NY, USA: IBM Corp.) were the programs used for statistical analysis. The presentation of continuous variables included the use of the mean and standard deviation (SD) if the variable followed a Gaussian distribution (Kolmogorov–Smirnov test). In order to determine the difference between the normally distributed variables, the Student's *t*-test was used in order to provide an estimate of the *p*-value. The Chi-square and Fisher's tests were carried out to investigate the proportional differences. A Mann–Whitney U-test was performed for the mMRC scale to compare the mean ranks. It was decided that a *p*-value of 0.05 was significant for statistical analysis.

3. Results

3.1. Comparison of Pre-Test and Post-Test Results in the Inpatient Setting

The current study enrolled a total of 72 patients in the inpatient setting and 58 in the online setting. The variables of interest from both study groups were measured before and after the intervention. As presented in Table 1, the average patient age in the inpatient setting was 64.9 years, while most of them were men (75.0%), with an average BMI of 25.4 kg/m^2. Regarding pulmonary parameters, the predicted FVC value was 4.1 L, with no significant difference in actual and (%) values. Similarly, the FEV1 predicted value was 3.0 L, with no significant difference in actual and (%) values. The MIP (%) and MEP (%) comparison between pre- and post-test results showed a difference from 53.8% to 60.8% (p-value = 0.006), respectively, from 72.8% to 76.9% (p-value = 0.038), the difference between these measurements being statistically significant, as observed in Figure 1. The CAT measurement was 19.5 before intervention and 14.7 after intervention (p-value $\leq$ 0.001). Lastly, the mMRC results also showed a statistically significant decrease from a mean rank of 45.25 pre-test to 27.75 post-test (p-value $\leq$ 0.001).

3.2. Comparison of Pre-Test and Post-Test Results in the Online Setting

As described in Table 2, the average patient age in the inpatient setting was 64.3 years, while most of them were men (72.4%), with an average BMI of 25.7 kg/m^2. Regarding pulmonary parameters, the predicted FVC value was 4.1 L, with no significant difference in actual and (%) values. Similarly, the predicted FEV1 value was 3.0 L, with no significant difference in actual and (%) values. The MIP (%) and MEP (%) comparison between pre- and post-test results showed a difference from 53.7% to 62.2% (p-value = 0.004), respectively, from an average of 70.9% to 74.1% (p-value = 0.145), as seen in Figure 2. The 6MWT levels were statistically significantly different between the pre-test and post-test measurement (342.9 vs. 387.2, p-value = 0.006). The CAT measurement was 20.1 before intervention and 13.9 after intervention (p-value < 0.001). Lastly, the mMRC results showed a statistically significant decrease from a mean rank of 39.48 pre-test to 19.52 post-test (p-value = 0.004).

3.3. Comparison of Pre-Test Results between Inpatients and Online Participants

The pre-test comparison between inpatients and online participants presented in Table 3 identified no statistically significant differences between the two study groups, providing an excellent basis for the post-test analysis by removing any suspicion that future changes might be caused by initial differences between groups. The actual FVC value in the inpatient group before intervention was 2.9 L compared with 3.0 L in the online group (p-value = 0.105). Similarly, the actual FEV1 value was 1.3 L in the inpatient group, compared with 1.4 L in the online group (p-value = 0.066). The comparison of mMRC pre-test results between patients in the inpatient and online settings did not show significant differences in mean ranks (33.71 vs. 32.12, p-value = 0.696).

Table 1. Comparison of pre-test and post-test results in the inpatient setting.

Variables *	Pre-Test (n = 72)	Post-Test (n = 72)	p-Value
Age, years (mean ± SD)	64.9 ± 5.7	64.9 ± 5.7	-
Sex (men) **	54 (75.0%)	54 (75.0%)	-
BMI, kg/m^2 (mean ± SD)	25.4 ± 3.3	25.4 ± 3.3	-
FVC (L) pred	4.1 ± 0.4	4.1 ± 0.4	-
FVC (L) actual	2.9 ± 0.4	3.0 ± 0.3	0.091
FVC (%)	70.8 ± 5.9	70.1 ± 5.9	0.477
FEV1 (L) pred	3.0 ± 0.3	3.0 ± 0.3	-
FEV1 (L) actual	1.4 ± 0.2	1.3 ± 0.3	0.200
FEV1 (%)	42.5 ± 4.6	43.1 ± 4.5	0.430
FEV1/FVC (%) pred	74.6 ± 1.1	74.6 ± 1.1	-
FEV1/FVC (%) actual	44.9 ± 5.7	45.2 ± 5.7	0.752
MIP (cmH2O) pred	103.3 ± 4.5	103.3 ± 4.5	-
MIP (cmH2O) actual	55.7 ± 15.8	62.5 ± 16.6	0.012
MIP (%)	53.8 ± 14.5	60.4 ± 15.1	0.008
MEP (cmH2O) pred	112.7 ± 4.6	112.7 ± 4.6	-
MEP (cmH2O) actual	82.2 ± 12.3	86.8 ± 12.5	0.027
MEP (%)	72.8 ± 9.9	76.9 ± 9.9	0.038
6MWT (m) pred	467.6 ± 35.0	467.6 ± 35.0	-
6MWT (m) actual	340.5 ± 85.0	371.5 ± 79.6	0.025
6MWT (%)	72.5 ± 15.6	79.2 ± 14.4	0.008
CAT	19.5 ± 5.1	14.7 ± 4.1	<0.001
mMRC (mean rank)	45.25	27.75	<0.001

* Data reported as mean ± SD and calculated using Student's t-test; ** Data reported as n (%), and calculated using Chi-square test; SD—standard deviation; BMI—body mass index; FVC—forced vital capacity; FEV1—forced expiratory volume in the first second; MIP—maximal inspiratory pressure; MEP—maximal expiratory pressure; 6MWT—6-min walking test; CAT—COPD assessment test; mMRC—modified Medical Research Council scale.

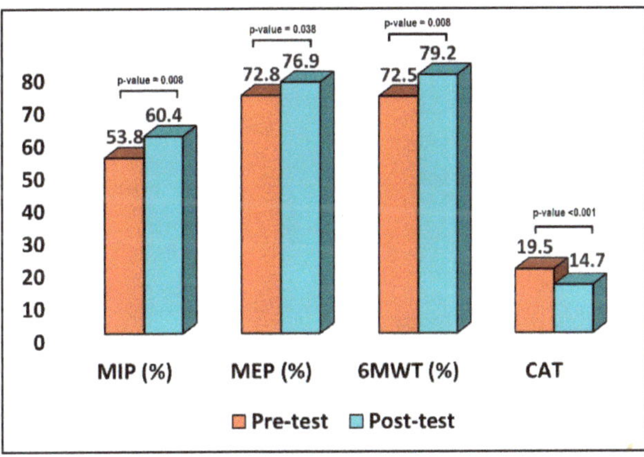

Figure 1. Comparison of pre-test and post-test results in the inpatient setting.

3.4. Comparison in Post-Test Results between Inpatients and Online Participants

Comparable to the pre-test measurements, the post-test measurements presented in Table 4 discovered statistically significant differences between inpatient and online participants with regard to the actual FVC and FEV1 levels. The FVC in the inpatient group was 2.9 L compared with 3.1 L (p-value = 0.004), and the actual FEV1 in the inpatient group was 1.2 L compared with 1.4 L (p-value = 0.010), respectively. The comparison of mMRC pre-test results between patients in the inpatient and online settings did not show significant differences in mean ranks (35.33 vs. 30.10, p-value = 0.222). Although the actual measured post-test results between patients undergoing the traditional and online rehabilitation methods did not show many significant differences, the calculated mean differences between pre-test and post-test results were significantly higher in favor of the online method, as seen in Table 5. Therefore, the most significant variations were encountered in MIP (6.6% vs. 8.5%, p-value < 0.001), 6MWT (6.7% vs. 9.4%, p-value < 0.001), CAT values (4.8 vs. 6.2, p-value < 0.001), respectively. However, the MEP (%) variation was significantly higher in patients undergoing the traditional rehabilitation method (4.1% vs. 3.2%, p-value < 0.001).

Table 2. Comparison of pre-test and post-test in the online setting.

Variables *	Pre-Test (n = 58)	Post-Test (n = 58)	p-Value
Age, years (mean ± SD)	64.3 ± 4.3	64.3 ± 4.3	-
Sex (men) **	42 (72.4%)	42 (72.4%)	-
BMI, kg/m^2 (mean ± SD)	25.7 ± 2.5	25.7 ± 2.5	-
FVC (L) pred	4.3 ± 0.3	4.3 ± 0.3	-
FVC (L) actual	3.0 ± 0.4	3.1 ± 0.4	0.896
FVC (%)	71.0 ± 6.8	71.4 ± 6.6	0.830
FEV1 (L) pred	3.3 ± 0.3	3.3 ± 0.3	-
FEV1 (L) actual	1.3 ± 0.2	1.4 ± 0.2	0.800
FEV1 (%)	41.7 ± 4.6	42.2 ± 4.6	0.674
FEV1/FVC (%) pred	74.8 ± 0.9	74.8 ± 0.9	-
FEV1/FVC (%) actual	44.2 ± 6.5	44.5 ± 6.2	0.894
MIP (cmH2O) pred	103.8 ± 3.4	103.8 ± 3.4	-
MIP (cmH2O) actual	55.7 ± 12.1	59.9 ± 12.3	0.194
MIP (%)	53.7 ± 11.6	62.2 ± 13.3	0.004
MEP (cmH2O) pred	113.2 ± 3.5	113.2 ± 3.5	-
MEP (cmH2O) actual	80.2 ± 13.6	83.3 ± 13.1	0.307
MEP (%)	70.9 ± 12.0	74.1 ± 11.5	0.145
6MWT (m) pred	473.0 ± 35.0	467.6 ± 35.0	-
6MWT (m) actual	342.9 ± 61.9	387.3 ± 56.3	0.006
6MWT (%)	72.5 ± 12.5	81.9 ± 11.3	<0.001
CAT	20.1 ± 5.3	13.9 ± 4.5	<0.001
mMRC (mean rank)	39.4	19.5	0.004

* Data reported as mean ± SD and calculated using Student's t-test; ** Data reported as n (%) and calculated using Chi-square test; SD—standard deviation; BMI—body mass index; FVC—forced vital capacity; FEV1—forced expiratory volume in the first second; MIP—maximal inspiratory pressure; MEP—maximal expiratory pressure; 6MWT—6-min walking test; CAT—COPD assessment test; mMRC—modified Medical Research Council scale.

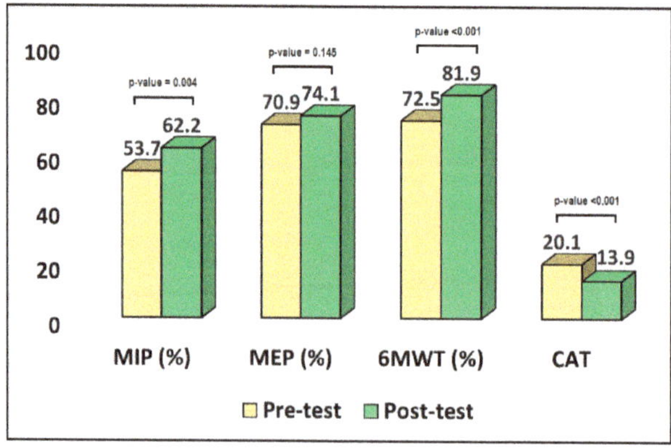

Figure 2. Comparison of pre-test and post-test results in the online setting.

Table 3. Comparison of pre-test results between inpatients and online participants.

Variables *	Inpatient (n = 72)	Online (n = 58)	*p*-Value
Age, years (mean ± SD)	64.9 ± 5.7	64.3 ± 4.3	0.659
Sex (men) **	54 (75.0%)	42 (72.4%)	0.727
BMI, kg/m^2 (mean ± SD)	25.4 ± 3.3	25.7 ± 2.5	0.689
FVC (L) pred	4.1 ± 0.4	4.3 ± 0.3	0.133
FVC (L) actual	2.9 ± 0.4	3.0 ± 0.4	0.105
FVC (%)	70.8 ± 5.9	71.0 ± 6.8	0.930
FEV1 (L) pred	3.0 ± 0.3	3.3 ± 0.3	0.299
FEV1 (L) actual	1.4 ± 0.2	1.3 ± 0.2	0.066
FEV1 (%)	42.5 ± 4.6	41.7 ± 4.6	0.479
FEV1/FVC (%) pred	74.6 ± 1.1	74.8 ± 0.9	0.639
FEV1/FVC (%) actual	44.9 ± 5.7	44.2 ± 6.5	0.654
MIP (cmH2O) pred	103.3 ± 4.5	103.8 ± 3.4	0.659
MIP (cmH2O) actual	55.7 ± 15.8	55.7 ± 12.1	0.978
MIP (%)	53.8 ± 14.5	53.7 ± 11.6	0.959
MEP (cmH2O) pred	112.7 ± 4.6	113.2 ± 3.5	0.662
MEP (cmH2O) actual	82.2 ± 12.3	80.2 ± 13.6	0.536
MEP (%)	72.8 ± 9.9	70.9 ± 12.0	0.482
6MWT (m) pred	467.6 ± 35.0	473.0 ± 35.0	0.496
6MWT (m) actual	340.5 ± 85.0	342.9 ± 61.9	0.899
6MWT (%)	72.5 ± 15.6	72.5 ± 12.5	0.967
CAT	19.5 ± 5.1	20.1 ± 5.3	0.608
mMRC (mean rank)	45.25	39.4	0.696

* Data reported as mean ± SD and calculated using Student's *t*-test; ** Data reported as n (%), and calculated using Chi-square test; SD—standard deviation; BMI—body mass index; FVC—forced vital capacity; FEV1—forced expiratory volume in the first second; MIP—maximal inspiratory pressure; MEP—maximal expiratory pressure; 6MWT—6-min walking test; CAT—COPD assessment test; mMRC—modified Medical Research Council scale.

Table 4. Comparison of post-test results between inpatients and online participants.

Variables *	Inpatient (n = 72)	Online (n = 58)	*p*-Value
Age, years (mean ± SD)	64.9 ± 5.7	64.3 ± 4.3	0.508
Sex (men) **	54 (75.0%)	42 (72.4%)	0.727
BMI, kg/m^2 (mean ± SD)	25.4 ± 3.3	25.7 ± 2.5	0.568
FVC (L) pred	4.1 ± 0.4	4.3 ± 0.4	0.502
FVC (L) actual	2.9 ± 0.4	3.1 ± 0.4	0.004
FVC (%)	71.3 ± 5.9	71.4 ± 6.6	0.927
FEV1 (L) pred	3.0 ± 0.3	3.2 ± 0.3	0.140
FEV1 (L) actual	1.2 ± 0.2	1.4 ± 0.2	0.010
FEV1 (%)	43.1 ± 4.5	42.2 ± 4.6	0.263
FEV1/FVC (%) pred	74.6 ± 1.2	74.8 ± 0.9	0.426
FEV1/FVC (%) actual	45.2 ± 5.7	44.5 ± 6.2	0.461
MIP (cmH2O) pred	103.3 ± 4.5	103.8 ± 3.4	0.639
MIP (cmH2O) actual	62.6 ± 16.6	59.9 ± 12.3	0.602
MIP (%)	60.4 ± 15.1	62.2 ± 13.2	0.659
MEP (cmH2O) pred	112.7 ± 4.6	113.2 ± 3.5	0.477
MEP (cmH2O) actual	86.9 ± 12.5	83.8 ± 13.1	0.614
MEP (%)	76.9 ± 9.9	74.1 ± 11.5	0.662
6MWT (m) pred	467.6 ± 35.0	473.0 ± 25.7	0.346
6MWT (m) actual	371.5 ± 79.6	387.3 ± 56.3	0.293
6MWT (%)	79.2 ± 14.4	81.9 ± 11.3	0.245
CAT	14.7 ± 4.1	13.9 ± 4.5	0.291
mMRC (mean rank)	35.33	30.10	0.222

* Data reported as mean ± SD and calculated using Student's *t*-test; ** Data reported as n (%), and calculated using Chi-square test; SD—standard deviation; BMI—body mass index; FVC—forced vital capacity; FEV1—forced expiratory volume in the first second; MIP—maximal inspiratory pressure; MEP—maximal expiratory pressure; 6MWT—6-min walking test; CAT—COPD assessment test; mMRC—modified Medical Research Council scale.

Table 5. Comparison of mean differences in rehabilitation results between inpatients and online participants.

Variables *	Inpatient (n = 72)	Online (n = 58)	p-Value
FVC (L) actual	0.1 ± 0.1	0.1 ± 0.1	1
FVC (%)	0.7 ± 0.1	0.4 ± 0.2	<0.001
FEV1 (L) actual	0.1 ± 0.1	0.1 ± 0.1	1
FEV1 (%)	0.6 ± 0.1	0.5 ± 0.1	<0.001
FEV1/FVC (%) actual	0.3 ± 0.1	0.3 ± 0.1	1
MIP (cmH2O) actual	6.8 ± 0.1	4.2 ± 0.3	<0.001
MIP (%)	6.6 ± 0.6	8.5 ± 1.3	<0.001
MEP (cmH2O) actual	4.6 ± 0.2	3.1 ± 0.5	<0.001
MEP (%)	4.1 ± 0.1	3.2 ± 0.1	<0.001
6MWT (m) actual	31.0 ± 5.4	44.4 ± 5.6	<0.001
6MWT (%)	6.7 ± 1.2	9.4 ± 1.2	<0.001
CAT	4.8 ± 1.0	6.2 ± 0.8	<0.001
mMRC (mean rank)	17.5	19.9	<0.001

* Data reported as mean ± SD and calculated using Student's t-test; SD—standard deviation; BMI—body mass index; FVC—forced vital capacity; FEV1—forced expiratory volume in the first second; MIP—maximal inspiratory pressure; MEP—maximal expiratory pressure; 6MWT—6-min walking test; CAT—COPD assessment test; mMRC—modified Medical Research Council scale.

4. Discussion

4.1. Important Findings

The lockdown during the COVID-19 pandemic had a major effect on patients with respiratory diseases, who were no longer able to access respiratory rehabilitation services with the same ease [21]. Moreover, due to the imposed governmental restrictions, the level of physical activity of these patients also suffered, since everyone was advised to stay at home. Considering these conditions, respiratory rehabilitation programs had no other option but to move to the online environment or to different mobile phone platforms.

Digitalized respiratory rehabilitation performed online or through various platforms is not new, having its birth in 2008, when Liu et al. tried using the mobile phone to provide exercises that improve walking exercise [22]. The same objective was followed by the current study in order to compare respiratory rehabilitation in hospitalized patients with online respiratory rehabilitation using a mobile phone application.

When we compared each group separately, we noticed that all patients showed significant improvements in all studied parameters. When comparing both groups, we observed that there were no significant differences after 21 days of pulmonary rehabilitation. Our findings support the results of other studies and the hypothesis that there is no difference between these two approaches to delivering pulmonary rehabilitation and that both can improve outcomes, in association with smoking cessation [23].

Compared to other studies that used online rehabilitation [22,24], interactive web-based applications [25], supervised telerehabilitation [26], and home-based telerehabilitation using video conference, we used an application on a mobile phone. The feasibility and utility of this application were previously demonstrated in other studies [18,19].

To our knowledge, this is the first study that, besides the conventional PR exercises, also used a medical exercise device for inspiratory muscle training (IMT) online through a mobile phone application.

In a study that used the same device for IMT, Langer et al. were the first to demonstrate that IMT with the POWERbreathe device reduced the proportion of inspiratory neural drive to the diaphragm. This has a favorable consequence for respiratory sensation and exercises tolerance, even in severe respiratory mechanical loading and tidal volume constraints [27].

The majority of the studies from the literature have a 6–12 weeks pulmonary rehabilitation design. In our country, the National Health System pays for only three weeks of hospitalized pulmonary rehabilitation. This is a major limitation on the patients and physical therapists who have to adapt to this reduced timeline.

In a study that compared online versus face-to-face PR, Bourne et al. demonstrated that online PR through a platform is non-inferior to traditional care [24]. His study duration was six weeks, and the most significant improvements were observed in the 6MWD and CAT scores. The authors exceeded the minimal important difference (MID) for the 6MWD, which is 25 m, and reduced the CAT score by 3.4 points [28]. Compared to his study, we also exceeded the MID for the 6MWD but reduced the CAT score by 4.5 points. One explanation for our findings could be that our patients used the IMT device, which reduces dyspnoea and chest tightness.

Tsai et al. also found a clinically relevant effect on 6MWD from his supervised pulmonary rehabilitation program when compared with no intervention [29]. By contrast, in a study of 22 weeks, Hansen et al. found that neither conventional PR nor supervised pulmonary telerehabilitation improved 6MWD above the MID. Explanations for his findings are that his patients had lower FEV_1, higher symptom burden, and more exacerbations [25].

Regarding the CAT score, Hansen et al. observed that the score was statistically different at the end of the intervention, with a greater symptom reduction difference of -1.6 points in the supervised pulmonary telerehabilitation group but did not exceed the MID [25]. The minimal important difference for the CAT score is -2 points [30].

In another study, Chaplin et al. compared the effect of unsupervised web-based individual exercise and education with conventional PR and found comparable between-group effects on walking tests [25].

An interesting finding of Chaplin et al. is that although the time spent in moderate-intensity physical activity was greater in the web-based group compared to the conventional PR group, this did not translate into an increase in the total amount of moderate to vigorously physical activity. The author suggests that a more supervised approach is needed to achieve longer bouts of physical activity at the level of $3 \geq$ METs [25].

In comparison to this, Loeckx et al., using a smartphone-based physical activity tele coaching approach, observed that patients requiring more contact from health care professionals experienced less physical activity benefits [31].

Compared to Loeckx's study [32], we observed that the online group had a better improvement in their 6MWD and CAT scores compared to the inpatient group. One explanation for our findings could be that the online group could leave their homes and perform their daily living activities, thus being more active and social.

4.2. Strengths and Limitations

One of the current study's strengths is that we used online IMT training using an application and thus had a better chance to improve the studied outcomes. A limitation of our study is the small number of patients and reduced days of pulmonary rehabilitation and the fact that the patients that used the application had to be connected online. Another important limitation is that we included patients who had a stationary bicycle at home for endurance training in the online PR group. Considering this factor, it would have been interesting to see what the evolution would have been for these patients if they could not perform endurance training. In the future, for those who want to perform online pulmonary rehabilitation, a pulse-oximeter, smartphone, and POWERbreathe device should be provided.

5. Conclusions

In conclusion, online pulmonary rehabilitation using a mobile phone application was not inferior to traditional inpatient pulmonary rehabilitation. As expected, improvements in all outcomes were found when comparing pre-test and post-test results of each of the two tests. In a direct comparison of pre-test and post-test variations, the online rehabilitation method showed better results regarding MIP (%), 6MWD (%), and CAT scores. However, the MEP (%) variation was significantly higher in patients undergoing the traditional rehabilitation method. Further studies are needed to demonstrate the utility and feasibility of mobile phone applications for pulmonary rehabilitation in patients with COPD.

Author Contributions: Conceptualization, P.I.B. and A.F.C.; methodology, C.O. and C.C.; software, F.B. and R.A.N.; validation, F.B. and R.A.N.; formal analysis, F.B. and C.C.; investigation, P.I.B. and A.F.C.; resources, C.O. and A.F.C.; data curation, A.M.; writing—original draft preparation, P.I.B. and A.F.C.; writing—review and editing, A.M. and O.R.; visualization, C.C. and F.B.; supervision, A.F.C. and C.O.; project administration, P.I.B. and C.O. All authors have read and agreed to the published version of the manuscript.

Funding: This research received no external funding.

Institutional Review Board Statement: The study was conducted according to the guidelines of the Declaration of Helsinki and approved by the Ethics Committee of the "Victor Babes" Hospital of Infectious Disease and Pneumophtisiology (nr.3209 5 April 2022).

Informed Consent Statement: Informed consent was obtained from all subjects involved in the study.

Data Availability Statement: The data presented in this study are available on request from the corresponding author.

Conflicts of Interest: The authors declare no conflict of interest.

References

1. Murray, C.; Kyu, H.; Abate, D.; Abate, K.; Abay, S.; Cristiana, A.; Abbasi, N.; Abbastabar, H.; Ebro, J.; Abdelalim, A.; et al. Global, regional, and national disability-adjusted life-years (DALYs) for 359 diseases and injuries and healthy life expectancy (HALE) for 195 countries and territories, 1990–2017: A systematic analysis for the Global Burden of Disease Study 2017. *Glob. Health Metr.* **2018**, *392*, 1859–1922.
2. Ramon, M.A.; Ter Riet, G.; Carsin, A.-E.; Gimeno-Santos, E.; Agustí, A.; Antó, J.M.; Donaire-Gonzalez, D.; Ferrer, J.; Rodríguez, E.; Rodriguez-Roisin, R.; et al. The dyspnoea-inactivity vicious circle in COPD: Development and external validation of a conceptual model. *Eur. Respir. J.* **2018**, *52*, 1800079. [CrossRef] [PubMed]
3. Christenson, S.A.; Smith, B.M.; Bafadhel, M.; Putcha, N. Chronic obstructive pulmonary disease. *Lancet* **2022**, *399*, 2227–2242. [CrossRef]
4. *Chronic Obstructive Pulmonary Disease in over 16s: Diagnosis and Management*; National Institute for Health and Care Excellence (NICE): London, UK, 2019; ISBN 978-1-4731-3468-3.
5. Vogiatzis, I.; Rochester, C.L.; Spruit, M.A.; Troosters, T.; Clini, E.M. Increasing implementation and delivery of pulmonary rehabilitation: Key messages from the new ATS/ERS policy statement. *Eur. Respir. J.* **2016**, *47*, 1336–1341. [CrossRef] [PubMed]
6. Méndez, A.; Labra, P.; Pizarro, R.; Baeza, N. Low rates of participation and completion of pulmonary rehabilitation in patients with chronic obstructive pulmonary disease in primary health care. *Rev. Med. Chil.* **2018**, *146*, 1304–1308. [CrossRef]
7. Cox, N.S.; Oliveira, C.C.; Lahham, A.; Holland, A.E. Pulmonary rehabilitation referral and participation are commonly influenced by environment, knowledge, and beliefs about consequences: A systematic review using the Theoretical Domains Framework. *J. Physiother.* **2017**, *63*, 84–93. [CrossRef]
8. Keating, A.; Lee, A.; Holland, A.E. What prevents people with chronic obstructive pulmonary disease from attending pulmonary rehabilitation? A systematic review. *Chron. Respir. Dis.* **2011**, *8*, 89–99. [CrossRef]
9. Fischer, M.J.; Scharloo, M.; Abbink, J.J.; van 't Hul, A.J.; van Ranst, D.; Rudolphus, A.; Weinman, J.; Rabe, K.F.; Kaptein, A.A. Drop-out and attendance in pulmonary rehabilitation: The role of clinical and psychosocial variables. *Respir. Med.* **2009**, *103*, 1564–1571. [CrossRef]
10. Rochester, C.L.; Vogiatzis, I.; Holland, A.E.; Lareau, S.C.; Marciniuk, D.D.; Puhan, M.A.; Spruit, M.A.; Masefield, S.; Casaburi, R.; Clini, E.M.; et al. An official American Thoracic Society/European Respiratory Society policy statement: Enhancing implementation, use, and delivery of pulmonary rehabilitation. *Am. J. Respir. Crit. Care Med.* **2015**, *192*, 1373–1386. [CrossRef]
11. Holland, A.E.; Mahal, A.; Hill, C.J.; Lee, A.L.; Burge, A.T.; Cox, N.S.; Moore, R.; Nicolson, C.; O'Halloran, P.; Lahham, A.; et al. Home-based rehabilitation for COPD using minimal resources: A randomised, controlled equivalence trial. *Thorax* **2017**, *72*, 57–65. [CrossRef]
12. Graham, B.L.; Steenbruggen, I.; Miller, M.R.; Barjaktarevic, I.Z.; Cooper, B.G.; Hall, G.L.; Hallstrand, T.S.; Kaminsky, D.A.; McCarthy, K.; McCormack, M.C.; et al. Standardization of Spirometry 2019 Update. An Official American Thoracic Society and European Respiratory Society Technical Statement. *Am. J. Respir. Crit. Care Med.* **2019**, *200*, e70–e88. [CrossRef] [PubMed]
13. Rabe, K.F.; Hurd, S.; Anzueto, A.; Barnes, P.J.; Buist, S.A.; Calverley, P.; Fukuchi, Y.; Jenkins, C.; Rodriguez-Roisin, R.; van Weel, C.; et al. Global strategy for the diagnosis, management, and prevention of chronic obstructive pulmonary disease: GOLD executive summary. *Am. J. Respir. Crit. Care Med.* **2007**, *176*, 532–555. [CrossRef] [PubMed]
14. Laveneziana, P.; Albuquerque, A.; Aliverti, A.; Babb, T.; Barreiro, E.; Dres, M.; Dubé, B.-P.; Fauroux, B.; Gea, J.; Guenette, J.A.; et al. ERS statement on respiratory muscle testing at rest and during exercise. *Eur. Respir. J.* **2019**, *53*, 1801214. [CrossRef] [PubMed]
15. Issues, S.; Test, M.W.; Equipment, R.; Preparation, P. American Thoracic Society ATS Statement: Guidelines for the Six-Minute Walk Test. *Am. J. Respir. Crit. Care Med.* **2002**, *166*, 111–117.

16. Jones, P.W.; Harding, G.; Berry, P.; Wiklund, I.; Chen, W.-H.; Kline Leidy, N. Development and first validation of the COPD Assessment Test. *Eur. Respir. J.* **2009**, *34*, 648–654. [CrossRef]
17. Borg, G.A. Psychophysical bases of perceived exertion. *Med. Sci. Sports Exerc.* **1982**, *14*, 377–381. [CrossRef]
18. Munari, A.B.; Gulart, A.A.; Dos Santos, K.; Venâncio, R.S.; Karloh, M.; Mayer, A.F. Modified Medical Research Council Dyspnea Scale in GOLD Classification Better Reflects Physical Activities of Daily Living. *Respir. Care* **2018**, *63*, 77–85. [CrossRef]
19. Munteanu, L.A.; Frandes, M.; Timar, B.; Tudorache, E.; Fildan, A.P.; Oancea, C.; Tofolean, D.E. The efficacy of a mobile phone application to improve adherence to treatment and self-management in people with chronic respiratory disease in Romanian population—A pilot study. *BMC Health Serv. Res.* **2020**, *20*, 475. [CrossRef]
20. Irina, B.P.; Steluta, M.M.; Emanuela, T.; Diana, M.; Cristina, O.D.; Mirela, F.; Cristian, O. Respiratory muscle training program supplemented by a cell-phone application in COPD patients with severe airflow limitation. *Respir. Med.* **2021**, *190*, 106679. [CrossRef]
21. Siddiq, M.A.B.; Rathore, F.A.; Clegg, D.; Rasker, J.J. Pulmonary Rehabilitation in COVID-19 patients: A scoping review of current practice and its application during the pandemic. *Turk. J. Phys. Med. Rehabil.* **2020**, *66*, 480–494. [CrossRef]
22. Liu, W.; Wang, C.; Lin, H.; Lin, S.; Lee, K.; Lo, Y.; Hung, S. Efficacy of a cell phone-based exercise programme for COPD. *Eur. Respir. J.* **2008**, *32*, 651–659. [CrossRef] [PubMed]
23. Pezzuto, A.; Carico, E. Effectiveness of smoking cessation in smokers with COPD and nocturnal oxygen desaturation: Functional analysis. *Clin. Respir. J.* **2020**, *14*, 29–34, PMID: 31613417. [CrossRef] [PubMed]
24. Wen, J.; Milne, S.; Sin, D.D. Pulmonary rehabilitation in a postcoronavirus disease 2019 world: Feasibility, challenges, and solutions. *Curr. Opin. Pulm. Med.* **2022**, *28*, 152–161. [CrossRef] [PubMed]
25. Bourne, S.; DeVos, R.; North, M.; Chauhan, A.; Green, B.; Brown, T.; Cornelius, V.; Wilkinson, T. Online versus face-to-face pulmonary rehabilitation for patients with chronic obstructive pulmonary disease: Randomised controlled trial. *BMJ Open* **2017**, *7*, e014580. [CrossRef] [PubMed]
26. Chaplin, E.; Hewitt, S.; Apps, L.; Bankart, J.; Pulikottil-Jacob, R.; Boyce, S.; Morgan, M.; Williams, J.; Singh, S. Interactive web-based pulmonary rehabilitation programme: A randomised controlled feasibility trial. *BMJ Open* **2017**, *7*, e013682. [CrossRef] [PubMed]
27. Hansen, H.; Bieler, T.; Beyer, N.; Kallemose, T.; Wilcke, J.T.; Østergaard, L.M.; Frost Andeassen, H.; Martinez, G.; Lavesen, M.; Frølich, A.; et al. Supervised pulmonary tele-rehabilitation versus pulmonary rehabilitation in severe COPD: A randomised multicentre trial. *Thorax* **2020**, *75*, 413–421. [CrossRef]
28. Langer, D.; Ciavaglia, C.; Faisal, A.; Webb, K.A.; Neder, J.A.; Gosselink, R.; Dacha, S.; Topalovic, M.; Ivanova, A.; O'Donnell, D.E. Inspiratory muscle training reduces diaphragm activation and dyspnea during exercise in COPD. *J. Appl. Physiol.* **2018**, *125*, 381–392. [CrossRef]
29. Holland, A.E.; Hill, C.J.; Rasekaba, T.; Lee, A.; Naughton, M.T.; McDonald, C.F. Updating the minimal important difference for six-minute walk distance in patients with chronic obstructive pulmonary disease. *Arch. Phys. Med. Rehabil.* **2010**, *91*, 221–225. [CrossRef]
30. Tsai, L.L.Y.; McNamara, R.J.; Moddel, C.; Alison, J.A.; McKenzie, D.K.; McKeough, Z.J. Home-based telerehabilitation via real-time videoconferencing improves endurance exercise capacity in patients with COPD: The randomized controlled TeleR Study. *Respirology* **2017**, *22*, 699–707. [CrossRef]
31. Kon, S.S.C.; Canavan, J.L.; Jones, S.E.; Nolan, C.M.; Clark, A.L.; Dickson, M.J.; Haselden, B.M.; Polkey, M.I.; Man, W.D.-C. Minimum clinically important difference for the COPD Assessment Test: A prospective analysis. *Lancet Respir. Med.* **2014**, *2*, 195–203. [CrossRef]
32. Loeckx, M.; Rabinovich, R.A.; Demeyer, H.; Louvaris, Z.; Tanner, R.; Rubio, N.; Frei, A.; De Jong, C.; Gimeno-Santos, E.; Rodrigues, F.M.; et al. Smartphone-Based Physical Activity Telecoaching in Chronic Obstructive Pulmonary Disease: Mixed-Methods Study on Patient Experiences and Lessons for Implementation. *JMIR Mhealth Uhealth* **2018**, *6*, e200. [CrossRef] [PubMed]

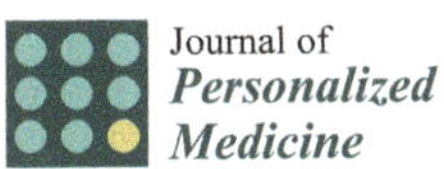
Journal of *Personalized Medicine*

MDPI

Review

Mycobacterium tuberculosis and Pulmonary Rehabilitation: From Novel Pharmacotherapeutic Approaches to Management of Post-Tuberculosis Sequelae

Andreea-Daniela Meca [1], Liliana Mititelu-Tarțău [2,*], Maria Bogdan [1,*], Lorena Anda Dijmarescu [3], Ana-Maria Pelin [4] and Liliana Georgeta Foia [5]

1 Department of Pharmacology, Faculty of Pharmacy, University of Medicine and Pharmacy, 200349 Craiova, Romania; andreea_mdc@yahoo.com
2 Department of Pharmacology, Faculty of Medicine, "Grigore T. Popa" University of Medicine and Pharmacy, 700115 Iasi, Romania
3 Department of Obstetrics-Gynecology, Faculty of Medicine, University of Medicine and Pharmacy, 200349 Craiova, Romania; lorenadijmarescu@yahoo.com
4 Department of Pharmaceutical Sciences, Faculty of Medicine and Pharmacy, "Dunarea de Jos" University, 800010 Galati, Romania; anapelin@gmail.com
5 Department of Biochemistry, Faculty of Medicine, "Grigore T. Popa" University of Medicine and Pharmacy, 700115 Iasi, Romania; lilifoia@yahoo.co.uk
* Correspondence: lylytartau@yahoo.com (L.M.-T.); bogdanfmaria81@yahoo.com (M.B.)

Abstract: Tuberculosis (TB) is still a worldwide public health burden, as more than 1.3 million deaths are expected to be reported in 2021. Even though almost 20 million patients have completed specific anti-TB treatment and survived in 2020, little information is known regarding their pulmonary sequelae, quality of life, and their need to follow rehabilitation services as researchers shifted towards proper diagnosis and treatment rather than analyzing post-disease development. Understanding the underlying immunologic and pathogenic mechanisms during mycobacterial infection, which have been incompletely elucidated until now, and the development of novel anti-TB agents could lead to the proper application of rehabilitation care, as TB sequelae result from interaction between the host and *Mycobacterium tuberculosis*. This review addresses the importance of host immune responses in TB and novel potential anti-TB drugs' mechanisms, as well as the assessment of risk factors for post-TB disease and usefulness of guidance and optimization of pulmonary rehabilitation. The use of rehabilitation programs for patients who successfully completed anti-tuberculotic treatment represents a potent multifaceted measure in preventing the increase of mortality rates, as researchers conclude that a patient with a TB diagnosis, even when properly completing pharmacotherapy, is threatened by a potential life loss of 4 years, in comparison to healthy individuals. Dissemination of pulmonary rehabilitation services and constant actualization of protocols could strengthen management of post-TB disease among under-resourced individuals.

Keywords: tuberculosis; antituberculotic drugs; host immune response; pulmonary rehabilitation

Citation: Meca, A.-D.; Mititelu-Tarțău, L.; Bogdan, M.; Dijmarescu, L.A.; Pelin, A.-M.; Foia, L.G. *Mycobacterium tuberculosis* and Pulmonary Rehabilitation: From Novel Pharmacotherapeutic Approaches to Management of Post-Tuberculosis Sequelae. *J. Pers. Med.* **2022**, *12*, 569. https://doi.org/10.3390/jpm12040569

Academic Editors: Ioannis Pantazopoulos and Ourania S. Kotsiou

Received: 9 March 2022
Accepted: 23 March 2022
Published: 2 April 2022

1. Introduction

The extension of rehabilitation programs as constant medical assistance can defy several obstacles in order to increase public health coverage [1]. Nevertheless, it is necessary to integrate these programs in accessible primary healthcare settings, not only in major urbanistic hospitals, for patients to benefit the full potential of rehabilitation [1,2]. Rehabilitation regimens could particularly improve the quality of life for individuals from low- and middle-income countries, taking into consideration that tuberculosis (TB) is the leading cause of death in those areas [2,3]. A holistic approach to TB management could prevent post-treatment complications [4]. The dissemination of rehabilitation services, as well as promoting equity and efficiency of public health measures, could strengthen worldwide health systems' capacity to ensure the needs of under-resourced populations [5].

The application of rehabilitation programs for patients diagnosed with TB represents a novel multifaceted healthcare service aiming to prevent chronic sequelae, organ failure, and death [6]. At present, there is a lack of protocols regarding pulmonary rehabilitation in TB [7–9], although the World Health Organization (WHO) estimated that there were more than 1.3 million deaths in HIV-negative individuals and an additional 214,000 deaths in HIV-positive people in 2020 [10]. An even greater number of deaths and rate of TB incidence is expected in 2021 [10]. Little information is reported regarding the millions of individuals who complete antituberculotic treatment and survive [4,11], more specifically, 19.8 million treated individuals of all ages [10].

In order to properly and equally apply rehabilitation care worldwide, it is imperative to understand the underlying immunologic and pathogenic mechanisms that appear in *Mycobacterium tuberculosis* (*M. tuberculosis*) infection to evaluate the risks of post-antituberculotic treatment complications and to synthesize existing rehabilitation health policies. Moreover, a major public health challenge consists of overcoming the emergence of drug-resistant mycobacterial strains, which can be kept under control through the development of novel anti-TB agents [12,13]. Long-term treatments, as well as mycobacterial survival, often lead to poor adherence, worse outcomes, and pulmonary consequences, even despite a complete pharmacotherapeutic procedure [14–17]. New therapeutic options and attractive drug targets are currently being analyzed worldwide by researchers and specialists in the field [18–22].

Even more, WHO published a concept note in 2019 recommending that the equity of rehabilitation services could be used as a unique optimization tool for human functioning, the third health indicator among mortality and morbidity [7]. Socioeconomic factors and nutritionally damaging behaviors (such as a poor diet or the absence of physical activity) increase the risk of morbidity in TB endemic regions [2,23–25]. A higher incidence of *M. tuberculosis* infection has been recorded in men, chronic smokers, alcohol consumers, and individuals with precarious socioeconomic status [2,10,26]. A delay in TB diagnosis also depends on the patient's socioeconomic status as it interferes with access to health services. Moreover, time prolongation prior to proper diagnosis directly increases the risk of tissular sequelae [26–28]. On the other hand, even though there are millions of patients who are cured and have survived mycobacterial infections, their life expectancy is reduced by four years, according to multiple researchers [23,29,30]. Hoger et al. warns that an average of 3.6 years of potential life loss occurs inpatients upon TB diagnosis, even when properly completing pharmacotherapy, in comparison with healthy humans [31]. Therefore, current re-evaluation of potential targets for novel antituberculotic drugs is crucial.

Even more, after 100 years of BCG (Bacille Calmette-Guerin) vaccine administration, a vaccine which is based on an attenuated strain of *Mycobacterium bovis* [32], more effective strategies are still required to reduce the TB burden [33]. BCG vaccination has proven to grant protection against bacillar dissemination, tuberculous meningitis, and death, rather than reducing the risk of infection, although it is the only vaccine approved until now in TB vaccination schemes [33]. Understanding mycobacterial adaptive and survival pathways in the host environment could lead not only to the development of therapeutic agents, but also to the discovery of novel vaccines [33].

International TB control programs have prioritized screening methods and effective treatment regimens in order to reduce the infection burden on public health systems. Researchers have shifted more towards proper diagnosis and effective treatment rather than understanding post-disease evolution [28,34]. Recovered patients have not been the main focus of intervention programs, although their long-term pulmonary sequelae directly affect their socioeconomic livelihood [35–37].

Therefore, the primary objective of this review is to highlight those patients who are not mentioned as often, but who need to benefit from various tools such as rehabilitation in order to improve their quality of life and life expectancy. Post-TB sequelae result from an interaction between the host, the bacillus, and the environment [29,38,39]. Implicitly, it becomes important to understand the specific immune mechanisms that appear during *M. tuberculosis* infection before and after the administration of specific pharmacological agents, in order to select the best rehabilitation program and the patients who would benefit the most.

This review focuses on (as shown in Figure 1):

- clarifications on the host immune responses in cases of *M. tuberculosis* infection, currently incompletely known;
- guidance on evaluation, future pharmacotherapy, and novel potential antimycobacterial drugs for patients diagnosed with TB after the assessment of risk factors for pulmonary sequelae;
- optimization of pulmonary rehabilitation.

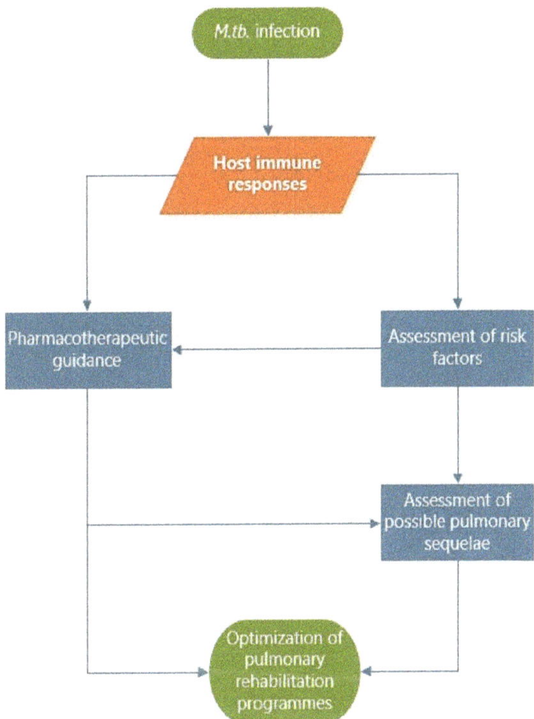

Figure 1. Multidisciplinary study purpose.

2. Pathogenesis and Immune Responses

A study conducted by Jesus and colleagues drew attention to the increased needs and various gaps in physical rehabilitation all over the globe. In 2017, more than 40% of impaired health conditions appeared from a lack of appropriate rehabilitation care [5]. Until now, official rehabilitation guidelines focused mainly upon chronic obstructive pulmonary disease and less on pulmonary TB [9,40]. However, after successful completion of anti-TB treatment, patients may present chronic obstructive respiratory symptoms such as wheezing, cough, sputum production, and dyspnea [3,26]. Recent data has confirmed that chronic lung symptoms among patients who have successfully completed anti-TB treatment increase their death rate and global healthcare burden [30,34].

De Souse Elias Nihues et al. conducted a cross-sectional study in cured TB patients and reported various pulmonary obstructive disorders in almost half of them, following the completion of therapy [26], a result also confirmed by other researchers [41,42]. Visca and colleagues mentioned the higher probability of clinical post-disease consequences from five to six times for patients diagnosed with pulmonary TB in comparison with those diagnosed with latent infections [30]. Based on the study of a cohort of immigrating individuals to Canada from 1985–2015, Basham et al. concluded that more that than 42% of *M. tuberculosis* infected people developed post-disease symptoms in the airways (emphysema, bronchitis, chronic respiratory obstruction) in high resource and low-TB incidence settings, despite the potential availability of pulmonary rehabilitation [43]. The researchers underlined higher social vulnerability due to pulmonary persistent heterogenous sequelae among individuals who successfully completed tuberculostatic treatment [26,27,29] and also reported repeated treatment courses as one of the most important risk factors for post-TB disease [30,44]. Chronic sequelae refer to various obstructive disorders with reduced expiratory capacity, non-responsiveness to bronchodilators, airflow obstruction, bronchiectasis, fibrotic changes, multiple non-tuberculous infections, and aspergillomas that can lead to abnormal spirometry results and impaired diffusing capacity [3,29,45]. Allwood et al. underlined the importance of post-TB lung disease assessment in order to extend life expectancy, although there are still no evidence-based recommendations or guidelines [46,47]. Despite the fact that exacerbations of post-TB pulmonary disease are poorly recognized, symptoms such as hemoptysis may derive from affected and infected parenchyma, pleura, and vasculature [42,45]. The pathogenic patterns of pulmonary post-TB symptoms are difficult to predict [38,42,48]; however, the first innate immune interactions between the bacilli and the human host, although yet poorly understood, are crucial for the outcome of the disease [48–51].

M. tuberculosis enters pulmonary macrophages after the inhalation of aerosolized droplets and encounters a beneficial long-term survival environment [38,44]. Mycobacteria are intriguing due to their remarkable ability to adapt to the human host after avoiding both the innate and adaptive immune responses [52]. After the epithelial recognition of bacilli (by toll-like receptors), signaling pathways and neutrophil migration are activated, triggering the synthesis of various chemokines and cytokines [49,53–55]. Dendritic cells and inflammatory mediators further recruit lymphocytes, monocytes, polymorphonuclear leukocytes, and phagocytes which proliferate and transform into a complex multicellular structure, the so-called histopathological hallmark of TB–granuloma, involved in both pathogenesis and immune protection (as depicted in Figure 2) [44,51,55,56].

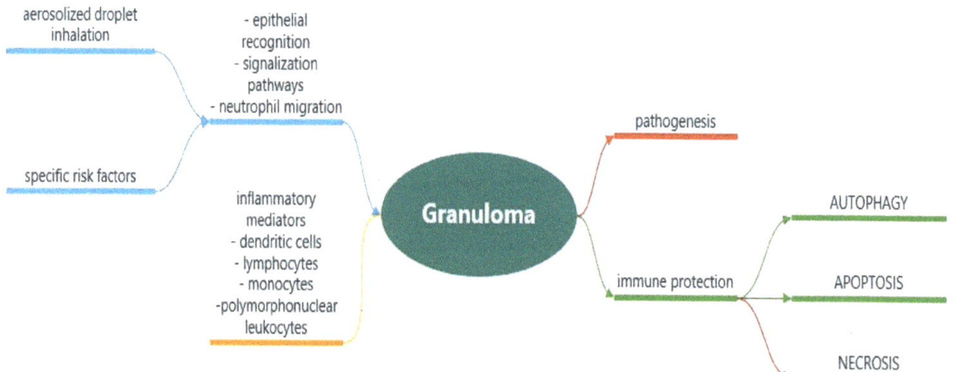

Figure 2. Immunologic pathways in *M. tuberculosis* infection. Color legend: blue and green represent the host innate and adaptive immune responses involved in mycobacterial recognition and removal; red represents mycobacterial survival and long-term tissue inflammation; and orange represents both pathways that can appear during *M. tuberculosis* infection: bacillar death or survival.

During granuloma formation, a protective initial response is observed subsequent to phagocytosis, the host's attempt to clear the pathogen [47,51]. Alveolar macrophages initiate proinflammatory responses after encountering *M. tuberculosis* in order to restrict its growth, while leucocytes generate pro-oxidative species such as nitric oxide and hydrogen peroxide in balance with antioxidant systems [52]. On the other side, mycobacteria inverts host immune activity through metabolic changes; more specifically, *M. tuberculosis* disrupts the production of $NADPH_2$-oxidase (reduced nicotinamide adenine dinucleotide phosphate), leading to granuloma formation, excessive synthesis of reactive oxygen species (ROS), and bacillar replication [47,52]. After bacillary replication, an adaptative immune response is initiated (autophagy), as shown in Figure 2 [47,51,57]. Nevertheless, various antituberculotic agents such as isoniazid and pyrazinamide can induce autophagy during *M. tuberculosis* infection [50,58,59]. Neutrophils are also able to secrete specific antimycobacterial enzymes to support the activity of other immune cells [49,54]. Neutrophils have been recently linked to pulmonary post-TB sequelae after stimulating the pro-inflammatory host response [47,60,61]. The resulted phagosomes represent the host's attempt at bacillar containment through oxidative burst sustained by neutrophil activity [47,62]. However, the oxidative burst promotes mycobacterial growth by down-regulating the synthesis of protective antioxidants, reducing the T-lymphocytes' inhibitory activity against *M. tuberculosis*, and by inducing necrosis (unprogrammed accidental cell death) instead of apoptosis (Figure 2) [57,62–64]. While apoptosis ensures programmed cellular death without the tissular spilling of cellular contents through nuclear envelope disassembly, cytoskeleton collapse, and inclusion of DNA fragments in specific apoptotic vesicles, necrosis leads to acute inflammation by releasing cellular components into the surrounding tissues [65–69]. *M. tuberculosis* has the ability to generate anti-apoptotic factors that combat specific host pro-apoptotic mechanisms, therefore evading the adaptive immune responses and managing survival [65,66,68]. Necrotic lesions also represent microenvironments for dormant bacilli, which are difficult to target and often resistant to standard pharmacotherapy [70–72]. Moreover, the dynamic interactions between the host's apoptotic immune responses and mycobacterial anti-apoptotic factors decide the outcome of infection [65]. In other words, *M. tuberculosis* disseminates and survives due to its ability to resist apoptosis.

However, Hunter recently argued that pulmonary TB actually begins as a macrophagic infection in individuals with a strong immune response, capable of healing granulomas [73]. The granuloma formation has been considered for many years to be a host protective response, although the mycobacteria manage to evade and to disseminate, even in case of administering proper pharmacotherapy [38,74], undergoing caseous necrosis with early obstructive pulmonary symptoms [73]. The enriched granulomatous center in macrophages which further differentiates into multinucleated giant cells, epithelioid macrophages are the main components of granuloma [51,57]. The immune cells are surrounded by T and B cells able to contain *M. tuberculosis* and prevent bacillar dissemination [49,51,55,57]. Nevertheless, tumor necrosis factor (TNF-α), produced by antigen-presenting cells in the early stages of mycobacterial infection, is essential in granuloma formation [51,75]. On the other hand, granuloma disruption and *M. tuberculosis* dissemination appear in the case of TNF-α blockade (initiated, for example, by anti-rheumatic agents such as adalimumab, infliximab, etanercept, and golimumab) [75,76]. A systematic review conducted by Sartori et al. underlined that the TB incidence in cases of rheumatic patients exposed to TNF-inhibitors was 9.62 per 1000 individuals, with pulmonary TB predominating [76]. Extracellular mycobacterial dissemination appears in cases of macrophage death [55,57,77]. This specific bronchial obstruction leads to macrophagic and lymphocytic dysfunctionalities that will further disrupt *M. tuberculosis* clearance [56,73,74]. Granuloma necrosis can also appear due to a high neutrophil and cytokine inflammatory response [55]. Even more, it seems that a higher cytokine synthesis as an innate immune activity predisposes individuals to an increased probability of a positive tuberculin skin test [49]. Muefong et al. underlined that the neutrophil count in patients with positive sputum-smear test points to a higher bacillary burden and correlates with unfavorable disease outcomes [47].

Although there are current guidelines that specifically recommend appropriate treatment strategies, some individuals develop fibrosis and irreversible tissular modifications [38,47,55]. A cross-sectional study conducted by Ngahane et al. concluded that the presence of fibrotic changes in patients diagnosed with pulmonary TB represents an independent risk factor for future organ impairment [78]. Moreover, the researchers reported lung function impairment in more than 45% of the study participants, despite completion of antituberculotic therapy in all subjects [78]. Calcification and fibrosis associated with a deficit in forced expiratory volume have been associated with increased activity of neutrophils [47,52]. Therefore, development of post-TB pulmonary lesions is related to the persistent host inflammatory responses, even after treatment completion and bacillar clearance [47,79,80]. Guidem et al. concluded that a pulmonary increase of neutrophils, monocytes, and lymphocytes is associated with a higher risk of developing chronic obstructive pulmonary disease (COPD) manifestations in patients who have successfully completed anti-TB treatment [79].

More than 70% of patients diagnosed with TB are malnourished [4,81], and therefore present reduced muscle functionality. Malnutrition also predisposes to unfavorable treatment outcomes and increases death rates among *M. tuberculosis* infected individuals [8,11,82]. Environmental factors such as air pollution, occupational risks, smoking, and alcohol consumption could also lead to unfavorable outcomes after anti-TB therapy due to immunosuppression [23,81]. Nevertheless, cigarette smoke can delay *M. tuberculosis* clearance after cilia paralyze and can interfere with granuloma formation [73]. Additionally, various studies have proven that urban air pollution directly modifies the innate immune response to *M. tuberculosis* infection by altering T-cell functionality and by increasing synthesis of pro-inflammatory cytokines [83,84]. The occurrence of subsequent life-threatening pulmonary infections (especially fungal diseases) after the completion of antituberculotic pharmacotherapy represents a burden among TB survivors, characterized by a slowly-progressive inflammatory response [34,85]. A background of TB is the first risk factor for chronic pulmonary aspergillosis [46,84,85]. Immunocompromised individuals with residual pulmonary cavitation after completion of anti-TB treatment are most likely to express saprophytic colonization and extensive pleural damage [86,87].

Hunter mentions that even though patients may survive after *M. tuberculosis* infection, a body can never recover, as the evolution of the mycobacteria within the host is difficult to predict [73]. A sustainable integrated approach regarding pulmonary rehabilitation plans [2] could improve long-term life quality in prior TB diagnostic and even multi-drug resistant TB (MDR-TB) patients [35,88]. Moreover, recent data confirm that preventing TB sequelae, rather than pharmacotherapeutic strategies, could better influence socioeconomic livelihood [82,88]. However, early TB diagnosis and effective pharmacotherapy are the main preventive methods for post-disease lesions [57,74,89].

Nevertheless, further assessment of rehabilitation programs should be intensively considered and hence, included in research in order to be implemented faster for better management of post-TB treatment patients with pulmonary sequelae. Last, but not least, it is worth mentioning that post-TB survivors may be permanently affected, not only due to pulmonary disease, but also due to other significant organ dysfunctionalities and psychological impact [35,45].

3. Pharmacotherapy in Patients Diagnosed with TB

Understanding the underlying immunological mechanisms in TB represents a key in opening the door to anti-TB drug discovery or repurposing pathways. One of the major burdens imposed by *M. tuberculosis* infection is developing novel antituberculotic agents that could further contribute to better outcomes in patients and increased adherence [90,91]. As patients' compliance increases, the risk of post-TB symptoms reduces [14,28]. This also appears as a worldwide critical demand due to rapid emergence of resistant bacillar strains [91], as no other first-line agent has been approved since the 1960s [92,93], when the combined schema of isoniazid (H), pyrazinamide (Z), rifampicin (R), and ethambutol (E) was completely discovered and introduced into the guidelines [72,90,94]. The minimum duration of first-line standard pharmacotherapy is 6 months, comprised of an intensive phase (HRZE for 2 months) and a continuation phase (HR regimen for 4 months) [14,95]. The first-line treatment targets drug-sensitive mycobacterial strains. Although it usually achieves more than an 80% success rate in cases of newly diagnosed individuals, it can lead to multiple adverse events specific to each active substance (hepatotoxicity, ototoxicity, flu-like syndrome, ocular or nervous toxicity, and much more) [96–98].

Although second-line pharmacotherapy is available and recommended to be followed for at least 20 months for patients infected with MDR strains, it has recently been reorganized based upon research regarding drug efficacy and adverse reactions [91,94,99–102]. The primary agents are clofazimine and linezolid, while p-aminosalicylic acid, one of the first discovered successful anti-TB agents [90], can be introduced as a supplementary drug when needed [91]. Macrolides have proven to have a reduced effectiveness in patients with MDR-TB or extensively drug-resistant (XDR)-TB and have been therefore excluded as second-line drugs [91].

The continuous research from the past years has led to the approval of novel effective anti-TB agents and new mechanisms that could further support lowering the necessity for future rehabilitation programs (Table 1).

Table 1. Novel antituberculotic drugs and their mechanisms of action.

Novel Anti-Tuberculotic Drugs	References	Mechanism of Action
Diarylquinolone Bedaquiline (R207910, TMC-207)	[92,102,103]	inhibits ATP-synthesis after binding to the c subunit of F_0F_1ATP synthase; prevents enzyme rotation and proton transfer within mycobacterial cell; acts on both replicating and dormant bacilli.
Nitroimidazoles Delamanid (OPC-67683) Pretomanid (PA-824)	[104–107] [71,108–110]	inhibits mycolic acids synthesis (ketomycolic and methoxymycolic acids) and targets mycobacterial wall; requires activation by a specific deazaflavin F420-dependent nitro-reductase (prodrug); potential decrease in fluoroquinolone resistance; additional activity–nitric oxide donor.
Oxazolidinones Sutezolid (PNU-100480) Delpazolid (LCB01-0371)	[111–113] [111–113]	inhibits mycobacterial protein synthesis; binds to 50 s ribosomal subunits; inhibits mitochondrial protein synthesis (responsible for adverse events such as myelotoxicity).
Imidazopyridine Telacebec (Q203)	[90,102,108,114]	inhibits ATP synthesis; binds to respiratory cytochrome bc_1 complex; its activity is independent of mycobacterial replication stage.
Benzothiazinones Benzothiazinone (BTZ-043) Macozinone (PBTZ-169, MCZ)	[115–118] [116,119,120]	DprE1 inhibitors (flavoenzyme decaprenyl-phosphoryl-β-d-ribose-20-oxidase inhibitors); inhibits arabinose synthesis and decreases synthesis of arabinogalactan and lipoarabinomannan (essential components of mycobacterial cellular wall); superior pharmacokinetics and lower risk of adverse events.
Indolcarboxamide (ethambutol derivate) SQ109	[13,116,119–122]	multitarget antituberculotic agent; Mmpl3 (Mycobacterial Membrane Protein Large 3)–primary target from respiratory chain; inhibits Mmpl3 transporter (trehalose mono-mycolate) and blocks protein membrane translocation; inhibits ATP synthesis; affects cell wall stability.

3.1. Bedaquiline

A lipophilic diarylquinolone called bedaquiline (R207910, TMC-207) was discovered in 2005 through phenotypic screening (a screening process among compound libraries, following antimycobacterial activity against mycobacterial culture cells) and approved in 2012 as a treatment for newly diagnosed patients with MDR-TB [90,92,102]. A total of 109 countries have used bedaquiline as part of their pharmacotherapeutic program for MDR-TB as of the end of 2020 [10]. The major mechanism of action for bedaquiline involves the *M. tuberculosis* proton pump of adenosine triphosphate (ATP) synthesis which subsequently leads to bacillar ATP impairment [92,103]. More specifically, bedaquiline binds with the c subunit of *M. tuberculosis* F_0F_1 ATP synthase, preventing the subunit rotation and proton transfer [103,123]. More interestingly, it acts in both replicating and dormant mycobacteria but it does not possess any substantial antimicrobial activity against other bacteria [102,103,107]. Bedaquiline has a risk of prolonging the cardiac QT interval [108,124–126]. It is also characterized by a long half-life (more than 150 days) [124–127]. The association between bedaquiline and other anti-TB drugs (such as fluoroquinolones) which involve risk of QT prolongation is not recommended [109]. Moreover, a significant interaction occurs between R and bedaquiline and their joint use is restricted, as the plasmatic concentration of bedaquiline could be reduced due to CYP3A4 induction [102,127,128]. Currently, phase 1 clinical trials are being conducted in order to identify safer and more potent diarylquinolines compared to bedaquiline, such as TBAJ-876, a 3,5-dialkoxypyridine analogue of bedaquiline, and TBAJ-587, which entered clinical trials in October 2020 [129,130].

3.2. Delamanid and Pretomanid

Delamanid (OPC-67683) and pretomanid (PA-824) have been analyzed as potent antituberculotic agents, with both bactericidal and sterilizing activities [130], added in MDR-TB regimens [90,107]. They are nitroimidazoles derivatives which inhibit mycolic acid synthesis (such as keto- and methoxy-mycolic acids [107]) and are able to improve outcomes in MDR-TB patients by affecting both replicating and dormant bacilli [104–106]. The mycobacterial cellular wall is crucial for long term survival and its synthesis depends on specific enzymes that are absent in humans. Therefore, it is considered as a potential target for new anti-TB agents [13,123]. Moreover, pretomanid acts as a nitric oxide donor, altering the oxidative mycobacterial balance [108]. Nitric oxide is a molecule which has a key role in the pathogenesis of inflammation. Under normal physiological conditions it shows an anti-inflammatory effect, but under pathological conditions, nitric oxide is considered to be a pro-inflammatory mediator that induces inflammation due to its over-production [131].

Delamanid was approved in 2014 as a treatment for MDR-TB for patients who cannot tolerate second-line regimen [71]. These antibacterial new drugs do not interact with P450 cytochrome and have shown no mutagenicity as of yet, which might minimize interactions with other anti-TB drugs and thus boost their use in individuals co-infected with HIV and *M. tuberculosis* [109,130,132]. However, a transient QTcF prolongation was also confirmed in case of delamanid administration [104], and therefore combination with bedaquiline is not recommended [110]. Nevertheless, an increased risk of cardiac events appears in cases of delamanid or bedaquiline combined with other second-line anti-TB drugs such as clofazimine and fluoroquinolones [110]. The most common claimed adverse reactions of delamanid include gastrointestinal disorders, insomnia, anxiety, tremor, paranesthesia, and migraines [133].

There is limited information regarding their pediatric use or association (trials no. 242-12-232, NCT01859923, NCT01856634) [107,130,132], although delamanid has not proven mutagenicity yet and was approved in 2014 as a potent dose-dependent antituberculotic agent [71,133]. Regarding of its mechanism of action, delamanid can attack residual *M. tuberculosis* from hypoxic and non-hypoxic lesions, as well as necrotizing and non-necrotizing tissues, because it is a prodrug that requires activation by a specific tuberculous deazaflavin (F420)-dependent nitroreductase [71,110,123]. Delamanid seems to be able to decrease fluoroquinolone resistance in mycobacterial strains as well, providing a status of useful associative drug among antituberculotic regimens [109].

The nitroimidazooxazine, pretomanid, has been quite recently approved by the FDA (granted limited population approval in 2019) for patients diagnosed with XDR-TB and intolerant or non-responsive MDR-TB, in combination with bedaquiline and linezolid [130].

Furthermore, pyrazinamide increased both pretomanid and bedaquiline activity when added to the treatment schema [92]. Quadruple therapy consisting of Z, pretomanid, bedaquiline, and moxifloxacin can reduce treatment duration to only three months, in patients diagnosed with MDR-TB [109,110].

3.3. Sutezolid and Other Oxazolidinones

Oxazolidinones (such as sutezolid, tedizolid, posizolid, delpazolid, and contezolid [111,112]) have been recently introduced in clinical trials as potent anti-TB drugs due to their inhibitory activity of protein synthesis after binding to the 50s ribosomal subunits [108]. Sutezolid (PNU-100480) and delpazolid (LCB01-0371) are currently in phase 2 clinical trials [111,113,130]. Myelotoxicity is their most important adverse effect besides cytopenia, lactic acidosis, and rhabdomyolysis (data obtained from randomized controlled trial NCT02540460 [113,134]), although sutezolid proved to be a more secure and efficient antituberculosis drug as compared to linezolid, which belongs to the same structural class and is already part of third-line regimens for MDR-TB and XDR-TB [115,135,136]. Another potential adverse event from sutezolid therapy was transient alanine transaminase (ALT) elevations, without life-threatening hepatotoxicity [92]. These adverse events appear to be due to the inhibition of mitochondrial protein synthesis [102]. Linezolid-bedaquiline-pretomanid regimen was approved by the FDA in 2019 [137], although mutations in the 23 rRNA gene seem to be involved in the mechanism of *M. tuberculosis* resistance to linezolid [13,138].

3.4. Telacebec (Q203)

Telacebec, a highly lipophilic antitubercular agent, consists of imidazopyridine, which operates independent of cellular oxygen deprivation and mycobacterial replication [90,102,123,139]. Telacebec in nanomolar concentrations restricts *M. tuberculosis* intra- and extra-cellular growth by interfering with ATP synthesis and, implicitly, cellular energy production [108,114]. Its principal target is the respiratory cytochrome bc_1 complex, which is essential for the respiratory electron transport chain involved in ATP synthesis [102,108]. Depletion of mycobacterial ATP leads to cellular death, independent of the replication stage [114,123]. Telacebec was proven to have a 90% oral bioavailability in mice, elevated serum protein binding ability, and a half-life of about 24 h [102]. No interactions with cytochrome P450 were recorded, making telacebec a safe, novel anti-TB drug [102].

3.5. Benzothiazinone (BTZ-043) and Macozinone (PBTZ-169, MCZ)

Benzothiazinone is currently advised as a potential antitubercular agent [90]. The primary target for bezothiazinone is the flavoenzyme decaprenyl-phosphoryl-β-d-ribose-20-oxidase (DprE1) [115,117]. DprE1 and DprE2 (decaprenylphosphoryl-2-keto-β-d-erythro-pentose reductase) are essential to the synthesis of arabinogalactan and lipoarabinomannan, main components of the mycobacterial cell wall [117,118]. DprE1 inhibitors block mycobacterial survival by leading to cellular lysis [120,140]. Macozinone is a piperazine derivative with a superior pharmacokinetics profile, security, and pharmacodynamic effect in comparison with the lipophilic benzothiazinone that is less effective in case of severe TB [119]. Moreover, macozinone has proven to have synergistic activity when administered along with bedaquiline and other anti-TB agents [119]. These agents are currently being investigated in phase 2 clinical trials [130]. Another inhibitor of DprE1 is the carbostyril derivate entitled OPC-167832, also currently being evaluated in phase 2 trials [90]. More than 15 compounds have been identified as potent mycobacterial DprE1 inhibitors, including triazoles (377790), nitroquinoxalines (VI-9376), dinitrobenzamides (DNB1), benzothiazoles (TCA1, 7a), carboxy-quinoxalines (Ty38c), thiadiazoles (GSK-710), azaindoles (TBA-7371, currently in phase 1 trials), and pyrazolopyridones [120,140–144].

3.6. SQ109

SQ109, a novel small molecule that can be orally administered, is currently being explored in phase 2 trials as a replacement for a first-line anti-TB agent, as it has already proved efficacy against both susceptible and resistant strains [130]. However, SQ109 did not show effectiveness when administered alone [92]. SQ109 (1,2-ethylendiamine derived from the first-line antituberculotic agent ethambutol) has displayed antimycobacterial activity upon ethambutol resistant strains, when administered concomitant with sutezolid and bedaquiline [145,146]. Nevertheless, when combined with standard regimen, SQ109 increased sputum conversion rate by 21% in a prospective randomized double-blind study that included 140 individuals [122]. SQ109 targets Mmpl3 (mycobacterial membrane protein large 3) within the mycobacterial respiratory chain and further manages intrusion in mycobacterial wall synthesis–a unique mechanism among anti-TB agents, as SQ109 is considered a multitarget antituberculotic [121,122]. The Mmpl3 transporter (trehalose mono-mycolate) is essential in mycobacterial wall stability and protein translocation among the membrane, further ensuring pathogenesis [121]. Mmpl3 belongs to a family of export bacterial proteins, but it represents the only protein from the MmpL (mycobacterial membrane protein large) family involved in *M. tuberculosis* survival; therefore, it is a very attractive drug target [120]. In other words, this indolcarboxamide is able to downregulate both the transport of metabolites from mycobacterial cytosol and ATP synthesis [13], with a minimal risk of adverse events (such as gastrointestinal dose-dependent effects) [92]. It could also shorten the average treatment duration [122]. Although SQ109 is structurally derived from ethambutol, it presents poly-pharmacologic properties and multiple bactericidal and antitubercular mechanisms [102]. These are due to the additional ability of SQ109 to inhibit menaquinone and ATP synthesis [102,147]. Both DprE1 and MmpL3 are regarded by researchers as promising antituberculotic drug targets, as several other MmpL3 inhibitors have been reported to have antimycobacterial activity: diarylpyrroles (BM212), adamantyl urea (AU1235), benzimidazoles (C215), indolcarboxamides (NIDT349), dihydrospiro(piperidine-4,4′-thieno(3,2-c)pyrans) (Spiro), tetrahydropyrazolo pyrimidine (THP P), acetamides (E11), piperidinols (PIPD1), and carboxamides (HC2091) [120].

However, it is still difficult to complete the pipeline for anti-TB drug development, as *M. tuberculosis* is a pretentious bacillus that requires environmental facilities and replicates very slowly [13,71]. Joseph and colleagues underlined the importance of the further evaluation and pulmonary care in individuals from their retrospective cohort study, as residual respiratory symptoms (such as chronic cough or breathlessness) were reported in almost 30% of patients although successfully completing first-line standard treatment [93]. Moreover, pathological modifications (cavitation, fibrosis) and hypoxic conditions in patients diagnosed with pulmonary TB may decrease drug bioavailability while allowing *M. tuberculosis* to reside and survive [13,71] and implicitly, to further increase the need of rehabilitation services among patients who may successfully complete pharmacotherapy. On the other hand, the promising activities of novel drugs are not only for their interesting mechanisms, but also for their ability to penetrate thick-walled pulmonary lesions where *M. tuberculosis* resides on long-term in case of telacebec and also for their bactericidal activity in case of MDR and XDR *M. tuberculosis* resistant strains in case of SQ109 [148]. However, are novel anti-TB agents enough for improving the quality of life and decreasing mortality rates in patients diagnosed with pulmonary TB? Matsuo et al. confirm that early interventions of pulmonary rehabilitation are associated with improved human quality of life and survival expectancy [45].

4. Pulmonary Rehabilitation

Post-TB sequelae and irreversible extensive pulmonary damage have become top priorities among researchers, as in 2020 more than 150 million *M. tuberculosis* infection survivors have been reported [43,86]. These individuals experienced long-term symptoms associated with aspergillosis, vascular pathologies [87], bronchiectasis, and COPD, in the absence of available pharmacological treatment that could reduce functional pulmonary decline [86,149,150]. The destruction of bronchial wall components during *M. tuberculosis* infection leads to airflow obstruction, bronchogenic spread of purulent sputum, hemoptysis, bronchiectasis, and pneumonia, with consequent symptoms worsening despite completing anti-TB pharmacotherapy [38,151]. Moreover, mixed patterns of ventilatory defects and airflow restrictions (quantified through an increased ratio of FEV_1/forced vital capacity or a decrease in forced vital capacity) were noted in individuals with TB who further experienced chronic cough, chest pains, and breathlessness [38]. Airflow obstruction appears in these patients due to abnormal healing processes and long-term inflammatory responses such as pleural thickening, bronchovascular distortion, and delimitation of specific fibrotic bands, despite completion of treatment [38].

Daniels et al., in their pilot study, found a decreased exercise capacity and quality of mental and physical life in patients who completed antituberculotic therapy [152]. Gupte et al. obtained abnormal pulmonary functionality in 77% of the patients included in their study, which is regarded as an alarming result after treatment completion [149]. Even more, Gupte et al. showed that only 21% of individuals with post-TB COPD pathogenesis had a beneficial bronchodilator response [149].

Therefore, effective non-pharmacological interventions such as exercise training, behavior management, and patient education are highly necessary [86], due to the lack of guidance regarding the management of post-TB disease [87,149,152]. Pulmonary rehabilitation can be a cost-effective measure, as programs can be held within hospital as well as within the patients' residence, although supplementary guidance and management of resistance and aerobic training is necessary to be developed for individuals who cannot access pulmonary rehabilitation centers [152].

Lung functionality in patients who completed successfully anti-TB cure can be assessed by performing:

- chest radiography and computed tomography,
- spirometry (including bronchodilator response),
- plethysmography (assessment of lung volumes),
- DLCO (diffusion for carbon oxide),
- arterial blood gas analyses (median arterial blood oxygen saturation and mean arterial oxygen partial pressure),
- evaluation of the capacity to perform exercise via the six minute walk test (6MWT) or the incremental shuttle walk test (ISWT) [4,31,149,150,152–155].

Radiographic monitoring in patients who completed antituberculotic treatment is useful to predict cavitary infectious diseases, pleural thickening and further colonization with *Aspergillus fumigatus* or other mycobacterial strains [150,156]. Various studies proved that 15% to 25% of patients who completed anti-TB therapy were diagnosed with cavitary aspergilloma [150,156,157]. In other words, management of possible fungal infections in those individuals could lead to higher rates of candidate identification for future pulmonary rehabilitation programs. Moreover, fibrotic patterns, revealed by chest X-rays, can lead to pain or dyspnea (specific symptoms of restrictive ventilatory pathogenesis) [154,158], further selecting post-TB survivors as possible rehabilitation recipients.

Spirometry tests could be used as predictor for post-TB sequelae because a positive response to bronchodilator therapy can prove impaired pulmonary function [149,155,159,160]. Therefore, spirometry monitoring may highlight the actual number of individuals who are in need of pulmonary rehabilitation programs. On the other hand, very recently, Patil and collaborators reported an obstructive pattern after spirometry assessment in 42% of individuals with symptomatic post-TB disease and 32% of individuals without a symptomatic burden after anti-TB treatment completion [161]. Therefore, asymptomatic post-TB survivors may also present defective pulmonary functionality [161,162]. Spirometry analysis is an effective tool in the evaluation of post-TB sequelae and should be included in the identification process of possible candidates for pulmonary rehabilitation, irrespective of symptomatology [161,162]. However, Radovic and collaborators mentioned that spirometry analysis only is not accurate in the detection of possible obstructive pathogenesis and hence, multiple rehabilitation strategies should be approached [163].

Approaching exercise training among patients who survived pulmonary TB requires analysis of patients' endurance and strength [86]. Several studies reported improvement in patients diagnosed with post-TB pathology after 6MWT and ISWT after measuring forced expiratory volume (FEV_1), forced vital capacity (FVC), median arterial blood oxygen saturation (SaO_2), and mean arterial oxygen partial pressure (PaO_2) [3,27,152]. Lower FEV_1/FVC ratios are correlated with chronic post-TB airflow obstruction [149,154,160], while lower a FVC result predicts restrictive symptoms [154,158,164]. Approximately 60% of participants from the study conducted by Jones et al. diagnosed with post-TB pathogenesis recorded improvement in the sit-to-stand test and in ISWT, as well as a reduction of restrictive ventilatory symptoms (hemoptysis and pain) [27]. Excessive fibrosis that appears as consequence of tissular healing [158,164] in patients who completed chemotherapy may lead to these restrictive pulmonary disorders [154]. Physical activity is reduced in case of post-TB fungal infections or bronchiectasis, also affecting quality of life [150]. Yang et al. also noticed that obstructive disorders are associated with both reduced quality of life and exercise tolerance, while restrictive ventilatory symptoms lead to lower training ability [154]. In order to limit bronchiectasis clinical symptoms (such as chest pain, respiratory deficiency, fatigue, and cough with hemoptysis), patients should follow rehabilitation programs that include physiotherapy (sputum clearance using hypertonic inhaled solutions) and physical training [150,164].

The recovery of muscle function after exercise training in malnourished subjects could also improve absorption of antituberculotic drugs concomitantly with prevention of unfavorable treatment outcomes [8]. Nevertheless, a higher body mass index before antituberculotic treatment onset lowers the risk of lung impairment [149,165]. Yang et al. reported a lesser body mass index as well as a higher rate of nicotine consumption in participants with obstructive ventilatory pathogenesis in comparison to those with normal or restrictive ventilatory symptoms [154]. Singh et al. obtained improvements in dyspnea score, 6MWT and quality of life for TB cured individuals, therefore recommending rehabilitation strategies for core management of post-pulmonary disease sequalae [158]. The recommendations for management of post-TB sequelae are summarized in Figure 3.

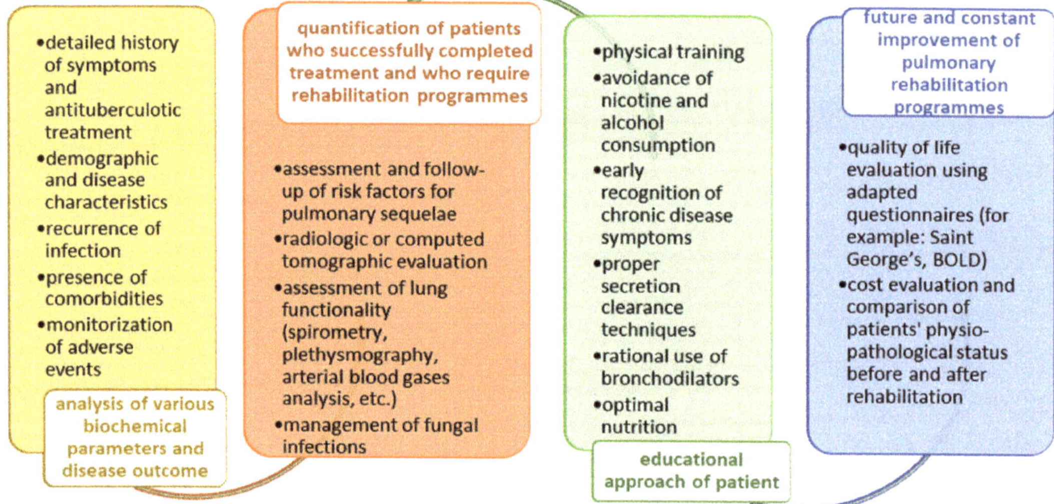

Figure 3. Recommendations for post-TB disease management.

Several researchers have recommended nutritional counselling among individuals with post-TB sequelae during rehabilitation programs [4,8], regardless of patients' age [149]. An impaired quality of life and decreased exercise tolerance are directly correlated with smoking [150,160,166,167]. However, young non-smoking individuals may not be screened for chronic post-TB disease, despite the research conducted by Gupte and collaborators which proved that this population has the highest risk of airflow obstruction development [78,149,166]. Furthermore, a complete pulmonary rehabilitation strategy should include smoking cessation recommendations and avoidance of air pollution [163,167]. Even more, researchers pointed out that irreversible pulmonary damage and various obstructive symptoms appear only if FEV_1 are lower than 50% [158], so multiple strategies should be followed in order to scale down morbidity and mortality rates in TB survivors [165]. In addition, the complex interactions between *M. tuberculosis* and the host immune response may include various impaired mechanisms in cases of individuals with poor nutritional status, exposed to air pollution or cigarette smoking. Pulmonary rehabilitation may improve host defense strategies by improving exercise ability and strength [27].

Nevertheless, airflow obstruction, excessive pulmonary tissue inflammation and injury, as well as lung functionality decline have been reported in HIV/TB co-infected patients [168,169]. Hoger and colleagues concluded that HIV infected individuals with a history of TB diagnosis were predicted to lose 16 potential years of life [31]. HIV status can therefore predict higher rates of expected life loss in fully treated TB patients [31].

Last, but not least, as we have experienced in the past years a pandemic caused by the severe acute respiratory syndrome coronavirus disease (COVID-19), it is essential to mention those individuals diagnosed with both TB and COVID-19 [170,171]. Although data are extremely limited, in TB patients, symptoms of COVID-19 infection were noted to be more severe and appeared rapidly due to increased host cytokine production, causing a synergistic socioeconomical worldwide burden [170,172,173]. Active TB has also been associated with a 2.1-fold increased risk of developing severe COVID-19; however, more studies with rigorously assessment of bias are necessary [173]. Tadolini et al. underlined that in the group of patients diagnosed with both post-TB sequelae (such as pulmonary infiltrates and cavities) and COVID-19 presented higher rates of mortality [170]. Therefore, it is urgent to gain data from clinical studies in order to predict the impact of this ongoing pandemic on individuals with post-TB disease.

5. Conclusions

Despite the constantly increasing efforts over the last years, *M. tuberculosis* infection continues to challenge researchers due to its underlying survival pathways and interactions with the host. The great variability and heterogeneity in pulmonary functionality among individuals who successfully complete anti-TB regimens (ranging from various grades of airflow obstruction and specific lung pathologies such as cavitation, nodular infiltrates, fibrosis, and combination) underlines the multitude of consequences that appear due to the immunologic interaction between the host response and mycobacteria, yet it has been incompletely elucidated. Significant advances have been noted regarding immunological implications and pharmacotherapeutic development, as the more we understand about TB and post-TB sequelae, the sooner novel mycobactericidal mechanisms could be investigated. Moreover, it is also crucial to detect and to quantify patients who require post-disease monitoring, despite completing antituberculotic regimens, as pulmonary symptoms seem to be mediated through host immune responses.

The importance of pulmonary rehabilitation services in individuals who have successfully completed anti-TB treatment has been discussed in this review and a guideline has been proposed. TB control programs and pulmonary rehabilitation services for patients are mandatory, along with the detection of novel, effective, anti-tuberculotic agents and an understanding of mycobacterial mechanisms in order to interrupt the worldwide transmission chain.

Author Contributions: Conceptualization, A.-D.M. and M.B.; writing—original draft preparation, A.-D.M., L.A.D. and A.-M.P.; writing—review and editing, M.B., A.-D.M., L.M.-T. and L.G.F.; supervision, L.M.-T. and L.G.F. All authors have read and agreed to the published version of the manuscript.

Funding: This research received no external funding.

Institutional Review Board Statement: Not applicable.

Informed Consent Statement: Not applicable.

Conflicts of Interest: The authors declare no conflict of interest.

References

1. Taking Rehabilitation Seriously. In *Bulletin of the World Health Organization;* World Health Organization: Geneva, Switzerland, 2019; Volume 97, pp. 519–520. [CrossRef]
2. Stubbs, B.; Siddiqi, K.; Elsey, H.; Siddiqi, N.; Ma, R.; Romano, E.; Siddiqi, S.; Koyanagi, A. Tuberculosis and Non-Communicable Disease Multimorbidity: An Analysis of the World Health Survey in 48 Low- and Middle-Income Countries. *Int. J. Environ. Res. Public Health* **2021**, *18*, 2439. [CrossRef] [PubMed]
3. Visca, D.; Zampogna, E.; Sotgiu, G.; Centis, R.; Saderi, L.; D'Ambrosio, L.; Pegoraro, V.; Pignatti, P.; Muñoz-Torrico, M.; Migliori, G.B.; et al. Pulmonary rehabilitation is effective in patients with tuberculosis pulmonary sequelae. *Eur. Respir. J.* **2019**, *53*, 1802184. [CrossRef] [PubMed]
4. Akkerman, O.W.; Ter Beek, L.; Centis, R.; Maeurer, M.; Visca, D.; Muñoz-Torrico, M.; Tiberi, S.; Migliori, G.B. Rehabilitation, optimized nutritional care, and boosting host internal milieu to improve long-term treatment outcomes in tuberculosis patients. *Int. J. Infect. Dis.* **2020**, *92S*, S10–S14. [CrossRef] [PubMed]
5. Jesus, T.S.; Hoenig, H.; Landry, M.D. Development of the Rehabilitation Health Policy, Systems, and Services Research Field: Quantitative Analyses of Publications over Time (1990–2017) and across Country Type. *Int. J. Environ. Res. Public Health* **2020**, *17*, 965. [CrossRef]
6. Chin, A.T.; Rylance, J.; Makumbirofa, S.; Meffert, S.; Vu, T.; Clayton, J.; Mason, P.; Woodruff, P.; Metcalfe, J. Chronic lung disease in adult recurrent tuberculosis survivors in Zimbabwe: A cohort study. *Int. J. Tuberc. Lung Dis.* **2019**, *23*, 203–211. [CrossRef]
7. Health Policy and Systems Research Agenda for Rehabilitation. Available online: https://www.who.int/rehabilitation/Global-HSPR-Rehabilitation-Concept-Note.pdf?ua=1 (accessed on 11 October 2021).
8. Ter Beek, L.; Alffenaar, J.C.; Bolhuis, M.S.; van der Werf, T.S.; Akkerman, O.W. Tuberculosis-related malnutrition: Public health implications. *J. Infect. Dis.* **2019**, *220*, 340–341. [CrossRef]
9. De la Mora, I.L.; Martínez-Oceguera, D.; Laniado-Laborín, R. Chronic airway obstruction after successful treatment of tuberculosis and its impact on quality of life. *Int. J. Tuberc. Lung Dis.* **2015**, *19*, 808–810. [CrossRef]
10. World Health Organization. *Global Tuberculosis Report 2021;* World Health Organization: Geneva, Switzerland, 2021. Available online: https://www.who.int/publications/i/item/9789240037021 (accessed on 25 November 2021).
11. Choi, R.; Jeong, B.H.; Koh, W.J.; Lee, S.Y. Recommendations for optimizing tuberculosis treatment: Therapeutic drug monitoring, pharmacogenetics, and nutritional status considerations. *Ann. Lab. Med.* **2017**, *37*, 97–107. [CrossRef]
12. Liu, X.; Blaschke, T.; Thomas, B.; De Geest, S.; Jiang, S.; Gao, Y.; Li, X.; Buono, E.W.; Buchanan, S.; Zhang, Z.; et al. Usability of a Medication Event Reminder Monitor System (MERM) by Providers and Patients to Improve Adherence in the Management of Tuberculosis. *Int. J. Environ. Res. Public Health* **2017**, *14*, 1115. [CrossRef]
13. Chetty, S.; Ramesh, M.; Singh-Pillay, A.; Soliman, M.E.S. Recent advancements in the development of anti-tuberculosis drugs. *Bioorg. Med. Chem. Lett.* **2017**, *27*, 370–386. [CrossRef]
14. Mazlan, M.K.N.; Mohd Tazizi, M.H.D.; Ahmad, R.; Noh, M.A.A.; Bakhtiar, A.; Wahab, H.A.; Mohd Gazzali, A. Antituberculosis Targeted Drug Delivery as a Potential Future Treatment Approach. *Antibiotics* **2021**, *10*, 908. [CrossRef]
15. Adane, A.A.; Alene, K.A.; Koye, D.N.; Zeleke, B.M. Non-adherence to anti-tuberculosis treatment and determinant factors among patients with tuberculosis in northwest Ethiopia. *PLoS ONE* **2013**, *8*, e78791. [CrossRef]
16. McLaren, Z.M.; Milliken, A.A.; Meyer, A.J.; Sharp, A.R. Does directly observed therapy improve tuberculosis treatment? More evidence is needed to guide tuberculosis policy. *BMC Infect. Dis.* **2016**, *16*, 537. [CrossRef]
17. Yellappa, V.; Lefèvre, P.; Battaglioli, T.; Narayanan, D.; Van der Stuyft, P. Coping with tuberculosis and directly observed treatment: A qualitative study among patients from South India. *BMC Health Serv. Res.* **2016**, *16*, 283. [CrossRef]
18. Falzon, D.; Jaramillo, E.; Schünemann, H.J.; Arentz, M.; Bauer, M.; Bayona, J.; Blanc, L.; Caminero, J.A.; Daley, C.L.; Duncombe, C.; et al. WHO Guidelines for the Programmatic Management of Drug-Resistant Tuberculosis: 2011 Update. *Eur. Respir. J.* **2011**, *38*, 516–528. [CrossRef]
19. Mori, M.; Stelitano, G.; Gelain, A.; Pini, E.; Chiarelli, L.R.; Sammartino, J.C.; Poli, G.; Tuccinardi, T.; Beretta, G.; Porta, A.; et al. Shedding X-ray Light on the Role of Magnesium in the Activity of *Mycobacterium tuberculosis* Salicylate Synthase (MbtI) for Drug Design. *J. Med. Chem.* **2020**, *63*, 7066–7080. [CrossRef]
20. Pini, E.; Poli, G.; Tuccinardi, T.; Chiarelli, L.; Mori, M.; Gelain, A.; Costantino, L.; Villa, S.; Meneghetti, F.; Barlocco, D. New Chromane-Based Derivatives as Inhibitors of *Mycobacterium tuberculosis* Salicylate Synthase (MbtI): Preliminary Biological Evaluation and Molecular Modeling Studies. *Molecules* **2018**, *23*, 1506. [CrossRef]

21. Mori, M.; Sammartino, J.C.; Costantino, L.; Gelain, A.; Meneghetti, F.; Villa, S.; Chiarelli, L.R. An Overview on the Potential Antimycobacterial Agents Targeting Serine/Threonine Protein Kinases from *Mycobacterium tuberculosis*. *Curr. Top. Med. Chem.* **2019**, *19*, 646–661. [CrossRef]
22. Meneghetti, F.; Villa, S.; Gelain, A.; Barlocco, D.; Chiarelli, L.R.; Pasca, M.R.; Costantino, L. Iron Acquisition Pathways as Targets for Antitubercular Drugs. *Curr. Med. Chem.* **2016**, *23*, 4009–4026. [CrossRef]
23. Harries, A.D.; Chakaya, J.M. Assessing and managing pulmonary impairment in those who have completed TB treatment in programmatic settings. *Int. J. Tuberc. Lung Dis.* **2019**, *23*, 1044–1045. [CrossRef]
24. Chushkin, M.I.; Ots, O.N. Impaired pulmonary function after treatment for tuberculosis: The end of the disease? *J. Bras. Pneumol.* **2017**, *43*, 38–43. [CrossRef]
25. Cai, H.; Chen, L.; Yin, C.; Liao, Y.; Meng, X.; Lu, C.; Tang, S.; Li, X.; Wang, X. The effect of micro-nutrients on malnutrition, immunity and therapeutic effect in patients with pulmonary tuberculosis: A systematic review and meta-analysis of randomised controlled trials. *Tuberculosis* **2020**, *125*, 101994. [CrossRef]
26. Nihues, S.D.S.E.; Mancuzo, E.V.; Sulmonetti, N.; Sacchi, F.P.C.; Viana, V.D.S.; Netto, E.M.; Miranda, S.S.; Croda, J. Chronic symptoms and pulmonary dysfunction in post-tuberculosis Brazilian patients. *Braz. J. Infect. Dis.* **2015**, *19*, 492–497. [CrossRef]
27. Jones, R.; Kirenga, B.J.; Katagira, W.; Singh, S.J.; Pooler, J.; Okwera, A.; Kasiita, R.; Enki, D.G.; Creanor, S.; Barton, A. A pre-post intervention study of pulmonary rehabilitation for adults with post-tuberculosis lung disease in Uganda. *Int. J. Chronic Obst. Pulm. Dis.* **2017**, *12*, 3533–3539. [CrossRef]
28. Lin, Y.; Liu, Y.; Zhang, G.; Cai, Q.; Hu, W.; Xiao, L.; Thekkur, P.; Golub, J.E.; Harries, A.D. Is It Feasible to Conduct Post-Tuberculosis Assessments at the End of Tuberculosis Treatment under Routine Programmatic Conditions in China? *Trop. Med. Infect. Dis.* **2021**, *6*, 164. [CrossRef]
29. Amaral, A.F.S.; Coton, S.; Kato, B.; Tan, W.C.; Studnicka, M.; Janson, C.; Gislason, T.; Mannino, D.; Bateman, E.D.; Buist, S.; et al. Tuberculosis associates with both airflow obstruction and low lung function: BOLD results. *Eur. Respir. J.* **2015**, *46*, 1104–1112. [CrossRef]
30. Visca, D.; Tiberi, S.; Centis, R.; D'Ambrosio, L.; Pontali, E.; Mariani, A.W.; Zampogna, E.; van den Boom, M.; Spanevello, A.; Migliori, G.B. Post-Tuberculosis (TB) Treatment: The Role of Surgery and Rehabilitation. *Appl. Sci.* **2020**, *10*, 2734. [CrossRef]
31. Hoger, S.; Lykens, K.; Beavers, S.F.; Katz, D.; Miller, T.L. Longevity loss among cured tuberculosis patients and the potential value of prevention. *Int. J. Tuberc. Lung Dis.* **2014**, *18*, 1347–1352. [CrossRef] [PubMed]
32. Bettencourt, P.J.G. The 100th anniversary of bacille Calmette-Guérin (BCG) and the latest vaccines against COVID-19. *Int. J. Tuberc. Lung Dis.* **2021**, *25*, 611–613. [CrossRef] [PubMed]
33. Medley, J.; Goff, A.; Bettencourt, P.J.G.; Dare, M.; Cole, L.; Cantillon, D.; Waddell, S.J. Dissecting the *Mycobacterium bovis* BCG Response to Macrophage Infection to Help Prioritize Targets for Anti-Tuberculosis Drug and Vaccine Discovery. *Vaccines* **2022**, *10*, 113. [CrossRef] [PubMed]
34. Allwood, B.W.; Byrne, A.; Meghji, J.; Rachow, A.; van der Zalm, M.M.; Schoch, O.D. Post-tuberculosis lung disease: Clinical review of an under-recognised global challenge. *Respiration* **2021**, *100*, 751–763. [CrossRef]
35. Sebio-García, R. Pulmonary Rehabilitation: Time for an Upgrade. *J. Clin. Med.* **2020**, *9*, 2742. [CrossRef]
36. Bansal, V.; Prasad, R. Pulmonary rehabilitation in chronic respiratory diseases. *Indian J. Chest Dis. Allied Sci.* **2014**, *56*, 147–148.
37. Spruit, M.A.; Singh, S.J.; Garvey, C.; Zu Wallack, R.; Nici, L.; Rochester, C.; Hill, K.; Holland, A.E.; Lareau, S.C.; Man, W.D.-C.; et al. An official American Thoracic Society/European Respiratory Society statement: Key concepts and advances in pulmonary rehabilitation. *Am. J. Respir. Crit. Care Med.* **2013**, *188*, e13–e64. [CrossRef]
38. Ravimohan, S.; Kornfeld, H.; Weissman, D.; Bisson, G.P. Tuberculosis and lung damage: From epidemiology to pathophysiology. *Eur. Respir. Rev.* **2018**, *27*, 170077. [CrossRef]
39. Stek, C.; Allwood, B.; Walker, N.F.; Wilkinson, R.J.; Lynen, L.; Meintjes, G. The immune mechanisms of lung parenchymal damage in tuberculosis and the role of host-directed therapy. *Front. Microbiol.* **2018**, *9*, 2603. [CrossRef]
40. Nahid, P.; Mase, S.R.; Migliori, G.B.; Sotgiu, G.; Bothamley, G.H.; Brozek, J.L.; Cattamanchi, A.; Cegielski, J.P.; Chen, L.; Daley, C.L.; et al. Treatment of drug-resistant tuberculosis. An official ATS/CDC/ERS/IDSA clinical practice guideline. *Am. J. Respir. Crit. Care Med.* **2019**, *200*, e93–e142. [CrossRef]
41. Chakaya, J.; Kirenga, B.; Getahun, H. Long term complications after completion of pulmonary tuberculosis treatment: A quest for a public health approach. *J. Clin. Tuberc. Other Mycobact. Dis.* **2016**, *3*, 10–12. [CrossRef]
42. Meghji, J.; Lesosky, M.; Joekes, E.; Banda, P.; Rylance, J.; Gordon, S.; Jacob, J.; Zonderland, H.; MacPherson, P.; Corbett, E.L.; et al. Patient outcomes associated with post-tuberculosis lung damage in Malawi: A prospective cohort study. *Thorax* **2020**, *75*, 269–278. [CrossRef]
43. Basham, C.A.; Karim, M.E.; Cook, V.J.; Patrick, D.M.; Johnston, J.C. Post-tuberculosis airway disease: A population-based cohort study of people immigrating to British Columbia, Canada, 1985–2015. *E Clinical Medicine* **2021**, *33*, 100752. [CrossRef]
44. De Martino, M.; Lodi, L.; Galli, L.; Chiappini, E. Immune response to *Mycobacterium tuberculosis*: A narrative review. *Front. Pediatr.* **2019**, *7*, 350. [CrossRef] [PubMed]
45. Matsuo, S.; Okamoto, M.; Ikeuchi, T.; Zaizen, Y.; Inomoto, A.; Haraguchi, R.; Mori, S.; Sasaki, R.; Nouno, T.; Tanaka, T.; et al. Early Intervention of Pulmonary Rehabilitation for Fibrotic Interstitial Lung Disease Is a Favorable Factor for Short-Term Improvement in Health-Related Quality of Life. *J. Clin. Med.* **2021**, *10*, 3153. [CrossRef] [PubMed]

46. Allwood, B.W.; Stolbrink, M.; Baines, N.; Louw, E.; Wademan, D.T.; Lupton-Smith, A.; Nel, S.; Maree, D.; Mpagama, S.; Osman, M.; et al. Persistent chronic respiratory symptoms despite TB cure is poorly correlated with lung function. *Int. J. Tuberc. Lung Dis.* **2021**, *25*, 262–270. [CrossRef] [PubMed]
47. Muefong, C.N.; Sutherland, J.S. Neutrophils in Tuberculosis-Associated Inflammation and Lung Pathology. *Front. Immunol.* **2020**, *11*, 962. [CrossRef]
48. Hunter, R.L.; Actor, J.K.; Hwang, S.-A.; Khan, A.; Urbanowski, M.E.; Kaushal, D.; Jagannath, C. Pathogenesis and Animal Models of Post-Primary (Bronchogenic) Tuberculosis, A Review. *Pathogens* **2018**, *7*, 19. [CrossRef]
49. Gupta, N.; Kumar, R.; Agrawal, B. New Players in Immunity to Tuberculosis: The Host Microbiome, Lung Epithelium, and Innate Immune Cells. *Front. Immunol.* **2018**, *9*, 709. [CrossRef]
50. O'Dwyer, D.N.; Dickson, R.P.; Moore, B.B. The lung microbiome, immunity, and the pathogenesis of chronic lung disease. *J. Immunol.* **2016**, *196*, 4839–4847. [CrossRef]
51. Amaral, E.P.; Vinhaes, C.L.; Oliveira-De-Souza, D.; Nogueira, B.; Akrami, K.M.; Andrade, B.B. The Interplay between Systemic Inflammation, Oxidative Stress, and Tissue Remodeling in Tuberculosis. *Antioxid. Redox Signal.* **2021**, *34*, 471–485. [CrossRef]
52. Pagán, A.J.; Ramakrishnan, L. Immunity and Immunopathology in the Tuberculous Granuloma. *Cold Spring Harb. Perspect. Med.* **2015**, *5*, a018499. [CrossRef]
53. Mortaz, E.; Adcock, I.M.; Tabarsi, P.; Masjedi, M.R.; Mansouri, D.; Velayati, A.A.; Casanova, J.-L.; Barnes, P.J. Interaction of pattern recognition receptors with *Mycobacterium tuberculosis*. *J. Clin. Immunol.* **2015**, *35*, 1–10. [CrossRef]
54. Stanke, F. The contribution of the airway epithelial cell to host defense. *Mediat. Inflamm.* **2015**, *2015*, 463016. [CrossRef]
55. Balcells, M.E.; Yokobori, N.; Hong, B.-Y.; Corbett, J.; Cervantes, J.L. The lung microbiome, vitamin D, and the tuberculous granuloma: A balance triangle. *Microb. Pathog.* **2019**, *131*, 158–163. [CrossRef]
56. Cella, M.; Miller, H.; Song, C. Beyond NK cells: The expanding universe of innate lymphoid cells. *Front. Immunol.* **2014**, *5*, 282. [CrossRef]
57. Meca, A.-D.; Turcu-Stiolica, A.; Stanciulescu, E.C.; Andrei, A.M.; Nitu, F.M.; Banita, I.M.; Matei, M.; Pisoschi, C.-G. Variations of Serum Oxidative Stress Biomarkers under First-Line Antituberculosis Treatment: A Pilot Study. *J. Pers. Med.* **2021**, *11*, 112. [CrossRef]
58. Moraco, A.H.; Kornfeld, H. Cell death and autophagy in tuberculosis. *Semin. Immunol.* **2014**, *26*, 497–511. [CrossRef]
59. Deretic, V. Autophagy in innate and adaptive immunity. *Trends Immunol.* **2005**, *26*, 523–528. [CrossRef]
60. Moideen, K.; Kumar, N.P.; Nair, D.; Banurekha, V.V.; Bethunaickan, R.; Babu, S. Heightened systemic levels of neutrophil and eosinophil granular proteins in pulmonary tuberculosis and reversal following treatment. *Infect. Immun.* **2018**, *86*, e00008-18. [CrossRef]
61. Vernon, P.J.; Schaub, L.J.; Dallelucca, J.J.; Pusateri, A.E.; Sheppard, F.R. Rapid detection of neutrophil oxidative burst capacity is predictive of whole blood cytokine responses. *PLoS ONE* **2015**, *10*, e0146105. [CrossRef]
62. Allen, M.; Bailey, C.; Cahatol, I.; Dodge, L.; Yim, J.; Kassissa, C.; Luong, J.; Kasko, S.; Pandya, S.; Venketaraman, V. Mechanisms of control of *Mycobacterium tuberculosis* by NK cells: Role of glutathione. *Front. Immunol.* **2015**, *6*, 508. [CrossRef]
63. Yang, C.T.; Cambier, C.J.; Davis, J.M.; Hall, C.J.; Crosier, P.S.; Ramakrishnan, L. Neutrophils exert protection in the early tuberculous granuloma by oxidative killing of mycobacteria phagocytosed from infected macrophages. *Cell Host Microbe* **2012**, *12*, 301–312. [CrossRef]
64. Robb, C.T.; Regan, K.H.; Dorward, D.A.; Rossi, A.G. Key mechanisms governing resolution of lung inflammation. *Semin. Immunopathol.* **2016**, *38*, 425–448. [CrossRef]
65. Mohareer, K.; Asalla, S.; Banerjee, S. Cell death at the cross roads of host-pathogen interaction in *Mycobacterium tuberculosis* infection. *Tuberculosis* **2018**, *113*, 99–121. [CrossRef]
66. Parandhaman, D.K.; Narayanan, S. Cell death paradigms in the pathogenesis of *Mycobacterium tuberculosis* infection. *Front. Cell. Infect. Microbiol.* **2014**, *4*, 31. [CrossRef]
67. Srinivasan, L.; Ahlbrand, S.; Briken, V. Interaction of *Mycobacterium tuberculosis* with host cell death pathways. *Cold Spring Harb. Perspect. Med.* **2014**, *4*, a022459. [CrossRef] [PubMed]
68. Sia, J.K.; Georgieva, M.; Rengarajan, J. Innate immune defenses in human tuberculosis: An overview of the interactions between *Mycobacterium tuberculosis* and innate immune cells. *J. Immunol. Res.* **2015**, *2015*, 747543. [CrossRef] [PubMed]
69. Dey, B.; Bishai, W.R. Crosstalk between *Mycobacterium tuberculosis* and the host cell. *Semin. Immunol.* **2014**, *26*, 486–496. [CrossRef]
70. Horsburgh, C.R., Jr.; Barry, C.E., 3rd; Lange, C. Treatment of Tuberculosis. *N. Engl. J. Med.* **2015**, *373*, 2149–2160. [CrossRef] [PubMed]
71. Liu, Y.; Matsumoto, M.; Ishida, H.; Ohguro, K.; Yoshitake, M.; Gupta, R.; Geiter, L.; Hafkin, J. Delamanid: From discovery to its use for pulmonary multidrug-resistant tuberculosis (MDR-TB). *Tuberculosis* **2018**, *111*, 20–30. [CrossRef]
72. Hughes, D.; Brandis, G. Rifampicin Resistance: Fitness Costs and the Significance of Compensatory Evolution. *Antibiotics* **2013**, *2*, 206–216. [CrossRef]
73. Hunter, R. The Pathogenesis of Tuberculosis–The Koch Phenomenon Reinstated. *Pathogens* **2020**, *9*, 813. [CrossRef]
74. Withers, D.R. Innate lymphoid cell regulation of adaptive immunity. *Immunology* **2016**, *149*, 123–130. [CrossRef] [PubMed]
75. Cantini, F.; Niccoli, L.; Capone, A.; Petrone, L.; Goletti, D. Risk of tuberculosis reactivation associated with traditional disease modifying anti-rheumatic drugs and non-anti-tumor necrosis factor biologics in patients with rheumatic disorders and suggestion for clinical practice. *Expert Opin. Drug Saf.* **2019**, *18*, 415–425. [CrossRef]

76. Sartori, N.S.; de Andrade, N.P.B.; da Silva Chakr, R.M. Incidence of tuberculosis in patients receiving anti-TNF therapy for rheumatic diseases: A systematic review. *Clin. Rheumatol.* **2020**, *39*, 1439–1447. [CrossRef]
77. Hong, B.-Y.; Maulén, N.P.; Adami, A.J.; Granados, H.; Balcells, M.E.; Cervantes, J. Microbiome changes during tuberculosis and antituberculous therapy. *Clin. Microbiol. Rev.* **2016**, *29*, 915–926. [CrossRef]
78. Ngahane, B.H.M.; Nouyep, J.; Motto, M.N.; Njankouo, Y.M.; Wandji, A.; Endale, M.; Ze, E.A. Post-tuberculous lung function impairment in a tuberculosis reference clinic in Cameroon. *Respir. Med.* **2016**, *114*, 67–71. [CrossRef]
79. Guiedem, E.; Ikomey, G.M.; Nkenfou, C.; Walter, P.-Y.E.; Mesembe, M.; Chegou, N.N.; Jacobs, G.B.; Assoumou, M.C.O. Chronic obstructive pulmonary disease (COPD): Neutrophils, macrophages and lymphocytes in patients with anterior tuberculosis compared to tobacco related COPD. *BMC Res. Notes* **2018**, *11*, 192. [CrossRef] [PubMed]
80. Bespyatykh, J.; Shitikov, E.; Bespiatykh, D.; Guliaev, A.; Klimina, K.; Veselovsky, V.; Arapidi, G.; Dogonadze, M.; Zhuravlev, V.; Ilina, E.; et al. Metabolic Changes of *Mycobacterium tuberculosis* during the Anti-Tuberculosis Therapy. *Pathogens* **2020**, *9*, 131. [CrossRef]
81. Gough, M.E.; Graviss, E.A.; Chen, T.-A.; Obasi, E.M.; May, E.E. Compounding effect of vitamin D3 diet, supplementation, and alcohol exposure on macrophage response to mycobacterium infection. *Tuberculosis* **2019**, *116*, S42–S58. [CrossRef]
82. Pasipanodya, J.G.; McNabb, S.J.; Hilsenrath, P.; Bae, S.; Lykens, K.; Vecino, E.; Munguia, G.; Miller, T.L.; Drewyer, G.; E Weis, S. Pulmonary impairment after tuberculosis and its contribution to TB burden. *BMC Public Health* **2010**, *10*, 259. [CrossRef] [PubMed]
83. Ibironke, O.; Carranza, C.; Sarkar, S.; Torres, M.; Choi, H.T.; Nwoko, J.; Black, K.; Quintana-Belmares, R.; Osornio-Vargas, Á.; Ohman-Strickland, P.; et al. Urban Air Pollution Particulates Suppress Human T-Cell Responses to *Mycobacterium tuberculosis*. *Int. J. Environ. Res. Public Health* **2019**, *16*, 4112. [CrossRef] [PubMed]
84. Rivas-Santiago, C.E.; Sarkar, S.; Cantarella, P.; Osornio-Vargas, Á.; Quintana-Belmares, R.; Meng, Q.; Kirn, T.J.; Strickland, P.O.; Chow, J.C.; Watson, J.G.; et al. Air pollution particulate matter alters antimycobacterial respiratory epithelium innate immunity. *Infect. Immun.* **2015**, *83*, 2507–2517. [CrossRef]
85. Rachow, A.; Ivanova, O.; Wallis, R.; Charalambous, S.; Jani, I.; Bhatt, N.; Kampmann, B.; Sutherland, J.; Ntinginya, N.E.; Evans, D.; et al. TB sequel: Incidence, pathogenesis and risk factors of long-term medical and social sequelae of pulmonary TB—A study protocol. *BMC Pulm. Med.* **2019**, *19*, 4. [CrossRef]
86. Bickton, F.M.; Fombe, C.; Chisati, E.; Rylance, J. Evidence for pulmonary rehabilitation in chronic respiratory diseases in sub-Saharan Africa: A systematic review. *Int. J. Tuberc. Lung Dis.* **2020**, *24*, 991–999. [CrossRef]
87. Bongomin, F. Post-tuberculosis chronic pulmonary aspergillosis: An emerging public health concern. *PLoS Pathog.* **2020**, *16*, e1008742. [CrossRef]
88. Vashakidze, S.A.; Kempker, J.A.; Jakobia, N.A.; Gogishvili, S.G.; Nikolaishvili, K.A.; Goginashvili, L.M.; Magee, M.J.; Kempker, R.R. Pulmonary function and respiratory health after successful treatment of drug-resistant tuberculosis. *Int. J. Infect. Dis.* **2019**, *82*, 66–72. [CrossRef]
89. Van Kampen, S.C.; Wanner, A.; Edwards, M.; Harries, A.D.; Kirenga, B.J.; Chakaya, J.; Jones, R. International research and guidelines on post-tuberculosis chronic lung disorders: A systematic scoping review. *BMJ Glob. Health* **2018**, *3*, e000745. [CrossRef]
90. Bandodkar, B.; Shandil, R.K.; Bhat, J.; Balganesh, T.S. Two Decades of TB Drug Discovery Efforts—What Have We Learned? *Appl. Sci.* **2020**, *10*, 5704. [CrossRef]
91. Pontali, E.; Visca, D.; Centis, R.; D'Ambrosio, L.; Spanevello, A.; Migliori, G.B. Multi and extensively drug-resistant pulmonary tuberculosis: Advances in diagnosis and management. *Curr. Opin. Pulm. Med.* **2018**, *24*, 1070–5287. [CrossRef]
92. Schito, M.; Migliori, G.B.; Fletcher, H.A.; McNerney, R.; Centis, R.; D'Ambrosio, L.; Bates, M.; Kibiki, G.; Kapata, N.; Corrah, T.; et al. Perspectives on Advances in Tuberculosis Diagnostics, Drugs, and Vaccines. *Clin. Infect. Dis.* **2015**, *61*, S102–S118. [CrossRef]
93. Joseph, M.R.; Thomas, R.A.; Nair, S.; Balakrishnan, S.; Jayasankar, S. Directly observed treatment short course for tuberculosis. What happens to them in the long term? *Indian J. Tuberc.* **2015**, *62*, 29–35. [CrossRef]
94. Alipanah, N.; Jarlsberg, L.; Miller, C.; Linh, N.N.; Falzon, D.; Jaramillo, E.; Nahid, P. Adherence interventions and outcomes of tuberculosis treatment: A systematic review and meta-analysis of trials and observational studies. *PLoS Med.* **2018**, *15*, e1002595. [CrossRef] [PubMed]
95. Heuvelings, C.C.; de Vries, S.G.; Grobusch, M.P. Tackling TB in low-incidence countries: Improving diagnosis and management in vulnerable populations. *Int. J. Infect. Dis.* **2017**, *56*, 77–80. [CrossRef] [PubMed]
96. Bhat, Z.S.; Rather, M.A.; Maqbool, M.; Ahmad, Z. Drug targets exploited in *Mycobacterium tuberculosis*: Pitfalls and promises on the horizon. *Biomed. Pharmacother.* **2018**, *103*, 1733–1747. [CrossRef] [PubMed]
97. Imam, F.; Sharma, M.; Khayyam, K.U.; Al-Harbi, N.O.; Rashid, M.K.; Ali, M.D.; Ahmad, A.; Qamar, W. Adverse drug reaction prevalence and mechanisms of action of first-line anti-tubercular drugs. *Saudi Pharm. J.* **2020**, *28*, 316–324. [CrossRef]
98. El Hamdouni, M.; Ahid, S.; Bourkadi, J.E.; Benamor, J.; Hassar, M.; Cherrah, Y. Incidence of adverse reactions caused by first-line anti-tuberculosis drugs and treatment outcome of pulmonary tuberculosis patients in Morocco. *Infection* **2020**, *48*, 43–50. [CrossRef]
99. Dalcolmo, M.; Gayoso, R.; Sotgiu, G.; D'Ambrosio, L.; Rocha, J.L.; Borga, L.; Fandinho, F.; Braga, J.U.; Sanchez, D.A.; Dockhorn, F.; et al. Resistance profile of drugs composing the 'shorter' regimen for multidrug-resistant tuberculosis in Brazil, 2000–2015. *Eur. Respir. J.* **2017**, *49*, 1602309. [CrossRef]

100. Mori, M.; Stelitano, G.; Chiarelli, L.R.; Cazzaniga, G.; Gelain, A.; Barlocco, D.; Pini, E.; Meneghetti, F.; Villa, S. Synthesis, Characterization, and Biological Evaluation of New Derivatives Targeting MbtI as Antitubercular Agents. *Pharmaceuticals* **2021**, *14*, 155. [CrossRef]
101. Aung, K.J.M.; Van Deun, A.; Declercq, E.; Sarker, M.R.; Das, P.K.; Hossain, M.A.; Rieder, H.L. Successful '9-month Bangladesh regimen' for multidrug-resistant tuberculosis among over 500 consecutive patients. *Int. J. Tuberc. Lung Dis.* **2014**, *18*, 1180–1187. [CrossRef]
102. Hoagland, D.; Liu, J.; Lee, R.B.; Lee, R.E. New agents for the treatment of drug-resistant *Mycobacterium tuberculosis*. *Adv. Drug Deliv. Rev.* **2016**, *102*, 55–72. [CrossRef]
103. Worley, M.V.; Estrada, S.J. Bedaquiline: A novel antitubercular agent for the treatment of multidrug-resistant tuberculosis. *Pharmacother. J. Hum. Pharmacol. Drug Ther.* **2014**, *34*, 1187–1197. [CrossRef]
104. Hewison, C.; Ferlazzo, G.; Avaliani, Z.; Hayrapetyan, A.; Jonckheere, S.; Khaidarkhanova, Z.; Mohr, E.; Sinha, A.; Skrahina, A.; Vambe, D.; et al. Six-month response to delamanid treatment in MDR TB patients. *Emerg. Infect. Dis.* **2017**, *23*, 1746–1748. [CrossRef]
105. Dawson, R.; Diacon, A.H.; Everitt, D.; van Niekerk, C.; Donald, P.R.; Burger, D.A.; Schall, R.; Spigelman, M.; Conradie, A.; Eisenach, K.; et al. Efficiency and safety of the combination of moxifloxacin, pretomanid (PA-824), and pyrazinamide during the first 8 weeks of antituberculosis treatment: A phase 2b, open-label, partly randomised trial in patients with drug-susceptible or drug-resistant pulmonary tuberculosis. *Lancet* **2015**, *385*, 1738–1747.
106. Diacon, A.H.; Dawson, R.; Von Groote-Bidlingmaier, F.; Symons, G.; Venter, A.; Donald, P.R.; Van Niekerk, C.; Everitt, D.; Hutchings, J.; Burger, D.A.; et al. Bactericidal activity of pyrazinamide and clofazimine alone and in combinations with pretomanid and bedaquiline. *Am. J. Respir. Crit. Care Med.* **2015**, *191*, 943–953. [CrossRef]
107. Gupta, R.; Wells, C.D.; Hittel, N.; Hafkin, J.; Geiter, L.J. Delamanid in the treatment of multidrug-resistant tuberculosis. *Int. J. Tuberc. Lung Dis.* **2016**, *20*, 33–37. [CrossRef]
108. AlMatar, M.; AlMandeal, H.; Var, I.; Kayar, B.; Köksal, F. New drugs for the treatment of *Mycobacterium tuberculosis* infection. *Biomed. Pharmacother.* **2017**, *91*, 546–558. [CrossRef]
109. Tiberi, S.; du Plessis, N.; Walzl, G.; Vjecha, M.J.; Rao, M.; Ntoumi, F.; Mfinanga, S.; Kapata, N.; Mwaba, P.; McHugh, T.D.; et al. Tuberculosis: Progress and advances in development of new drugs, treatment regimens, and host-directed therapies. *Lancet Infect. Dis.* **2018**, *18*, e183–e198. [CrossRef]
110. Maryandyshev, A.; Pontali, E.; Tiberi, S.; Akkerman, O.; Ganatra, S.; Sadutshang, T.D.; Alffenaar, J.-W.; Amale, R.; Mullerpattan, J.; Topgyal, S.; et al. Bedaquiline and Delamanid Combination Treatment of 5 Patients with Pulmonary Extensively Drug-Resistant Tuberculosis. *Emerg. Infect. Dis.* **2017**, *23*, 1718–1721. [CrossRef]
111. Yu, X.; Huo, F.; Wang, F.; Wen, S.; Jiang, G.; Xue, Y.; Dong, L.; Zhao, L.; Zhu, R.; Huang, H. In vitro Antimicrobial Activity Comparison of Linezolid, Tedizolid, Sutezolid and Delpazolid against Slowly Growing Mycobacteria Isolated in Beijing, China. *Infect. Drug Resist.* **2021**, *14*, 4689–4697. [CrossRef]
112. Ying, R.; Huang, X.; Gao, Y.; Wang, J.; Liu, Y.; Sha, W.; Yang, H. In vitro Synergism of Six Antituberculosis Agents against Drug-Resistant *Mycobacterium tuberculosis* Isolated from Retreatment Tuberculosis Patients. *Infect. Drug Resist.* **2021**, *14*, 3729–3736. [CrossRef]
113. Choi, Y.; Lee, S.W.; Kim, A.; Jang, K.; Nam, H.; Cho, Y.L.; Yu, K.-S.; Jang, I.-J.; Chung, J.-Y. Safety, tolerability and pharmacokinetics of 21day multiple oral administration of a new oxazolidinone antibiotic, LCB01-0371, in healthy male subjects. *J. Antimicrob. Chemother.* **2018**, *73*, 183–190. [CrossRef]
114. De Jager, V.R.; Dawson, R.; Van Niekerk, C.; Hutchings, J.; Kim, J.; Vanker, N.; Van Der Merwe, L.; Choi, J.; Nam, K.; Diacon, A.H. Telacebec (Q203), a New Antituberculosis Agent. *N. Engl. J. Med.* **2020**, *382*, 1280–1281. [CrossRef]
115. Stephanie, F.; Saragih, M.; Tambunan, U.S.F. Recent Progress and Challenges for Drug-Resistant Tuberculosis Treatment. *Pharmaceutics* **2021**, *13*, 592. [CrossRef]
116. Degiacomi, G.; Benjak, A.; Madacki, J.; Boldrin, F.; Provvedi, R.; Palù, G.; Kordulákova, J.; Cole, S.T.; Manganelli, R. Essentiality of *mmpL3* and impact of its silencing on *Mycobacterium tuberculosis* gene expression. *Sci. Rep.* **2017**, *7*, 43495. [CrossRef]
117. Landge, S.; Mullick, A.B.; Nagalapur, K.; Neres, J.; Subbulakshmi, V.; Murugan, K.; Ghosh, A.; Sadler, C.; Fellows, M.D.; Humnabadkar, V.; et al. Discovery of benzothiazoles as antimycobacterial agents: Synthesis, structure-activity relationships and binding studies with *Mycobacterium tuberculosis* decaprenylphosphoryl-β-d-ribose 20-oxidase. *Bioorg. Med. Chem.* **2015**, *23*, 7694–7710. [CrossRef]
118. Abrahams, K.A.; Besra, G.S. Mycobacterial cell wall biosynthesis: A multifaceted antibiotic target. *Parasitology* **2018**, *145*, 116–133. [CrossRef]
119. Lupien, A.; Vocat, A.; Foo, C.S.; Blattes, E.; Gillon, J.Y.; Makarov, V.; Cole, S.T. Optimized background regimen for treatment of active tuberculosis with the next-generation benzothiazinone Macozinone (PBTZ169). *Antimicrob. Agents Chemother.* **2018**, *62*, e00840-18. [CrossRef]
120. Degiacomi, G.; Belardinelli, J.M.; Pasca, M.R.; De Rossi, E.; Riccardi, G.; Chiarelli, L.R. Promiscuous Targets for Antitubercular Drug Discovery: The Paradigm of DprE1 and MmpL3. *Appl. Sci.* **2020**, *10*, 623. [CrossRef]
121. Stelitano, G.; Sammartino, J.C.; Chiarelli, L.R. Multitargeting Compounds: A Promising Strategy to Overcome Multi-Drug Resistant Tuberculosis. *Molecules* **2020**, *25*, 1239. [CrossRef] [PubMed]

122. Borisov, S.; Bogorodskaya, E.M.; Volchenkov, G.V.; Kulchavenya, E.V.; Maryandyshev, A.O.; Skornyakov, S.N.; Talibov, O.; Tikhonov, A.M.; Vasilyeva, I.A.; Dispensary, V.R.T.; et al. Efficiency and safety of chemotherapy regimen with SQ109 in those suffering from multiple drug resistant tuberculosis. *Tuberc. Lung Dis.* **2018**, *96*, 6–18. [CrossRef]
123. Campaniço, A.; Moreira, R.; Lopes, F. Drug discovery in tuberculosis. New drug targets and antimycobacterial agents. *Eur. J. Med. Chem.* **2018**, *150*, 525–545. [CrossRef] [PubMed]
124. Pontali, E.; Sotgiu, G.; D'Ambrosio, L.; Centis, R.; Migliori, G.B. Bedaquiline and multidrug-resistant tuberculosis: A systematic and critical analysis of the evidence. *Eur. Respir. J.* **2016**, *47*, 394–402. [CrossRef]
125. Pontali, E.; Sotgiu, G.; Tiberi, S.; D'Ambrosio, L.; Centis, R.; Migliori, G.B. Cardiac safety of bedaquiline: A systematic and critical analysis of the evidence. *Eur. Respir. J.* **2017**, *50*, 1701462. [CrossRef]
126. Wallis, R.S. Cardiac safety of extensively drug-resistant tuberculosis regimens including bedaquiline, delamanid and clofazimine. *Eur. Respir. J.* **2016**, *48*, 1526–1527. [CrossRef]
127. Van Heeswijk, R.P.; Dannemann, B.; Hoetelmans, R.M.W. Bedaquiline: A review of human pharmacokinetics and drug–drug interactions. *J. Antimicrob. Chemother.* **2014**, *69*, 2310–2318. [CrossRef]
128. Svensson, E.M.; Murray, S.; Karlsson, M.O.; Dooley, K.E. Rifampicin and rifapentine significantly reduce concentrations of bedaquiline, a new anti-TB drug. *J. Antimicrob. Chemother.* **2015**, *70*, 1106–1114. [CrossRef]
129. Sutherland, H.S.; Tong, A.S.; Choi, P.; Blaser, A.; Conole, D.; Franzblau, S.; Lotlikar, M.U.; Cooper, C.B.; Upton, A.M.; Denny, W.A.; et al. 3,5-Dialkoxypyridine analogues of bedaquiline are potent antituberculosis agents with minimal inhibition of the hERG channel. *Bioorg. Med. Chem.* **2019**, *27*, 1292–1307. [CrossRef]
130. Working Group on New TB Drugs—Stop TB Partnership. Clinical Pipeline. Available online: https://www.newtbdrugs.org/pipeline/clinical (accessed on 23 November 2021).
131. Buca, B.R.; Tartau Mititelu, L.; Rezus, C.; Filip, C.; Pinzariu, A.C.; Rezus, E.; Popa, G.E.; Panainte, A.; Lupusoru, C.E.; Bogdan, M.; et al. The Effects of Two Nitric Oide Donors in Acute Inflammation in Rats Experimental data. *Rev. Chim.* **2018**, *69*, 2899–2903. [CrossRef]
132. Diacon, A.H.; Dawson, R.; Hanekom, M.; Narunsky, K.; Maritz, S.J.; Venter, A.; Donald, P.R.; van Niekerk, C.; Whitney, K.; Rouse, D.J.; et al. Early Bactericidal Activity and Pharmacokinetics of PA-824 in Smear-Positive Tuberculosis Patients. *Antimicrob. Agents Chemother.* **2010**, *54*, 3402–3407. [CrossRef]
133. Ryan, N.J.; Lo, J.H. Delamanid: First global approval. *Drugs* **2014**, *74*, 1041–1045. [CrossRef]
134. Sunwoo, J.; Kim, Y.K.; Choi, Y.; Yu, K.-S.; Nam, H.; Cho, Y.L.; Yoon, S.; Chung, J.-Y. Effect of food on the pharmacokinetic characteristics of a single oral dose of LCB01-0371, a novel oxazolidinone antibiotic. *Drug Des. Dev. Ther.* **2018**, *12*, 1707–1714. [CrossRef]
135. Gualano, G.; Capone, S.; Matteelli, A.; Palmieri, F. New antituberculosis drugs: From clinical trial to programmatic use. *Infect. Dis. Rep.* **2016**, *8*, 6569. [CrossRef] [PubMed]
136. Lee, M.; Song, T.; Kim, Y.; Jeong, I.; Cho, S.N.; E Barry, C. Linezolid for XDR-TB—Final study outcomes. *N. Engl. J. Med.* **2015**, *373*, 290–291. [CrossRef] [PubMed]
137. FDA Approves New Drug for Treatment-Resistant Forms of Tuberculosis That Affects the Lungs. Available online: https://www.fda.gov/news-events/press-announcements/fda-approves-new-drug-treatment-resistant-forms-tuberculosis-affects-lungs (accessed on 20 November 2021).
138. Zong, Z.; Jing, W.; Shi, J.; Wen, S.; Zhang, T.; Huo, F.; Shang, Y.; Liang, Q.; Huang, H.; Pang, Y. Comparison of in vitro activity and MIC distributions between the novel oxazolidinone delpazolid and linezolid against multidrug-resistant and extensively drug-resistant *Mycobacterium tuberculosis* in China. *Antimicrob. Agents Chemother.* **2018**, *62*, e00165-18. [CrossRef] [PubMed]
139. Pethe, K.; Bifani, P.; Jang, J.; Kang, S.; Park, S.; Ahn, S.; Jiricek, J.; Jung, J.; Jeon, H.K.; Cechetto, J.; et al. Discovery of Q203, a potent clinical candidate for the treatment of tuberculosis. *Nat. Med.* **2013**, *19*, 1157–1160. [CrossRef]
140. Batt, S.M.; Cacho Izquierdo, M.; Castro Pichel, J.; Stubbs, C.J.; Del Peral, L.V.-G.; Pérez-Herrán, E.; Dhar, N.; Mouzon, B.; Rees, M.; Hutchinson, J.P.; et al. Whole cell target engagement identifies novel inhibitors of *Mycobacterium tuberculosis* decaprenylphosphoryl-β-d-ribose oxidase. *ACS Infect. Dis.* **2015**, *1*, 615–626. [CrossRef]
141. Robertson, G.T.; Ramey, M.E.; Massoudi, L.M.; Carter, C.L.; Zimmerman, M.; Kaya, F.; Graham, B.G.; Gruppo, V.; Hastings, C.; Woolhiser, L.K.; et al. Comparative Analysis of Pharmacodynamics in the C3HeB/FeJ. Mouse Tuberculosis Model for DprE1 Inhibitors TBA-7371, PBTZ169, and OPC-167832. *Antimicrob. Agents Chemother.* **2021**, *65*, e0058321. [CrossRef]
142. Naik, M.; Humnabadkar, V.; Tantry, S.J.; Panda, M.; Narayan, A.; Guptha, S.; Panduga, V.; Manjrekar, P.; Jena, L.K.; Koushik, K.; et al. 4-Aminoquinolone piperidine amides: Noncovalent inhibitors of DprE1 with long residence time and potent antimycobacterial activity. *J. Med. Chem.* **2014**, *57*, 5419–5434. [CrossRef]
143. Panda, M.; Ramachandran, S.; Ramachandran, V.; Shirude, P.S.; Humnabadkar, V.; Nagalapur, K.; Sharma, S.; Kaur, P.; Guptha, S.; Narayan, A.; et al. Discovery of pyrazolopyridones as a novel class of noncovalent DprE1 inhibitor with potent anti-mycobacterial activity. *J. Med. Chem.* **2014**, *57*, 4761–4771. [CrossRef]
144. Chatterji, M.; Shandil, R.; Manjunatha, M.R.; Solapure, S.; Ramachandran, V.; Kumar, N.; Saralaya, R.; Panduga, V.; Reddy, J.; Kr, P.; et al. 1,4-azaindole, a potential drug candidate for treatment of tuberculosis. *Antimicrob. Agents Chemother.* **2014**, *58*, 5325–5331. [CrossRef]

145. Heinrich, N.; Dawson, R.; Du Bois, J.; Narunsky, K.; Horwith, G.; Phipps, A.J.; Nacy, C.A.; Aarnoutse, R.E.; Boeree, M.J.; Gillespie, S.; et al. Early phase evaluation of SQ109 alone and in combination with rifampicin in pulmonary TB patients. *J. Antimicrob. Chemother.* **2015**, *70*, 1558–1566. [CrossRef]
146. Tahlan, K.; Wilson, R.; Kastrinsky, D.B.; Arora, K.; Nair, V.; Fischer, E.; Barnes, S.W.; Walker, J.R.; Alland, D.; Barry, C.E.; et al. SQ109 targets *MmpL3*, a membrane transporter of trehalosemonomycolate involved in mycolic acid donation to the cell wall core of *Mycobacterium tuberculosis*. *Antimicrob. Agents Chemother.* **2012**, *56*, 1797–1809. [CrossRef]
147. Egbelowo, O.; Sarathy, J.P.; Gausi, K.; Zimmerman, M.D.; Wang, H.; Wijnant, G.-J.; Kaya, F.; Gengenbacher, M.; Van, N.; Degefu, Y.; et al. Pharmacokinetics and target attainment of SQ109 in plasma and human-like tuberculosis lesions in rabbits. *Antimicrob. Agents Chemother.* **2021**, *65*, e00024-21. [CrossRef]
148. Bahuguna, A.; Rawat, D.S. An overview of new antitubercular drugs, drug candidates, and their targets. *Med. Res. Rev.* **2020**, *40*, 263–292. [CrossRef]
149. Gupte, A.N.; Paradkar, M.; Selvaraju, S.; Thiruvengadam, K.; Shivakumar, S.V.B.Y.; Sekar, K.; Marinaik, S.; Momin, A.; Gaikwad, A.; Natrajan, P.; et al. Assessment of lung function in successfully treated tuberculosis reveals high burden of ventilatory defects and COPD. *PLoS ONE* **2019**, *14*, e0217289. [CrossRef]
150. Hsu, D.; Irfan, M.; Jabeen, K.; Iqbal, N.; Hasan, R.; Migliori, G.B.; Zumla, A.; Visca, D.; Centis, R.; Tiberi, S. Post tuberculosis treatment infectious complications. *Int. J. Infect. Dis.* **2020**, *92S*, S41–S45. [CrossRef]
151. Ko, J.M.; Kim, K.J.; Park, S.H.; Park, H.J. Bronchiectasis in active tuberculosis. *Acta Radiol.* **2013**, *54*, 412–417. [CrossRef]
152. Daniels, K.J.; Irusen, E.; Pharaoh, H.; Hanekom, S. Post-tuberculosis health-related quality of life, lung function and exercise capacity in a cured pulmonary tuberculosis population in the Breede Valley District, South Africa. *S. Afr. J. Physiother.* **2019**, *75*, 1319. [CrossRef]
153. Datta, S.; Gilman, R.H.; Montoya, R.; Cruz, L.Q.; Valencia, T.; Huff, D.; Saunders, M.J.; Evans, C.A. Quality of life, tuberculosis and treatment outcome; a case–control and nested cohort study. *Eur. Respir. J.* **2020**, *56*, 1900495. [CrossRef]
154. Yang, B.; Choi, H.; Shin, S.H.; Kim, Y.; Moon, J.-Y.; Park, H.Y.; Lee, H. Association of Ventilatory Disorders with Respiratory Symptoms, Physical Activity, and Quality of Life in Subjects with Prior Tuberculosis: A National Database Study in Korea. *J. Pers. Med.* **2021**, *11*, 678. [CrossRef]
155. Báez-Saldaña, R.; López-Arteaga, Y.; Bizarrón-Muro, A.; Ferreira-Guerrero, E.; Ferreyra-Reyes, L.; Delgado-Sánchez, G.; Cruz-Hervert, L.P.; Mongua-Rodríguez, N.; García-García, L. A novel scoring system to measure radiographic abnormalities and related spirometric values in cured pulmonary tuberculosis. *PLoS ONE* **2013**, *8*, e78926. [CrossRef]
156. Rozaliyani, A.; Rosianawati, H.; Handayani, D.; Agustin, H.; Zaini, J.; Syam, R.; Adawiyah, R.; Tugiran, M.; Setianingrum, F.; Burhan, E.; et al. Chronic Pulmonary Aspergillosis in Post Tuberculosis Patients in Indonesia and the Role of LDBio *Aspergillus* ICT as Part of the Diagnosis Scheme. *J. Fungi* **2020**, *6*, 318. [CrossRef]
157. Page, I.D.; Byanyima, R.; Hosmane, S.; Onyachi, N.; Opira, C.; Richardson, M.; Sawyer, R.; Sharman, A.; Denning, D.W. Chronic Pulmonary Aspergillosis Commonly Complicates Treated Pulmonary Tuberculosis with Residual Cavitation. *Eur. Respir. J.* **2019**, *53*, 1801184. [CrossRef]
158. Singh, S.K.; Naaraayan, A.; Acharya, P.; Menon, B.; Bansal, V.; Jesmajian, S. Pulmonary Rehabilitation in Patients with Chronic Lung Impairment from Pulmonary Tuberculosis. *Cureus* **2018**, *10*, e3664. [CrossRef]
159. Sailaja, K.; Nagasreedhar Rao, H. Study of pulmonary function impairment by spirometry in post pulmonary tuberculosis. *J. Evol. Med. Dent Sci.* **2015**, *4*, 7365–7370. [CrossRef]
160. Jung, J.-W.; Choi, J.-C.; Shin, J.-W.; Kim, J.-Y.; Choi, B.-W.; Park, I.-W. Pulmonary Impairment in Tuberculosis Survivors: The Korean National Health and Nutrition Examination Survey 2008–2012. *PLoS ONE* **2015**, *10*, e0141230. [CrossRef] [PubMed]
161. Patil, S.; Patil, R.; Jadhav, A. Pulmonary Functions' Assessment in Post-tuberculosis Cases by Spirometry: Obstructive Pattern is Predominant and Needs Cautious Evaluation in all Treated Cases Irrespective of Symptoms. *Int. J. Mycobacteriol.* **2018**, *7*, 128–133. [CrossRef] [PubMed]
162. Orme, M.W.; Free, R.C.; Manise, A.; Jones, A.V.; Akylbekov, A.; Barton, A.; Emilov, B.; Girase, B.; Jayamaha, A.R.; Jones, R.; et al. Global RECHARGE: Establishing a standard international data set for pulmonary rehabilitation in low and middle-income countries. *J. Glob. Health* **2020**, *10*, 020316. [CrossRef] [PubMed]
163. Radovic, M.; Ristic, L.; Ciric, Z.; Radovic, V.D.; Stankovic, I.; Pejcic, T.; Rancic, M.; Bogdanovic, D. Changes in respiratory function impairment following the treatment of severe pulmonary tuberculosis—Limitations for the underlying COPD detection. *Int. J. Chronic Obstr. Pulm. Dis.* **2016**, *11*, 1307–1316. [CrossRef]
164. Powers, M.; Sanchez, T.R.; Welty, T.K.; Cole, S.A.; Oelsner, E.C.; Yeh, F.; Turner, J.; O'Leary, M.; Brown, R.H.; O'Donnell, M.; et al. Lung Function and Respiratory Symptoms after Tuberculosis in an American Indian Population—The Strong Heart Study. *Ann. Am. Thorac. Soc.* **2020**, *17*, 38–48. [CrossRef]
165. Shuldiner, J.; Leventhal, A.; Chemtob, D.; Mor, Z. Mortality after anti-tuberculosis treatment completion: Results of long-term follow-up. *Int. J. Tuberc. Lung Dis.* **2016**, *20*, 43–48. [CrossRef]
166. Ko, Y.; Lee, Y.-M.; Lee, H.-Y.; Lee, Y.S.; Song, J.-W.; Hong, G.-Y.; Kim, M.-Y.; Lee, H.-K.; Choi, S.J.; Shim, E.-J. Changes in lung function according to disease extent before and after pulmonary tuberculosis. *Int. J. Tuberc. Lung Dis.* **2015**, *19*, 589–595. [CrossRef]
167. Christensen, A.S.; Roed, C.; Andersen, P.H.; Andersen, A.B.; Obel, N. Long-term mortality in patients with pulmonary and extrapulmonary tuberculosis: A Danish nationwide cohort study. *Clin. Epidemiol.* **2014**, *6*, 405–421. [CrossRef]

168. Van Riel, S.E.; Klipstein-Grobusch, K.; Barth, R.E.; Grobbee, D.E.; Feldman, C.; Shaddock, E.; Stacey, S.L.; Venter, W.D.F.; Vos, A.G. Predictors of impaired pulmonary function in people living with HIV in an urban African setting. *S. Afr. J. HIV Med.* **2021**, *22*, 1252. [CrossRef]
169. Kayongo, A.; Wosu, A.C.; Naz, T.; Nassali, F.; Kalyesubula, R.; Kirenga, B.; Wise, R.A.; Siddharthan, T.; Checkley, W. Chronic Obstructive Pulmonary Disease Prevalence and Associated Factors in a Setting of Well-Controlled HIV, A Cross-Sectional Study. *COPD J. Chronic Obstr. Pulm. Dis.* **2020**, *17*, 297–305. [CrossRef]
170. Tadolini, M.; Codecasa, L.; García-García, J.-M.; Blanc, F.-X.; Borisov, S.; Alffenaar, J.-W.; Andréjak, C.; Bachez, P.; Bart, P.-A.; Belilovski, E.; et al. Active tuberculosis, sequelae and COVID-19 co-infection: First cohort of 49 cases. *Eur. Respir. J.* **2020**, *56*, 2001398. [CrossRef]
171. Bandyopadhyay, A.; Palepu, S.; Bandyopadhyay, K.; Handu, S. COVID-19 and tuberculosis co-infection: A neglected paradigm. *Monaldi Arch. Chest Dis.* **2020**, *90*, 3. [CrossRef]
172. Feldman, C.; Anderson, R. The role of co-infections and secondary infections in patients with COVID-19. *Pneumonia* **2021**, *13*, 5. [CrossRef]
173. Crisan-Dabija, R.; Grigorescu, C.; Pavel, C.A.; Artene, B.; Popa, I.V.; Cernomaz, A.; Burlacu, A. Tuberculosis and COVID-19: Lessons from the Past Viral Outbreaks and Possible Future Outcomes. *Can. Respir. J.* **2020**, *2020*, 1401053. [CrossRef]

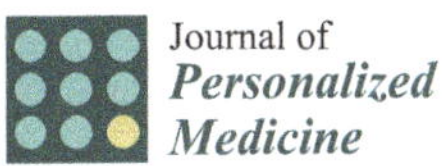
Journal of *Personalized Medicine*
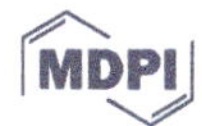

Article

Respiratory Muscle Training Can Improve Cognition, Lung Function, and Diaphragmatic Thickness Fraction in Male and Non-Obese Patients with Chronic Obstructive Pulmonary Disease: A Prospective Study

Yuan-Yang Cheng [1,2,3], Shih-Yi Lin [3,4], Chiann-Yi Hsu [5] and Pin-Kuei Fu [2,6,7,8,*]

1 Department of Physical Medicine and Rehabilitation, Taichung Veterans General Hospital, Taichung 407219, Taiwan; rifampin@gmail.com
2 Department of Post-Baccalaureate Medicine, College of Medicine, National Chung Hsing University, Taichung 402010, Taiwan
3 School of Medicine, National Yang Ming Chiao Tung University, Taipei 11221, Taiwan; sylin@vghtc.gov.tw
4 Center for Geriatrics and Gerontology, Taichung Veterans General Hospital, Taichung 40705, Taiwan
5 Biostatistics Task Force of Taichung Veterans General Hospital, Taichung 407219, Taiwan; chiann@vghtc.gov.tw
6 Department of Critical Care Medicine, Taichung Veterans General Hospital, Taichung 407219, Taiwan
7 Integrated Care Center of Interstitial Lung Disease, Taichung Veterans General Hospital, Taichung 407219, Taiwan
8 College of Human Science and Social Innovation, Hungkuang University, Taichung 433304, Taiwan
* Correspondence: yetquen@gmail.com; Tel.: +886-937-701-592

Citation: Cheng, Y.-Y.; Lin, S.-Y.; Hsu, C.-Y.; Fu, P.-K. Respiratory Muscle Training Can Improve Cognition, Lung Function, and Diaphragmatic Thickness Fraction in Male and Non-Obese Patients with Chronic Obstructive Pulmonary Disease: A Prospective Study. *J. Pers. Med.* **2022**, *12*, 475. https://doi.org/10.3390/jpm12030475

Academic Editors: Ioannis Pantazopoulos and Ourania S. Kotsiou

Received: 9 February 2022
Accepted: 13 March 2022
Published: 16 March 2022

Publisher's Note: MDPI stays neutral with regard to jurisdictional claims in published maps and institutional affiliations.

Abstract: Patients with chronic obstructive pulmonary disease (COPD) are frequently comorbid with mild cognitive impairment (MCI). Whether respiratory muscle training (RMT) is helpful for patients with COPD comorbid MCI remains unclear. Inspiratory muscle training (IMT) with or without expiratory muscle training (EMT) was performed. Patients were randomly assigned to the full training group (EMT + IMT) or the simple training group (IMT only). A total of 49 patients completed the eight-week course of RMT training. RMT significantly improved the maximal inspiratory pressure (MIP), the diaphragmatic thickness fraction and excursion, lung function, scores in the COPD assessment test (CAT), modified Medical Research Council (mMRC) scale scores, and MMSE. The between-group difference in the full training and single training group was not significant. Subgroup analysis classified by the forced expiratory volume in one second (FEV1) level of patients showed no significant differences in MIP, lung function, cognitive function, and walking distance. However, a significant increase in diaphragmatic thickness was found in patients with FEV1 $\geq$ 30%. We suggest that patients with COPD should start RMT earlier in their disease course to improve physical activity.

Keywords: COPD; respiratory muscle training; cognitive impairment; inspiratory muscle training; expiratory muscle training; FEV1; diaphragmatic thickness fraction

1. Introduction

Chronic obstructive pulmonary disease (COPD) is characterized by chronic airway inflammation, which causes obstructed airflow from the lungs, resulting in muscle wasting and respiratory failure [1]. Currently, approximately 300 million people world-wide have COPD, contributing to approximately 64 million disability-adjusted life years [2]. In addition to smoking cessation, oxygen therapy, and long-acting bronchodilator therapy, comprehensive pulmonary rehabilitation programs involving aerobic exercise, cough technique education, and respiratory muscle training (RMT) are crucial in the management of COPD [3]. Inspiratory muscle training (IMT), the major method of RMT, can improve inspiratory muscle strength, exercise capacity, quality of life, and dyspnea [4]. Therefore, IMT has been recommended as a part of pulmonary rehabilitation programs for patients with COPD [5,6]. Expiratory muscle training (EMT) can improve vital capacity and peak expiratory flow [7,8], which are also beneficial for cough function. In addition, the improvement in cough function is a vital part of pulmonary rehabilitation; therefore, RMT including IMT and EMT plays a critical role in the management of COPD [9].

Mild cognitive impairment (MCI) is defined based on the following four criteria [10]: (1) a change in cognition reported by the patient, caregiver, or clinician; (2) objective evidence of impairment in one or more cognitive domains, which typically includes memory; (3) preservation of independence in functional abilities; and (4) absence of dementia. Mini-Mental State Examination (MMSE) scores of 23–27 indicate MCI [11]. Many studies have revealed an association between COPD and MCI [12–15], and a dose–response relationship between the duration of COPD and the risk of MCI [13,14]. Furthermore, forced expiratory volume in one second (FEV1) is positively correlated with cognitive function throughout adulthood [16] because of the higher risk of neuronal injury in patients with chronic hypoxemia [17]. The chronic generalized inflammatory status of patients with COPD can affect MCI pathogenesis [18]. Although aerobic exercise can improve the cognitive function of patients with dementia [19–21], only one study has evaluated the effect of IMT on cognitive function [22]. Because FEV1 is associated with cognitive function, and RMT can improve FEV1 performance, RMT may improve cognitive function. However, whether RMT provides additional benefits for the cognitive function of patients with COPD whose MMSE scores are within the range of MCI remains unclear.

Because RMT is an important part of pulmonary rehabilitation, the aim of the current study investigated the improvement of cognition, lung function, clinical scores, and diaphragmatic muscle performance before and after the introduction of RMT in populations of COPD comorbid with mild cognitive impairment. In subgroup analysis, we want to compare the training efficacy between the full training group (EMT + IMT) and the single training group (IMT only) on cognition, lung function test, clinical scores, and diaphragmatic muscle performance. Finally, we will evaluate the RMT efficacy on patients with different severities of lung function impairment classified by the forced expiratory volume in one second (FEV1) level less than 30%.

2. Materials and Methods

2.1. Participants

Our study was a prospective study that was approved by the Institutional Review Board-I (107-A-09 Board Meeting) of Taichung Veterans General Hospital (protocol code: CF18259A; date of approval: 4 October 2018; clinical trial number: NCT04929990). Participants were recruited from the outpatient department of chest medicine in a tertiary referral center, and written informed consent was obtained from them or their authorized representatives before enrolment. Patients with the following criteria were enrolled: (1) a definitive diagnosis of COPD based on a FEV1/forced vital capacity (FVC) value of less than 0.7 at 10–15 min after short-acting beta-2 agonist (SABA) inhalation, and (2) an MMSE score between 23 and 27. The exclusion criteria were as follows: (1) being unable to follow RMT instructions or complete the questionnaires of our study due to cognitive impairment; (2) difficulty in completing cardiopulmonary exercise testing (CPET) or the 6 min walking test (6MWT) due to high-risk cardiopulmonary diseases or orthopedic conditions, such as critical aortic stenosis, early stage of post myocardial infarction, or lower limb amputation; (3) a diagnosis of lung cancer or a history of thoracoabdominal surgery; and (4) a body mass index (BMI) of $\geq$30.

2.2. Protocol of Intervention

After signing the informed consent form, the participants were assigned to the full RMT training group (EMT + IMT) or the single RMT training group (IMT only) through simple randomization (i.e., tossing a coin). Neither the participants nor the examiner were blinded. The patients enrolled into the current study performed both full RMT training or single RMT training using a threshold-type breathing trainer (Dofin DT11/14, Galemed,

Taipei, Taiwan) at the hospital, and the RMT program included 30 breaths two times a day, 5 days a week, for a total of 8 weeks at home. IMT was performed after complete and slow air expiration, followed by quick and forceful air inspiration to overcome the threshold resistance of the device. By contrast, EMT was performed after complete and slow air inspiration, followed by quick and forceful air expiration. In the full RMT training group (IMT + EMT), before training, maximal inspiratory pressure (MIP) and maximal expiratory pressure (MEP) were measured using a digital pressure gauge (GB60, Jitto International, Taipei, Taiwan), and the best performance of the three trials was recorded. The procedure of MIP/MEP measurement resembled that of IMT/EMT training, except the breathing trainer was replaced with the digital pressure gauge. The initial intensity of training was set at 30% of MIP and MEP. The intensity was adjusted with the addition of 5% resistance each week, and a well-trained assistant contacted the participants telephonically to remind them to adjust the intensity every week.

In the simple RMT training group, only IMT was performed using the same type of Dofin DT11/14 breathing trainer. The initial resistance of the breathing trainer was set at 30% of MIP, and subsequent adjustments were made in accordance with the protocol of the experimental group. The participants were instructed to perform training for 30 breaths twice daily for 8 weeks at home, and they were also telephonically supervised by the same assistant every week.

2.3. Parameter Measures

Parameter measures in the current study were MMSE score; diaphragmatic thickness fraction and excursion examined through ultrasound; scores of the COPD assessment test (CAT) and modified Medical Research Council (mMRC) scale; percentage of predicted FVC, FEV1, FEV1/FVC, diffusing capacity of the lung for carbon monoxide (DLCO), and DLCO divided by alveolar volume (VA) examined using a pulmonary function test; dead space fraction (Vd/Vt) and minute ventilation to CO_2 output (VE/VCO_2) slope examined using the cardiopulmonary exercise test (CPET); and distance walked and changes in oxygen saturation (SpO_2) and perceived exertion (Borg scale) during six-minute walking test (6MWT). All these measures were assessed the day before the initiation of the RMT program and again 8 weeks later at the end of the program.

Diaphragmatic thickness fraction and excursion were measured using an ultrasound machine (Alpinion E-cube i7, who Medical Co., Ltd., Taipei, Taiwan). With the participant in the supine position, diaphragmatic thickness at the intercostal space between the 7th and 8th or the 8th and 9th ribs in the anterior axillary line was examined using a high-frequency ultrasound probe (10–15 MHz). The thickness of the diaphragmatic apposition zone was visualized below the intercostal muscles (Figure 1). The diaphragmatic thickness fraction was calculated as follows: (end-inspiration thickness—end-expiration thickness)/end-expiration thickness [23]. Diaphragmatic excursion was measured by placing a 2–6-MHz ultrasound probe at the right mid-clavicular line, and the amount of movement of the posterior edge of the liver was traced and measured using M mode ultra-sonography [24]. Limitations, such as the variations of probe tilting angle and the impact of the increased echogenicity of the liver, were considered in our study. The sonographic measurements were performed by one single examiner, which could reduce the inter-observer variability, and none of our participants' liver echogenicity was too high to clearly identify the posterior edge of liver.

CAT consists of eight questions, each scored from 0 to 5. mMRC only has one question, which is graded from 0 to 4. Both questionnaires are useful in discerning the respiratory difficulty encountered in daily life for patients with COPD, and in categorizing them for guiding treatment [25]. Regarding the assessment of dementia severity, the MMSE is one of the most widely adopted questionnaires in health care settings. The highest total score on the MMSE is 30, and a score of 23–27 indicates MCI [11], which was used in our study.

For patients with COPD, the pulmonary function test is crucial for grading disease severity, and predicting prognosis. In patients with FEV1/FVC < 0.7 [26], COPD severity can be further categorized into four groups according to the extent to which FEV1 reaches the predicted level: <30%, 30–50%, 50–80%, and >80%. In addition to spirometry data, a diffusion study, including DLCO and DLCO/VA, was conducted using a pulmonary function measurement machine (Vmax Encore VS229, Carefusion Co., Ltd., San Diego, CA, USA).

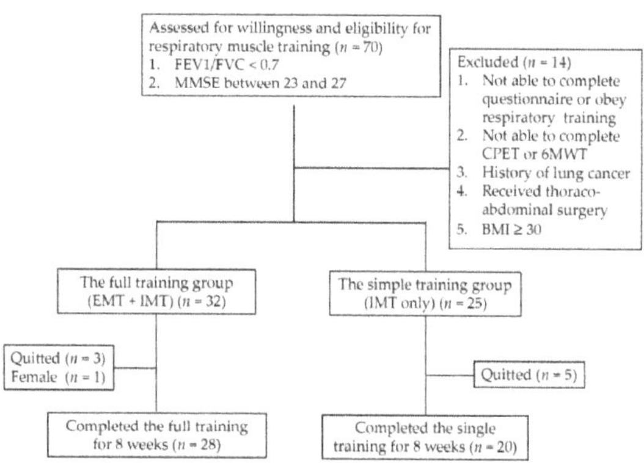

Figure 1. Participant recruitment flowchart: BMI: body mass index; CPET: cardiopulmonary exercise test; IMT: inspiratory muscle training; EMT: expiratory muscle training; 6MWT: six-minute walking test.

In patients with COPD, exercise performance and cardiopulmonary endurance frequently worsen as the disease progresses. Moreover, 6MWT involves walking as far as possible for 6 min, and is a common indicator of oxidative capacity in patients with cardiopulmonary diseases [27]. We established 6MWT distance by having our participants walk back and forth on a 30 m-long walkway with two cones placed at both ends, and we recorded changes in oxygen saturation and perceived exertion on the Borg scale during 6MWT. In addition, a cardiopulmonary exercise test can detect any gas exchange abnormalities during exercise in patients with COPD [28,29]. Patients with COPD have a higher VE/VCO_2 slope [29] and Vd/Vt [28] during exercise. In this study, we measured these parameters during peak exercise. CPET was performed using an electro-magnetically braked cycle ergometer, and a mask was used to collect the partial pressure of O_2 and CO_2 simultaneously; a 10 W/min ramp protocol was used. All the testing procedures followed the guidelines of the American Heart Association [30].

2.4. Statistical Analysis

SPSS 17.0 (IBM, Chicago, IL, USA) was used to perform the statistical analysis. Categorical variables were presented as frequency and percent, and analyzed using the chi-squared test to determine significance. For nonparametric data distribution, differences between groups were assessed using the nonparametric Mann–Whitney U test or Wilcoxon signed ranks test. Results are presented as the mean and standard deviation (SD). To determine the sample size, we adopted G*Power 3.1.9.7 (Heinrich-Heine-Universität Düsseldorf, Germany) to analyze improvements in the MMSE score after physical exercise training, as described previously [21]. With a difference in the improvement of MMSE between 2.67 ± 1.88 and 0.2 ± 2.87 under the setting of $\alpha = 0.05$ and power $-1 - \beta) = 0.8$, the effect size was 1.018, and at least 36 cases were deemed necessary to achieve sufficient statistical power. All tests were two-sided, with $p < 0.05$ considered significant.

3. Results

3.1. Patients' Clinical and Demographic Characteristics

From June 2019 to February 2021, a total of 70 patients were enrolled into the study, and 49 participants completed the 8-week course of the RMT program for the final analysis.

Because there was only one female patient, the study also excluded her data to reduce the effect of gender difference. Table 1 presents a summary of the demographic characteristics, and clinical and physiological parameters of all participants. Among them, 29 and 20 participants were included in the full RMT training group (IMT + EMT) and the single training group (IMT only), respectively. Figure 1 presents the flowchart of participant recruitment and the case numbers in the subgroup of RMT training. Classified by the FEV1 level, 28.6% of participants were <30% (n = 14), and 71.4% of patients were ≥30% (n = 35).

Table 1. Demographic characteristics, and clinical and physiological parameters in patients with COPD enrolled into respiratory muscle training program (n = 48).

Characteristics	Mean ± SD (n, %)
Age (years)	67.23 ± 7.32
Body mass index (kg/m^2)	23.02 ± 3.89
Pulmonary function test	
FVC (%)	78.77 ± 21.36
FEV1 (%)	41.08 ± 15.26
FEV1/FVC (%)	42.83 ± 14.19
DLCO (%)	78.05 ± 24.63
DLCO/VA	83.76 ± 25.82
Clinical score	
CAT score	14.17 ± 8.39
mMRC score	1.63 ± 0.98
MMSE	24.39 ± 2.50
MIP (cmH_2O)	69.41 ± 28.02
MEP (cmH_2O)	85.30 ± 18.07
6MWT	
6MWT distance (m)	328.25 ± 71.72
SpO_2 at rest (%)	95.19 ± 4.98
Nadir SpO_2 in 6MWT	92.69 ± 7.97
Borg scale at rest	1.17 ± 1.32
Borg scale after 6MWT	2.89 ± 1.83
Sonography evaluation	
Diaphragmatic thickness fraction	39.38 ± 28.50
Diaphragmatic excursion (cm)	3.00 ± 1.10
CPET	
Vd/Vt	32.80 ± 7.04
VE/VCO_2 slope	36.81 ± 6.34
FEV1 subgroup	
<30%	14 (29.17%)
≥30%	34 (70.83%)
Respiratory training subgroup	
IMT	20 (41.67%)
IMT + EMT	28 (58.33%)

IMT, inspiratory muscle training; EMT, expiratory muscle training; CAT, chronic obstructive pulmonary disease assessment test; mMRC, modified Medical Research Council; 6MWT, 6-min walking test; Vd/Vt, dead space fraction; VE/VCO_2, minute ventilation to CO_2 output; FVC, forced vital capacity; FEV1, forced expiratory volume in 1 s; DLCO, diffusing capacity of the lung for carbon monoxide; VA, alveolar volume; MMSE, Mini-Mental State Examination.

3.2. Differences between before and after RMT Program

Before and after RMT were compared with respect to all parameters (Table 2). After RMT, patients exhibited significant improvements in FEV1 (%), CAT score, mMRC score, MMSE score, MIP (cmH_2O), MEP (cmH_2O), SpO_2 at rest (%), diaphragmatic thickness fraction, and diaphragmatic excursion (all $p < 0.01$). In addition, the Borg scale after 6MWT was significantly decreased after the RMT program ($p = 0.016$). No significant differences were observed in DLCO (%), 6MWT distance (m), and CPET test after RMT program (all $p > 0.05$).

Table 2. Comparison of the difference of parameters between before and after RMT program implementation.

Characteristics	before RMT	after RMT	p Value
Pulmonary function test			
FVC (%)	78.25 ± 20.68	81.93 ± 19.14	0.318
FEV1 (%)	40.05 ± 15.09	43.75 ± 15.72	0.002 **
FEV1/FVC (%)	42.05 ± 14.27	41.81 ± 15.82	0.372
DLCO (%)	79.83 ± 26.93	80.33 ± 22.62	0.969
DLCO/VA	86.42 ± 31.44	84.67 ± 27.47	0.563
Clinical score			
CAT score	14.17 ± 8.39	9.06 ± 6.06	<0.001 **
mMRC score	1.63 ± 0.98	1.13 ± 0.67	<0.001 **
MMSE	24.39 ± 2.50	26.00 ± 4.13	0.002 **
MIP (cmH_2O)	64.08 ± 30.42	80.79 ± 36.93	0.001 **
MEP (cmH_2O)	80.86 ± 23.48	99.81 ± 34.57	0.036 *
6MWT			
6MWT distance (m)	331.28 ± 70.05	338.80 ± 68.91	0.381
SpO_2 at rest (%)	95.19 ± 4.98	96.67 ± 2.77	0.005 *
Nadir SpO_2 in 6MWT	92.69 ± 7.97	93.78 ± 4.11	0.466
SpO_2 change in 6MWT	2.50 ± 5.82	2.89 ± 3.34	0.174
Borg scale at rest	1.17 ± 1.32	0.83 ± 0.97	0.167
Borg scale after 6MWT	2.89 ± 1.83	2.19 ± 1.65	0.020 *
Borg scale change in 6MWT	1.72 ± 1.61	1.36 ± 1.22	0.232
Sonography evaluation			
Diaphragmatic thickness fraction	39.38 ± 28.50	56.40 ± 28.16	<0.001 **
Diaphragmatic excursion	3.00 ± 1.10	3.83 ± 1.31	<0.001 **
CPET			
Vd/Vt	32.83 ± 7.18	32.98 ± 6.54	0.576
VE/VCO_2 slope	36.63 ± 6.41	36.51 ± 5.62	1.000

CAT, chronic obstructive pulmonary disease assessment test; DLCO, diffusing capacity of the lung for carbon monoxide; EMT, expiratory muscle training; FVC, forced vital capacity; FEV1, forced expiratory volume in 1 s; IMT, inspiratory muscle training; MIP: maximal inspiratory pressure; MEP: maximal expiratory pressure; mMRC, modified Medical Research Council; MMSE, Mini-Mental State Examination; 6MWT, 6-min walking test; SpO_2, oxygen saturation; Vd/Vt, dead space fraction; VE/VCO_2, minute ventilation to CO_2 output; VA, alveolar volume; * $p < 0.05$, ** $p < 0.01$.

3.3. Differences between the Full RMT Training and Single RMT Training Group

The characteristics of the full RMT training and single RMT training groups were compared (Table 3). After 8 weeks, both groups exhibited increases in lung function, MIP, diaphragmatic excursion, and thickness fraction (Figure 2). However, the between-group difference in the full training (IMT + EMT) and single training (IMT only) groups was not significant in all parameters listed in Table 3.

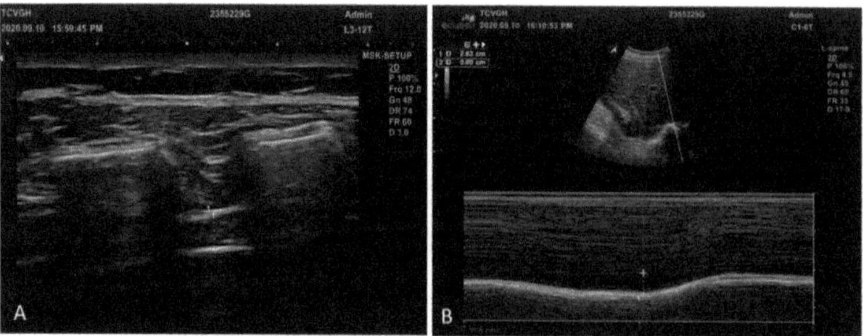

Figure 2. Ultrasonographic evaluation of diaphragm. (**A**) Diaphragmatic thickness was measured below the intercostal muscles between the ribs. +: Markers of the anterior and posterior edges of diaphragm. (**B**) Amount of diaphragmatic excursion was measured using the M mode to trace the movement of the posterior edge of liver. +: Markers of the posterior edge of liver during respiration.

Table 3. The differences between the single training group (IMT only) and the full training group (IMT + EMT) in patients with COPD after RMT program implementation.

	IMT Only (n = 20)	IMT + EMT (n = 28)	p Value
Pulmonary function test			
FVC (%)	83.11 ± 19.54	80.86 ± 19.20	0.722
FEV1 (%)	46.32 ± 16.93	41.43 ± 14.56	0.371
FEV1/FVC (%)	43.55 ± 18.88	40.24 ± 12.72	0.386
DLCO (%)	80.00 ± 27.95	72.29 ± 15.13	0.624
DLCO/VA	90.00 ± 28.66	83.36 ± 25.68	0.711
Clinical score			
CAT score	7.75 ± 4.46	10.00 ± 6.91	0.396
mMRC score	1.20 ± 0.62	1.07 ± 0.72	0.667
MMSE	25.78 ± 5.47	26.14 ± 3.23	0.585
MIP (cmH_2O)	75.25 ± 38.30	83.82 ± 37.69	0.714
MEP (cmH_2O)		99.81 ± 34.57	---
6MWT			
6MWT distance (m)	321.75 ± 73.09	351.92 ± 63.83	0.166
SpO_2 at rest (%)	95.95 ± 2.67	96.16 ± 3.45	0.289
Nadir SpO_2 in 6MWT	92.25 ± 4.89	92.72 ± 4.93	0.680
SpO_2 change in 6MWT	3.70 ± 3.15	3.44 ± 3.88	0.549
Borg scale at rest	0.95 ± 0.89	0.64 ± 0.95	0.160
Borg scale after 6MWT	2.30 ± 1.98	2.60 ± 1.80	0.523
Borg scale change in 6MWT	1.35 ± 1.63	1.96 ± 1.43	0.076
Sonography evaluation			
Diaphragmatic thickness fraction	50.74 ± 28.74	60.44 ± 27.55	0.098
Diaphragmatic excursion (cm)	4.00 ± 1.17	3.72 ± 1.40	0.523
CPET			
Vd/Vt	31.70 ± 8.52	33.96 ± 4.40	0.230
VE/VCO_2 slope	36.21 ± 5.75	36.75 ± 5.62	0.991

Mann–Whitney U test.

3.4. Differences of RMT Training Effect between FEV1 < 30% and FEV1 ≥ 30% among Patients with COPD

The subgroup analysis of the RMT training effect between different severities of FEV1 in patients with COPD was compared (Table 4). After 8 weeks, both groups exhibited increases in FVC (%), FEV1 (%), and the distance of 6MWT; and decreases in CAT score, mMRC score, and Borg scale sore (Table 4). In addition, cognitive function in terms of the MMSE score improved in both groups. However, only diaphragmatic thickness fraction exhibited significant between-group differences in improvement (p = 0.044) (Figure 3).

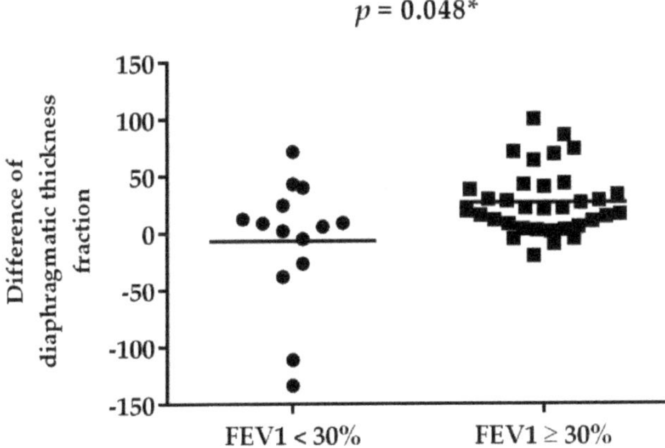

Figure 3. Difference of diaphragmatic thickness fraction before and after RMT. * $p < 0.05$.

Table 4. Comparison of the RMT training effect between FEV1 < 30% and FEV1 ≥ 30% in patients with COPD.

	FEV1 < 30%	FEV1 ≥ 30%	*p* Value
Pulmonary function test			
ΔFVC (%)	3.33 ± 17.41	3.82 ± 18.62	0.821
ΔFEV1 (%)	3.00 ± 5.22	4.00 ± 7.32	0.666
ΔFEV1/FVC (%)	−1.80 ± 13.23	0.43 ± 7.34	0.867
ΔDLCO (%)	9.33 ± 5.03	−2.44 ± 20.28	0.195
ΔDLCO/VA	0.00 ± 6.08	−2.33 ± 10.99	0.864
Clinical score			
ΔCAT score	−6.86 ± 7.49	−4.38 ± 6.92	0.265
ΔmMRC score	−0.86 ± 1.10	−0.35 ± 0.69	0.074
ΔMMSE	2.00 ± 1.87	1.50 ± 2.48	1.000
ΔMIP (cmH2O)	8.33 ± 15.64	15.79 ± 23.35	0.549
ΔMEP (cmH2O)	18.80 ± 6.08	19.00 ± 23.27	1.000
6MWT			
Δ6MWT distance (m)	15.92 ± 65.42	4.21 ± 29.50	0.951
ΔSpO_2 at rest (%)	1.86 ± 1.21	1.38 ± 4.03	0.152
ΔNadir SpO_2 in 6MWT	1.57 ± 2.70	0.97 ± 7.20	0.302
ΔBorg scale at rest	0.29 ± 0.76	−0.48 ± 1.43	0.122
ΔBorg scale after 6MWT	−0.71 ± 1.70	−0.69 ± 1.71	0.922
Sonography evaluation			
ΔDiaphragmatic thickness fraction	−6.84 ± 56.35	26.84 ± 28.55	0.048 *
ΔDiaphragmatic excursion (cm)	1.09 ± 1.50	0.73 ± 1.14	0.734
CPET			
ΔVd/Vt	0.46 ± 5.92	0.02 ± 4.94	0.565
ΔVE/VCO_2 slope	−0.38 ± 3.71	−0.01 ± 5.18	0.678

Mann–Whitney U test. * $p < 0.05$, Δ: value of parameter after training—value of parameter before training.

4. Discussion

This study yielded three major findings. First, the results of our study indicated that RMT, both in the full training group (IMT + EMT) and simple training group (only IMT), could significantly improve not only cognition, but also inspiratory strength, diaphragmatic performance, FEV1, and dyspnea scores in the patients with COPD comorbid with mild cognitive impairment. Second, we observed that even with a baseline FEV1 of <30%, benefits could be derived from RMT in terms of the outcome measures. Third, we found that patients with preserved lung function (FEV1 ≥ 30%) significantly increased in diaphragmatic thickness fraction after RMT training. The strength of current study is that it is the first to use not only clinical score and lung function test, but also apply both diaphragmatic ultrasonography and the cardiopulmonary exercise test to evaluate the effect of RMT. To the best of our knowledge, this is the first study to evaluate the different RMT training models and the impact of RMT in different severities of patients with COPD.

IMT was necessary in both full and simple RMT training groups in the current study, and the FEV1 was improved after RMT training. Several studies have demonstrated that IMT can elevate FEV1 [31–34] due to the improvement in trunk control, with more favorable respiratory biomechanics [35]. In addition, IMT can improve cognitive function, as reported in a previous study [22]. Many studies have demonstrated the relationship between hypoxemia and cognitive impairment [36,37]; however, we cannot conclude that the cognition improvement of our patients was due to the increase of resting SpO_2. That is because the level of SpO_2 in our participants never reached the threshold level of hypoxemia. Since FEV1 level was positively correlated with cognitive function [16], we suggest that the cognition improvement of this cohort was due to the increase in FEV1 rather than the increase of resting SpO_2 after RMT implementation. However, the underlying mechanism requires further study.

Our study revealed that RMT implementation, both in the simple and full training group, improved not only cognition, and FEV1 and SpO_2 at rest, but also MIP, diaphragmatic thickness fraction, diaphragmatic excursion, and CAT and mMRC scores. The results are consistent with those of previous studies [9,38,39]. Weiner et al. reported that dyspnea was alleviated in IMT-only and IMT + EMT groups, but not in the EMT-only group [38]. Weiner and McConnell concluded that no additional benefit was obtained by adding EMT to IMT [39]. Xu et al. revealed improved scores of mMRC, CAT, and St George's Respiratory Questionnaire in both IMT and IMT + EMT groups, with no significant between-group differences [9]. One important reason is that expiration is predominantly accomplished by elastic recoil instead of active muscle contraction, and therefore, the improvement of inspiratory capacity can also facilitate the performance of expiration. On the contrary, the improvement of expiratory strength may not be so practical in daily respiration, and thus, the indicators of life quality, such as CAT and mMRC scores, cannot be further improved through EMT. Our results also showed that the between-group difference in the full training (IMT + EMT) and single training (IMT only) groups was not significant in all parameters. In addition, our study further provided the image evidence of ultrasonography in diaphragmatic excursion and thickness fraction to support the viewpoint that IMT is the most important part of RMT.

In the current study, the VE/VCO_2 slope and Vd/Vt during peak exercise did not significantly change after the training program in either group. The VE/VCO_2 slope, also known as exercise ventilatory efficiency, is an essential prognostic factor in COPD. Vd/Vt, also called the dead space fraction, is considered a comprehensive marker of gas exchange in patients with COPD [40]. RMT cannot enhance ventilator efficiency, and the dead space fraction is probably because RMT can only improve respiratory muscle strength, and not alveolar function of gas exchange.

Most of the previous studies recruited patients with higher FEV1, as easy fatigue during training and poor compliance of training protocol are more common in patients with FEV1 < 30% [41–43]. However, the subgroup analysis of the current study revealed no significant between-group difference exhibited in patients with FEV1 < 30% and $\geq$30%. A study compared the effect of IMT between patients with baseline FEV1 < 50% and $\geq$50%, and revealed that patients with poor lung function (FEV1 < 50%) demonstrated significant improvement in the sensation of dyspnea after 3 weeks of respiratory training [44]. In our study, we found that the decreases of CAT score and mMRC score were larger in patients with FEV1 < 30%, although it did not reach the statistical difference, which may owe to the small case numbers in the FEV1 < 30% group. A recent meta-analysis demonstrated the benefit of IMT in improving COPD parameters; the authors reported that a shorter intervention time ($\leq$4 weeks) improved MIP only, and a longer training period (6–8 weeks) also improved functional capacity, such as 6MWT distance [45]. Although the training period of our study was up to 8 weeks, no significant change was found in the 6MWT distance. One primary reason for this may be that our participants' MMSE scores were in the range of MCI, which may affect their ability to achieve full exertion during 6MWT. On the other hand, 6MWT distance reflects cardiopulmonary aerobic capacity, which could be improved only after aerobic exercise training theoretically. RMT, which is a form of strength training, can produce little effect on aerobic capacity. Therefore, inconsistent results were also mentioned in the past meta-analysis regarding the effect of RMT on 6MWT distance [45]. Further studies may be required to elucidate it.

A major strength of our study is that we incorporated the result of diaphragmatic ultrasonography to validate improvements in MIP and MEP. Furthermore, parameters including the VE/VCO_2 slope and Vd/Vt obtained in CPET were analyzed to determine the reason for the change. However, our study has some limitations. First, although the total number of participants was as per the required sample size for this study, only 14 patients had a baseline FEV1 < 30%, which may have been too few to achieve sufficient statistical power. The data of the improvement of diaphragmatic thickness fraction from two patients with FEV1 < 30% even became outliers. The data of the improvement of diaphragmatic thickness fraction from two patients with FEV1 < 30% even became outliers. Future studies should include more patients with COPD and a baseline FEV1 < 30% to validate our findings. Second, MMSE has limited sensitivity and specificity for diagnosing

MCI against healthy controls [46]. Our participants only had MCI according to MMSE scores, but they did not have a confirmed diagnosis of MCI. Third, our participants had MMSE scores suggestive of MCI, which may have affected their compliance with the RMT program at home, despite us having assigned an assistant to contact and encourage the participants every week via telephone. Finally, we excluded those with BMI $\geq$ 30 to improve the reliability of ultrasonographic results, and none of our participants were female. Therefore, our results may only be applicable to male and non-obese patients with COPD.

5. Conclusions

Our study results revealed that the 8-week RMT program improved not only cognitive function, but also CAT score, mMRC score, and diaphragmatic thickness in male and non-obese patients with COPD comorbid mild cognitive impairment. In addition, we found that IMT is the most important part of RMT, as the combination of EMT with IMT was not superior to IMT alone. Furthermore, even patients with a baseline FEV1 of <30% derive benefits from RMT. Patients with preserved lung function (FEV1 $\geq$ 30%) significantly increased in diaphragmatic thickness fraction after RMT training. We suggest that patients with COPD should start to receive IMT earlier in their disease course to increase their respiratory strength, and thus, achieve a high quality of life.

Author Contributions: Conceptualization, Y.-Y.C., S.-Y.L., C.-Y.H. and P.-K.F.; data curation, Y.-Y.C. and P.-K.F.; formal analysis, Y.-Y.C. and C.-Y.H.; funding acquisition, P.-K.F.; investigation, Y.-Y.C. and P.-K.F.; writing—original draft, Y.-Y.C. and P.-K.F.; writing—review and editing, Y.-Y.C., S.-Y.L., C.-Y.H. and P.-K.F. All authors have read and agreed to the published version of the manuscript.

Funding: The authors sincerely appreciate funding in part by the Department of Medical Research of Taichung Veterans General Hospital (TCVGH-1104401B) and the Ministry of Science and Technology (Taiwan) (MOST109-2410-H-075A-001-SSS; MOST 110-2410-H-075A-001& MOST-1102622H075A001) for the supporting of study manpower, materials, and the publication fees in the open access journal.

Institutional Review Board Statement: The study was conducted according to the guidelines of the Declaration of Helsinki, and approved by the Institutional Review Board of Taichung Veterans General Hospital (IRB number: CF18259A, date of approval, 4 October 2018; clinical trial number: NCT04929990).

Informed Consent Statement: Informed consent was obtained from all subjects involved in the study. Written informed consent has been obtained from the patients to publish this paper.

Data Availability Statement: The data presented in this study are available on request from the corresponding author. The data are not publicly available due to the regulation of the Institutional Review Board of Taichung Veterans General Hospital in Taiwan.

Conflicts of Interest: The authors declare no conflict of interest.

References

1. Rabe, K.F.; Watz, H. Chronic obstructive pulmonary disease. *Lancet* **2017**, *389*, 1931–1940. [CrossRef]
2. Ruvuna, L.; Sood, A. Epidemiology of Chronic Obstructive Pulmonary Disease. *Clin. Chest Med.* **2020**, *41*, 315–327. [CrossRef]
3. McCarthy, B.; Casey, D.; Devane, D.; Murphy, K.; Murphy, E.; Lacasse, Y. Pulmonary rehabilitation for chronic obstructive pulmonary disease. *Cochrane Database Syst. Rev.* **2015**, *2*, CD003793. [CrossRef]
4. Beaumont, M.; Forget, P.; Couturaud, F.; Reychler, G. Effects of inspiratory muscle training in COPD patients: A systematic review and meta-analysis. *Clin. Respir. J.* **2018**, *12*, 2178–2188. [CrossRef]
5. Hill, K.; Cecins, N.M.; Eastwood, P.R.; Jenkins, S.C. Inspiratory muscle training for patients with chronic obstructive pulmonary disease: A practical guide for clinicians. *Arch. Phys. Med. Rehabil.* **2010**, *91*, 1466–1470. [CrossRef]
6. Frangogiannis, N.G.; Dewald, O.; Xia, Y.; Ren, G.; Haudek, S.; Leucker, T.; Kraemer, D.; Taffet, G.; Rollins, B.J.; Entman, M.L. Critical role of monocyte chemoattractant protein-1/CC chemokine ligand 2 in the pathogenesis of ischemic cardiomyopathy. *Circulation* **2007**, *115*, 584–592. [CrossRef]
7. Chigira, Y.; Miyazaki, I.; Izumi, M.; Oda, T. Effects of expiratory muscle training on the frail elderly's respiratory function. *J. Phys. Ther. Sci.* **2018**, *30*, 286–288. [CrossRef]

8. Kim, J.; Davenport, P.; Sapienza, C. Effect of expiratory muscle strength training on elderly cough function. *Arch. Gerontol. Geriatr.* **2009**, *48*, 361–366. [CrossRef]
9. Xu, W.; Li, R.; Guan, L.; Wang, K.; Hu, Y.; Xu, L.; Zhou, L.; Chen, R.; Chen, X. Combination of inspiratory and expiratory muscle training in same respiratory cycle versus different cycles in COPD patients: A randomized trial. *Respir. Res.* **2018**, *19*, 225. [CrossRef]
10. Albert, M.S.; DeKosky, S.T.; Dickson, D.; Dubois, B.; Feldman, H.H.; Fox, N.C.; Gamst, A.; Holtzman, D.M.; Jagust, W.J.; Petersen, R.C.; et al. The diagnosis of mild cognitive impairment due to Alzheimer's disease: Recommendations from the National Institute on Aging-Alzheimer's Association workgroups on diagnostic guidelines for Alzheimer's disease. *Alzheimers Dement.* **2011**, *7*, 270–279. [CrossRef]
11. Zaudig, M. A new systematic method of measurement and diagnosis of "mild cognitive impairment" and dementia according to ICD-10 and DSM-III-R criteria. *Int. Psychogeriatr.* **1992**, *4* (Suppl. S2), 203–219. [CrossRef]
12. Kakkera, K.; Padala, K.P.; Kodali, M.; Padala, P.R. Association of chronic obstructive pulmonary disease with mild cognitive impairment and dementia. *Curr. Opin. Pulm. Med.* **2018**, *24*, 173–178. [CrossRef]
13. Singh, B.; Mielke, M.M.; Parsaik, A.K.; Cha, R.H.; Roberts, R.O.; Scanlon, P.D.; Geda, Y.E.; Christianson, T.J.; Pankratz, V.S.; Petersen, R.C. A prospective study of chronic obstructive pulmonary disease and the risk for mild cognitive impairment. *JAMA Neurol.* **2014**, *71*, 581–588. [CrossRef]
14. Singh, B.; Parsaik, A.K.; Mielke, M.M.; Roberts, R.O.; Scanlon, P.D.; Geda, Y.E.; Pankratz, V.S.; Christianson, T.; Yawn, B.P.; Petersen, R.C. Chronic obstructive pulmonary disease and association with mild cognitive impairment: The Mayo Clinic Study of Aging. *Mayo Clin. Proc.* **2013**, *88*, 1222–1230. [CrossRef]
15. Ranzini, L.; Schiavi, M.; Pierobon, A.; Granata, N.; Giardini, A. From Mild Cognitive Impairment (MCI) to Dementia in Chronic Obstructive Pulmonary Disease. Implications for Clinical Practice and Disease Management: A Mini-Review. *Front. Psychol.* **2020**, *11*, 337. [CrossRef]
16. Anstey, K.J.; Windsor, T.D.; Jorm, A.F.; Christensen, H.; Rodgers, B. Association of pulmonary function with cognitive performance in early, middle and late adulthood. *Gerontology* **2004**, *50*, 230–234. [CrossRef]
17. de la Torre, J.C. Critical threshold cerebral hypoperfusion causes Alzheimer's disease? *Acta Neuropathol.* **1999**, *98*, 1–8. [CrossRef]
18. Koyama, A.; O'Brien, J.; Weuve, J.; Blacker, D.; Metti, A.L.; Yaffe, K. The role of peripheral inflammatory markers in dementia and Alzheimer's disease: A meta-analysis. *J. Gerontol. A Biol. Sci. Med. Sci.* **2013**, *68*, 433–440. [CrossRef]
19. Venturelli, M.; Scarsini, R.; Schena, F. Six-month walking program changes cognitive and ADL performance in patients with Alzheimer. *Am. J. Alzheimers Dis. Other Demen.* **2011**, *26*, 381–388. [CrossRef]
20. Vreugdenhil, A.; Cannell, J.; Davies, A.; Razay, G. A community-based exercise programme to improve functional ability in people with Alzheimer's disease: A randomized controlled trial. *Scand. J. Caring Sci.* **2012**, *26*, 12–19. [CrossRef]
21. Van de Winckel, A.; Feys, H.; De Weerdt, W.; Dom, R. Cognitive and behavioural effects of music-based exercises in patients with dementia. *Clin. Rehabil.* **2004**, *18*, 253–260. [CrossRef]
22. Ferreira, L.; Tanaka, K.; Santos-Galduroz, R.F.; Galduroz, J.C. Respiratory training as strategy to prevent cognitive decline in aging: A randomized controlled trial. *Clin. Interv. Aging* **2015**, *10*, 593–603. [CrossRef]
23. Sarwal, A.; Walker, F.O.; Cartwright, M.S. Neuromuscular ultrasound for evaluation of the diaphragm. *Muscle Nerve* **2013**, *47*, 319–329. [CrossRef]
24. Epelman, M.; Navarro, O.M.; Daneman, A.; Miller, S.F. M-mode sonography of diaphragmatic motion: Description of technique and experience in 278 pediatric patients. *Pediatr. Radiol.* **2005**, *35*, 661–667. [CrossRef]
25. Halpin, D.M.G.; Criner, G.J.; Papi, A.; Singh, D.; Anzueto, A.; Martinez, F.J.; Agusti, A.A.; Vogelmeier, C.F. Global Initiative for the Diagnosis, Management, and Prevention of Chronic Obstructive Lung Disease. The 2020 GOLD Science Committee Report on COVID-19 and Chronic Obstructive Pulmonary Disease. *Am. J. Respir. Crit. Care Med.* **2021**, *203*, 24–36. [CrossRef]
26. Burkhardt, R.; Pankow, W. The diagnosis of chronic obstructive pulmonary disease. *Dtsch. Arztebl. Int.* **2014**, *111*, 834–845, quiz 846. [CrossRef]
27. Rasekaba, T.; Lee, A.L.; Naughton, M.T.; Williams, T.J.; Holland, A.E. The six-minute walk test: A useful metric for the cardiopulmonary patient. *Intern. Med. J.* **2009**, *39*, 495–501. [CrossRef]
28. Chuang, M.L. Combining Dynamic Hyperinflation with Dead Space Volume during Maximal Exercise in Patients with Chronic Obstructive Pulmonary Disease. *J. Clin. Med.* **2020**, *9*, 1127. [CrossRef]
29. Boutou, A.K.; Zafeiridis, A.; Pitsiou, G.; Dipla, K.; Kioumis, I.; Stanopoulos, I. Cardiopulmonary exercise testing in chronic obstructive pulmonary disease: An update on its clinical value and applications. *Clin. Physiol. Funct. Imaging* **2020**, *40*, 197–206. [CrossRef]
30. Guazzi, M.; Arena, R.; Halle, M.; Piepoli, M.F.; Myers, J.; Lavie, C.J. 2016 Focused Update: Clinical Recommendations for Cardiopulmonary Exercise Testing Data Assessment in Specific Patient Populations. *Circulation* **2016**, *133*, e694–e711. [CrossRef]
31. Weiner, P.; Man, A.; Weiner, M.; Rabner, M.; Waizman, J.; Magadle, R.; Zamir, D.; Greiff, Y. The effect of incentive spirometry and inspiratory muscle training on pulmonary function after lung resection. *J. Thorac. Cardiovasc. Surg.* **1997**, *113*, 552–557. [CrossRef]
32. Abodonya, A.M.; Abdelbasset, W.K.; Awad, E.A.; Elalfy, I.E.; Salem, H.A.; Elsayed, S.H. Inspiratory muscle training for recovered COVID-19 patients after weaning from mechanical ventilation: A pilot control clinical study. *Medicine* **2021**, *100*, e25339. [CrossRef]
33. El-Deen, H.A.B.; Alanazi, F.S.; Ahmed, K.T. Effects of inspiratory muscle training on pulmonary functions and muscle strength in sedentary hemodialysis patients. *J. Phys. Ther. Sci.* **2018**, *30*, 424–427. [CrossRef]

34. Bostanci, O.; Mayda, H.; Yilmaz, C.; Kabadayi, M.; Yilmaz, A.K.; Ozdal, M. Inspiratory muscle training improves pulmonary functions and respiratory muscle strength in healthy male smokers. *Respir. Physiol. Neurobiol.* **2019**, *264*, 28–32. [CrossRef]
35. Aydogan Arslan, S.; Ugurlu, K.; Sakizli Erdal, E.; Keskin, E.D.; Demirguc, A. Effects of Inspiratory Muscle Training on Respiratory Muscle Strength, Trunk Control, Balance and Functional Capacity in Stroke Patients: A single-blinded randomized controlled study. *Top. Stroke Rehabil.* **2022**, *29*, 40–48. [CrossRef]
36. Findley, L.J.; Barth, J.T.; Powers, D.C.; Wilhoit, S.C.; Boyd, D.G.; Suratt, P.M. Cognitive impairment in patients with obstructive sleep apnea and associated hypoxemia. *Chest* **1986**, *90*, 686–690. [CrossRef]
37. Areza-Fegyveres, R.; Kairalla, R.A.; Carvalho, C.R.R.; Nitrini, R. Cognition and chronic hypoxia in pulmonary diseases. *Dement. Neuropsychol.* **2010**, *4*, 14–22. [CrossRef]
38. Weiner, P.; Magadle, R.; Beckerman, M.; Weiner, M.; Berar-Yanay, N. Comparison of specific expiratory, inspiratory, and combined muscle training programs in COPD. *Chest* **2003**, *124*, 1357–1364. [CrossRef]
39. Weiner, P.; McConnell, A. Respiratory muscle training in chronic obstructive pulmonary disease: Inspiratory, expiratory, or both? *Curr. Opin. Pulm. Med.* **2005**, *11*, 140–144. [CrossRef]
40. Chuang, M.L.; Hsieh, B.Y.; Lin, I.F. Resting Dead Space Fraction as Related to Clinical Characteristics, Lung Function, and Gas Exchange in Male Patients with Chronic Obstructive Pulmonary Disease. *Int. J. Gen. Med.* **2021**, *14*, 169–177. [CrossRef]
41. Garcia, S.; Rocha, M.; Pinto, P.; Lopes, A.M.; Bárbara, C. Inspiratory muscle training in COPD patients. *Rev. Port. Pneumol.* **2008**, *14*, 177–194. [CrossRef]
42. Petrovic, M.; Reiter, M.; Zipko, H.; Pohl, W.; Wanke, T. Effects of inspiratory muscle training on dynamic hyperinflation in patients with COPD. *Int. J. Chron. Obstruct. Pulmon. Dis.* **2012**, *7*, 797–805. [CrossRef] [PubMed]
43. Hill, K.; Jenkins, S.C.; Philippe, D.L.; Cecins, N.; Shepherd, K.L.; Green, D.J.; Hillman, D.R.; Eastwood, P.R. High-intensity inspiratory muscle training in COPD. *Eur. Respir. J.* **2006**, *27*, 1119–1128. [CrossRef] [PubMed]
44. Beaumont, M.; Mialon, P.; Le Ber-Moy, C.; Lochon, C.; Peran, L.; Pichon, R.; Gut-Gobert, C.; Leroyer, C.; Morelot-Panzini, C.; Couturaud, F. Inspiratory muscle training during pulmonary rehabilitation in chronic obstructive pulmonary disease: A randomized trial. *Chron. Respir. Dis.* **2015**, *12*, 305–312. [CrossRef] [PubMed]
45. Figueiredo, R.I.N.; Azambuja, A.M.; Cureau, F.V.; Sbruzzi, G. Inspiratory Muscle Training in COPD. *Respir. Care* **2020**, *65*, 1189–1201. [CrossRef] [PubMed]
46. Mitchell, A.J. A meta-analysis of the accuracy of the mini-mental state examination in the detection of dementia and mild cognitive impairment. *J. Psychiatr. Res.* **2009**, *43*, 411–431. [CrossRef] [PubMed]

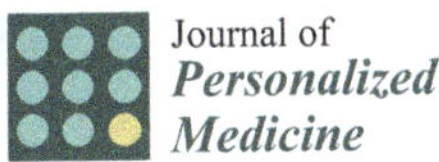
Journal of *Personalized Medicine*

MDPI

Review

Elements of Sleep Breathing and Sleep-Deprivation Physiology in the Context of Athletic Performance

Dimitra D. Papanikolaou [1], Kyriaki Astara [1,2], George D. Vavougios [1,3], Zoe Daniil [1], Konstantinos I. Gourgoulianis [1] and Vasileios T. Stavrou [1,*]

1 Laboratory of Cardio-Pulmonary Testing and Pulmonary Rehabilitation, Department of Respiratory Medicine, Faculty of Medicine, University of Thessaly, 41110 Larissa, Greece; dimitra.papanikolaoy2001@gmail.com (D.D.P.); kyriakiastarara@gmail.com (K.A.); dantevavougios@hotmail.com (G.D.V.); zdaniil@uth.gr (Z.D.); kgourg@uth.gr (K.I.G.)
2 Department of Neurology, 417 Army Equity Fund Hospital (NIMTS), 11521 Athens, Greece
3 Department of Neurology, Faculty of Medicine, University of Cyprus, Nicosia 2029, Cyprus
* Correspondence: vasileiosstavrou@hotmail.com; Tel.: +30-241-350-2157

Abstract: This review summarizes sleep deprivation, breathing regulation during sleep, and the outcomes of its destabilization. Breathing as an automatically regulated task consists of different basic anatomic and physiological parts. As the human body goes through the different stages of sleep, physiological changes in the breathing mechanism are present. Sleep disorders, such as obstructive sleep apnea-hypopnea syndrome, are often associated with sleep-disordered breathing and sleep deprivation. Hypoxia and hypercapnia coexist with lack of sleep and undermine multiple functions of the body (e.g., cardiovascular system, cognition, immunity). Among the general population, athletes suffer from these consequences more during their performance. This concept supports the beneficial restorative effects of a good sleeping pattern.

Keywords: sleep deprivation; exercise; cardiovascular; cognitive

Citation: Papanikolaou, D.D.; Astara, K.; Vavougios, G.D.; Daniil, Z.; Gourgoulianis, K.I.; Stavrou, V.T. Elements of Sleep Breathing and Sleep-Deprivation Physiology in the Context of Athletic Performance. *J. Pers. Med.* **2022**, *12*, 383. https://doi.org/10.3390/jpm12030383

Academic Editor: Kentaro Inamura

Received: 28 January 2022
Accepted: 1 March 2022
Published: 2 March 2022

1. Sleep-Disordered Breathing Physiology

1.1. Respiratory Aspect

The mechanism of breathing includes air flow through the passages of the respiratory system due to pressure gradients that are formed by contraction of the diaphragm and the thoracic muscles. Air flows from a region of higher pressure to a region of lower pressure. Respiration involves the interplay between three different pressures: the atmospheric, the interalveolar, and the intrapleural pressure. Inspiration is the active phase of respiration and the result of muscle contraction, and expiration is the passive phase in calm state. Regulation of respiratory system is subconscious and determines rhythmic rotation between inspiration and expiration and ventilation (breathing frequency and depth) [1].

Sleep state is associated with significant changes in respiratory physiology, including ventilatory responses to hypoxia and hypercapnia, upper airway, and intercostal muscle tone, and tidal volume and minute ventilation. These changes are further magnified in certain disease states, such as chronic obstructive pulmonary disease, restrictive respiratory disorders, neuromuscular conditions, and cardiac diseases [2]. Sleep-disordered breathing (SDB), which causes sleep deprivation and intermittent hypoxia, encompasses a broad spectrum of sleep-related breathing disorders, including obstructive sleep apnea (OSA), central sleep apnea (CSA), as well as sleep-related hypoventilation and hypoxemia. Relative hypotonia of respiratory muscles, body posture changes, and altered ventilatory control result in additional physiologic changes contributing to hypoventilation [3]. Hypercapnia, hypoxemia, and negative intrathoracic pressure swings lead to increased sympathetic response in order to maintain the normal air flow followed by hyperventilation.

1.2. Neural Aspect

Breathing is an automatic function and is regulated, according to the metabolic demands, by the autonomic nervous system (ANS) and, more specifically, by the respiratory center (RC), a central pattern generator (CPG) located in medulla oblongata along with the other vital reflexes. Cortical–medullary circuits furthermore guarantee that voluntary control of breathing is possible [4]. Upon loss of cortical functions without the loss of the medullary CPG, however, control is maintained by the latter.

1.3. Input Sensors

Wakefulness, non-rapid eye-movement sleep (NREM), and rapid eye-movement sleep (REM) sleep represent three distinct states during the sleep–wake cycle [5]. Breathing is maintained during sleep, but its regulation differs from wakefulness [6]. The progression through sleep stages is accompanied by a sequence of physiological changes based on chemoreceptor and baroreceptor reflexes [7]. Chemoreceptors are divided into peripheral and central. Chemoreflex input consist of peripheral (carotid and aortic bodies), which reflect the concentrations of arterial O_2, and of central receptors, which are sensitive to CO_2 and H^+ changes in the CSF [8]. Consequently, the ventilatory feedback control system of the chemoreflex is vulnerable to rapid fluctuations of this input, similar to those that occur during NREM sleep [9].

Two additional respiratory control centers exist in the medulla: the vasomotor (VMC) that regulates blood pressure and the cardiac center (cardioinhibitory and cardioacceleratory centers) for the regulation of heart rate. The three centers are interconnected to function coordinately for the release not only of the chemoreflex but also for the baroreflex [10]. The baroreceptor reflex is activated when blood pressure is found increased by the baroreceptors in walls of carotid internal artery and of aorta and vasodilation occurs (inhibition of VMC) as well as decreased heart rate (stimulation of cardioinhibitory centers).

In sleep-disordered breathing, the circle of intermittent hypoxia–hypercapnia stimulates chemoreflex entirely, which in turn overstimulates SNS, attenuates baroreflex, and enhances hyperventilation after arousal [11]. Arousal occurs in order to increase the muscle tone and compensate for hypoventilation. Interestingly, the increased tone of SNS persists during daytime, too. As baroreflex is desensitized, the PNS is incapable of antagonizing the detrimental effects of SNS overstimulation, demonstrating mainly hypertension and tachycardia.

1.4. Output Mediators

The mutable environment of respiratory regulation during sleep affects multiple systems and structures: the ANS as well as lungs, chest wall, and upper airway [12]. During wakefulness and REM, sympathetic tone is dominant, whereas during NREM sleep, parasympathetic tone prevails to create a state of reduced activity [13]. Therefore, blood pressure and heart rate are reduced during NREM, whereas in REM sleep, the pulses of sympathetic activity induce tachycardia and relatively increase blood pressure [14].

During sleep, ventilation and functional residual capacity decrease slightly [15]. In stage I of NREM sleep, sufficient muscle tone is maintained, and frequent body posture changes occur. Respiratory pattern is more regular, while minute ventilation is progressively reduced, resulting in an increase of end-tidal carbon dioxide ($ETCO_2$) compared to a waking state. During REM, respiratory pattern varies while ventilation further drops, accompanied by a slight reduction in oxygen saturation [16].

These fluctuations of arterial blood pressure, heart rate, and respiration occur in NREM and REM sleep and during transitions between sleep and arousal [17]; they may explain the sensitivity differences in hypoxia–hypercapnia, a major pathophysiologic element in sleep-disordered breathing [5]. Pulmonary stretch receptors work in coordination with central and peripheral chemoreceptors as the corresponding reflexes affect upper airway and respiratory pump muscles. The relationship is displayed in detail in Figure 1. A reduction in respiratory muscle tone occurs during NREM sleep but is more prominent during

REM [18], attenuating the occlusion pressure responses to both hypoxia and hypercapnia in REM sleep stage, a clinical phenomenon consistent with emerging even in normal people [19]. In this context, arousals emerge, fragmenting sleep architecture. A protective reflex is activated by local upper airway (UA) mechanoreceptors due to the negative pressure in the UA, preventing its collapse by enhancing activity of UA dilators [20]. This reflex re-establishes ventilation in an alternative-to-arousal manner.

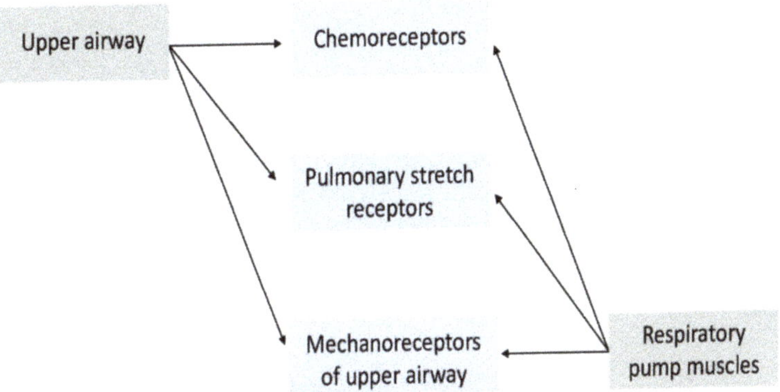

Figure 1. All the reflexes that take part in the control of respiratory rate during sleep. As inspiration occurs, upper airway muscles are activated by the mechanoreceptors, resulting in a protective reflex that prevents occlusion of airflow without arousals. However, inspiratory activation may become insufficient in terms of timing and magnitude due to stronger activation of respiratory pump muscles that lead to inadequate compensation for the airway-collapsing effect of negative inspiratory pressure.

2. Sleep Deprivation

Sleep-disordered breathing is associated with sleep deprivation. This sleep disruption interferes with the normal restorative functions of NREM and REM sleep, resulting in disruptions of breathing and cardiovascular function, changes in emotional reactivity, and cognitive decline in attention, memory, and decision making [21]. Sleep-disordered breathing is common among overweight and obese children. It is a risk factor for several health complications, including cardiovascular disease. Inflammatory processes leading to endothelial dysfunction are a possible mechanism linking SDB and cardiovascular disease [22,23].

2.1. Sleep Deprivation and CO_2 Retention

Disordered breathing is commonly associated with hypercapnia, which is followed by sufficient CO_2 retention. This phenomenon leads to various impairments due to dangerous levels of hypercapnia. Acute responses to CO_2 affect breathing primarily via central chemoreceptors [24]. Retention of CO_2 not only contributes to chemoreflex via hypercapnia and acidosis but also serves as a powerful stimulus to increase respiration. Hypoxia potentiates the effects of CO_2, resulting in a stronger ventilatory response. Through various mechanisms, retention of CO_2 can persist during daytime, too [25].

Carbon dioxide retention is related to oxidative stress and increased sympathetic activity with subsequent effects, such as hypertension. Recent evidence has now implicated a role for oxidative stress in sleep and sleep loss [26]. Oxidative stress is defined by increased oxygen reactive species (ROS) production and inability of the cell to alienate them. Prolonged wakefulness/sleep deprivation activates an adaptive stress pathway termed the unfolded protein response, which temporarily guards against the deleterious consequences of reactive oxygen species [24,26]. The elevated sympathetic response also triggers a generalized inflammatory cascade that is associated with the pathophysiology of multiple comorbidities, including insulin resistance, hypertension, diabetes, atherosclerosis, and metabolic syndrome [27]. Epidemiologic studies in adults and children and laboratory studies in young adults indicate that sleep deprivation may be associated with several relevant impairments: decreased glucose tolerance, decreased insulin sensitivity, increased evening concentrations of cortisol, increased levels of ghrelin, decreased levels of leptin, and increased hunger and appetite (Table 1). Nevertheless, the current epidemic of obesity could be partly attenuated by better sleep regulation [28]. In healthy adults who are chronically sleep restricted, a simple, low-cost intervention, such as sleep extension, is feasible and is associated with improvements in fasting insulin sensitivity [29]. In the matter of inflammatory system, sleep loss triggers signaling pathways in the brain and periphery. The Toll-like receptor 4 (TLR4) activates inflammatory signaling cascades in response to endogenous and pathogen-associated ligands known to be elevated in association with sleep deprivation. TLR4 is therefore a possible mediator of some of the inflammation-related effects of sleep loss [30]. Furthermore, total sleep loss produces significant increases in plasma levels of sTNF-alpha receptor I and IL-6, messengers that connect the nervous, endocrine, and immune systems [31].

Table 1. Responses and sleep deprivation.

References	Participants	Intervention Protocol	Results
Chapman et al. [32]	Healthy adults (age: 26.0 ± 4.0 yrs, M: n = 7, F: n = 7)	Blood velocity was measured in the renal and segmental arteries with Doppler ultrasound while subjects breathed room air and while they breathed a 3% CO_2, 21% O_2, 76% N_2 gas mixture for 5 min	CO_2 decreased blood velocity in the renal and segmental arteries and increased vascular resistance in the renal and segmental arteries (kidneys are hemodynamically responsive to a mild and acute hypercapnic stimulus in healthy humans)
Lei et al. [33]	14 healthy and right-handed adult males (mean age: 25.9 years) with normal or corrected-to-normal vision	fMRI study during RW and after 36 h of TSD	Self-reported scores of sleepiness were higher for TSD than for RW. A subsequent working memory task showed that memory performance was lower after 36 h of TSD. Significant increase of sleep pressure index was observed after 36 h of TSD
Van Eyck et al. [22]	120 children; control (age: 12.0 ± 3.0 y, M: n = 30, F: n = 55), mild OSAS (age: 11.0 ± 3.0 y, M: n = 9, F: n = 11), and moderate-to-severe OSAS (age: 12.0 ± 3.0 y, M: n = 10, F: n = 5)	PSG and a blood sample was taken to determine CRP levels	Relationship between CRP and BMI and between CRP and fat mass
Jones et al. [34]	OSAHS patients (age: 44.0 ± 7.0 y, M: n = 13, F: n = 7, AHI: ≥15/h and ESS score ≥ 11) vs. controls (age: 44.0 ± 7.0 y, M: n = 13, F: n = 7)	Evaluation of arterial stiffness (applanation tonometry and cardiovascular MRI) and endothelial function (measuring vascular reactivity after administration of glyceryl trinitrate and salbutamol)	Subjects with OSAHS had increased arterial stiffness and impaired endothelial function and were at increased risk for cardiovascular disease
Robertson et al. [35]	Healthy and normal-weight male students aged 20–30 y, BMI: 19–26 kg/m^2. They were randomized to either sleep restriction (habitual bedtime minus 1.5 h) or a control condition (habitual bedtime) for three weeks	Weekly assessments of insulin sensitivity by hyperinsulinemic-euglycemic clamp, anthropometry, vascular function, leptin, and adiponectin were made. Sleep was assessed continuously using actigraphy and diaries.	Sleep restriction led to changes in insulin sensitivity, body weight, and plasma concentrations of leptin, which varied during the 3-week period. There was no effect on plasma adiponectin or vascular function. Even minor reductions in sleep duration led to changes in insulin sensitivity, body weight, and other metabolic parameters, which vary during the exposure period.

Abbreviations: AHI, apnea–hypopnea index; BMI, body mass index; CO_2, carbon dioxide; CRP, C-reactive protein; ESS, Epworth Sleepiness Scale; F, female; fMRI, functional magnetic resonance imaging; M, male; n, number; N_2, nitrogen; O_2, oxygen; OSAHS, obstructive sleep apnea–hypopnea syndrome; OSAS, obstructive sleep apnea syndrome; PSG, polysomnography study; RW, rested wakefulness; TSD, total sleep deprivation.

2.2. Sleep Deprivation and Exercise: Cognitive Implications

A sleep-deprived brain fails to recuperate neurons, undermining cognitive performance. General cognitive assessment tests unveil the cognitive phenotype of SD, especially in attention and short-term memory, as they anatomically overlap [36,37]. Furthermore, SD, in the context of sleep apnea, affects learning and memory [38,39] (Table 1). Furthermore, other daytime consequences, such as excessive sleepiness and fatigue, coexist and interact with cognitive impairment [40]. These are linked with various effects on exercise, including athletic performance, reaction time, accuracy, strength and endurance [41]. Alertness, judgment, and decision making suffer due to SD, shifting motivational behaviors towards sleep-promoting goals [42,43].

Sleep deprivation of 30 to 72 h consecutively does not affect cardiovascular and respiratory responses to exercise of varying intensity or the aerobic and anaerobic performance capability of individuals. Muscle strength and electromechanical responses are also not affected. Time to exhaustion, however, is decreased by sleep deprivation [44]. Research indicates that some maximal physical efforts and gross motor performances can be maintained. Effects on cognitive function consist of slower and less accurate cognitive performance. Reduction in sleep quality and quantity could result in an autonomic nervous system imbalance, simulating symptoms of the overtraining syndrome [45]. The integrity of sleep architecture seems to determine subjective sleep quality and waking performance. The effects of insufficient sleep primarily concern subjective and objective sleepiness as well as attention, whereas performance on higher cognitive functions appears to be better preserved albeit at the cost of increased effort [46]. All in all, sleep deprivation induces a vulnerability in various domains of cognition, leading to overall suboptimal performance.

This vulnerability to cognitive impairment due to sleep deprivation is conjoined with mood disorders and particularly symptom severity [47]. Emotional information is misinterpreted, making sleep-deprived subjects prone to anxiety [48] and depressive symptoms [49] as well as altered reward-seeking and impulsive behaviors [50]. Stress is one of the main factors influencing sleep. Hyperarousal is a key component in all modern etiological models of insomnia disorder. Overactive neurobiological and psychological systems contribute to sleep onset disorders. Sleep reactivity is the degree to which stress disrupts sleep, manifesting as difficulty falling and staying asleep. Individuals with highly reactive sleep systems experience drastic deterioration of sleep when stressed, whereas those with low sleep reactivity proceed largely unperturbed during stress. Research points to genetics, family history of insomnia, gender, and environmental stress as factors that influence sleep reactivity. High sleep reactivity is also linked to risk of shift-work disorder, depression, and anxiety [51–53] (Figure 2).

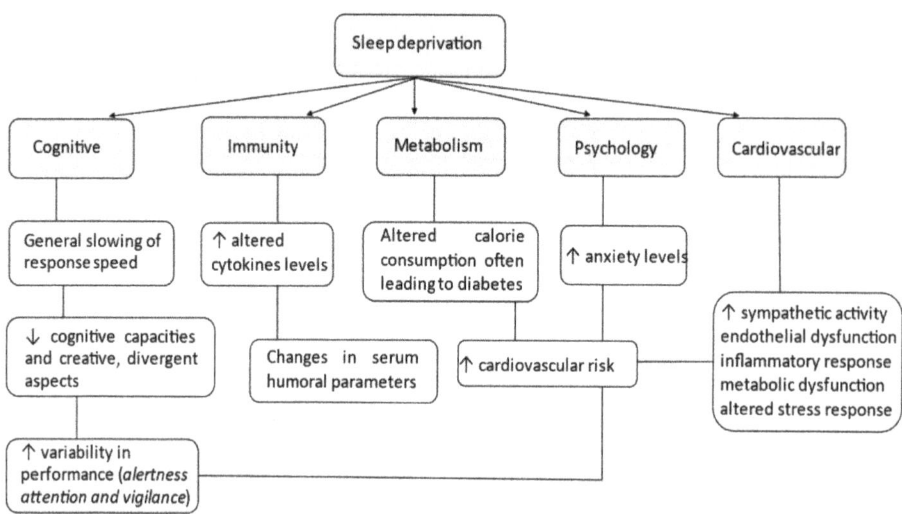

Figure 2. Sleep deprivation on general population.

Exercise could improve to one extent cognitive performance. High-intensity resistance training has shown to enhance memory and critical thinking while ameliorating the symptomatology of mood disorders [54]. Concomitantly, aerobic exercise prevented further cognitive deterioration in cases of mild cognitive impairment [55]. The advancement in understanding and implementing exercise in patients with underlying pathology has supplemented training programs for professional athletes with techniques to reinforce cognitive performance along with athletic [56]. Due to the great variety of sports, there are different requirements that presuppose the existence of individualized programs. Therefore, future studies could focus on specific groups of athletes and highlight personalized programs centered on sleep hygiene.

2.3. *Sleep Deprivation and Exercise: Cardiovascular Implications—The Example of Sleep Apnea*

Recent epidemiological studies have revealed relationships between sleep deprivation and hypertension, coronary heart disease, and diabetes mellitus due to increased activity of sympathetic system [57,58]. Obstructive sleep apnea–hypopnoea syndrome (OSAHS) is associated with increased cardiovascular morbidity and mortality. Subjects with OSAHS and no known cardiovascular disease had increased arterial stiffness and impaired endothelial function compared to controls [34] (Table 1). A brief, mild hypercapnic exposure increases vascular resistance in the renal and segmental arteries [32]. Sleep-disordered breathing, short sleep time, and low sleep quality are frequently reported by patients with heart failure (HF). Sleep-disordered breathing, which includes OSA and CSA, is common in patients with HF and has been suggested to increase the morbidity and mortality in these patients. Both OSA and CSA are associated with increased sympathetic activation, vagal withdrawal, altered hemodynamic loading conditions, and hypoxemia [59].

There are several parameters that describe the mechanism that leads to increased risk of cardiovascular impairment. Sleep-disordered breathing, such as in OSA, activates the sympathetic system and contributes to systemic inflammation, metabolic dysregulation, vascular endothelial dysfunction, and uncoupling of myocardial workload [5,7]. Moreover, high blood pressure and increased heart rate combined with increased oxygen demand, accompanying hypertension and dyslipidemia, lead to variety of cardiovascular diseases, such as atherosclerosis and even heart failure [5,7]. Chronic sleep deprivation is associated with increased risk of cardiometabolic disease (Figure 2). Laboratory studies demonstrate that sleep deprivation causes impaired whole-body insulin sensitivity and glucose disposal. Evidence suggests that inadequate sleep also impairs adipose tissue insulin sensitivity and the NEFA rebound during intravenous glucose-tolerance tests [60]. In addition, muscle recovery is hindered when athletes are sleep deprived through inflammatory exacerbation [61].

In conclusion, potential mechanisms of influence on quality and quantity of sleep may allow scientists to positively influence sleep in athletes and maximize their performance and health [41]. Exercise itself may result in a fundamental therapeutic approach, as preliminary data have shown that it restabilizes sleep architecture and quality [62]. In fact, some novel therapeutic strategies have emerged related to inspiratory muscle training. Inspiratory muscle strength training (IMT) has shown promising results in managing both sleep apneas and arterial hypertension [63,64]. Assessing and training inspiratory strength in athletes could prove beneficial in counteracting the detrimental effects of the aforementioned sleep disturbances [65].

2.4. Sleep Deprivation and Performance

Sleep optimization via sleep extension has been shown to enhance athletic performance and provide increased benefits regarding aerobic function and metabolism [66]. Beneficial effects attributed to longer sleep periods have also been observed in basketball [67], handball [68], and rugby players [69], among others. Aside from general aspects of health and performance, sleep optimization has shown to improve specific aspects of the athlete's performance, i.e., serve accuracy in tennis and stroke performance in swimming [42], as well as cognitive aspects [70], with a high dependency on the quality of sleep and its architecture [71]. Notably, sleep extension may be achieved by supplementing sleep with fixed naps, shown to significantly diminish sleep inertia and promote overall better performance [72].

Conversely, diminished sleep may be detrimental not only performance-wise but as a contributor to training and performance-related injuries [73]. A study in elite female football athletes has shown that there is significant inter-individual variability, and hence, personalized approaches in promoting sleep health should be adopted [74]. The latter concept can be generalized in several sports and with expert recommendations clearly advocating a case-based approach to sleep optimization [75].

3. Beneficial Sleep Effects

Sleep, in particular slow-wave sleep, is a restorative state that enables recovery from prior wakefulness and fatigue by repairing processes and repleting energy [76]. Sleep has also been shown to have a restorative effect on the immune system and the endocrine system, facilitate the recovery of the nervous system and metabolic cost of the waking state, and play an integral role in learning, memory and synaptic plasticity, all of which can impact both athletic recovery and performance [77]. Adequate sleep duration and consistency with its internal organization, namely four to ix NREM/REM cycles, each lasting approximately 90 to 110 min [78], as well as quality may be important for preventing cardiovascular diseases in modern society [58]. Even midday, short-term breaks of napping have been proved to be as valuable as extending nighttime sleep [79], in particular when combined with exercise [80]. Wakefulness results in an oxidative burden, and sleep provides a protective mechanism against these harmful effects [26].

4. Conclusions

Optimal sleep extends its benefits to all systems, exerting its main effect on cognition and the cardiovascular and respiratory system. Adequate sleep quality and quantity consist of the two components crucial for the effective human function and restitution. Conversely, sleep deprivation undermines these effects with significant declines in cognitive tasks and hindered cardiovascular adaptability and responses. It is possible that an extension of sleep duration could prevent these detrimental effects and enhance its efficient role.

Author Contributions: D.D.P., K.A., G.D.V., Z.D., K.I.G. and V.T.S. conceived and designed the review and wrote and edited the paper. All authors have read and agreed to the published version of the manuscript.

Funding: This research received no external funding.

Institutional Review Board Statement: Not applicable.

Informed Consent Statement: Not applicable.

Data Availability Statement: All data are available after request.

Conflicts of Interest: The authors declare no conflict of interest.

References

1. Patwa, A.; Shah, A. Anatomy and physiology of respiratory system relevant to anaesthesia. *Indian J. Anaesth.* **2015**, *59*, 533–541. [CrossRef] [PubMed]
2. Newton, K.; Malik, V.; Lee-Chiong, T. Sleep and breathing. *Clin. Chest Med.* **2014**, *35*, 451–456. [CrossRef]
3. Sowho, M.; Amatoury, J.; Kirkness, J.P.; Patil, S.P. Sleep and respiratory physiology in adults. *Clin. Chest Med.* **2014**, *35*, 469–481. [CrossRef] [PubMed]
4. Dutschmann, M.; Dick, T.E. Pontine mechanisms of respiratory control. *Comprehensive Physiol.* **2012**, *2*, 2443–2469.
5. Stavrou, V.T.; Astara, K.; Tourlakopoulos, K.N.; Papayianni, E.; Boutlas, S.; Vavougios, G.D.; Daniil, Z.; Gourgoulianis, K.I. Obstructive Sleep Apnea Syndrome: The Effect of Acute and Chronic Responses of Exercise. *Front. Med.* **2021**, *8*, 806924. [CrossRef] [PubMed]
6. Stavrou, V.T.; Astara, K.; Karetsi, E.; Daniil, Z.; Gourgoulianis, K.I. Respiratory Muscle Strength as an Indicator of the Severity of the Apnea-Hypopnea Index: Stepping Towards the Distinction between Sleep Apnea and Breath Holding. *Cureus* **2021**, *13*, e14015. [CrossRef]
7. Stavrou, V.; Bardaka, F.; Karetsi, E.; Daniil, Z.; Gourgoulianis, K.I. Brief Review: Ergospirometry in Patients with Obstructive Sleep Apnea Syndrome. *J. Clin. Med.* **2018**, *31*, 191. [CrossRef]
8. Iturriaga, R. Translating carotid body function into clinical medicine. *J. Physiol.* **2018**, *596*, 3067–3077. [CrossRef]
9. Yumino, D.; Bradley, T.D. Central sleep apnea and Cheyne-Stokes respiration. *Proc. Am. Thorac. Soc.* **2008**, *5*, 226–236. [CrossRef]
10. Halliwill, J.R.; Morgan, B.J.; Charkoudian, N. Peripheral chemoreflex and baroreflex interactions in cardiovascular regulation in humans. *J. Physiol.* **2003**, *552*, 295–302. [CrossRef]
11. Marcus, N.J.; Li, Y.L.; Bird, C.E.; Schultz, H.D.; Morgan, B.J. Chronic intermittent hypoxia augments chemoreflex control of sympathetic activity: Role of the angiotensin II type 1 receptor. *Respir. Physiol. Neurobiol.* **2010**, *171*, 36–45. [CrossRef] [PubMed]
12. Krimsky, W.R.; Leiter, J.C. Physiology of breathing and respiratory control during sleep. *Semin. Respir. Crit. Care Med.* **2005**, *26*, 5–12. [CrossRef] [PubMed]
13. Harris, C.D. Neurophysiology of sleep and wakefulness. *Respir. Care Clin. N. Am.* **2005**, *11*, 567–586. [PubMed]
14. Penzel, T.; Kantelhardt, J.W.; Lo, C.C.; Voigt, K.; Vogelmeier, C. Dynamics of heart rate and sleep stages in normals and patients with sleep apnea. *Neuropsychopharmacology* **2003**, *28* (Suppl. 1), S48–S53. [CrossRef]
15. Appelberg, J.; Pavlenko, T.; Bergman, H.; Rothen, H.U.; Hedenstierna, G. Lung aeration during sleep. *Chest* **2007**, *131*, 122–129. [CrossRef]
16. Krieger, J. Breathing during sleep in normal subjects. *Clin. Chest Med.* **1985**, *6*, 577–594. [CrossRef]
17. Benarroch, E.E. Control of the cardiovascular and respiratory systems during sleep. *Auton. Neurosci.* **2019**, *218*, 54–63. [CrossRef]
18. Giglio, P.; Lane, J.T.; Barkoukis, T.J.; Dumitru, I. CHAPTER 3-Sleep Physiology. In *Review of Sleep Medicine*, 2nd ed.; Barkoukis, T.J., Avidan, A.Y., Eds.; Butterworth-Heinemann: Philadelphia, PA, USA, 2007; pp. 29–41.
19. Han, F.; Chen, E.; Wei, H.; Ding, D.; He, Q. Influence of different sleep stages on respiratory regulation in normal humans. *Zhongguo Yi Xue Ke Xue Yuan Xue Bao* **2004**, *26*, 237–240.
20. Wirth, K.J.; Steinmeyer, K.; Ruetten, H. Sensitization of upper airway mechanoreceptors as a new pharmacologic principle to treat obstructive sleep apnea: Investigations with AVE0118 in anesthetized pigs. *Sleep* **2013**, *36*, 699–708. [CrossRef]
21. Brown, R.E.; Basheer, R.; McKenna, J.T.; Strecker, R.E.; McCarley, R.W. Control of sleep and wakefulness. *Physiol. Rev.* **2012**, *92*, 1087–1187. [CrossRef]
22. Van Eyck, A.; Van Hoorenbeeck, K.; De Winter, B.Y.; Ramet, J.; Van Gaal, L.; De Backer, W.; Verhulst, S.L. Sleep-disordered breathing and C-reactive protein in obese children and adolescents. *Sleep Breath.* **2014**, *18*, 335–340. [CrossRef]
23. Yoshihisa, A.; Takeishi, Y. Sleep Disordered Breathing and Cardiovascular Diseases. *J. Atheroscler. Thromb.* **2019**, *26*, 315–327. [CrossRef]
24. Cummins, E.P.; Keogh, C.E. Respiratory gases and the regulation of transcription. *Exp. Physiol.* **2016**, *101*, 986–1002. [CrossRef]
25. Plataki, M.; Sands, S.A.; Malhotra, A. Clinical consequences of altered chemoreflex control. *Respir. Physiol. Neurobiol.* **2013**, *189*, 354–363. [CrossRef] [PubMed]
26. Brown, M.K.; Naidoo, N. The UPR and the anti-oxidant response: Relevance to sleep and sleep loss. *Mol. Neurobiol.* **2010**, *42*, 103–113. [CrossRef]

27. Yun, A.J.; Lee, P.Y.; Bazar, K.A. Autonomic dysregulation as a basis of cardiovascular, endocrine, and inflammatory disturbances associated with obstructive sleep apnea and other conditions of chronic hypoxia, hypercapnia, and acidosis. *Med. Hypotheses* **2004**, *62*, 852–856.
28. Leproult, R.; Van Cauter, E. Role of sleep and sleep loss in hormonal release and metabolism. *Endocr Dev.* **2010**, *17*, 11–21. [PubMed]
29. Leproult, R.; Deliens, G.; Gilson, M.; Peigneux, P. Beneficial impact of sleep extension on fasting insulin sensitivity in adults with habitual sleep restriction. *Sleep* **2015**, *38*, 707–715. [CrossRef] [PubMed]
30. Wisor, J.P.; Clegern, W.C.; Schmidt, M.A. Toll-like receptor 4 is a regulator of monocyte and electroencephalographic responses to sleep loss. *Sleep* **2011**, *34*, 1335–1345. [CrossRef] [PubMed]
31. Shearer, W.T.; Reuben, J.M.; Mullington, J.M.; Price, N.J.; Lee, B.N.; Smith, E.O.; Szuba, M.P.; Van Dongen, H.P.; Dinges, D.F. Soluble TNF-alpha receptor 1 and IL-6 plasma levels in humans subjected to the sleep deprivation model of spaceflight. *J. Allergy Clin. Immunol.* **2001**, *107*, 165–170. [CrossRef]
32. Chapman, C.L.; Schlader, Z.J.; Reed, E.L.; Worley, M.L.; Johnson, B.D. Renal and segmental artery hemodynamic response to acute, mild hypercapnia. *Am. J. Physiol. Regul. Integr. Comp. Physiol.* **2020**, *318*, R822–R827. [CrossRef] [PubMed]
33. Lei, Y.; Shao, Y.; Wang, L.; Zhai, T.; Zou, F.; Ye, E.; Jin, X.; Li, W.; Qi, J.; Yang, Z. Large-Scale Brain Network Coupling Predicts Total Sleep Deprivation Effects on Cognitive Capacity. *PLoS ONE* **2015**, *10*, e0133959. [CrossRef] [PubMed]
34. Jones, A.; Vennelle, M.; Connell, M.; McKillop, G.; Newby, D.E.; Douglas, N.J.; Riha, R.L. Arterial stiffness and endothelial function in obstructive sleep apnoea/hypopnoea syndrome. *Sleep Med.* **2013**, *14*, 428–432. [CrossRef] [PubMed]
35. Robertson, M.D.; Russell-Jones, D.; Umpleby, A.M.; Dijk, D.-J. Effects of three weeks of mild sleep restriction implemented in the home environment on multiple metabolic and endocrine markers in healthy young men. *Metabolism* **2013**, *62*, 204–211. [CrossRef] [PubMed]
36. Astara, K.; Siachpazidou, D.; Vavougios, G.D.; Ragias, D.; Vatzia, K.; Rapti, G.; Alexopoulos, E.; Gourgoulianis, K.I.; Xiromerisiou, G. Sleep disordered breathing from preschool to early adult age and its neurocognitive complications: A preliminary report. *Sleep Sci.* **2021**, *14*, 140–149. [CrossRef]
37. Alhola, P.; Polo-Kantola, P. Sleep deprivation: Impact on cognitive performance. *Neuropsychiatr. Dis. Treat.* **2007**, *3*, 553–567.
38. Martella, D.; Plaza, V.; Estévez, A.F.; Castillo, A.; Fuentes, L.J. Minimizing sleep deprivation effects in healthy adults by differential outcomes. *Acta Psychol.* **2012**, *139*, 391–396. [CrossRef]
39. Pollicina, I.; Maniaci, A.; Lechien, J.R.; Iannella, G.; Vicini, C.; Cammaroto, G.; Cannavicci, A.; Magliulo, G.; Pace, A.; Cocuzza, S.; et al. Neurocognitive Performance Improvement after Obstructive Sleep Apnea Treatment: State of the Art. *Behav. Sci.* **2021**, *11*, 180. [CrossRef]
40. Roth, T. Effects of excessive daytime sleepiness and fatigue on overall health and cognitive function. *J. Clin. Psychiatry* **2015**, *76*, e1145. [CrossRef]
41. Stavrou, V.T.; Astara, K.; Tourlakopoulos, K.N.; Daniil, Z.; Gourgoulianis, K.I.; Kalabakas, K.; Karagiannis, D.; Basdekis, G. Sleep Quality's Effect on Vigilance and Perceptual Ability in Adolescent and Adult Athletes. *J. Sports Med.* **2021**, *2021*, 5585573. [CrossRef]
42. Vitale, K.C.; Owens, R.; Hopkins, S.R.; Malhotra, A. Sleep Hygiene for Optimizing Recovery in Athletes: Review and Recommendations. *Int. J. Sports Med.* **2019**, *40*, 535–543. [CrossRef]
43. Axelsson, J.; Ingre, M.; Kecklund, G.; Lekander, M.; Wright, K.P.; Sundelin, T. Sleepiness as motivation: A potential mechanism for how sleep deprivation affects behavior. *Sleep* **2020**, *43*, zsz291. [CrossRef]
44. VanHelder, T.; Radomski, M.W. Sleep deprivation and the effect on exercise performance. *Sports Med.* **1989**, *7*, 235–247. [CrossRef]
45. Fullagar, H.H.K.; Skorski, S.; Duffield, R.; Hammes, D.; Coutts, A.J.; Meyer, T. Sleep and athletic performance: The effects of sleep loss on exercise performance, and physiological and cognitive responses to exercise. *Sports Med.* **2015**, *45*, 161–186. [CrossRef] [PubMed]
46. Dijk, D.-J.; Landolt, H.-P. Sleep Physiology, Circadian Rhythms, Waking Performance and the Development of Sleep-Wake Therapeutics. *Handb. Exp. Pharmacol.* **2019**, *253*, 441–481. [PubMed]
47. Marvel, C.L.; Paradiso, S. Cognitive and neurological impairment in mood disorders. *Psychiatr. Clin. N. Am.* **2004**, *27*, 19–36. [CrossRef]
48. Pires, G.N.; Bezerra, A.G.; Tufik, S.; Andersen, M.L. Effects of acute sleep deprivation on state anxiety levels: A systematic review and meta-analysis. *Sleep Med.* **2016**, *24*, 109–118. [CrossRef]
49. Riemann, D.; Krone, L.B.; Wulff, K.; Nissen, C. Sleep, insomnia, and depression. *Neuropsychopharmacology* **2020**, *45*, 74–89. [CrossRef]
50. Franken, I.H.; van Strien, J.W.; Nijs, I.; Muris, P. Impulsivity is associated with behavioral decision-making deficits. *Psychiatry Res.* **2008**, *158*, 155–163. [CrossRef] [PubMed]
51. Strygin, K.N. Sleep and stress. *Ross Fiziol Zh Im I M Sechenova* **2011**, *97*, 422–432. [PubMed]
52. Kalmbach, D.A.; Anderson, J.R.; Drake, C.L. The impact of stress on sleep: Pathogenic sleep reactivity as a vulnerability to insomnia and circadian disorders. *J. Sleep Res.* **2018**, *27*, 12710. [CrossRef] [PubMed]
53. Kalmbach, D.A.; Cuamatzi-Castelan, A.S.; Tonnu, C.V.; Tran, K.M.; Anderson, J.R.; Roth, T.; Drake, C.L. Hyperarousal and sleep reactivity in insomnia: Current insights. *Nat. Sci. Sleep* **2018**, *10*, 193–201. [CrossRef]

54. MacQueen, G.M.; Memedovich, K.A. Cognitive dysfunction in major depression and bipolar disorder: Assessment and treatment options. *Psychiatry Clin. Neurosci.* **2017**, *71*, 18–27. [CrossRef] [PubMed]
55. Baker, L.D.; Frank, L.L.; Foster-Schubert, K.; Green, P.S.; Wilkinson, C.W.; McTiernan, A.; Plymate, S.R.; Fishel, M.A.; Watson, G.S.; Cholerton, B.A.; et al. Effects of aerobic exercise on mild cognitive impairment: A controlled trial. *Arch. Neurol.* **2010**, *67*, 71–79. [CrossRef] [PubMed]
56. Hernández-Mendo, A.; Reigal, R.E.; López-Walle, J.M.; Serpa, S.; Samdal, O.; Morales-Sánchez, V.; Juárez-Ruiz de Mier, R.; Tristán-Rodríguez, J.L.; Rosado, A.F.; Falco, C. Physical Activity, Sports Practice, and Cognitive Functioning: The Current Research Status. *Front. Psychol.* **2019**, *10*, 2658. [CrossRef] [PubMed]
57. Stavrou, V.; Boutou, A.K.; Vavougios, G.D.; Pastaka, C.; Gourgoulianis, K.I.; Koutedakis, Y.; Daniil, Z.; Karetsi, E. The use of cardiopulmonary exercise testing in identifying the presence of obstructive sleep apnea syndrome in patients with compatible symptomatology. *Respir. Physiol. Neurobiol.* **2019**, *262*, 26–31. [CrossRef]
58. Nagai, M.; Hoshide, S.; Kario, K. Sleep duration as a risk factor for cardiovascular disease- a review of the recent literature. *Curr. Cardiol. Rev.* **2010**, *6*, 54–61. [CrossRef]
59. Parati, G.; Lombardi, C.; Castagna, F.; Mattaliano, P.; Filardi, P.P.; Agostoni, P.; Italian Society of Cardiology (SIC); Working Group on Heart Failure members. Heart failure and sleep disorders. *Nat. Rev. Cardiol.* **2016**, *13*, 389–403. [CrossRef]
60. Ness, K.M.; Strayer, S.M.; Nahmod, N.G.; Schade, M.M.; Chang, A.M.; Shearer, G.C.; Buxton, O.M. Four nights of sleep restriction suppress the postprandial lipemic response and decrease satiety. *J. Lipid Res.* **2019**, *60*, 1935–1945. [CrossRef]
61. Dáttilo, M.; Antunes, H.K.M.; Galbes, N.M.N.; Mônico-Neto, M.; DE Sá Souza, H.; Dos Santos Quaresma, M.V.L.; Lee, K.S.; Ugrinowitsch, C.; Tufik, S.; DE Mello, M.T. Effects of Sleep Deprivation on Acute Skeletal Muscle Recovery after Exercise. *Med. Sci. Sports Exerc.* **2020**, *52*, 507–514. [CrossRef]
62. Alves, E.S.; Lira, F.S.; Santos, R.V.; Tufik, S.; de Mello, M.T. Obesity, diabetes and OSAS induce of sleep disorders: Exercise as therapy. *Lipids Health Dis.* **2011**, *23*, 148. [CrossRef] [PubMed]
63. Vranish, J.R.; Bailey, E.F. Inspiratory Muscle Training Improves Sleep and Mitigates Cardiovascular Dysfunction in Obstructive Sleep Apnea. *Sleep* **2016**, *39*, 1179–1185. [CrossRef] [PubMed]
64. Craighead, D.H.; Heinbockel, T.C.; Freeberg, K.A.; Rossman, M.J.; Jackman, R.A.; Jankowski, L.R.; Hamilton, M.N.; Ziemba, B.P.; Reisz, J.A.; D'Alessandro, A.; et al. Time-Efficient Inspiratory Muscle Strength Training Lowers Blood Pressure and Improves Endothelial Function, NO Bioavailability, and Oxidative Stress in Midlife/Older Adults With Above-Normal Blood Pressure. *J. Am. Heart Assoc.* **2021**, *10*, e020980. [CrossRef] [PubMed]
65. Stavrou, V.T.; Tourlakopoulos, K.N.; Daniil, Z.; Gourgoulianis, K.I. Respiratory Muscle Strength: New Technology for Easy Assessment. *Cureus* **2021**, *13*, e14803. [CrossRef] [PubMed]
66. Simpson, N.S.; Gibbs, E.L.; Matheson, G.O. Optimizing sleep to maximize performance: Implications and recommendations for elite athletes. *Scand. J. Med. Sci. Sports* **2017**, *27*, 266–274. [CrossRef] [PubMed]
67. Mah, C.D.; Mah, K.E.; Kezirian, E.J.; Dement, W.C. The effects of sleep extension on the athletic performance of collegiate basketball players. *Sleep* **2011**, *34*, 943–950. [CrossRef]
68. Nishida, M.; Yamamoto, K.; Murata, Y.; Ichinose, A.; Shioda, K. Exploring the Effect of Long Naps on Handball Performance and Heart Rate Variability. *Sports Med. Int. Open.* **2021**, *5*, E73–E80. [CrossRef]
69. Teece, A.R.; Argus, C.K.; Gill, N.; Beaven, M.; Dunican, I.C.; Driller, M.W. Sleep and Performance during a Preseason in Elite Rugby Union Athletes. *Int. J. Environ. Res. Public Health* **2021**, *18*, 4612. [CrossRef]
70. Lever, J.R.; Murphy, A.P.; Duffield, R.; Fullagar, H.H.K. A Combined Sleep Hygiene and Mindfulness Intervention to Improve Sleep and Well-Being during High-Performance Youth Tennis Tournaments. *Int. J. Sports Physiol. Perform.* **2020**, *16*, 250–258. [CrossRef]
71. Edinger, J.D.; Marsh, G.R.; McCall, W.V.; Erwin, C.W.; Lininger, A.W. Daytime functioning and nighttime sleep before, during, and after a 146-hour tennis match. *Sleep* **1990**, *13*, 526–532. [CrossRef]
72. Lastella, M.; Halson, S.L.; Vitale, J.A.; Memon, A.R.; Vincent, G.E. To Nap or Not to Nap? A Systematic Review Evaluating Napping Behavior in Athletes and the Impact on Various Measures of Athletic Performance. *Nat. Sci. Sleep* **2021**, *13*, 841–862. [CrossRef]
73. Haraldsdottir, K.; Sanfilippo, J.; McKay, L.; Watson, A.M. Decreased Sleep and Subjective Well-Being as Independent Predictors of Injury in Female Collegiate Volleyball Players. *Orthop. J. Sports Med.* **2021**, *9*, 23259671211029285. [CrossRef] [PubMed]
74. Costa, J.; Figueiredo, P.; Nakamura, F.; Rago, V.; Rebelo, A.; Brito, J. Intra-individual variability of sleep and nocturnal cardiac autonomic activity in elite female soccer players during an international tournament. *PLoS ONE* **2019**, *14*, e0218635. [CrossRef] [PubMed]
75. Walsh, N.P.; Halson, S.L.; Sargent, C.; Roach, G.D.; Nédélec, M.; Gupta, L.; Leeder, J.; Fullagar, H.H.; Coutts, A.J.; Edwards, B.J.; et al. Sleep and the athlete: Narrative review and 2021 expert consensus recommendations. *Br. J. Sports Med.* **2020**, *55*, 356–368. [CrossRef] [PubMed]
76. Halson, S.L.; Juliff, L.E. Sleep, sport, and the brain. *Prog. Brain Res.* **2017**, *234*, 13–31.
77. Doherty, R.; Madigan, S.; Warrington, G.; Ellis, J. Sleep and Nutrition Interactions: Implications for Athletes. *Nutrients* **2019**, *11*, 822. [CrossRef]
78. Luyster, F.S.; Strollo, P.J., Jr.; Zee, P.C.; Walsh, J.K. Boards of Directors of the American Academy of Sleep Medicine and the Sleep Research Society. Sleep: A health imperative. *Sleep* **2012**, *35*, 727–734. [CrossRef]

79. Vgontzas, A.N.; Pejovic, S.; Zoumakis, E.; Lin, H.M.; Bixler, E.O.; Basta, M.; Fang, J.; Sarrigiannidis, A.; Chrousos, G.P. Daytime napping after a night of sleep loss decreases sleepiness, improves performance, and causes beneficial changes in cortisol and interleukin-6 secretion. *Am. J. Physiol. Endocrinol. Metab.* **2007**, *292*, E253–E261. [CrossRef]
80. Mograss, M.; Crosetta, M.; Abi-Jaoude, J.; Frolova, E.; Robertson, E.M.; Pepin, V.; Dang-Vu, T.T. Exercising before a nap benefits memory better than napping or exercising alone. *Sleep* **2020**, *43*, zsaa062. [CrossRef]

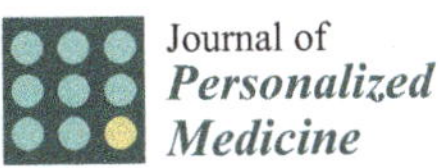
Journal of *Personalized Medicine*

MDPI

Review

Dental and Skeletal Side Effects of Oral Appliances Used for the Treatment of Obstructive Sleep Apnea and Snoring in Adult Patients—A Systematic Review and Meta-Analysis

Ioannis A. Tsolakis [1,*], Juan Martin Palomo [2], Stefanos Matthaios [2] and Apostolos I. Tsolakis [3]

1 Department of Orthodontics, School of Dentistry, Aristotle University of Thessaloniki, 541 24 Thessaloniki, Greece
2 Department of Orthodontics, Case Western Reserve University School of Dental Medicine, Cleveland, OH 44106, USA; palomo@case.edu (J.M.P.); stefmattheos@hotmail.com (S.M.)
3 Department of Orthodontics, School of Dentistry, National and Kapodistrian, University of Athens, 157 72 Athens, Greece; apostso@otenet.gr
* Correspondence: tsolakisioannis@gmail.com

Abstract: Background: Mandibular advancement devices for obstructive sleep apnea treatment are becoming increasingly popular among patients who do not prefer CPAP devices or surgery. Our study aims to evaluate the literature regarding potential dental and skeletal side effects caused by mandibular advancement appliances used for adult OSA treatment. Methods: Electronic databases were searched for published and unpublished literature along with the reference lists of the eligible studies. Randomized clinical trials and non-randomized trials assessing dental and skeletal changes by comparing cephalometric radiographs were selected. Study selection, data extraction, and risk of bias assessment were performed individually and in duplicate. Fourteen articles were finally selected (two randomized clinical trials and 12 non-randomized trials). Results: The results suggest that mandibular advancement devices used for OSA treatment increase the lower incisor proclination by $1.54 \pm 0.16°$, decrease overjet by 0.89 ± 0.04 mm and overbite by 0.68 ± 0.04 mm, rotate the mandible downward and forward, and increase the SNA angle by to $0.06 \pm 0.03°$. The meta-analysis revealed high statistical heterogeneity. Conclusions: The MADs affect the lower incisor proclination, overjet, overbite, the rotation of the mandible and the SNA angle. More randomized clinical trials providing high-quality evidence are needed to support those findings.

Keywords: mandibular advancement devices (MADs); obstructive sleep apnea (OSA); dental effects; skeletal effects; adults

Citation: Tsolakis, I.A.; Palomo, J.M.; Matthaios, S.; Tsolakis, A.I. Dental and Skeletal Side Effects of Oral Appliances Used for the Treatment of Obstructive Sleep Apnea and Snoring in Adult Patients—A Systematic Review and Meta-Analysis. *J. Pers. Med.* **2022**, *12*, 483. https://doi.org/10.3390/jpm12030483

Academic Editor: Ioannis Pantazopoulos

Received: 25 February 2022
Accepted: 14 March 2022
Published: 16 March 2022

1. Introduction

Obstructive sleep apnea syndrome (OSAS) is a sleep breathing disorder characterized by a periodic collapse of the upper airway during sleep. OSAS is diagnosed when there are five or more obstructive respiratory events per hour of sleep and signs/symptoms (i.e., snoring, and daytime sleepiness) or related medical/psychiatric disorders (i.e., hypertension). A sleep breathing disorder can also be considered as obstructive sleep apnea when 15 or more respiratory events occur in an hour of sleep without any signs/symptoms or disorders [1]. Although snoring is its primary symptom, some patients have less than five respiratory events per hour of sleep, and thus they are considered non-apnoeic snorers [2]. Respiratory events include obstructive and mixed apneas, hypopneas, and respiratory effort-related arousals, according to the American Academy of Sleep Medicine (AASM).

OSAS prevalence is high in adults, as it is thought to affect 14% of men and 5% of women. Its consequences, such as cardiovascular conditions, neurocognitive and mental health problems, decrease patients' quality of life and can be lethal in some cases [3–6].

OSAS therapies include conservative measures (i.e., weight loss, better sleeping position, and alcohol avoidance), upper airway surgery, nasal continuous positive airway pressure (CPAP), and oral appliances [6]. Although CPAP, a device that continuously pressures the upper airway and prevents its collapse during sleep, is considered the gold standard for obstructive sleep apnea (OSA) treatment, oral appliances can be used as an alternative, and are often preferred by the patients. Oral appliances (OAs) are also proposed for apnoeic patients with intolerance to CPAP or non-apnoeic snorers who have failed conservative lifestyle changes (i.e., weight loss) [7].

Nearly 100 different oral appliances are currently available, and they can be divided into three main groups: mandibular advancement devices (MADs), tongue retaining devices (TRD), and soft palate lifting devices. All of them intend to maintain the airway open, preventing its collapse. MADs which are the most commonly used, advance the mandible in order to increase the airway space and reduce pharyngeal collapsibility [8].

Custom, titratable MADs are the most effective OAs for OSAS and snoring, according to the AASM. These MADs can reduce the apnea-hypopnea index (AHI), oxygen desaturation, arousal index, and increase oxygen saturation, although to a lower extent than CPAP in patients with OSAS. On the other hand, they have equivalent effectiveness compared with CPAP in the reduction in daytime sleepiness and hypertension and quality of life improvement. Furthermore, they have greater device adherence and less possibility of treatment discontinuation due to side effects (odds ratio of discontinuation of treatment due to the use of an OA vs. CPAP: 0.54:1). These oral appliances can also be useful in primary snoring, as they improve sleep quality and quality of life (QOL) and reduce snoring frequency and intensity [9,10].

In the past decades, many studies have examined the adverse effects of oral appliance use in OSAS/snoring treatment. These include subjective side effects, such as mouth dryness and temporomandibular dysfunction, examined through questionnaires and objective side effects assessed by dental casts and cephalometric analysis [11,12].

To our knowledge, there are some literature reviews, assessing the dental and skeletal side effects of mandibular protruding devices for the treatment of adult obstructive sleep apnea and snoring. In 2004, Hoekema et al. stated that there were predominantly occlusal changes, but they could not conclude about long term side effects [13]. More recently, Araie et al. (2018) found significant dental changes, regarding overjet and overbite decrease and lower incisor axis-mandibular plane angle (L1-MP) increase, but no skeletal changes [14]. Patel et al. (2019) also reported that there was a significant reduction in overjet and overbite [15]. On the other hand, Bartolucci et al. (2019) were the first to report significant skeletal changes in point A-nasion-point B angle (ANB) and anterior facial height, except for dental changes in overjet, overbite, and incisor inclination [16]. Moreover, Mendes Martins et al. (2019) concluded that there were mainly long-term dental changes. The treatment duration and the population sample in some of the included studies for these reviews were small [17]. Furthermore, a cephalometric analysis, for assessing skeletal changes was not performed in all their included studies. A cephalometric analysis is based on the lateral X-ray tracing anatomic landmarks. The angles of these anatomic landmarks can conclude in valuable and accurate information for the skeletal and dental changes. Some of the most important landmarks for this research are the SNA angle that refers to the relationship of maxilla to the cranial base, the SNB angle that reveals the relationship of mandible to the cranial base, the ANB that refers to the relationship between maxilla and mandible, and the L1-MP angle that refers to the angulation of the lower incisors to the mandibular plane.

Our study aims to systematically review the most up-to-date scientific literature related with dental and skeletal changes caused by mandibular advancement devices used for the adult OSAS/snoring treatment, and perform a meta-analysis, in order to strengthen the current knowledge and help sleep physicians and qualified dentists/orthodontists to improve treatment's efficacy and prevent discontinuation due to side effects.

2. Materials and Methods

2.1. Protocol and Registration

The protocol for this present systematic review was registered on the National Institute of Health Research Database (Protocol: CRD42020169736).

2.2. Eligibility Criteria

The following selection criteria were applied for the review:

1. Study design: randomized clinical trials (RCTs), quasi-randomized clinical trials, and non-randomized prospective and retrospective trials (non-RCTs), without any restriction in language and time of publication, were considered eligible for inclusion in this review;
2. Participants: adult patients with obstructive sleep apnea syndrome or snoring;
3. Interventions: studies that treated obstructive sleep apnea and/or snoring patients with an oral appliance that protruded the mandible forward;
4. Comparisons: comparisons were made between baseline and follow-up patient characteristics;
5. Outcomes measures: any objective dental and skeletal change, in the treated patients.

2.3. Information Sources, Search Strategy and Study Selection

A literature search was carried out in the following electronic databases: Medline database (via PubMed), Embase (via Ovid), Scopus, CENTRAL, Google Scholar, and the Cochrane Oral Health Group's Trial Register. Language restrictions were not applied. Unpublished literature was searched on ClinicalTrials.gov (accessed on 24 February 2022) and the National Research Register. The Medical Subject Heading (MeSH) terms used for this study were "sleep apnea syndromes", "adverse effects", "jaw", and "tooth". Conference proceedings and abstracts were also accessed when possible. The authors were contacted to identify unpublished or ongoing clinical trials and to clarify data as required. Reference lists of the included studies were screened for relevant research. Finally, hand-searching was performed. The search strategy for PubMed is presented in Table 1.

Table 1. The search strategy for PubMed. Abbreviations: Mesh—Medical Subject Headings.

(("Sleep Apnea Syndromes"(Mesh)) AND "adverse effects" (Subheading))	2163 results
((("Sleep Apnea Syndromes" (Mesh)) AND "adverse effects" (Subheading)) AND "Jaw" (Mesh))	94 results
(("Sleep Apnea Syndromes" (Mesh)) AND "Jaw" (Mesh) AND "Tooth" (Mesh))	33 results
(((("Sleep Apnea Syndromes" (Mesh)) AND "adverse effects" (Subheading)) AND "Jaw" (Mesh)) AND "Tooth" (Mesh))	7 results

Studies were selected independently and in duplicate by two authors (I.A.T., S.M.). Any inconsistencies were resolved by discussion with the other two authors (J.M.P., A.I.T.). They were not blinded while identifying the authors of the studies, their institutions, or their research findings. After the identification of potentially relevant studies by title, abstracts were read, and non-eligible studies were eliminated. After this stage, hand-searching of the references of the eligible studies was performed to find additional articles, which were not previously found. Finally, after reading the articles in full, the choice was made according to our inclusion and exclusion criteria (Table 2).

Table 2. Inclusion and exclusion criteria.

Inclusion Criteria	Exclusion Criteria
Studies that refer to oral appliance use for the treatment of OSA/snoring and its side effects in occlusion and skeletal tissues.	Studies that refer to non-specific side effects of oral appliance use or treatment of OSA/snoring, such as tooth discomfort and increased salivation.
RCTs, non-randomized trials (prospective or retrospective).	Studies that refer to side effects of oral appliance use for other reasons, than to treat OSA/snoring.
Studies in humans.	Case reports, case series, reviews, guidelines, and authors' opinion.
Studies in adults with sufficient number of teeth to retain the oral appliance.	

2.4. Data Items and Collection Extraction and Management

Two review authors (I.A.T., S.M.) performed data extraction independently and in duplicate. The information that was extracted included participants, intervention/appliance, treatment duration/observational period, outcomes, methods of outcome assessment, results, and conclusions. In case of no access to the missing data, only the existing data were reported and analyzed.

2.5. Risk of Bias/Quality Assessment in Individual Studies

The quality assessment of the included studies was performed using the ACROBAT-NRSI tool of Cochrane for non-randomized clinical trials and the Cochrane handbook for systematic reviews (chapter 8) for randomized clinical trials. Two review authors (I.A.T., S.M.) assessed the articles individually and then compared their findings. Any disagreements were resolved by discussion with the other two authors (J.M.P., A.I.T.). Regarding the randomized clinical trials, seven domains of bias were assessed: random sequence generation, allocation concealment, performance bias, detection bias, attrition bias, bias due to selective outcome reporting, and other sources of bias. A judgment of 'low', 'high', or 'unclear' risk of bias was made for each domain, while a final overall judgment was assessed based on the following:

1. Low risk of bias if all key domains of the study were at low risk of bias;
2. Unclear risk of bias if one or more key domains of the study were unclear;
3. High risk of bias if one or more key domains were at high risk of bias.

Concerning the non-randomized trials, bias due to confounding, bias in the selection of participants, bias in the measurement of interventions, bias due to departures from intended interventions, bias due to missing data, bias in the measurement of outcomes, and bias in the selection of the reported result were assessed for the qualitative evaluation of the study. Possible results for each domain and hence the overall evaluation of each study was: 'low', 'moderate', 'serious' risk of bias, and 'no information'. We used the GRADE approach to interpret the results of this review.

2.6. Additional Analyses

Meta-analyses were undertaken using individual results on the change from the baseline in the parameters under study. They were summarized over all studies providing appropriate statistics (i.e., standard error/deviation for the change or p-value from a parametric test) using fixed or random-effects meta-analysis. Heterogeneity between studies was assessed using I2, and in the presence of significant heterogeneity, a random-effects model was used [18]. Stata command, metan, in Stata v13 was used for the analysis (StataCorp. 2013. Stata Statistical Software: Release 13. College Station, TX, USA: StataCorp LP).

3. Results

3.1. Study Selection and Characteristics

Our search resulted in 2297 articles. After title and abstract reading, irrelevant articles and duplicates were excluded, and 155 articles were read in full. Finally, 14 articles were selected for final analysis (two RCTs and 12 non-RCTs), based on our inclusion/exclusion criteria (Table 1) [19–32]. The procedure of article selection is presented on a flow diagram (Figure 1), and data are briefly presented in Table 3.

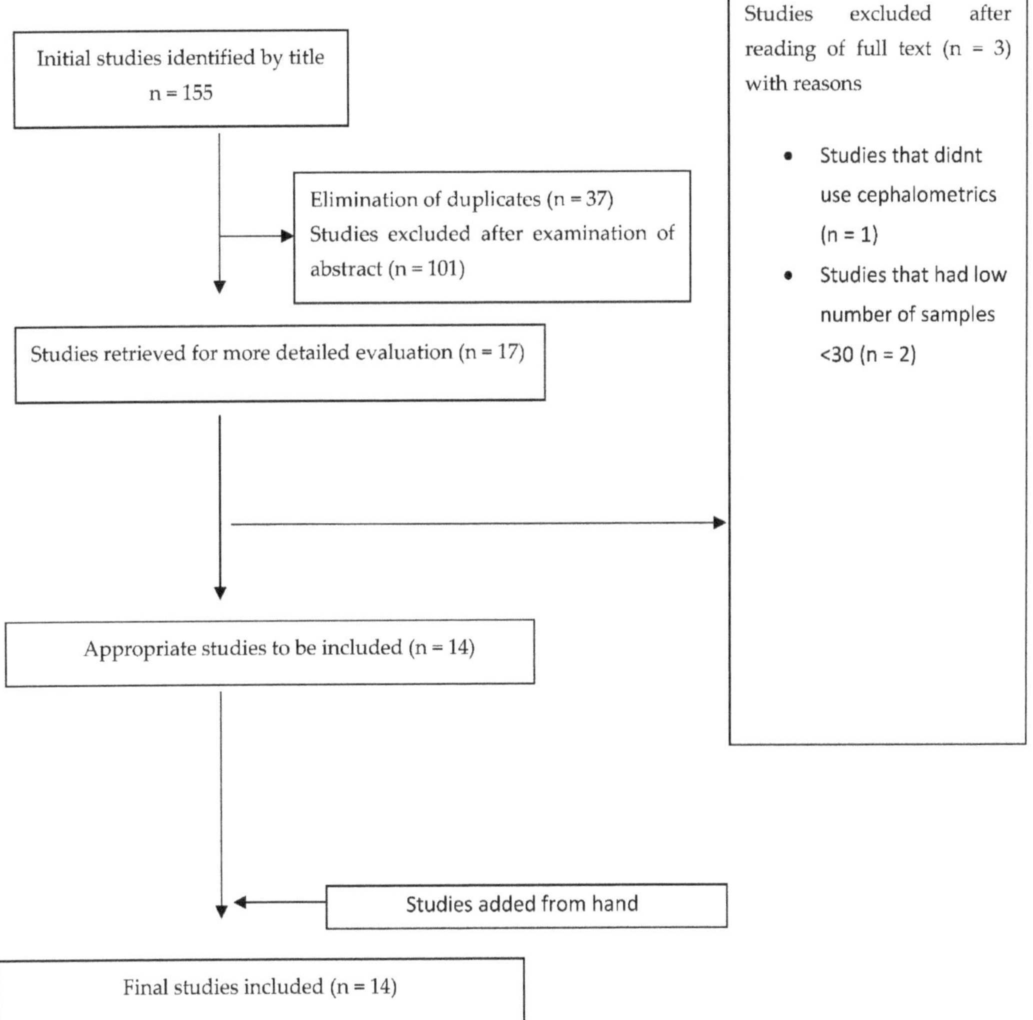

Figure 1. Flow diagram, selection of studies.

Table 3. Data extraction.

Authors/ Publication Year	Study Design	Participants (Number-Age-Gender-AHI)	Intervention/Appliance	Treatment Duration/ Observational Period	Outcomes	Method of Outcome Assessment	Results	Conclusion
Bondemark [19] (1999)	Prospective	30 obstructive sleep apnea (OSA)/snoring patients (21 males (M), 9 females (F), mean age 55.3 ± 8.61 months)	Monobloc acrylic mandibular advancement splint, with 8 posterior stainless steel caps and full tooth coverage	2 years (y)	• Sagittal and vertical, dental, and skeletal measurements • Mandibular length measurements • Angle measurements	Baseline and follow-up cephalometric radiographs	• Decreased overjet (OJ) and overbite (OB) • Increased sella-nasion-pointB angle (SNB), mandibular plane to cranial base angle (ML/NSL) and decreased pointA-nasion-pointB angle (ANB) • Increased mandibular length and more forward and downward mandibular position • Forward mandibular movement correlated with mandibular length change and SNB	Forward and downward change in mandibular position, due to increase in mandibular length
Robertson [20] (2001)	Prospective	100 OSA/snoring patients (87M, 13F, mean age 49 ± 8.5 years)	Non-adjustable mandibular advancement splint with full tooth coverage	6–30 months (6 months intervals)	• Dentoalveolar and skeletal measurements	Baseline and follow-up cephalometric radiographs	• Increased sella-nasion-pointA angle (SNA), ANB, anterior nasal spine to posterior nasal spine distance (ANS-PNS), vertical condylar position relative to cranial base (Cd-vert), lower and total anterior and posterior facial height • Decrease in OJ and OB • Decreased angle of upper incisor axis to anterior nasal spine/posterior nasal spine line (Ui/ANS-PNS) (palatal tipping) and increased angle of lower incisor axis to mandibular plane (Li/Me-Go) (labial tipping) • Changes over time	Mainly minor skeletal and dental changes
Fransson et al. [21]. (2002)	Prospective	65 patients (52M, 13F, mean age 54.8 ± 9.0 years, 44 OSA, 21 snoring)	Monobloc heat-cured methyl methacrylate mandibular protruding device with 4 metal caps for molars and full tooth coverage	2 years	• Dentofacial measurements • Pharyngeal measurements	Baseline and follow-up cephalometric radiographs	• Increased cranial base to occlusal plane SN/OL, anterior facial height and decreased SNB • Increased lower incisor axis to mandibular line angle (ILi/ML) (proclination of lower incisors) • Increased distance between the hyoid bone, maxilla (hy-NL) and mandible (hy-ML)	Posterior rotation of the mandible and proclination of mandibular incisors

Table 3. *Cont.*

Authors/ Publication Year	Study Design	Participants (Number-Age-Gender-AHI)	Intervention/Appliance	Treatment Duration/ Observational Period	Outcomes	Method of Outcome Assessment	Results	Conclusion
Rose et al. [22] (2002)	Retrospective	34 mild–moderate OSA patients (mean age 52.9 ± 9.6 years, mean body mass index (BMI) 28.6 ± 4.2 kg/m^2)	Mandibular advancement device (MAD) consisted of 2 hard acrylic plates joined by U-shaped clasps (Karwwetzky U-clasp activator)	29.6 ± 5.1 months	• Dentofacial cephalometric measurements • Dental cast analysis	Baseline and follow-up dental casts and cephalometric radiographs	• OJ and OB decrease • Is-SN decrease (retroclination of upper incisors) • Ii-Me-Go increase (proclination of lower incisors) • Dental cast analysis • Decrease in OJ, OB, posterior OB (bilaterally), molar relationship (bilaterally) • Increase in anterior arch length and overlaps/spaces reduction	Incisor inclination and mesial shift of the occlusion
Robertson et al. [23] (2003)	Longitudinal, observational study	100 OSA/snoring patients (87M, 13F, mean age 49 ± 8.5 years)	Non-adjustable mandibular advancement splint ith full tooth coverage	6–30 months (6 months intervals)	• Dentoalveolar skeletal measurements	Baseline and follow-up cephalometric radiographs	Combined group: increase in SNA, ANB, anterior facial height, posterior and mainly in lower facial height, maxillary length, vertical mandibular position. Mandibular first molars and maxillary first premolars overeruption, retroclination of upper incisors and proclination of lower incisors, reduction in OJ, OB and maxillary arch length. Positive correlation between device advancement and ANB angle. 6 months: facial height increase, downward mandibular position, OJ and OB decrease 12 months: vertical mandibular position increase 18 months: total and lower facial height increase, vertical mandibular position, OJ and OB decrease 24 months: increase in facial height, SNA, vertical mandibular position. Over-eruption of mandibular first molars and maxillary premolars and proclination of mandibular incisors 30 months: proclination of mandibular incisors, OJ and OB decrease. Reduced lower facial height compared with 18 and 24 months. Positive correlation of MAD anterior opening and OB change.	Changes in facial height, overjet, overbite, and position of the mandible even before 6 months of device use. Over-eruption of upper first premolars and lower first molars and proclination of lower incisors occurred after 2 years of device use. Overbite changes might be decreased by keeping a minimum bite opening

Table 3. *Cont.*

Authors/ Publication Year	Study Design	Participants (Number-Age-Gender-AHI)	Intervention/Appliance	Treatment Duration/ Observational Period	Outcomes	Method of Outcome Assessment	Results	Conclusion
Ringqvist [24] (2003)	Randomized clinical trial	45 OSA patients treated with MAD (mean age 48.9 years, mean weight 87.8 kg, mean BMI 27.0 kg/m^2) 43 OSA patients treated with uvu-lopalatopharungo-plasty (UPPP): mean age 51 years, mean weight 87.8 kg, mean BMI 27.1 kg/m^2	MAD was a mono-bloc device consisted of heat-cured methyl methacrylate.	MAD patients (4.1 years, 30 patients completed the follow-up and 27 were only treated with MAD) UPPP patients (4.3 years, 37 completed the follow-up and 27 were only treated with UPPP)	O1: MAD group dental and skeletal measurements O2: UPPP group dental and skeletal measurements	Lateral cephalometric radiographs with the patient in supine position.	O1: • Significant alterations in horizontal (Is-NSL) and vertical upper incisor position (Is-ML), and in horizontal position of lower incisors (Ii-NSL) • No significant changes in overjet, overbite, and mandibular length • Significant change in horizontal position (B-B′) and inclination of the mandible (ML-NSL) • Increase in the Is-NSL, Is-ML and Ii-NSL distances was correlated with an increased angle ML/NSL O2: • Significant increase in Ii-NSL	Minor dental and skeletal changes after 4 years of MAD use. No clinically important differences between MAD and UPPP groups
Hou et al. [25] (2006)	Prospective	67 Chinese OSA patients (50M, 17F, mean age 46.9 ± 8.9 years)	modified Harvold monobloc type of functional appliance	1–3 years 1 year: $n = 63$ 2 years: $n = 43$ 3 years: $n = 30$	• Dental and skeletal measurements	Baseline and follow-up cephalometric radiographs	• Increased mandibular plane to cranial base angle (MnPl/SN) • Increased lower (LFH) and total anterior and posterior facial height (TFH) • Decreased OJ and OB • Changes over time	Small dentofacial changes and main OJ and OB reduction during early treatment
Almeida et al. [26] (2006)	Retrospective	71 OSA patients (63M, 8F, mean age 49.7 ± 9.7 years, respiratory disturbance index 28.9 ± 17.0/h, BMI 29.3 ± 5.9 kg/m^2)	Klearway oral appliance	7.3 ± 2.1 years on average	• Dental, skeletal, and upper airway measurements • Changes over time	Baseline and follow-up cephalometric radiographs	• Decreased upper incisor (U1-SN and U1-PP) and upper molar inclination (U6-SN and U6-PP), upper to lower molar distance projected to cranial base (U6-L6-SN), OJ, and OB • Increased L1-MP, lower molar to mandibular plane angle (L6-MP), cranial base to mandibular plane angle (SN-MP) and palatal plane to mandibular plane angle (PP-MP), maxillary molar height (MXMH) and mandibular molar height (MDMH), ANB, LFH and TFH • Changes according to baseline Angle classification • Changes according to baseline OB • Correlations	Craniofacial and dental changes occur after long-term OA use

Table 3. *Cont.*

Authors/ Publication Year	Study Design	Participants (Number-Age-Gender-AHI)	Intervention/Appliance	Treatment Duration/ Observational Period	Outcomes	Method of Outcome Assessment	Results	Conclusion
Hammond et al. [27] (2007)	Retrospective	64 OSA patients (50M, 14F)	2-piece acrylic appliance with full occlusal coverage and a screw that titrates the device (Mehta et al.)	25.1 ± 11.8 months on average	• Dental, skeletal, and anthropometric measurements • Subjective side effects and satisfaction with the oral appliance	Baseline and follow-up cephalometric radiographs, study model analysis and anthropometric measurements Questionnaire	Cephalometric analysis on 46 patients (34M, 12F): • Sagittal changes: vertical upper incisor position (ii-OLp: mean 0.52 mm), vertical lower incisor position (mi-OLP: mean 0.26 mm) • Increased upper incisor to cranial base angle (ii/MP: mean 0.96°) • Decreased interincisal angle (ii/is: mean −1.69°), and upper incisor to occlusal plane angle (ii/OL: mean −1.02°)	Minor dental and skeletal side effects
Doff et al. [28] (2010)	Randomized clinical trial	103 OSA patients (51 with MAD)	Thorton Adjustable positioner	2.3 ± 0.2 years on average	• Dental and skeletal measurements	Baseline and follow-up cephalometric radiographs	• Decreased OJ, OB, SNB, upper incisor to palatal plane angle, interincisal angle, and anterior facial height ratio • Increased ANB, lower incisor to mandibular plane angle, LFH and TFH • Downward and backward rotation of the mandible • Decreased shortest linear distance menton line SN-perpendicular (Me-hor) and increased shortest linear distance menton line SN	Mainly dental changes
Wang et al. [29] (2015)	Prospective	42 patients OSA patients (31M, 11F, mean age 47 ± 10 years, mean AHI 27 ± 19)	Silensor appliance	4 ± 3 years on average	• Dental and skeletal measurements • Changes over time • Subjective side effects	Questionnaire and baseline and follow-up cephalometric radiographs	• Decreased OJ, OB, U1-SN and upper incisor axis to nasion-pointA line (U1-NA) angle, U1-NA distance • Increased L1-MP and lower incisor to nasion-pointB line (L1-NB) angle, mandibular plane to Franfort horizontal plane, anterior LFH and TFH • Changes prior to and over 3 years of treatment • Reduction in most subjective side effects at follow-up	Minor dental and skeletal side effects (1–3 years of treatment mainly skeletal changes, after 3 years of treatment dental and skeletal changes)

Table 3. *Cont.*

Authors/ Publication Year	Study Design	Participants (Number-Age-Gender-AHI)	Intervention/Appliance	Treatment Duration/ Observational Period	Outcomes	Method of Outcome Assessment	Results	Conclusion
Minagi et al. [30] (2018)	Retrospective	64 OSA patients (44M, 20F, mean age 57.7 ± 14.2 years, mean BMI 23.9 ± 3.6 kg/m^2, mean apnea-hypopnea index (AHI) 24.9 ± 14.7	Mad consisted of two separate acrylic monoblock modified plates (ERKODRNT)	4.3 ± 2.1 years on average	• Dental and skeletal measurements • Rate of changes • Predictors of changes	Baseline and follow-up cephalometric radiographs	• Decreased OJ, OB and L1-MP angle • Great OJ decrease (≥1 mm) correlated with treatment duration, MAD use frequency and mandibular advancement rate. • Weak negative correlation between total number of teeth and decrease in OJ • Weak negative correlation between maxillary teeth and decrease in OJ	Dental side effects (low number of maxillary teeth and MAD treatment duration, use frequency and mandibular advancement correlated with OJ reduction)
Hamoda et al. [31] (2018)	Retrospective	62 patients with primary snoring or mild to severe OSA (52M, 10F, mean age 49 ± 8.6 years, mean BMI 29.1 ± 6.9 kg/m^2, mean AHI 30.0 ± 14.6 for 56 patients, Angle Class I/Class II/ Class III 31/26/4)	Klearway® or SomnoDent®	12.6 ± 3.9 years on average	• Dental and skeletal measurements • Rate of changes • Predictors of changes	Baseline and follow-up cephalometric radiographs (up to 9 cephalometric radiographs for some patients)	• Decreased OJ, OB and L1-MP angle • Greater OJ decrease (≥1 mm) correlated with treatment duration, MAD use frequency and mandibular advancement rate. • Upper incisor retroclination (U1-SN, U1-PP, U1-NA) with constant rate over the years (U1-SN reduction of 0.49°/year) • Lower incisor proclination (L1-NB, L1-MP) with declining and not constant rate over the years • Minor posterior and downward mandibular movement (decrease: in SNB 0.7° with a constant rate of 0.05°/year and mean ANB reduction of 0.43° and mean increase in: mandibular plane to Frankfort horizontal plane angle (MPFH) 1.1° and in cranial base to gonion-gnathion line angle (SNGoGn) 0.9°) • Treatment duration correlated with all the cephalometric variables that changed • Greater baseline BMI correlated with greater upper incisor retroclination and higher baseline ANB angle with greater mandibular incisor proclination	Dental changes happen progressively and duration of mandibular advancement device treatment is the greatest factor of their magnitude Minor skeletal changes that occur are not clinically significant
Fransson et al. [32] (2020)	Prospective	65 patients (52M, 13F, mean age 54.8 ± 9.0 years, 44 OSA, 21 snoring)	Monobloc heat-cured methyl methacrylate mandibular protruding device with 4 metal caps for molars and full tooth coverage	10 years	• Dentofacial measurements • Pharyngeal measurements	Baseline and follow-up cephalometric radiographs	• Increased SN/OL, SN/ML, anterior facial height and decreased SNB • Increased ILi/ML (proclination of lower incisors) • Increased distance between the hyoid bone, maxilla (hy-NL) and mandible (hy-ML)	Posterior rotation of the mandible and proclination of mandibular incisors

3.2. Risk of Bias within Studies

The seven criteria for the RCT bias assessment were random sequence generation, allocation concealment, performance bias, detection bias, attrition bias, selective reporting, and additional bias. One of the RCTs presented low risk of bias in all seven criteria, while the other study presented serious risk of bias due to random sequence generation, allocation concealment, attrition bias, and additional bias (Table 4).

The seven criteria for the non-RCT studies were: bias due to confounding, bias in the selection participants into the study, bias in the measurement of interventions, bias due to departures from intended interventions, bias due to missing data, bias in measurement outcomes and bias in the selection of the reported result. Seven studies presented a low risk of bias. None of the 12 studies showed bias in the selection of the reported result. One study presented a serious risk of bias due to confounding and in the measurement of intervention, while two studies presented a serious risk of bias due to confounding, in the selection of participants, in the measurement of intervention and the measurement of outcomes. Another study showed a serious risk of bias. Finally, one study presented bias in the selection of participants and the measurement of outcomes. Another study showed a serious risk of bias in five out of seven criteria. This study presented a serious risk of bias: due to confounding, in the selection of participants, in the measurement of intervention, due to missing data and in the measurement of outcomes (Table 5).

3.3. Results of Meta-Analysis

A meta-analysis was performed for the outcomes of sella-nasion-pointA angle (SNA), sella-nasion-pointB angle (SNB), ANB angle, overjet, overbite, and L1-MP angle. (Table 6) There was no significant heterogeneity in SNA results (I2 = 14.8%, $p = 0.31$). An overall statistically significant positive change from baseline was found in SNA when studies were combined: 0.06 with 95% confidence interval (CI) (0.007, 0.116) (Figure 2). The SNB results were heterogeneous (I2 = 90.8%, $p < 0.001$). Overall estimated change from baseline in SNB was not statistically significant ($p = 0.436$): −0.099 with 95% CI (−0.347, 0.150) (Figure 3). Furthermore, the ANB results were heterogeneous (I2 = 82.2%, $p < 0.001$). Overall estimated change from baseline in ANB was not statistically significant ($p = 0.360$): 0.09 with 95% CI (−0.107, 0.296) (Figure 4). Overjet results were also heterogeneous (I2 = 94.5%, $p < 0.001$). An overall statistically significant decrease compared with baseline was found in overjet when studies were combined: −0.89 with 95% CI (−1.334, −0.459) (Figure 5). Overbite results were also heterogeneous (I2 = 93.3%, $p < 0.001$). An overall statistically significant decrease compared with baseline was found in overjet when studies were combined: −0.68 with 95% CI (−1.016, −0.344) (Figure 6). Finally, heterogeneity was found in L1-MP, between studies (I2 = 96.9%, $p < 0.001$). An overall positive and statistically significant change from baseline was found in L1-MP when studies were combined: 2.97 with 95% CI (0.993, 4.954) (Figure 7).

Table 4. Risk of bias assessment for randomized clinical trials. Abbreviations: CPAP—continuous positive airway pressure, MAD(s)—mandibular advancement device(s), UPPP—uvulopalatopharyngoplasty.

Author (Year)	Outcomes	Random Sequence Generation	Allocation Concealment	Performance Bias	Detection Bias	Attrition Bias	Selective Reporting	Other	Overall
Ringqvist et al. [24] (2003)	O1: dental and skeletal measurements on MAD patients O2: dental and skeletal measurements on UPPP patients	Unclear for all outcomes ('... 45 were randomly assigned to treatment with the mandibular advancement device (MAD) group and 43 to treatment with UPPP') not possible to conclude if randomization was successful	Unclear for all outcomes (not mentioned concealment of allocation, probably not performed)	Low for all outcomes (not mentioned blinding of participants/personnel but the outcome is not likely to be affected)	Unclear for all outcomes (blinding of outcome assessor is not mentioned)	High for all outcomes (patients that did not attend the 4-year follow-up were 15 in the MAD group and 6 in the UPPP group)	Low for all outcomes (all pre-specified variables were measured)	High for all outcomes (patients received both treatments, 3 patients in the MAD group and 10 in the UPPP group)	High for all outcomes (patients not attending the follow-up and patients receiving both treatments can affect the outcomes)
Doff et al. [28] (2010)	Craniofacial changes	Unclear for all outcomes ('... patients were randomized') not possible to conclude if randomization was successful	Unclear for all outcomes (not mentioned concealment of allocation, probably not performed)	Low for all outcomes (not mentioned blinding of participants/personnel but the outcome is not likely to be affected)	Low for all outcomes ('... one blinded observer (MD) performed all tracings')	Low for all outcomes (number of missing outcome data balanced among groups-reasons not related to outcome)	Low for all outcomes (all pre-specified variables were measured)	Low for all outcomes (patients that randomized in oral appliance treatment, and after treated for 3 months, changed to CPAP treatment were excluded)	Low for all outcomes (no concealed allocation but baseline characteristics that can affect the outcome -AHI, BMI, number of teeth, appliance usage, were similar among groups)

Table 5. Risk of bias assessment for non-randomized controlled trials.

Author (Year)	Outcomes	Bias Due to Confounding	Bias in Selection of Participants into the Study	Bias in Measurement of Interventions	Bias Due to Departures from Intended Interventions	Bias Due to Missing Data	Bias in Measurement of Outcomes	Bias in Selection of the Reported Result	Overall Bias
Bondemark [19] (1999)	Mandibular and dentofacial changes	Low for all outcomes	Low for all outcomes (all eligible participants were included and start of intervention and follow-up coincide)	Low for all outcomes (well-defined intervention status)	Low for all outcomes (no bias due to departure from intervention is expected)	Low for all outcomes (data were reasonably complete)	Low for all outcomes (objective method of outcome assessment, any error is unrelated to intervention status)	Low for all outcomes (all reported results correspond to intended outcome)	Low for all outcomes
Robertson [20] (2001)	Dentoalveolar and skeletal changes	Low for all outcomes	Low for all outcomes	Low for all outcomes	Low for all outcomes	Low for all outcomes (no missing outcome data)	Low for all outcomes (all pre-specified variables were measured)	Low for all outcomes (no possible risk of bias from other source)	Low for all outcomes
Robertson et al. [23] (2003)	Dentoalveolar and skeletal changes	Low for all outcomes	Low for all outcomes	Low for all outcomes	Low for all outcomes	Low for all outcomes (no missing outcome data)	Low for all outcomes (all pre-specified variables were measured)	Low for all outcomes (no possible risk of bias from other source)	Low for all outcomes
Rose et al. [22] (2002)	Dentofacial cephalometric and dental casts measurements	Low for all outcomes	Low for all outcomes	Low for all outcomes	Low for all outcomes	Low for all outcomes	Low for all outcomes	Low for all outcomes	Low for all outcomes

Table 5. *Cont.*

Author (Year)	Outcomes	Bias Due to Confounding	Bias in Selection of Participants into the Study	Bias in Measurement of Interventions	Bias Due to Departures from Intended Interventions	Bias Due to Missing Data	Bias in Measurement of Outcomes	Bias in Selection of the Reported Result	Overall Bias
Fransson et al. [21] (2002)	O_1: airway changes O_2: skeletal, dental, soft tissue changes	Low for all outcomes	Low for all outcomes (all eligible participants were included and start of intervention and follow-up coincide)	Serious for all outcomes (intervention status regarding usage frequency not well-defined)	Low for all outcomes (no bias due to departure from intervention is expected)	Low for all outcomes (data were reasonably complete)	Low for all outcomes (objective method of outcome assessment, any error is unrelated to intervention status, outcome assessor was blinded during cephalometric analysis.)	Low for all outcomes (all reported results correspond to intended outcome)	Low for all outcomes
Hou et al. [25] (2006)	Long-term dento-facial changes	Serious for all outcomes (at least one critically important domain not appropriately measured or not adjusted for)	Low for all outcomes (all eligible participants were included and start of intervention and follow-up coincide)	Serious for all outcomes (intervention status not well-defined)	Serious for all outcomes (switches in treatment is apparent and are not adjusted in for the analysis)	Low for all outcomes (data were reasonably complete)	Low for all outcomes (objective method of outcome assessment, any error is unrelated to intervention status)	Low for all outcomes (all reported results correspond to intended outcome)	Serious for all outcomes (the study is judged to be in serious risk of bias in at least one domain)
Almeida et al. [26] (2006)	Skeletal, dental, and occlusal changes	Serious for all outcomes (at least one critically important domain not appropriately measured or not adjusted for)	Serious for all outcomes (retrospective study (start follow-up did not coincide) selection into the study was related to intervention and possibly to outcome)	Serious for all outcomes (intervention status not well-defined)	Low for all outcomes (no bias due to departure from intervention is expected)	Low for all outcomes (data were reasonably complete)	Serious for all outcomes (outcome assessor was aware of the intervention received by the participants)	Low for all outcomes (all reported results correspond to intended outcome)	Serious for all outcomes (the study is judged to be in serious risk of bias in at least one domain)
Hammond et al. [27] (2007)	O_1: long-term subjective side-effects O_2: long-term dental and skeletal effects side-effects	Serious for all outcomes (at least one critically important domain not appropriately measured or not adjusted for)	Serious for all outcomes (inception bias)	Serious for all outcomes (intervention status not well-defined)	Low for O_1 outcomes Serious for O_2 outcomes (switches in treatment)	Serious for all outcomes (missing data-baseline characteristics; the risk of bias cannot be removed trough appropriate analysis)	Serious for O_1 (subjective method of outcome assessment) Serious for O_2 (outcome assessor was aware of the intervention received by the participants)	Low for all outcomes (all reported results correspond to intended outcome)	Serious for all outcomes (the study is judged to be in serious risk of bias in at least one domain)
Wang et al. [29] (2015)	O_1: long-term subjective side-effects O_2: long-term dental and skeletal effects side-effects	Serious for all outcomes (at least one critically important domain not appropriately measured or not adjusted for)	Low for all outcomes (all eligible participants were included and start of intervention and follow-up coincide)	Low for all outcomes (well-defined intervention status)	Low for all outcomes (no bias due to departure from intervention is expected)	Low for all outcomes (data were reasonably complete)	Serious for O_1 outcome (subjective method of outcome assessment) Low for O_2 outcomes (objective method of outcome assessment, any error is unrelated to intervention status, outcome assessor was blinded during cephalometric analysis.)	Low for all outcomes (all reported results correspond to intended outcome)	Serious for all outcomes (the study is judged to be in serious risk of bias in at least one domain)

Table 5. *Cont.*

Author (Year)	Outcomes	Bias Due to Confounding	Bias in Selection of Participants into the Study	Bias in Measurement of Interventions	Bias Due to Departures from Intended Interventions	Bias Due to Missing Data	Bias in Measurement of Outcomes	Bias in Selection of the Reported Result	Overall Bias
Minagi et al. [30] (2018)	causing factors and predictors of orthodontic changes after long-term use	Low for all outcomes	Low for all outcomes (all eligible participants were included and start of intervention and follow-up coincide)	Low for all outcomes (well-defined intervention status)	Low for all outcomes (no bias due to departure from intervention is expected)	Low for all outcomes (data were reasonably complete)	Low for all outcomes (objective method of outcome assessment, any error is unrelated to intervention status, outcome assessor was blinded during cephalometric analysis.)	Low for all outcomes (all reported results correspond to intended outcome)	Low for all outcomes
Hamoda et al. [31] (2018)	O1: dental and skeletal changes O2: Rate and predictors of changes	Serious for all outcomes (at least one critically important domain not appropriately measured or not adjusted for)	Serious for all outcomes (retrospective study)	Serious for all outcomes (intervention status regarding usage frequency not well-defined)	Low for all outcomes (no bias due to departure from intervention is expected)	Low for all outcomes (data were reasonably complete)	Low for all outcomes (objective method of outcome assessment)	Low for all outcomes (all reported results correspond to intended outcome)	Serious for all outcomes (the study is judged to be in serious risk of bias in at least one domain)
Fransson et al. [32] (2020)	O_1: airway changes O_2: skeletal, dental, soft tissue changes	Serious for all outcomes (at least one critically important domain not appropriately measured or not adjusted for)	Low for all outcomes (all eligible participants were included and start of intervention and follow-up coincide)	Low for all outcomes (well-defined intervention status)	Low for all outcomes (no bias due to departure from intervention is expected)	Low for all outcomes (data were reasonably complete)	Low for all outcomes (objective method of outcome assessment, any error is unrelated to intervention status, outcome assessor was blinded during cephalometric analysis.)	Low for all outcomes (all reported results correspond to intended outcome)	Low for all outcomes

Table 6. Overall results of meta-analysis. Mean difference, upper limit, and standard deviation.

Parameters	ES (Mean Diff.)	Upper Limit	SD
SNA	0.061	0.116	0.028
SNB	0.019	0.088	0.035
ANB	0.067	0.143	0.039
Overjet	−0.506	−0.420	0.044
Overbite	−0.326	−0.255	0.036
L1-MP	1.535	1.838	0.155

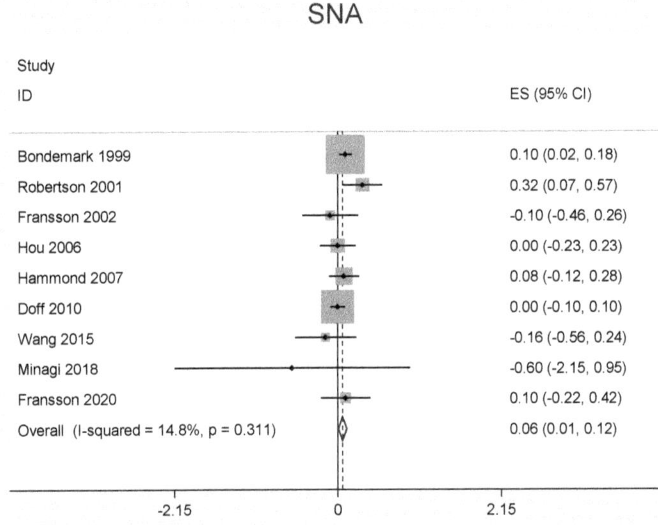

Figure 2. Forest plot of the results of SNA changes using the random-effects model.

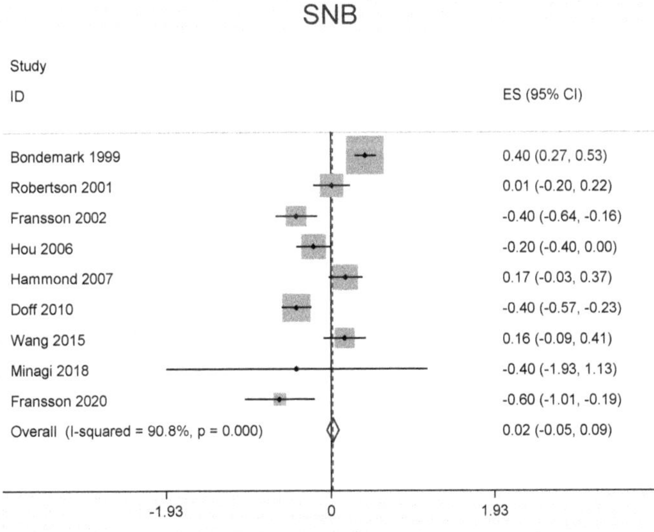

Figure 3. Forest plot of the results of SNB changes using the random-effects model.

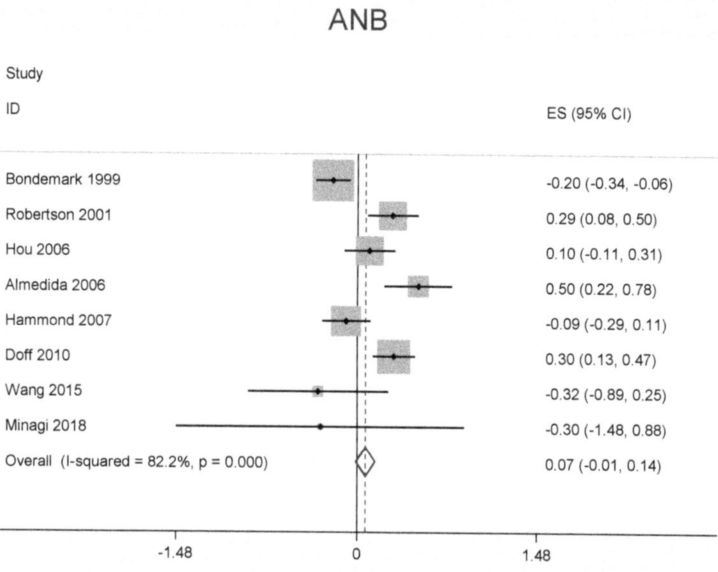

Figure 4. Forest plot of the results of ANB changes using the random-effects model.

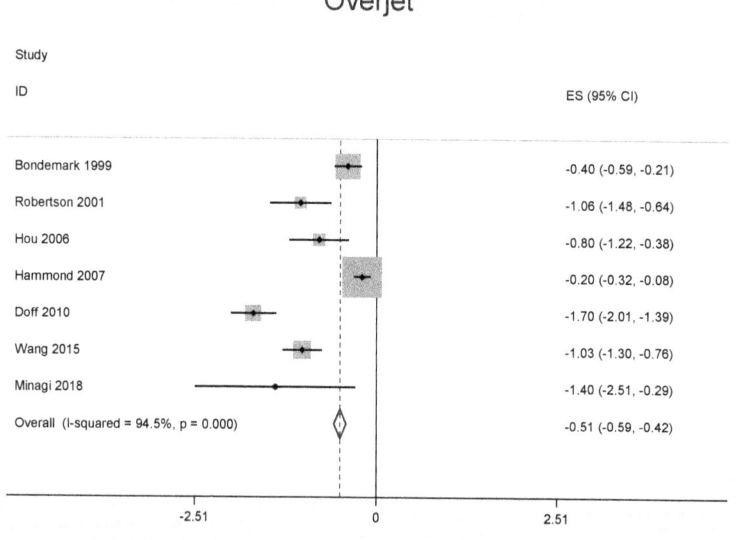

Figure 5. Forest plot of the results of overjet changes using the random-effects model.

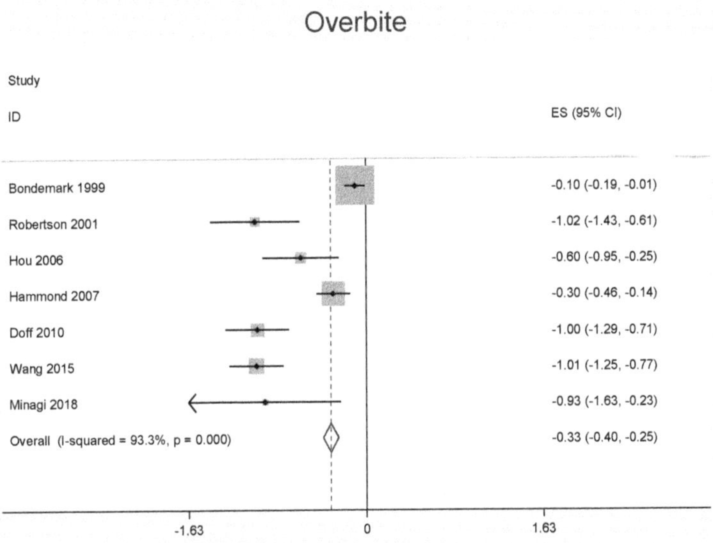

Figure 6. Forest plot of the results of overbite changes using the random-effects model.

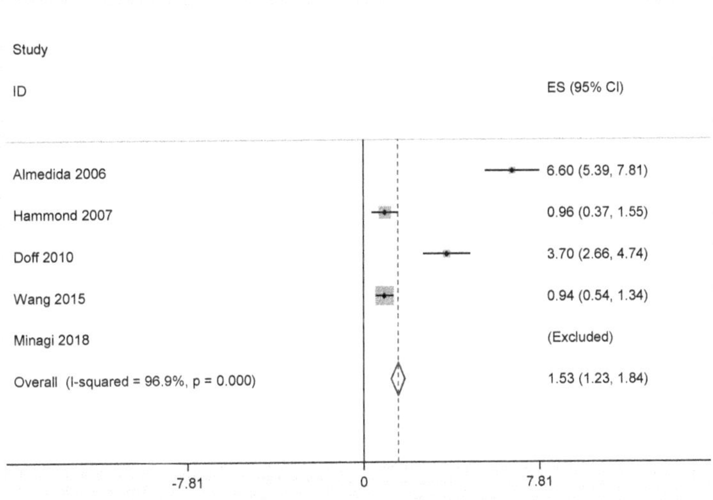

Figure 7. Forest plot of the results of L1-MP changes using the random-effects model.

3.4. Dental Changes

Bondemark et al. found a reduction in overjet and overbite, but no significant changes in incisor inclination or interincisal angle [19]. A few years later, Rose et al. and Robertson et al. found that maxillary incisors were retroclined, mandibular incisors were proclined, and thus overjet and overbite were reduced [20,22,23]. Still, according to Rose et al., the interincisal angle was not altered [22]. Conversely, Fransson et al. observed a reduction in the interincisal angle, because only the lower incisors were proclined, without a significant inclination change in upper incisors [21]. On the other hand, in the RCT of Ringqvist et al., incisor inclination changed only vertically, without any further alteration in overjet, overbite, and interincisal angle [24].

In the following years, the studies of Almeida et al., Doff et al., and Wang et al. showed that both, proclination of lower incisors and retroclination of the upper incisors, led to overjet and overbite reduction [26,28,29]. Moreover, Hou et al. found a decrease in overjet and overbite without examining incisor inclination, and Hammond et al. observed only upper incisor posterior tipping [25,27]. Although the interincisal angle was reduced, according to Almeida et al., Doff et al., and Hammond et al., it did not change significantly in Wang et al. study [26–29].

More recently, Minagi et al. showed a significant decrease in overjet and overbite because of mandibular incisor proclination, while the interincisal angle remained unchanged [30]. Furthermore, Hamoda et al. found that both upper and lower incisors were tipped backward and forward, respectively [31]. Finally, Fransson et al. observed overjet and overbite reduction due to altered inclination of upper and lower incisors, after 10 years of mandibular protruding device use [32].

Regarding posterior teeth changes, Robertson et al. found that the upper first premolars and lower first molars had over-erupted while, Almeida et al. found that first upper and lowers molars, except from over-erupting, had also moved distally and mesially [23,26]. Moreover, Hammond et al. showed a mesial tip of the lower first molars, but without a change in the upper first molars [27].

3.5. Skeletal Changes

Regarding changes in mandibular position relative to the cranial base, in most studies, the mandibular plane angle was significantly increased, and thus the mandible had a more downward position [20,21,23,25,26,28–30]. Bondemark found a more downward and forward position and Ringqvist et al. a more downward and backward position [19,24]. On the other hand, Rose et al., Hammond et al., and Minagi et al. found no significant changes in mandibular position [22,27,30]. The vertical condylar position was also observed to be more downward by Robertson et al., but not in Almeida et al. study, in which there were no condylar changes [23,26]. Regarding the relation between the maxilla and the mandible and each jaw relationship with the cranial base, the ANB angle was found slightly reduced by Bondemark, because the SNB angle was increased, and the SNA angle did not change [19]. Robertson et al., also observed a decrease in ANB angle, because the SNA angle was reduced and SNB was not altered significantly [23]. On the other hand, the ANB angle was increased in the study by Hamoda et al., due to a decrease in the SNB angle and no significant change in the SNA angle [31]. Moreover, according to Doff et al., the ANB angle was increased, while the SNB angle was reduced, and the SNA angle did not change [28]. Conversely, some studies showed no significant change in the ANB angle [22,25,27,29,30]. Furthermore, the SNB angle was found slightly reduced by Fransson et al. [21,32].

Alterations in facial height were also observed in many studies. An increase in lower anterior facial height and thus an increase in total anterior facial height was found by most researchers, except Minagi et al. that found no significant change [19,21,23–26,28–30]. On the other hand, lower posterior facial height and total posterior facial height was found significantly increased only in two studies [23,25], while four other studies showed no significant change [19,21,28,29].

Bondemark also observed a significant increase in mandibular length [19]. On the contrary, a significant alteration in mandibular length was not found by others [21,24–28]. Although Fransson et al. did not find a significant change after 2 years of treatment, they observed a significant increase in patients that continued the treatment for 10 years as well as in patients that stopped the treatment [21,32].

The maxillary length was also increased in the studies by Robertson and Robertson et al. [20,23], but no significant change was observed in any other study [25,28,29].

Frasson et al. also observed an alteration in the hyoid bone position. More specifically, the distance between the hyoid bone and mandibular plane and between the hyoid bone and occlusal line was increased [21]. Moreover, a more downward hyoid bone position was observed by Fransson et al. after 10 years of oral appliance use, but it was also evident in patients that had stopped using the device [32].

4. Discussion

Summary of Evidence

Different outcomes were searched among studies, the quality of which was also variable, according to the risk of bias assessment.

The two existing RCT studies were reported in 2003 by Ringvist et al. and in 2010 by Doff et al. [24,28]. The study of Ringvist et al. in 2003 presented a high risk of attrition bias [24]. In this study, patients that used two different methods of treatment at the same time were included in the final sample. Furthermore, this study presented a high risk of bias due to additional bias. In the study, a high number of patients did not attend the 4-year follow-up (15 in the MAD group and 6 in the uvulopalatopharyngoplasty -UPPP- group). On the other hand, the study of Doff et al. appeared to have a low risk of bias in all seven criteria for the outcome assessment [28]. Consequently, the statement that the use of MAD appliances leads to a decrease in overjet and overbite as well as results in shorter a downward and backward rotation of the mandible considered conclusions with a high level of evidence.

Twelve non-RCT studies were reported for the assessment of dental and skeletal effects from the long-term use of mandibular advancement devices. The study of Hou et al. showed a serious risk of bias due to confounding and in the measurement of intervention [25]. More specifically, the intervention status was not well-defined, and there were patients that switched treatment, which was not adjusted in the final analysis. The study of Almeida et al. presented a serious risk of bias due to confounding, in the selection of participants, in the measurement of intervention and the measurement of outcomes [26]. In this study, the start and follow-up measurements did not coincide, and the intervention status was not well-defined. The study of Hamoda et al. showed a serious risk of bias in those three criteria as well [31]. The most important bias in this study was the absence of the intervention status regarding the usage frequency of the devices. Hammond et al. showed a serious risk of bias in five out of seven criteria [27]. This study presented a serious risk of bias: due to confounding, in the selection of participants, in the measurement of intervention, due to missing data and in the measurement of outcomes. According to this study, there were patients that switched treatment, there were missing data, and the outcome assessor was aware of the intervention received by the participants (not blinded). The study by Wang et al. showed a serious risk of bias in the selection of participants and the measurement of outcomes [29]. The method of outcome assessment was subjective.

The remaining seven studies showed a low risk of bias in all criteria. Bondemark found that the use of MADs appliances resulted in decreased overjet and overbite, increased mandibular length, and the mandible moved forward and downwards [19]. Robertson in 2001 showed decreased overjet and overbite, increased lower incisor proclination, SNA, and ANB [20]. Robertson et al. in 2003 found that the use of MAD appliances resulted in over eruption of upper first premolars and lower first molars and proclination of the lower incisors [23]. Rose et al. showed an increase in incisor inclination, a mesial shift of the occlusion, and a decreased overjet and overbite [22]. Fransson et al. in 2002 found an increase in the posterior rotation of the mandible as long as an increased proclination of the mandibular incisors [21]. The study of Minagi et al. resulted in decreased overjet and overbite [30]. In 2020 Fransson et al. concluded that the use of MADs resulted in proclination of the mandibular incisors with consequent decreased overjet and overbite [32]. All these statements are considered to be strong since those researches had a low risk of bias.

The heterogeneity was high for all the outcomes in this meta-analysis. A possible explanation for this might be the different treatment duration among the included studies. The mean treatment duration was less or equal to 3 years in most studies [19–23,25,27,28], 4 years for two studies [29,30], 7 years in one study [26], and over 10 years in two studies [31,32].

Moreover, the design of the mandibular advancement devices was different in most of the studies [19–32]. All the oral appliances protruded the mandible and provided full occlusal coverage [19–23,25–32], except for one that provided occlusal coverage only for the posterior teeth [24]. There was also variation in the amount of protrusion for each oral appliance. A 65–75% of the maximum protrusion with a small vertical opening was used in most studies [19–23,25–32], but 50% of the maximum protrusion was chosen by one study [24]. In the study by Ringvist et al. that used the appliance that provided only posterior occlusal coverage and protruded the mandible, only 50% showed no change in overjet and overbite. On the other hand, a systematic review and meta-analysis found no significant difference between the side effects caused by 50% and 75% of maximum protrusion [33].

Furthermore, adherence to the oral appliance daily wear might be a factor that increased outcome heterogeneity. All studies required the patients to wear the oral appliances at least 5 h a day and at least 4 days per week. The non-adherent patients were also excluded from all studies. Nevertheless, no objective method was used to record patient total wear time and thus evaluate true patient compliance.

Finally, one of the outcomes that was controversial is the extrusion of the molars as an effect of the MADs use. An explanation on that disagreement between the studies can be that MADs design differs on the occlusal coverage. More specific, the studies that used appliances with occlusal coverage could prevent dental extrusion while the ones that do not have the coverage could not. In the near future, 3D printing technology can be helpful in order to fabricate those appliances and possibly be delivered the same day to the patient's mouth. There are lots of other appliances in the field of orthodontics that have been fabricated with 3D printing technology and proved to be significantly successful for the treatment outcome [34]. The limitation of this study is the small number of randomized clinical trials in the present literature.

5. Conclusions

Regarding dental and skeletal side effects caused by mandibular advancement appliances used for adult OSA treatment, the current level of evidence is weak. The meta-analysis results suggest that mandibular advancement devices used for OSA treatment increase the lower incisor proclination by $1.54 \pm 0.16°$, decrease overjet by 0.89 ± 0.04 mm, decrease overbite by 0.68 ± 0.04 mm, rotate the mandible downward and forward, and increase SNA angle by to $0.06 \pm 0.03°$. Some of those results are clearly not clinically significant. More randomized clinical trials providing high-quality evidence are needed.

Author Contributions: I.A.T., data curation, formal analysis, investigation, methodology, resources, software, validation, visualization, roles/writing—original draft; J.M.P., project administration, supervision, writing—review and editing; S.M., data curation, formal analysis, investigation, resources, writing—review and editing; A.I.T., conceptualization, methodology, project administration, supervision, validation, writing—review and editing. All authors have read and agreed to the published version of the manuscript.

Funding: This research received no external funding.

Institutional Review Board Statement: Not applicable.

Informed Consent Statement: Not applicable.

Data Availability Statement: Not applicable.

Conflicts of Interest: The authors declare no conflict of interest.

References

1. Sateia, M.J. International classification of sleep disorders-third edition: Highlights and modifications. *Chest* **2014**, *146*, 1387–1394. [CrossRef] [PubMed]
2. Koutsourelakis, I.; Perraki, E.; Zakynthinos, G.; Minaritzoglou, A.; Vagiakis, E.; Zakynthinos, S. Clinical and polysomnographic determinants of snoring. *J. Sleep Res.* **2012**, *21*, 693–699. [CrossRef]
3. Tsolakis, I.A.; Venkat, D.; Hans, M.G.; Alonso, A.; Palomo, J.M. When static meets dynamic: Comparing cone-beam computed tomography and acoustic reflection for upper airway analysis. *Am. J. Orthod Dentofac. Orthop.* **2016**, *150*, 643–650. [CrossRef]
4. Rohra, A.K., Jr.; Demko, C.A.; Hans, M.G.; Rosen, C.; Palomo, J.M. Sleep disordered breathing in children seeking orthodontic care. *Am. J. Orthod Dentofac. Orthop.* **2018**, *154*, 65–71. [CrossRef] [PubMed]
5. Caples, S.M.; Gami, A.S.; Somers, V.K. Obstructive sleep apnea. *Ann. Intern. Med.* **2005**, *142*, 187–197. [CrossRef] [PubMed]
6. Behrents, R.G.; Shelgikar, A.V.; Conley, R.S.; Flores-Mir, C.; Hans, M.; Levine, M.; McNamara, J.A.; Palomo, J.M.; Pliska, B.; Stockstill, J.W.; et al. Obstructive sleep apnea and orthodontics: An American Association of Orthodontists White Paper. *Am. J. Orthod Dentofac. Orthop.* **2019**, *156*, 13–28.e1. [CrossRef] [PubMed]
7. Punjabi, N.M. The epidemiology of adult obstructive sleep apnea. *Proc. Am. Thorac. Soc.* **2008**, *5*, 136–143. [CrossRef] [PubMed]
8. Williams, S.K.; Ravenell, J.; Jean-Louis, G.; Zizi, F.; Underberg, J.A.; McFarlane, S.I.; Ogedegbe, G. Resistant hypertension and sleep apnea: Pathophysiologic insights and strategic management. *Curr. Diab. Rep.* **2011**, *11*, 64–69. [CrossRef] [PubMed]
9. Usmani, Z.A.; Chai-Coetzer, C.L.; Antic, N.A.; McEvoy, R.D. Obstructive sleep apnoea in adults. *Postgrad. Med. J.* **2013**, *89*, 148–156. [CrossRef]
10. Ramar, K.; Dort, L.C.; Katz, S.G.; Lettieri, C.J.; Harrod, C.G.; Thomas, S.M.; Chervin, R.D. Clinical Practice Guideline for the Treatment of Obstructive Sleep Apnea and Snoring with Oral Appliance Therapy: An Update for 2015. *J. Clin. Sleep Med.* **2015**, *11*, 773–827. [CrossRef] [PubMed]
11. Marklund, M.; Braem, M.J.A.; Verbraecken, J. Update on oral appliance therapy. *Eur. Respir. Rev.* **2019**, *28*, 190083. [CrossRef] [PubMed]
12. Chen, A.; Burger, M.S.; Rietdijk-Smulders, M.A.W.J.; Smeenk, F.W.J.M. Mandibular advancement device: Effectiveness and dental side effects. A real-life study. *Cranio* **2020**, *40*, 97–106. [CrossRef] [PubMed]
13. Hoekema, A.; Stegenga, B.; De Bont, L.G. Efficacy and co-morbidity of oral appliances in the treatment of obstructive sleep apnea-hypopnea: A systematic review. *Crit Rev. Oral Biol. Med.* **2004**, *15*, 137–155. [CrossRef] [PubMed]
14. Araie, T.; Okuno, K.; Ono Minagi, H.; Sakai, T. Dental and skeletal changes associated with long-term oral appliance use for obstructive sleep apnea: A systematic review and meta-analysis. *Sleep Med. Rev.* **2018**, *41*, 161–172. [CrossRef] [PubMed]
15. Patel, S.; Rinchuse, D.; Zullo, T.; Wadhwa, R. Long-term dental and skeletal effects of mandibular advancement devices in adults with obstructive sleep apnoea: A systematic review. *Int. Orthod.* **2019**, *17*, 3–11. [CrossRef] [PubMed]
16. Bartolucci, M.L.; Bortolotti, F.; Martina, S.; Corazza, G.; Michelotti, A.; Alessandri-Bonetti, G. Dental and skeletal long-term side effects of mandibular advancement devices in obstructive sleep apnea patients: A systematic review with meta-regression analysis. *Eur. J. Orthod.* **2019**, *41*, 89–100. [CrossRef] [PubMed]
17. Martins, O.F.M.; Chaves Junior, C.M.; Rossi, R.R.P.; Cunali, P.A.; Dal-Fabbro, C.; Bittencourt, L. Side effects of mandibular advancement splints for the treatment of snoring and obstructive sleep apnea: A systematic review. *Dent. Press J. Orthod.* **2018**, *23*, 45–54. [CrossRef]
18. DerSimonian, R.; Laird, N. Meta-analysis in clinical trials. *Control Clin. Trials* **1986**, *7*, 177–188. [CrossRef]
19. Bondemark, L. Does 2 years' nocturnal treatment with a mandibular advancement splint in adult patients with snoring and OSAS cause a change in the posture of the mandible? *Am. J. Orthod. Dentofac. Orthop.* **1999**, *116*, 621–628. [CrossRef]
20. Robertson, C.J. Dental and skeletal changes associated with long-term mandibular advancement. *Sleep* **2001**, *24*, 531–537. [CrossRef]
21. Fransson, A.M.; Tegelberg, A.; Svenson, B.A.; Lennartsson, B.; Isacsson, G. Influence of mandibular protruding device on airway passages and dentofacial characteristics in obstructive sleep apnea and snoring. *Am. J. Orthod. Dentofac. Orthop.* **2002**, *122*, 371–379. [CrossRef] [PubMed]
22. Rose, E.C.; Staats, R.; Virchow, C., Jr.; Jonas, I.E. Occlusal and skeletal effects of an oral appliance in the treatment of obstructive sleep apnea. *Chest* **2002**, *122*, 871–877. [CrossRef]
23. Robertson, C.; Herbison, P.; Harkness, M. Dental and occlusal changes during mandibular advancement splint therapy in sleep disordered patients. *Eur. J. Orthod.* **2003**, *25*, 371–376. [CrossRef] [PubMed]
24. Ringqvist, M.; Walker-Engström, M.L.; Tegelberg, A.; Ringqvist, I. Dental and skeletal changes after 4 years of obstructive sleep apnea treatment with a mandibular advancement device: A prospective, randomized study. *Am. J. Orthod. Dentofac. Orthop.* **2003**, *124*, 53–60. [CrossRef]
25. Hou, H.M.; Sam, K.; Hägg, U.; Rabie, A.B.M.; Bendeus, M.; Yam, L.Y.C.; Ip, M.S. Long-term dentofacial changes in Chinese obstructive sleep apnea patients after treatment with a mandibular advancement device. *Angle Orthod.* **2006**, *76*, 432–440. [PubMed]
26. Almeida, F.R.; Lowe, A.A.; Sung, J.O.; Tsuiki, S.; Otsuka, R. Long-term sequellae of oral appliance therapy in obstructive sleep apnea patients: Part 1. Cephalometric analysis. *Am. J. Orthod. Dentofac. Orthop.* **2006**, *129*, 195–204. [CrossRef] [PubMed]

27. Hammond, R.J.; Gotsopoulos, H.; Shen, G.; Petocz, P.; Cistulli, P.A.; Darendeliler, M.A. A follow-up study of dental and skeletal changes associated with mandibular advancement splint use in obstructive sleep apnea. *Am. J. Orthod. Dentofac. Orthop.* **2007**, *132*, 806–814. [CrossRef]
28. Doff, M.H.; Hoekema, A.; Pruim, G.J.; Huddleston Slater, J.J.; Stegenga, B. Long-term oral-appliance therapy in obstructive sleep apnea: A cephalometric study of craniofacial changes. *J. Dent.* **2010**, *38*, 1010–1018. [CrossRef]
29. Wang, X.; Gong, X.; Yu, Z.; Gao, X.; Zhao, Y. Follow-up study of dental and skeletal changes in patients with obstructive sleep apnea and hypopnea syndrome with long-term treatment with the Silensor appliance. *Am. J. Orthod. Dentofac. Orthop.* **2015**, *147*, 559–565. [CrossRef] [PubMed]
30. Minagi, H.O.; Okuno, K.; Nohara, K.; Sakai, T. Predictors of Side Effects with Long-Term Oral Appliance Therapy for Obstructive Sleep Apnea. *J. Clin. Sleep Med.* **2018**, *14*, 119–125. [CrossRef] [PubMed]
31. Hamoda, M.M.; Almeida, F.R.; Pliska, B.T. Long-term side effects of sleep apnea treatment with oral appliances: Nature, magnitude and predictors of long-term changes. *Sleep Med.* **2019**, *56*, 184–191. [CrossRef]
32. Fransson, A.M.C.; Benavente-Lundahl, C.; Isacsson, G. A prospective 10-year cephalometric follow-up study of patients with obstructive sleep apnea and snoring who used a mandibular protruding device. *Am. J. Orthod. Dentofac. Orthop.* **2020**, *157*, 91–97. [CrossRef] [PubMed]
33. Sakamoto, Y.; Furuhashi, A.; Komori, E.; Ishiyama, H.; Hasebe, D.; Sato, K.; Yuasa, H. The Most Effective Amount of forwarding Movement for Oral Appliances for Obstructive Sleep Apnea: A Systematic Review. *Int. J. Environ. Res. Public Health* **2019**, *16*, 3248. [CrossRef] [PubMed]
34. Thurzo, A.; Urbanová, W.; Novák, B.; Waczulíková, I.; Varga, I. Utilization of a 3D Printed Orthodontic Distalizer for Tooth-Borne Hybrid Treatment in Class II Unilateral Malocclusions. *Materials* **2022**, *15*, 1740. [CrossRef] [PubMed]

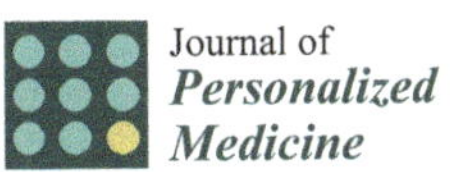
Journal of
Personalized
Medicine

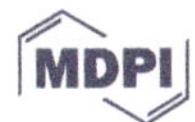

Article

Effect of PM2.5 Levels on ED Visits for Respiratory Causes in a Greek Semi-Urban Area

Maria Mermiri [1,2,*], Georgios Mavrovounis [1], Nikolaos Kanellopoulos [3], Konstantina Papageorgiou [1], Michalis Spanos [1], Georgios Kalantzis [4], Georgios Saharidis [4], Konstantinos Gourgoulianis [3] and Ioannis Pantazopoulos [1]

[1] Department of Emergency Medicine, Faculty of Medicine, University of Thessaly, BIOPOLIS, 41110 Larissa, Greece
[2] Department of Anesthesiology, Faculty of Medicine, University of Thessaly, BIOPOLIS, 41110 Larissa, Greece
[3] Department of Respiratory Medicine, Faculty of Medicine, University of Thessaly, BIOPOLIS, 41110 Larissa, Greece
[4] Department of Mechanical Engineering, University of Thessaly, Leoforos Athinon, 8 Pedion Areos, 38334 Volos, Greece
* Correspondence: mmermiri@gmail.com

Abstract: Fine particulate matter that have a diameter of <2.5 μm (PM2.5) are an important factor of anthropogenic pollution since they are associated with the development of acute respiratory illnesses. The aim of this prospective study is to examine the correlation between PM2.5 levels in the semi-urban city of Volos and Emergency Department (ED) visits for respiratory causes. ED visits from patients with asthma, pneumonia and upper respiratory infection (URI) were recorded during a one-year period. The 24 h PM2.5 pollution data were collected in a prospective manner by using twelve fully automated air quality monitoring stations. PM2.5 levels exceeded the daily limit during 48.6% of the study period, with the mean PM2.5 concentration being 30.03 ± 17.47 μg/m^3. PM2.5 levels were significantly higher during winter. When PM2.5 levels were beyond the daily limit, there was a statistically significant increase in respiratory-related ED visits (1.77 vs. 2.22 visits per day; p: 0.018). PM2.5 levels were also statistically significantly related to the number of URI-related ED visits (0.71 vs. 0.99 visits/day; $p = 0.01$). The temperature was negatively correlated with ED visits (r: −0.21; $p < 0.001$) and age was found to be positively correlated with ED visits (r: 0.69; $p < 0.001$), while no statistically significant correlation was found concerning humidity (r: 0.03; $p = 0.58$). In conclusion, PM2.5 levels had a significant effect on ED visits for respiratory causes in the city of Volos.

Keywords: PM2.5; air pollution; respiratory diseases; asthma; pneumonia; upper respiratory infections; emergency department

Citation: Mermiri, M.; Mavrovounis, G.; Kanellopoulos, N.; Papageorgiou, K.; Spanos, M.; Kalantzis, G.; Saharidis, G.; Gourgoulianis, K.; Pantazopoulos, I. Effect of PM2.5 Levels on ED Visits for Respiratory Causes in a Greek Semi-Urban Area. *J. Pers. Med.* **2022**, *12*, 1849. https://doi.org/10.3390/jpm12111849

Academic Editor: Eumorfia Kondili

Received: 30 July 2022
Accepted: 31 October 2022
Published: 5 November 2022

1. Introduction

Anthropogenic air pollution is a major cause of environmental pollution, which can have detrimental effects on human health [1]. Fine particle matter 2.5 (PM2.5) are fine particles that have an aerodynamic diameter of less than 2.5 μm, which are produced mainly by wood and fuel combustion [2]. Because of their small diameters, they are able to infiltrate through the nose into the lower respiratory system, accumulating in respiratory bronchioles [2]. Alveolar damage may consequently occur due to the production of free radicals, imbalanced intracellular homeostasis and inflammation [2].

High levels of PM2.5 have been previously associated with several respiratory diseases, as well as increased morbidity and mortality due to respiratory causes [3]. In a meta-analysis of 16 studies, short-term exposure to increased PM2.5 levels were shown to precipitate asthma attacks leading to increased hospitalizations in patients suffering from severe respiratory disorders [4]. Moreover, a prospective study of 431 patients suffering from Chronic Obstructive Pulmonary Disease (COPD) in a highly polluted city of Italy showcased that high PM10 and PM2.5 levels may precipitate COPD exacerbations and increase hospital admissions in these patients. Furthermore, several prospective studies and a meta-analysis by Kim et al. proved that elevated PM2.5 levels have been associated with a surge in Emergency Department (ED) visits for respiratory causes, such as asthma attacks and respiratory infections [4–6].

While the connection between PM2.5 pollution and respiratory diseases has been extensively researched, there is a lack of studies pertaining to the relationship between air pollution and health in rural or semi-urban areas. Although these areas may have lower exposure to industrial and motor vehicle pollution [7], studies have shown that several non-urban regions are greatly exposed to pollution produced by agriculture, coal burning and mining and wood burning [8,9]. The semi-urban city of Volos is a medium-size coastal city in Greece, where high levels of PM10 and PM2.5 pollution have been previously recorded [10,11]. Moustris et al. studied the effect of PM10 pollution in hospital admissions for respiratory diseases during a five-year period in Volos [10]. Their results showcased that increased PM10 levels were associated with an 25% increase in hospital admissions. Later, our team in a similarly designed study studied the effect of PM2.5 levels in pediatric ED visits for respiratory causes during a one-year period [11]. Likewise, elevated PM2.5 levels resulted in an increase in pediatric ED visits for respiratory causes.

The aim of the present study was to investigate the relationship between daily PM2.5 levels in the semi-urban Greek city of Volos and the number of adult ED visits for respiratory causes.

2. Materials and Methods

2.1. Study Design and Population

This study retrospectively analysed a prospectively collected database. The study was approved by the local scientific committee (2/7-2-2019). The methodology has been previously described in detail for our pediatric ED visits study [11].

Data were collected for adult patients visiting the ED of Volos with respiratory symptoms, including asthma, pneumonia, COPD and upper respiratory tract infection (URI)-related visits between 1 March 2019 and 29 February 2020. We used the following inclusion criteria: (1) residents of Volos city, (2) those who visited the adult ED and (3) those with respiratory conditions (URI, COPD exacerbation, asthma exacerbation and pneumonia). The following data were collected for all patients: age, gender, address of residence, main complaint/diagnosis and date of visit.

2.2. Network of Sensors

The GreenYourAir research group established a fully automated network for monitoring air pollution in the city of Volos. Twelve stations located throughout the central and greater Volos areas collected the data prospectively during the entire study period. The locations were chosen based on a mathematical formula and an optimization model developed by the GreenYourAir team that parcellated the city into smaller areas. Briefly, the team divided the city into five distinct areas, namely the commercial and recreational zone; the industrial zone; and the high-density, medium-density and low-density residential zones, while the traffic jam of the city was divided into three categories (high, medium and low). Furthermore, additional information regarding the city was taken into consideration, such as the geographical and geomorphological characteristics of the area, the commercial port, the passenger port, the urban and intercity bus stations, the train station, the main roads, the recreational parks, the sport facilities, the schools and other academic institutions and two big industrial plants located just outside the city (one cement company and one petroleum company). It should be mentioned that the residents of the city use oil, natural gas and fireplaces for heating during the winter. The exact location of the sensors throughout the city of Volos is presented in Figure 1.

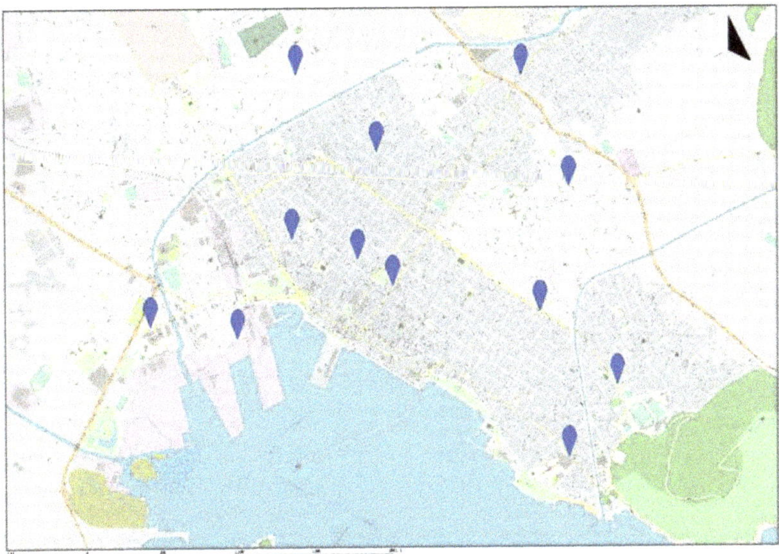

Figure 1. Map of the city of Volos presenting the location of sensors. Markers indicate the location of the sensors.

The devices that were used for monitoring (GreenYourAir Device 1178/PM2.5) used light-scattering methods for data collection, as described previously in the literature [12,13]. The devices consist of a sensor, an expansion shield and an Arduino YUN rev. 2. The sensor collects data regarding PM2.5 concentration, temperature and humidity in the area. The collection of data was performed automatically every second for the entire 24 h of the day. The programming language used for the devices was C++.

A two-phase calibration methodology was implemented to check the accuracy of the devices. During the first stage development and testing period, the sensors were validated in laboratory conditions using reference equipment that followed EU standards EN 14907:2005 (gravimetric device with filters that collects PM2.5). Later, during the second stage, the sensors were validated in real-life conditions.

The network created started operating on 1 March 2019 and is still working 24/7 at the time of writing this manuscript. The real-time data for the city of Volos can be found at http://greenyourair.org/ (accessed on 30 October 2022).

2.3. Statistical Analysis

The independent samples t-test and analysis of variance were used for the between groups comparisons of continuous variables as appropriate. The chi-square test was used to identify possible relationships between categorical variables. We used regression analysis and Pearson's correlation in order to describe the relationship between the number of ED visits and temperature, humidity, age and PM2.5 levels. The significance for all tests was set at p values < 0.05 and all tests were two-tailed. The SPSS statistical package was used for all statistical analyses (IBM Corp. Released 2016. IBM SPSS Statistics for Windows, Version 24.0. Armonk, NY, USA; IBM Corp).

3. Results

3.1. Patient Characteristics

During our study period, a total of 728 patients visited the adult ED for respiratory causes. The male to female ratio was 1.05 (373 male and 355 female patients), while the mean age for male patients was 64.50 ± 19.69, and for female patients, it was 61.43 ± 20.52.

A total of 310 patients (mean age (standard deviation): 66.35 ± 20.77; male gender: 166 (54%)) were diagnosed with an URI, 202 patients were diagnosed with a lower respiratory tract infection/pneumonia (mean age (standard deviation): 52.41 ± 20.70; male gender: 106(52%)), 53 patients were diagnosed with asthma exacerbation (mean age (standard deviation): 50.39 ± 20.05; male gender: 15(28%)) and 163 patients were diagnosed with COPD exacerbation (mean age (standard deviation): 69.49 ± 12.20; male gender: 85(52%)).

3.2. *PM2.5 Levels*

In the city of Volos, the mean annual PM2.5 concentration during the study period was calculated to be 30.03 ± 17.47 μg/m^3 compared to WHO's yearly limit of 10 μg/m^3. Overall, the suggested daily limit of PM2.5 (25 μg/m^3) was exceeded for 178 days, which was 48.60% of the study period. The recorded levels of PM2.5 were found to be higher in winter when compared with summer (mean difference: 25.64, p: < 0.001), autumn (mean difference: 20.20, p: < 0.001) and spring (mean difference: 17.71, p: < 0.001).

3.3. *PM2.5 Levels, Humidity, Temperature, Age and ED Visits*

The mean number of daily ED visits for respiratory causes was 1.99 ± 1.81. The number of monthly ED alongside the corresponding monthly PM2.5 levels are presented in Figure 2. As shown in Table 1, a 25.42% increase in daily ED visits for all respiratory causes was identified when PM2.5 levels exceeded the daily limit (1.77 vs. 2.22 visits per day; p: 0.018). Further analyses performed by season (Table 2) illustrated that the increase in ED visits was more pronounced during winter (34.08%) and autumn (29.40%), although the difference was non-statistically significant. Moreover, there was statistically significant elevation in ED visits when PM2.5 levels of the previous day were higher than the proposed limit 25 μg/m^3 (p = 0.018).

Additionally, we identified that temperature was negatively correlated with ED visits (r: −0.21; p < 0.001), while humidity did not exhibit any statistically significant correlation (r: 0.03; p = 0.58). Finally, age was found to be positively correlated with ED visits (r: 0.69; p < 0.001).

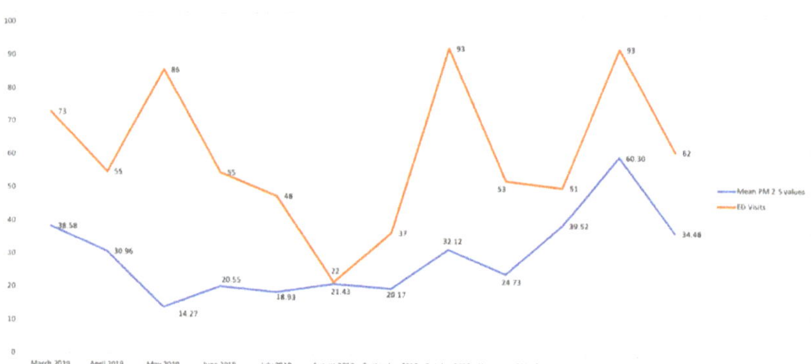

Figure 2. Monthly PM2.5 levels and ED visits.

Table 1. Table presenting the number of ED visits in relation to daily PM2.5 levels.

	PM2.5 Level	Total Days N = 366	Number of ED Visits N = 728	Mean ED Visits/Day ± SD	% Increase in Mean ED Visits	*p* Value
All patients	<25 μg/m³ ≥25 μg/m³	188 178	333 395	1.77 ± 1.81 2.22 ± 1.77	25.42%	0.018
URI	<25 μg/m³ ≥25 μg/m³	188 178	134 176	0.71 ± 1.03 0.99 ± 1.03	38.72%	0.011
Pneumonia	<25 μg/m³ ≥25 μg/m³	188 178	93 109	0.49 ± 0.91 0.61 ± 0.94	23.79%	0.224
Asthma exacerbation	<25 μg/m³ ≥25 μg/m³	188 178	30 23	0.16 ± 0.43 0.13 ± 0.35	−19.03%	0.465
COPD exacerbation	<25 μg/m³ ≥25 μg/m³	188 178	76 87	0.40 ± 0.68 0.49 ± 0.75	20.90%	0.261

Abbreviations: ED: emergency department; SD: standard deviation; URI: upper respiratory tract infection; COPD: Chronic Obstructive Pulmonary Disease.

Table 2. Table presenting the number of ED visits in relation to mean PM2.5 levels of each season.

	PM2.5 Level	Total Days	Number of ED Visits	Mean ED Visits/Day ± SD	% Increase in Mean ED Visits	*p* Value
Winter	<25 μg/m³ ≥25 μg/m³	18 73	32 174	1.78 ± 1.48 2.38 ± 1.77	34.08%	0.12
Spring	<25 μg/m³ ≥25 μg/m³	42 50	102 112	2.43 ± 2.32 2.24 ± 1.67	−7.76%	0.65
Summer	<25 μg/m³ ≥25 μg/m³	74 18	102 23	1.38 ± 1.41 1.28 ± 1.13	−7.30%	0.78
Autumn	<25 μg/m³	54	97	1.80 ± 1.86	29.40%	0.21

Abbreviations: ED: emergency department; SD: standard deviation.

3.4. *Specific Conditions and PM2.5 Levels*

A statistically significant increase in ED visits for URI was noted during the days that PM2.5 levels exceeded the limit of 25 μg/m³, when compared to the days when PM2.5 levels were below 25 μg/m³ (0.71 vs. 0.99 visits/day; $p = 0.01$). Table 1 presents the comparisons for all studied conditions. No statistically significant differences were identified when a further analysis was performed based on the season (Supplementary File S1). Finally, no statistically significant differences in mean ED visits were observed for all studied conditions (URI: $p = 0.05$; Pneumonia: $p = 0.42$; Asthma: $p = 0.28$; COPD: $p = 0.47$) when comparing males and females.

In regression analysis, a linear correlation (r square: 0.022; $p < 0.001$) was noted between the levels of PM2.5 and the total number of daily ED visits. This is described by the following equation: total number of ED visits = 1.524 + 0.015 × PM2.5 levels (Figure 3). When we included temperature and humidity in the model's parameters, the model was still statistically significant (r square: 0.047; $p < 0.001$) although the only parameter with statistical significance was temperature.

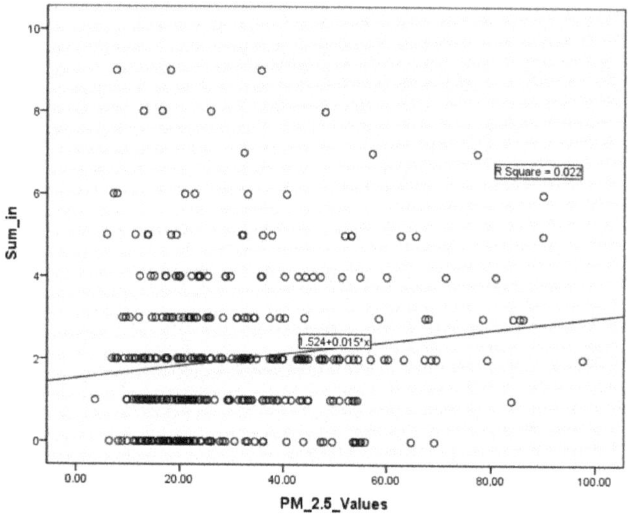

Figure 3. Correlation between daily PM2.5 levels and daily ED visits.

4. Discussion

In our study, PM2.5 levels exceeded the daily limit of 10 μg/m^3 during 48.6% of the study period, with the mean PM2.5 concentration being 30.03 ± 17.47 μg/m^3. PM2.5 levels were higher during the winter compared to autumn, spring, and summer. ED visits were significantly higher on days when PM2.5 concentrations exceeded the daily limit, or the day after. Although age and temperature had a significant correlation with ED visits, humidity did not play a role in the number of daily ED visits. Moreover, high PM2.5 levels were associated with an increase in URI-related ED visits.

Air pollution has become increasingly prevalent during the last decades, since many global areas are exposed daily to high levels of air pollutants [14]. While large metropolises suffer greatly [15], semi-urban and rural areas can also be affected [8]. Research pertaining to the relationship between air pollution and human health in rural and semi-urban areas may further highlight the importance of air pollutants on respiratory health.

Despite the fact that the city of Volos is a semi-urban area, high levels of air pollutants have been previously recorded [10,11]. In accordance with our study, Moustris et al. [10] reported elevated levels of PM10 pollution in the city of Volos, with PM10 levels regularly exceeding the daily and annual proposed limits by WHO. In the study by Moustris et al., an increase in the annual PM10 concentration in the city of Volos resulted in an increase in the annual hospital admissions for respiratory diseases. However, in our study, we researched the relationship between daily PM2.5 concentrations and ED visits for respiratory causes, which further highlights the direct effect of PM2.5 pollution and respiratory health.

PM2.5 production is mainly anthropogenic [14]. Fine particle matter is produced primarily through fuel and wood combustion, mainly deriving from vehicle and biofuel emissions [16]. A meta-analysis of PM source apportionment in Europe revealed that traffic, as well as wood burning during the cold months, were the most important factors in PM production [16]. In the last decade, the number of Greek households using wood burning as a means of heating during the winter rapidly increased due to the high petrol prices and economic crisis [17]. This increase in wood burning has subsequently led to an increase in fine PM levels, which are significantly higher during the cold months [17]. Likewise, the present study indicates that PM2.5 levels in the city of Volos are higher during winter compared to other seasons. This relationship may indicate that the production of PM2.5 by wood burning may be a significant component of environmental pollution in semi-urban or rural areas, where pollutant production by industrial processes is less prominent.

Approximately 4.2 premature million deaths annually can be attributed to PM2.5 pollution, placing fine particle pollution as the fifth most common cause of death worldwide [18]. Exposure to elevated PM2.5 levels has been associated with increased Out-of-Hospital Cardiac Arrests (OHCAs), as well as a variety of cardiovascular and respiratory diseases [19–21]. Interestingly, a meta-analysis by Atkinson et al. [20] demonstrated that PM2.5 pollution is more strongly associated with mortality due to respiratory causes [20]. Indeed, high PM2.5 levels are associated with increased rates of respiratory infections and asthma or COPD exacerbations, leading to an increase in ED visits for respiratory causes [22,23].

According to our findings, in the semi-urban city of Volos, there was a statistically significant association between PM2.5 levels and ED visits for respiratory causes. These findings are in accordance with two similar studies conducted in the city of Volos, which demonstrated that fine particulate matter pollution is associated with increased hospital admissions for respiratory causes in both adult and pediatric patients [10,11]. As previously mentioned, high levels of PM2.5 can precipitate a variety of respiratory diseases, such as respiratory infections and asthma and COPD exacerbations, as well as increased hospital admissions and mortality due to respiratory causes [20,22]. Specifically, our research team, using the model developed by the GreenYourAir research group, discovered that pediatric ED visits in the city of Volos were linearly correlated with PM2.5 levels [11]. In our study, the same research group discovered that a similar relationship exists in adult patients. Furthermore, our results revealed a significant correlation between age and ED visits for respiratory causes. As showcased in previous studies, the effect of PM2.5 on respiratory diseases seems to be more pronounced in children and adults [7,24] According to previous studies, the effect of PM2.5 on respiratory-related conditions is more significant in adults more than 65 years old [7].

Several meteorological factors have been shown to influence the concentration of PM2.5 and its effect on human health [25,26]. In our study, a decrease in the mean daily temperature resulted in an increase in daily ED visits while humidity did not have a statistically significant correlation with ED visits. Similarly, a study by Wang et al. in 28 Chinese cities showcased that low temperatures during winter were correlated with higher PM2.5 concentrations [25]. The researchers hypothesized that this effect may be due to the increased coal and wood burning during the cold months. Moreover, low temperature has been associated with an increased susceptibility to URIs [27], which may increase respiratory-related ED visits. However, a study in Lima, Peru, showcased that the effect of PM2.5 concentrations in respiratory and cardiac mortality was more pronounced when the mean daily temperature was higher than 23.8 °C [28]. A similar relationship between PM10 and respiratory disease was found in a systematic review and meta-analysis by Chen et al. [29], which found that the effect of air pollution on respiratory diseases is more significant when the temperature is higher. These conflicting results prove that more research is necessary in order to accurately understand the complicated effects of meteorological factors in fine particulate matter concentrations and their effects on human health. Moreover, while our results did not reveal a significant correlation between humidity and ED visits, it is important to note that several researchers proved that high relative humidity may be accompanied by higher PM2.5 and PM10 concentrations, which may have a negative effect on respiratory-related ED visits [30,31].

In our study, there was a statistically significant association between URI-related ED visits and PM2.5 levels. The association between PM2.5 levels and respiratory infections has been proved by numerous studies, which showcase that increased PM2.5 levels lead to increased ED visits and hospital admissions for upper and lower respiratory infections [7,32]. The study by our research team in the city of Volos, also indicated that high daily PM2.5 levels are correlated with increased pediatric ED visits for URI [11]. This effect has been attributed to increased susceptibility to infections [33] based on experimental animal models [34,35]. While the exact mechanism remains unknown, it is speculated that PM2.5 impairs the host's defense of the respiratory system by altering epithelial cell functions and immune cell activity [33]. This effect is more pronounced in pediatric and elderly patients [33].

The association between PM2.5 pollution and chronic respiratory diseases has been well documented. Both PM2.5 and PM10 may cause COPD exacerbations, leading to more ED visits for respiratory causes and increased morbidity and mortality in COPD patients [22,36]. Interestingly, it has been demonstrated that PM2.5 exposure may cause chronic respiratory dysfunction, creating emphysematous lesions and chronic inflammation, which in turn may lead to COPD developments [36]. Moreover, PM2.5 pollution can aggravate the effects of smoking on lung function, increasing the likelihood of COPD [36]. In contrast to the existing literature, no statistically significant association between PM2.5 levels and COPD association was noted in our study. However, this discrepancy may be attributed to the small number of patients presenting to the ED with respiratory symptoms due to COPD exacerbation.

PM2.5 pollution may also worsen asthma symptoms, leading to increased ED visits and hospital admissions for asthma exacerbations [4,37,38]. A meta-analysis by Fan et al. demonstrated that asthma-related ED visits increased proportionally to PM2.5 levels [4]. The effect was more pronounced in pediatric patients. Moreover, asthma exacerbations are most likely to occur during spring possibly due to the prevalence of allergens, such as pollen [37]. The association between PM2.5 pollution and asthma can be attributed to the increased inflammation of airway epithelial cells and the increased secretion of inflammatory cytokines [39,40]. Our study did not reveal a statistically significant association between PM2.5 levels and asthma-related ED visits. Moreover, our team in a similar study in pediatric patients did not discover a statistically significant relationship between asthma-related ED visits and PM2.5 levels. Similarly to COPD cases, this could be explained by the small number of asthma-related ED visits during our study period.

Limitations

Our study has some limitations that should be acknowledged. Firstly, is it a single-center study that collected data from a single ED; thus, our results should be interpreted with caution. Moreover, the diagnoses were made in an emergency setting; therefore, there may have been some misdiagnoses. It is also important to note that our analysis was conducted based on the mean PM2.5 levels of each day and may not accurately reflect patient exposure, since no regional analysis was conducted.

5. Conclusions

In our study, high PM2.5 levels were associated with an increase in adult ED visits for respiratory causes. PM2.5 pollution was statistically significantly related to the number of URI-related visits but not COPD or asthma-related visits. Moreover, low temperatures and increased age increased ED visits for respiratory causes. While the association between fine particle pollution and respiratory illnesses has been well documented, more studies are necessary in order to ascertain the pathophysiological mechanisms leading to respiratory dysfunction, as well as individual factors that may predispose certain patients to PM2.5-related respiratory symptoms.

Supplementary Materials: The following supporting information can be downloaded at: https://www.mdpi.com/article/10.3390/jpm12111849/s1.

Author Contributions: Conceptualization, N.K., G.S., G.K. and K.G.; methodology, N.K., G.S., G.K. and K.G.; software, G.S. and G.K.; formal analysis, G.S., GK. and M.S.; data curation, G.S., G.K., M.S. and K.P.; writing—original draft preparation, M.M., G.M. and K.P.; writing—review and editing, N.K., I.P., K.G. and M.M.; visualization, G.S. and G.K.; supervision, I.P. and K.G.; project ad-ministration, I.P. and K.G.; funding acquisition, K.G. All authors have read and agreed to the published version of the manuscript.

Funding: This research received no external funding.

Institutional Review Board Statement: The study was conducted according to the guidelines of the Declaration of Helsinki and approved by the Institutional Review Board of the University of Thessaly (2/7-2-2019).

Informed Consent Statement: Patient consent was waived due to the retrospective nature of the data analysis. Patient anonymity and confidentiality were maintained through all stages of the data analysis process.

Data Availability Statement: The data that support the findings of this study are available from the corresponding author (MM) upon reasonable request.

Conflicts of Interest: The authors declare no conflict of interest.

References

1. Kampa, M.; Castanas, E. Human Health Effects of Air Pollution. *Environ. Pollut.* **2008**, *151*, 362–367. [CrossRef] [PubMed]
2. Xing, Y.-F.; Xu, Y.-H.; Shi, M.-H.; Lian, Y.-X. The Impact of PM2.5 on the Human Respiratory System. *J. Thorac. Dis.* **2016**, *8*, E69–E74. [CrossRef] [PubMed]
3. Brunekreef, B.; Holgate, S.T. Air Pollution and Health. *Lancet* **2002**, *360*, 1233–1242. [CrossRef]
4. Fan, J.; Li, S.; Fan, C.; Bai, Z.; Yang, K. The Impact of PM2.5 on Asthma Emergency Department Visits: A Systematic Review and Meta-Analysis. *Environ. Sci. Pollut. Res. Int.* **2016**, *23*, 843–850. [CrossRef]
5. Krall, J.R.; Mulholland, J.A.; Russell, A.G.; Balachandran, S.; Winquist, A.; Tolbert, P.E.; Waller, L.A.; Sarnat, S.E. Associations between Source-Specific Fine Particulate Matter and Emergency Department Visits for Respiratory Disease in Four U.S. Cities. *Environ. Health Perspect.* **2017**, *125*, 97–103. [CrossRef] [PubMed]
6. Alhanti, B.A.; Chang, H.H.; Winquist, A.; Mulholland, J.A.; Darrow, L.A.; Sarnat, S.E. Ambient Air Pollution and Emergency Department Visits for Asthma: A Multi-City Assessment of Effect Modification by Age. *J. Expo. Sci. Environ. Epidemiol.* **2016**, *26*, 180–188. [CrossRef]
7. Strosnider, H.M.; Chang, H.H.; Darrow, L.A.; Liu, Y.; Vaidyanathan, A.; Strickland, M.J. Age-Specific Associations of Ozone and Fine Particulate Matter with Respiratory Emergency Department Visits in the United States. *Am. J. Respir. Crit. Care Med.* **2019**, *199*, 882–890. [CrossRef]
8. Yang, T. Association between Perceived Environmental Pollution and Health among Urban and Rural Residents—A Chinese National Study. *BMC Public Health* **2020**, *20*, 194. [CrossRef]
9. Hendryx, M.; Fedorko, E.; Halverson, J. Pollution Sources and Mortality Rates across Rural-Urban Areas in the United States. *J. Rural Health* **2010**, *26*, 383–391. [CrossRef]
10. Moustris, K.P.; Proias, G.T.; Larissi, I.K.; Nastos, P.T.; Koukouletsos, K.V.; Paliatsos, A.G. Health Impacts Due to Particulate Air Pollution in Volos City, Greece. *J. Environ. Sci. Health A Tox. Hazard Subst. Environ. Eng.* **2016**, *51*, 15–20. [CrossRef]
11. Kanellopoulos, N.; Pantazopoulos, I.; Mermiri, M.; Mavrovounis, G.; Kalantzis, G.; Saharidis, G.; Gourgoulianis, K. Effect of PM2.5 Levels on Respiratory Pediatric ED Visits in a Semi-Urban Greek Peninsula. *Int. J. Environ. Res. Public Health* **2021**, *18*, 6384. [CrossRef] [PubMed]
12. Rogulski, M. Low-Cost PM Monitors as an Opportunity to Increase the Spatiotemporal Resolution of Measurements of Air Quality. *Energy Procedia* **2017**, *128*, 437–444. [CrossRef]
13. Tagle, M.; Rojas, F.; Reyes, F.; Vásquez, Y.; Hallgren, F.; Lindén, J.; Kolev, D.; Watne, Å.K.; Oyola, P. Field Performance of a Low-Cost Sensor in the Monitoring of Particulate Matter in Santiago, Chile. *Environ. Monit. Assess.* **2020**, *192*, 171. [CrossRef] [PubMed]
14. Xu, Z.; Ding, W.; Deng, X. PM2.5, Fine Particulate Matter: A Novel Player in the Epithelial-Mesenchymal Transition? *Front. Physiol.* **2019**, *10*, 1404. [CrossRef]
15. Shahrabi, N.S.; Pourezzat, A.; Fayaz-Bakhsh, A.; Mafimoradi, S.; Poursafa, P. Pathologic Analysis of Control Plans for Air Pollution Management in Tehran Metropolis: A Qualitative Study. *Int. J. Prev. Med.* **2013**, *4*, 995–1003. [PubMed]
16. Belis, C.A.; Karagulian, F.; Larsen, B.R.; Hopke, P.K. Critical Review and Meta-Analysis of Ambient Particulate Matter Source Apportionment Using Receptor Models in Europe. *Atmos. Environ.* **2013**, *69*, 94–108. [CrossRef]
17. Fourtziou, L.; Liakakou, E.; Stavroulas, I.; Theodosi, C.; Zarmpas, P.; Psiloglou, B.; Sciare, J.; Maggos, T.; Bairachtari, K.; Bougiatioti, A.; et al. Multi-Tracer Approach to Characterize Domestic Wood Burning in Athens (Greece) during Wintertime. *Atmos. Environ.* **2017**, *148*, 89–101. [CrossRef]
18. Nazarenko, Y.; Pal, D.; Ariya, P.A. Air Quality Standards for the Concentration of Particulate Matter 2.5, Global Descriptive Analysis. *Bull. World Health Organ.* **2021**, *99*, 125–137D. [CrossRef]
19. Gentile, F.R.; Primi, R.; Baldi, E.; Compagnoni, S.; Mare, C.; Contri, E.; Reali, F.; Bussi, D.; Facchin, F.; Currao, A.; et al. Out-of-Hospital Cardiac Arrest and Ambient Air Pollution: A Dose-Effect Relationship and an Association with OHCA Incidence. *PLoS ONE* **2021**, *16*, e0256526. [CrossRef]
20. Atkinson, R.W.; Kang, S.; Anderson, H.R.; Mills, I.C.; Walton, H.A. Epidemiological Time Series Studies of PM2.5 and Daily Mortality and Hospital Admissions: A Systematic Review and Meta-Analysis. *Thorax* **2014**, *69*, 660–665. [CrossRef]

21. Tian, Y.; Liu, H.; Wu, Y.; Si, Y.; Song, J.; Cao, Y.; Li, M.; Wu, Y.; Wang, X.; Chen, L.; et al. Association between Ambient Fine Particulate Pollution and Hospital Admissions for Cause Specific Cardiovascular Disease: Time Series Study in 184 Major Chinese Cities. *BMJ* **2019**, *367*, l6572. [CrossRef] [PubMed]
22. Pini, L.; Giordani, J.; Gardini, G.; Concoreggi, C.; Pini, A.; Perger, E.; Vizzardi, E.; Di Bona, D.; Cappelli, C.; Ciarfaglia, M.; et al. Emergency Department Admission and Hospitalization for COPD Exacerbation and Particulate Matter Short-Term Exposure in Brescia, a Highly Polluted Town in Northern Italy. *Respir. Med.* **2021**, *179*, 106334. [CrossRef] [PubMed]
23. Pennington, A.F.; Strickland, M.J.; Gass, K.; Klein, M.; Sarnat, S.E.; Tolbert, P.E.; Balachandran, S.; Chang, H.H.; Russell, A.G.; Mulholland, J.A.; et al. Source-Apportioned PM2.5 and Cardiorespiratory Emergency Department Visits: Accounting for Source Contribution Uncertainty. *Epidemiology* **2019**, *30*, 789–798. [CrossRef]
24. Vu, B.N.; Tapia, V.; Ebelt, S.; Gonzales, G.F.; Liu, Y.; Steenland, K. The Association between Asthma Emergency Department Visits and Satellite-Derived PM2.5 in Lima, Peru. *Environ. Res.* **2021**, *199*, 111226. [CrossRef]
25. Wang, S.; Gao, J.; Guo, L.; Nie, X.; Xiao, X. Meteorological Influences on Spatiotemporal Variation of PM2.5 Concentrations in Atmospheric Pollution Transmission Channel Cities of the Beijing–Tianjin–Hebei Region, China. *Int. J. Environ. Res. Public Health* **2022**, *19*, 1607. [CrossRef] [PubMed]
26. Wang, J.; Ogawa, S. Effects of Meteorological Conditions on PM2.5 Concentrations in Nagasaki, Japan. *Int. J. Environ. Res. Public Health* **2015**, *12*, 9089–9101. [CrossRef] [PubMed]
27. Tchicaya, A.; Lorentz, N.; Omrani, H.; de Lanchy, G.; Leduc, K. Impact of Long-Term Exposure to PM2.5 and Temperature on Coronavirus Disease Mortality: Observed Trends in France. *Environ. Health* **2021**, *20*, 101. [CrossRef] [PubMed]
28. Steenland, K.; Vu, B.; Scovronick, N. Effect Modification by Maximum Temperature of the Association between PM2.5 and Short-Term Cardiorespiratory Mortality and Emergency Room Visits in Lima, Peru, 2010–2016. *J. Expo. Sci. Environ. Epidemiol.* **2022**, *32*, 590–595. [CrossRef]
29. Chen, F.; Fan, Z.; Qiao, Z.; Cui, Y.; Zhang, M.; Zhao, X.; Li, X. Does Temperature Modify the Effect of PM10 on Mortality? A Systematic Review and Meta-Analysis. *Environ. Pollut.* **2017**, *224*, 326–335. [CrossRef]
30. Cheng, Y.; He, K.; Du, Z.; Zheng, M.; Duan, F.; Ma, Y. Humidity Plays an Important Role in the PM2.5 Pollution in Beijing. *Environ. Pollut.* **2015**, *197*, 68–75. [CrossRef]
31. Lou, C.; Liu, H.; Li, Y.; Peng, Y.; Wang, J.; Dai, L. Relationships of Relative Humidity with PM2.5 and PM10 in the Yangtze River Delta, China. *Environ. Monit Assess.* **2017**, *189*, 582. [CrossRef] [PubMed]
32. Xia, X.; Zhang, A.; Liang, S.; Qi, Q.; Jiang, L.; Ye, Y. The Association between Air Pollution and Population Health Risk for Respiratory Infection: A Case Study of Shenzhen, China. *Int. J. Environ. Res. Public Health* **2017**, *14*, 950. [CrossRef] [PubMed]
33. Yang, L.; Li, C.; Tang, X. The Impact of PM2.5 on the Host Defense of Respiratory System. *Front. Cell Dev. Biol.* **2020**, *8*. [CrossRef] [PubMed]
34. Sigaud, S.; Goldsmith, C.-A.W.; Zhou, H.; Yang, Z.; Fedulov, A.; Imrich, A.; Kobzik, L. Air Pollution Particles Diminish Bacterial Clearance in the Primed Lungs of Mice. *Toxicol. Appl. Pharm.* **2007**, *223*, 1–9. [CrossRef] [PubMed]
35. Zhao, H.; Li, W.; Gao, Y.; Li, J.; Wang, H. Exposure to Particular Matter Increases Susceptibility to Respiratory Staphylococcus Aureus Infection in Rats via Reducing Pulmonary Natural Killer Cells. *Toxicology* **2014**, *325*, 180–188. [CrossRef]
36. Zhao, J.; Li, M.; Wang, Z.; Chen, J.; Zhao, J.; Xu, Y.; Wei, X.; Wang, J.; Xie, J. Role of PM2.5 in the Development and Progression of COPD and Its Mechanisms. *Respir. Res.* **2019**, *20*, 120. [CrossRef]
37. Williams, A.M.; Phaneuf, D.J.; Barrett, M.A.; Su, J.G. Short-Term Impact of PM2.5 on Contemporaneous Asthma Medication Use: Behavior and the Value of Pollution Reductions. *Proc. Natl. Acad. Sci. USA* **2019**, *116*, 5246–5253. [CrossRef]
38. Wu, J.; Zhong, T.; Zhu, Y.; Ge, D.; Lin, X.; Li, Q. Effects of Particulate Matter (PM) on Childhood Asthma Exacerbation and Control in Xiamen, China. *BMC Pediatr.* **2019**, *19*, 194. [CrossRef]
39. Iskandar, A.; Andersen, Z.J.; Bønnelykke, K.; Ellermann, T.; Andersen, K.K.; Bisgaard, H. Coarse and Fine Particles but Not Ultrafine Particles in Urban Air Trigger Hospital Admission for Asthma in Children. *Thorax* **2012**, *67*, 252–257. [CrossRef]
40. Senthil Kumar, S.; Muthuselvam, P.; Pugalenthi, V.; Subramanian, N.; Ramkumar, K.M.; Suresh, T.; Suzuki, T.; Rajaguru, P. Toxicoproteomic Analysis of Human Lung Epithelial Cells Exposed to Steel Industry Ambient Particulate Matter (PM) Reveals Possible Mechanism of PM Related Carcinogenesis. *Environ. Pollut.* **2018**, *239*, 483–492. [CrossRef]

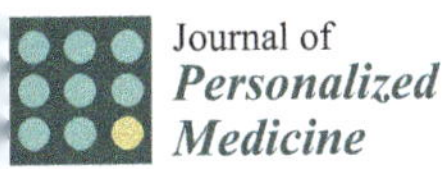
Journal of *Personalized Medicine*

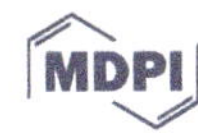

Brief Report

Serum Levels of Urokinase Plasminogen Activator Receptor (suPAR) Discriminate Moderate Uncontrolled from Severe Asthma

Ourania S. Kotsiou [1,*], Ioannis Pantazopoulos [2], Georgios Mavrovounis [3], Konstantinos Marsitopoulos [3], Konstantinos Tourlakopoulos [3], Paraskevi Kirgou [3], Zoe Daniil [3] and Konstantinos I. Gourgoulianis [3]

1 Department of Human Pathophysiology, Faculty of Nursing, University of Thessaly, 41110 Larissa, Greece
2 Department of Internal Medicine, University of Thessaly, 41500 Larissa, Greece
3 Department of Respiratory Medicine, University of Thessaly, 41500 Larissa, Greece
* Correspondence: raniakotsiou@gmail.com

Abstract: Introduction: The most clinically useful concept in asthma is based on the intensity of treatment required to achieve good asthma control. Biomarkers to guide therapy are needed. Aims: To investigate the role of circulating levels of soluble urokinase plasminogen activator receptor suPAR as a marker for asthma severity. Methods: We recruited patients evaluated at the Asthma Clinic, University of Thessaly, Greece. Asthma severity and control were defined according to the GINA strategy and Asthma Contro Test (ACT). Anthropometrics, spirometry, fractional exhaled nitric oxide (FeNO), suPAR, blood cell count, c-reactive protein (CRP), and analyses of kidney and liver function were obtained. Patients with a history of inflammatory, infectious, or malignant disease or other lung disease, more than 5 pack years of smoking history, or corticosteroid therapy were excluded. Results: We evaluated 74 asthma patients (69% female, mean age 57 ± 17 years, mean body mass index (BMI) 29 ± 6 kg/m^2). In total, 24%, 13%, 6%, 5%, 29% and 23% of the participants had mild well-controlled, mild uncontrolled, moderate well-controlled, moderate uncontrolled, severe well-controlled, and severe uncontrolled asthma, respectively. Overall, 67% had T2-high asthma, 26% received biologics (15% and 85% received omalizumab and mepolizumab, respectively), and 34% had persistent airway obstruction. suPAR levels were significantly lower in asthmatics with moderate uncontrolled asthma than in patients with severe uncontrolled asthma without (2.1 ± 0.4 vs. 3.3 ± 0.7 ng/mL, p = 0.023) or with biologics (2.1 ± 0.4 vs. 3.6 ± 0.8 ng/mL, p = 0.029). No correlations were found between suPAR levels and age, BMI, T2 biomarkers, CRP, or spirometric parameters. Conclusions: suPAR levels were higher in asthmatics with severe disease than in those with moderate uncontrolled asthma.

Keywords: asthma; control; severity; urokinase plasminogen activator receptor

Citation: Kotsiou, O.S.; Pantazopoulos, I.; Mavrovounis, G.; Marsitopoulos, K.; Tourlakopoulos, K.; Kirgou, P.; Daniil, Z.; Gourgoulianis, K.I. Serum Levels of Urokinase Plasminogen Activator Receptor (suPAR) Discriminate Moderate Uncontrolled from Severe Asthma. *J. Pers. Med.* **2022**, *12*, 1776. https://doi.org/10.3390/jpm12111776

Academic Editor: Bruno Mégarbané

Received: 21 September 2022
Accepted: 24 October 2022
Published: 28 October 2022

1. Introduction

The soluble urokinase plasminogen activator receptor (suPAR) is the circulating form of the cell surface receptor urokinase plasminogen activator receptor (uPAR) (CD87), which is expressed by a plethora of cells ranging from mono- and lymphocytes to endothelial and smooth muscle cells [1]. suPAR is a novel biomarker playing an important role in many physiological and pathological processes, including endothelial dysfunction, thrombosis [2], inflammation [1–4], chemotaxis [1,2], tissue remodeling [1–4], and tumorigenesis [1,2]. suPAR's high stability in plasma samples makes it an ideal candidate biomarker in patients with inflammatory, infectious, and malignant diseases [1–7]. Recently, a position statement on the prognostic role of suPAR in the screening of patients admitted to the emergency department was issued by the Hellenic Sepsis Study Group.

A remarkable role for suPAR serum levels has been demonstrated in airway diseases. It has been reported that suPAR can be used to evaluate stable chronic obstructive disease (COPD) [3] as a predictor of acute exacerbation and in monitoring response to treatment [3]. Moreover, suPAR has a significant role in increased systemic inflammation associated with coexisting COPD and bronchiectasis [4].

Evidence has shown that airway inflammation might spread into the circulatory system and cause systemic inflammatory injuries. In that context, emerging data support asthma associated with chronic low-grade systemic inflammation, a prothrombotic state, and premature atherosclerosis, even in clinically stable asthma patients [5]. Asthma is also characterized by endothelial dysfunction related to airway obstruction [5]. There is evidence of an abnormal amount of endothelial tissue in asthma and that this tissue and its progenitor cells behave in a dysfunctional manner [6]. Sputum, biopsy and serum suPAR levels were elevated in stable asthma patients compared to controls [7]. Moreover, in asthmatic patients, high suPAR indicated impaired lung function and was shown to correlate with airway resistance [1]. However, no data on the potential role of circulating suPAR as a marker for asthma severity and prognosis according to severity have been reported so far.

Patients with severe asthma are at a particularly high risk of exacerbations, hospitalization and death and have severely impaired quality of life. On the other hand, patients with mild asthma (the silent majority of asthmatics) account for the majority of the morbidity and healthcare resource utilization associated with asthma [1,8].

The aim of this study was to investigate the effectiveness of suPAR as an indicator of the severity of asthma.

2. Methods

2.1. Study Design

The recruitment period of the study lasted 6 months. Detailed lung function tests were performed in severe asthmatic patients and control groups in the following order: measurement of the fraction of exhaled nitric oxide (FeNO and spirometry) [9]. Severe asthmatics and controls had a set of standard blood tests analyzed, including suPAR, blood cell count (white blood cell count, eosinophils %, absolute eosinophil count), C-reactive protein (CRP), electrolytes (sodium, potassium), and analyses of the kidney (urea, creatinine) and liver function (aspartate transaminase (AST), alanine transaminase (ALT), gamma-glutamyl transpeptidase (γGT), and alkaline phospatase (ALP)) at baseline. The Ethics Committee of the University of Thessaly approved the protocol. Written informed consent was obtained.

2.2. Participants

All patients were well-defined regarding asthma severity as they were managed by an experienced pulmonologist in the external Unit of Asthma of the University of Thessaly in Greece for at least one year prior to recruitment. Exclusion criteria were: any history of acute (within four weeks of recruitment) or chronic inflammatory, infectious or malignant disease, COPD and/or other relevant lung diseases causing alternating impairment in lung function, current smoking or more than 5 pack years of smoking history, hypertension, diabetes mellitus, angiopathy, renal disorder, or corticosteroid therapy.

2.3. Assessment of the Severity of Asthma

The severity of asthma was assessed according to the level of treatment required to control symptoms and exacerbations according to GINA 2022 [8]. Mild asthma was defined as asthma that was well controlled while treated with as-needed inhaled corticosteroids (ICS)/formoterol or with low-dose ICSs, plus an as-needed short-acting bronchodilator (SABA) [8]. Moderate asthma was defined as asthma that was well-controlled with a low- or medium-dose ICS-long-acting bronchodilator (LABA) (with step 3 or step 4 treatment) [8]. Severe asthma was defined as asthma that required high-dose ICS/LABA to prevent it from becoming uncontrolled or asthma that remained uncontrolled despite this treatment [8].

2.4. Asthma Control Evaluation

Asthma control was assessed according to the level of symptom control [8]. Symptom control was determined using the Asthma Control Test (ACT) [10] and discriminated as well-controlled or uncontrolled [8]. In the ACT, scores range from 5–25. Scores of 20–25 were classified as controlled and 5–19 as not well-controlled [10].

2.5. Fraction of Exhaled Nitric Oxide (FeNO)

The FeNO (MEDISOFT, MEDICAL GRAPHICS CORP, Minnesota, USA) was performed according to recommendations [11]. Recommended cut-off values for normal FeNO levels were <25 parts per billion (ppb) [11].

2.6. Spirometry

Lung function was measured by means of an electronic spirometer (Spirolab FCC ID: TUK-MIR045) according to the American Thoracic Society (ATS) guidelines [12]. Persistent airflow limitation was defined as forced expiratory volume in the first second (FEV1)/forced vital capacity (FVC) ratio consistently < 70% despite irreversibility in asthma expressed as an increase in FEV1 $\geq$ 12% and 200 mL [8].

2.7. Blood Sample Collection

Peripheral venous blood samples were collected in sterile, pro-coagulation tubes and centrifuged immediately; the resulting serum samples were stored at −80 °C until analysis. Plasma suPAR levels were measured using the suPARnostic AUTO Flex ELISA kit (ViroGates A/S, Birkerød, Denmark) as described in detail previously [13]. The suPARnostic ELISA measures the full-length suPAR molecule (D1D2D3) and the cleaved suPAR molecule (D2D3). CRP was measured using a COBAS 6000 analyzer (Roche Diagnostics, Mannheim, Germany).

2.8. Statistical Analyses

The Pearson correlation method was used for correlation analysis between pairs of continuous variables. To identify differences between two independent groups, an unpaired t-test was used. Parametric data comparing three or more groups were analyzed with one-way ANOVA and Tukey's multiple comparisons test, while non-parametric data were analyzed with the Kruskal–Wallis test and Dunn's multiple comparison test. Pearson's chi-squared test was used to determine whether there was a statistically significant difference between frequencies. A result was considered statistically significant when the p-value was <0.05. Data were analyzed and visualized using SPSS Statistics v. 23 (Armonk, NY, USA, IBM Corp.) and GraphPad Prism 8.

3. Results

We evaluated 74 asthma patients. A total of 69% of them were female. The mean age of the population was 57 ± 17 years. The mean body mass index (BMI) was 29 ± 6 kg/m^2 (Table 1).

Overall, 24%, 13%, 6%, 5%, 29% and 23% of the participants had mild well-controlled, mild uncontrolled, moderate well-controlled, moderate uncontrolled, severe well-controlled, and severe uncontrolled asthma, respectively.

Furthermore, 67% of the population had T2-high asthma according to the measured T2 high biomarkers (blood eosinophil count $\geq$ 150 cells/μL and FeNO $\geq$ 20 ppb). Overall, 26% received biologics (15% and 85% received omalizumab and mepolizumab, respectively), while 34% had persistent airway obstruction. The demographic, clinical and spirometric characteristics of the study population are presented in Table 1. Females had significantly less symptom control than males (Table 1).

Abbreviations: BMI, body mass index; FeNO, fraction of exhaled nitric oxide; FEV1, forced expiratory volume in the first second; FVC, forced vital capacity. No significant differences regarding the measured laboratory parameters (white blood cell count, CRP, sodium, potassium, urea, creatinine, AST, ALT, γGT, and ALP were detected among genders. The comparison of serum suPAR levels among groups of asthmatics is presented in Table 1.

Table 1. Demographic, clinical and spirometric characteristics of the asthmatics (n = 74).

Parameter	Study Population (n = 75)	Males (n = 23)	Females (n = 52)	p-Value
Age (years)	57 ± 17	52 ± 18	59 ± 16	0.089
BMI (kg/m^2)	29 ± 6	28 ± 6	29 ± 6	0.758
T2 high phenotype	50 (67)	19 (83)	31 (60)	0.042
Eosinophils (cells per μL)	199 ± 171	194 ± 130	202 ± 185	0.869
FeNO (ppb)	10 ± 3	13 ± 2	9 ± 5	0.216
Mean FEV1/FVC	74 ± 9	73 ± 7	74 ± 9	0.566
Obstruction in spirometry (FEV1/FVC < 70)	25 (34)	7 (30)	18 (34)	0.354
ACT	20 ± 6	22 ± 2	19 ± 5	0.005
Biologics (yes)	19 (26)	6 (26)	13 (25)	0.585

Note: Data are expressed as mean ± SD or as frequencies (percentages).

suPAR levels were significantly higher in asthmatics with severe uncontrolled asthma not receiving biologics than in patients with moderate uncontrolled asthma (3.3 ± 0.7 vs. 2.1 ± 0.4 ng/mL, p = 0.023) (Figure 1). Moreover, suPAR levels were significantly lower in asthmatics with moderate uncontrolled asthma than in patients with severe uncontrolled asthma without (2.1 ± 0.4 vs. 3.3 ± 0.7 ng/mL, p = 0.023) or with biologics (2.1 ± 0.4 vs. 3.6 ± 0.8 ng/mL, p = 0.029) (Figure 2).

No correlations were found between suPAR levels and age, BMI, T2 biomarkers, white blood cell count, CRP, electrolytes, parameters of the kidney and liver function, or spirometric parameters (Supplementary Table S1). The correlation analysis between suPAR levels and the most important parameters is shown in Figure 3.

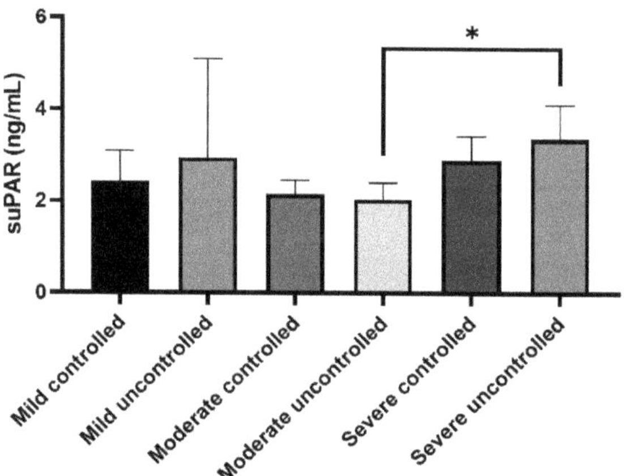

Note: * p = 0.023

Figure 1. Comparison of serum soluble urokinase plasminogen activator receptor (suPAR) levels between groups of asthmatics.

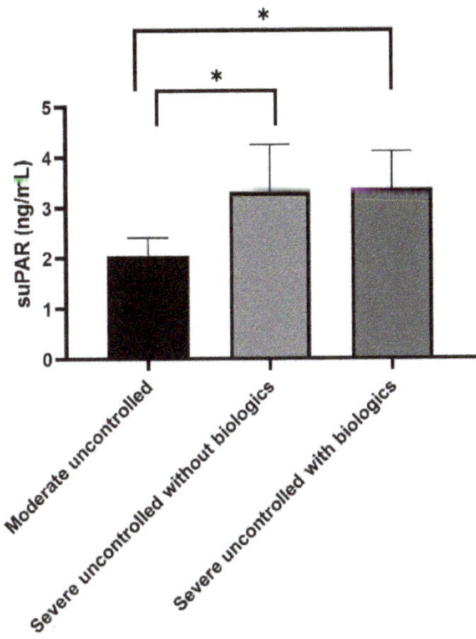

Note: * $p < 0.05$

Figure 2. Comparison of serum ssoluble urokinase plasminogen activator receptor (suPAR) levels between moderate uncontrolled and severe uncontrolled asthmatics.

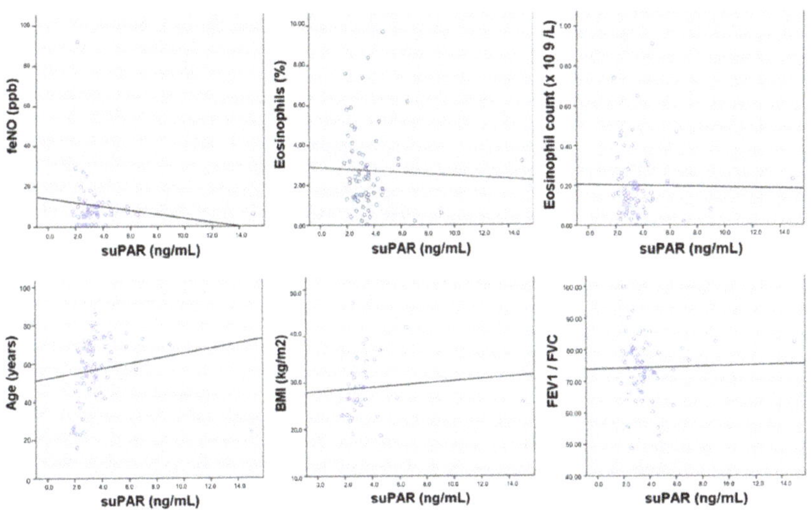

Figure 3. Correlation analysis between suPAR levels and age, body mass index (BMI), T2 biomarkers, and forced expiratory volume in the first second (FEV1)/ forced vital capacity (FVC). Note: No correlation was found between suPAR levels and fractional exhaled nitric oxide (FeNO) (r = −0.014, p = 0.308), eosinophils % (r = −0.037, p = 0.767), eosinophil count (r = −0.016, p = 0.895), age (r = 0.14, p = 0.238), BMI (r = 0.079, p = 0.646)), and FeV1/FVC (r = 0.020, p = 0.870). Abbreviations: BMI, body mass index; FeNO, fractional exhaled nitric oxide; FeV1/FVC, forced expiratory volume in the first second/forced vital capacity.

4. Discussion

This study found that suPAR levels were significantly higher in asthmatics with severe uncontrolled asthma with or without biologics than in patients with moderate uncontrolled asthma. No correlations were found between suPAR levels and age, BMI, T2 biomarkers, white blood cell count, CRP, electrolytes, kidney and liver function parameters, CRP, or spirometric parameters.

Previous studies have shown that suPAR is associated with disease progression and severity in multiple diseases. Thus far, few studies have explored suPAR's role in asthma outcomes [1]. More specifically, elevated suPAR levels have been associated with hospital all-cause readmission and all-cause mortality in hospitalized patients with a diagnosis of asthma made as soon as they were acutely admitted to the emergency department [8]. Another study found that suPAR concentrations were increased in a small cohort of asthmatics with poor disease control compared to patients with well-controlled asthma [1].

In this study, we found no correlation between age and suPAR levels. Nevertheless, there is evidence that age is a non-modifiable risk factor that correlates with an increase in suPAR levels [14]. A previous study in a population of 182 generally healthy individuals aged 74–89 years found that those aged 24–66 years had higher suPAR levels than younger controls: 3.79 ng/mL (95% CI 3.64–3.96 ng/mL) vs. 3.16 ng/mL (95% CI 2.86–3.45 ng/mL) [14]. These levels increased further with advancing age and were similar in women and men. Aging is associated with systematic cardiac and vascular structure alterations due to immunological responses and natural hormonal changes, resulting in a gradual decline in organ function [14]. However, in our study, we excluded asthmatics with comorbidities associated with low-grade chronic inflammation processes such as diabetes, heart failure, and malignant and inflammatory systemic diseases; this could explain the fact that we did not find any association between age and suPAR levels.

Although obesity is considered a low-grade inflammatory disease, or parainflammation, in this study, we found no association between suPAR levels and BMI. Limited data investigate suPAR as an inflammatory biomarker in obesity. More specifically, Kosecik et al. reported that suPAR has no predictive value for future atherosclerosis in obese children after investigating 136 participants with a median age of 12.05 years [15].

We found no association between suPAR levels and T2-high biomarkers. A previous study documented that in patients acutely admitted with asthma, elevated suPAR concentrations together with blood eosinophil count < 150 cells/μL at the time of hospital admission were associated with both 365-day all-cause readmission and mortality, implying that in asthma, the uPAR pathway associates with non-T2 asthma but is implicated in neutrophils and T1/T17 T-cells that are thought to be part of the pathogenesis of the non-T2 asthma endotypes [14,16,17].

Neutrophils are a primary source of circulating suPAR [18]. Studies report the usefulness of suPAR in predicting severe outcomes in critical illness related to inflammatory and infectious diseases [18], along with CRP and leukocytes. In this study, we found no correlation between suPAR and other inflammatory markers, such as white blood cell count or CRP, given that we excluded patients with significant comorbidities. In the same context, no correlation was detected between suPAR and kidney parameters and liver function parameters. However, there is evidence that suPAR plasma levels were significantly higher in patients with chronic kidney disease (7.9 ± 3.82 ng/mL) than in controls (1.76 ± 0.77 ng/mL, $p < 0.001$) and correlated with disease severity [19]. Similar to its prognostic properties in patients with sepsis, serum suPAR concentrations might serve as an interesting biomarker in cirrhosis and acute liver failure [19].

FEV1 levels are not the only factor taken into account to classify disease severity [16]; they have long been known to be one of the major predictors of mortality among individuals with asthma [16]. However, lung function deficits with magnitudes insufficient to cause clinically manifest functional impairments found in mild asthma are also related to molecular pathways that increase susceptibility to the pulmonary effects of exposures. Furthermore, small airway disease (SAD) is highly prevalent in asthma, even in patients with milder disease. Structural alterations at the peribronchiolar level contribute to the pathogenesis of functional abnormalities observed in patients with asthma [16]. Remodeling can affect small airway wall stiffness, thereby changing their distensibility. Given the clinical impact of SAD, its presence should not be underestimated or overlooked as part of the daily management of patients with asthma. SAD is likely to be directly or indirectly captured by combinations of physiological tests, such as spirometry. Notably, suPAR levels have been previously linked to impaired lung function and airway resistance [1]. This study found no correlation between suPAR levels and airway obstruction. Further research is needed to evaluate any potential correlation between suPAR levels and SAD using more detailed techniques.

In asthma, a panel of several cytokines, chemokines, and granule proteins induce airway inflammation and hyperresponsiveness through enhancing innate and type 2 (T2) or non-T2 immune responses [1,8,16]. Although disease severity-related airway inflammation is found in asthma, new evidence has documented persistent chronic airway inflammation and remodeling in mild asthma, except for those with severe asthma, as defined by the treatment step [8]. Neutrophilic asthma is the lesser-known asthma phenotype and is characterized by severe refractory disease. Airway neutrophilia is associated with asthma severity, acute asthma exacerbation, and airflow limitation. However, neutrophils can also be detected in the airways of mild asthmatics [8,16]. Interestingly, studies suggest that the inflammation reflected in circulating suPAR concentrations in part stems from neutrophil activity [9], commonly considered to be non-T2 inflammation [16]. Accordingly, this study found no correlation between suPAR concentrations and T2 biomarkers such as eosinophils and FeNO.

Our study's findings should be interpreted within the context of its limitations. As such, when considering absolute numbers, our study's population is small, in a single center with patients from the same population in terms of geo-ethnicity, limiting our findings' generalizability. Larger multi-center and multi-nation studies are needed to confirm our results. However, other factors could not have confounded our findings, given that we carefully excluded patients with comorbidities associated with high suPAR levels.

5. Conclusions

suPAR levels were higher in asthmatics with severe disease receiving or not receiving biologics than in those with moderate uncontrolled asthma. suPAR's high stability in plasma samples and its noninvasiveness make it an ideal candidate for the management of asthma and the prediction of worse outcomes. The findings of this study suggested a prognostic value of suPAR that would translate into clinical practice in asthma patients and might predict step-up treatment benefits across the spectrum of asthma severity. Furthermore, the information can be used to develop targeted interventions aimed at the risks of so-called mild asthma. An important practical implication is that suPAR might be a useful addition to existing stratification algorithms for identifying patients that particularly benefit from step-up treatment. This study also indicates that suPAR levels might be effective for clinical use associated with specific clinical features, inflammatory phenotypes of asthma, or impaired lung function.

Supplementary Materials: The following supporting information can be downloaded at: https://www.mdpi.com/article/10.3390/jpm12111776/s1.

Author Contributions: Conceptualization, O.S.K.; methodology, O.S.K. and I.P.; validation, O.S.K.; I.P.; formal analysis, O.S.K.; investigation, G.M., K.T., K.M., P.K.; data curation, O.S.K.; writing—original draft preparation, O.S.K.; writing—review and editing, O.S.K.; supervision, O.S.K., K.I.G., Z.D.; project administration, O.S.K. All authors have read and agreed to the published version of the manuscript.

Funding: This work is supported by a Grant from the Hellenic Thoracic Society. The funders had no role in study design, data collection, and analysis, decision to publish, or preparation of the manuscript. (Grant Number: 17/2020).

Institutional Review Board Statement: The study was conducted in accordance with the Declaration of Helsinki and approved by the Ethics Committee of the University of Thessaly (No. 2800-01/11/2020; approved on 1 November 2020).

Informed Consent Statement: Patient consent was waived due to the retrospective nature of this study, and the analysis used anonymous clinical data.

Data Availability Statement: The data that support the findings of this study are available on request from the corresponding author, O.S.K.

Conflicts of Interest: The authors declare no conflict of interest.

References

1. Ivancsó, I.; Toldi, G.; Bohács, A.; Eszes, N.; Müller, V.; Rigó, J., Jr.; Vásárhelyi, B.; Losonczy, G.; Tamási, L. Relationship of Circulating Soluble Urokinase Plasminogen Activator Receptor (suPAR) Levels to Disease Control in Asthma and Asthmatic Pregnancy. *PLoS ONE* **2013**, *8*, e60697. [CrossRef] [PubMed]
2. Luo, Q.; Ning, P.; Zheng, Y.; Shang, Y.; Zhou, B.; Gao, Z. Serum suPAR and syndecan-4 levels predict severity of community-acquired pneumonia: A prospective, multi-centre study. *Crit Care* **2018**, *22*, 15. [CrossRef] [PubMed]
3. Can, Ü.; Güzelant, A.; Yerlikaya, F.H.; Yosunkaya, Ş. The role of serum soluble urokinase-type plasminogen activator receptor in stable chronic obstructive pulmonary disease. *J. Investig. Med.* **2014**, *62*, 938–943. [CrossRef] [PubMed]
4. Sever, Z.K.; Bircan, H.A.; Sirin, F.B.; Evrimler, S.; Celik, S.; Merd, N. Serum biomarkers in patients with stable and exacerbated COPD-bronchiectasis overlap syndrome. *Clin. Respir. J.* **2020**, *14*, 1032–1039. [CrossRef] [PubMed]
5. Pacholczak-Madej, R.; Kuszmiersz, P.; Iwaniec, T.; Zaręba, L.; Zarychta, J.; Walocha, J.A.; Dropiński, J.; Bazan-Socha, S. Endothelial Dysfunction and Pentraxin-3 in Clinically Stable Adult Asthma Patients. *J. Investig. Allergol. Clin. Immunol.* **2021**, *31*, 417–425. [CrossRef] [PubMed]
6. Green, C.E.; Turner, A.M. The role of the endothelium in asthma and chronic obstructive pulmonary disease (COPD). *Respir. Res.* **2017**, *18*, 20. [CrossRef] [PubMed]
7. Portelli, M.A.; Moseley, C.; Stewart, C.E.; Postma, D.S.; Howarth, P.; Warner, J.A.; Holloway, J.W.; Koppelman, G.H.; Brightling, C.; Sayers, I. Airway and peripheral urokinase plasminogen activator receptor is elevated in asthma, and identifies a severe, nonatopic subset of patients. *Allergy* **2017**, *72*, 473–482. [CrossRef] [PubMed]
8. FitzGerald, J.M.; Barnes, P.J.; Chipps, B.E.; Jenkins, C.R.; O'Byrne, P.M.; Pavord, I.D.; Reddel, H.K. The burden of exacerbations in mild asthma: A systematic review. *ERJ Open Res.* **2020**, *6*, 00359–02019. [CrossRef] [PubMed]
9. Global Initiative for Asthma. 2020 GINA Main Report. Available online: https://ginasthma.org/gina-reports/ (accessed on 20 October 2022).
10. Dweik, R.A.; Boggs, P.B.; Erzurum, S.C.; Irvin, C.G.; Leigh, M.W.; Lundberg, J.O.; Olin, A.C.; Plummer, A.L.; Taylor, D.R.; American Thoracic Society Committee on Interpretation of Exhaled Nitric Oxide Levels (FENO) for Clinical Applications. An official ATS clinical practice guideline: Interpretation of exhaled nitric oxide levels (FENO) for clinical applications. *Am. J. Respir. Crit. Care Med.* **2011**, *184*, 602–615. [CrossRef] [PubMed]
11. Rasmussen, L.J.; Ladelund, S.; Haupt, T.H.; Ellekilde, G.; Poulsen, J.H.; Iversen, K.; Eugen-Olsen, J.; Andersen, O. Soluble urokinase plasminogen activator receptor (suPAR) in acute care: A strong marker of disease presence and severity, readmission and mortality. A retrospective cohort study. *Emerg. Med. J.* **2016**, *33*, 769–775. [CrossRef] [PubMed]
12. Håkansson, K.E.J.; Rasmussen, L.J.H.; Godtfredsen, N.S.; Tupper, O.D.; Eugen-Olsen, J.; Kallemose, T.; Andersen, O.; Ulrik, C.S. The biomarkers suPAR and blood eosinophils are associated with hospital readmissions and mortality in asthma—A retrospective cohort study. *Respir. Res.* **2019**, *20*, 258. [CrossRef] [PubMed]
13. Wlazel, R.N.; Szwabe, K.; Guligowska, A.; Kostka, T. Soluble urokinase plasminogen activator receptor level in individuals of advanced age. *Sci. Rep.* **2020**, *10*, 15462. [CrossRef] [PubMed]
14. Kosecik, M.; Dervisoglu, P.; Koroglu, M.; Isguven, P.; Elmas, B.; Demiray, T.; Altindis, M. Usefulness of soluble urokinase plasminogen activator receptor (suPAR) as an inflammatory biomarker in obese children. *Int. J. Cardiol.* **2017**, *228*, 158–161. [CrossRef] [PubMed]
15. Ricciardolo, F.L.M.; Sorbello, V.; Folino, A.; Gallo, F.; Massaglia, G.M.; Favatà, G.; Conticello, S.; Vallese, D.; Gani, F.; Malerba, M.; et al. Identification of IL-17F/frequent exacerbator endotype in asthma. *J. Allergy Clin. Immunol.* **2017**, *140*, 395–406. [CrossRef] [PubMed]
16. Håkansson, K.E.J.; Ulrik, C.S.; Godtfredsen, N.S.; Kallemose, T.; Andersen, O.; Eugen-Olsen, J.; Marsaa, K.; Rasmussen, L.J.H. High suPAR and Low Blood Eosinophil Count are Risk Factors for Hospital Readmission and Mortality in Patients with COPD. *Int. J. Chronic Obstruct. Pulm. Dis.* **2020**, *15*, 733–743. [CrossRef] [PubMed]
17. Gussen, H.; Hohlstein, P.; Bartneck, M.; Warzecha, K.T.; Buendgens, L.; Luedde, T.; Trautwein, C.; Koch, A.; Tacke, F. Neutrophils are a main source of circulating suPAR predicting outcome in critical illness. *J. Intensive Care* **2019**, *7*, 26. [CrossRef] [PubMed]
18. Ahmed, R.M.; Khalil, M.A.; Ibrahim, A.H.; Eid, H.M.; Abdelbasset, W.K.; Soliman, G.S. Clinical value of soluble urokinase type plasminogen activator receptors in chronic kidney disease. *Medicine* **2019**, *98*, e17146. [CrossRef] [PubMed]
19. Koch, A.; Zimmermann, H.W.; Gassler, N.; Jochum, C.; Weiskirchen, R.; Bruensing, J.; Buendgens, L.; Dückers, H.; Bruns, T.; Gerken, G.; et al. Clinical relevance and cellular source of elevated soluble urokinase plasminogen activator receptor (suPAR) in acute liver failure. *Liver Int.* **2014**, *34*, 1330–1339. [CrossRef] [PubMed]

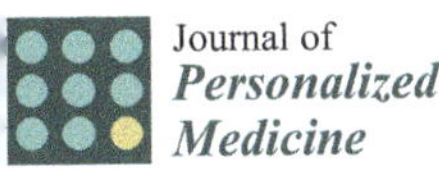
Journal of *Personalized Medicine*

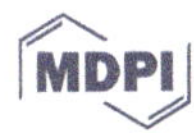

Review

Contemporary Biomarkers in Pulmonary Embolism Diagnosis: Moving beyond D-Dimers

Androniki Gkana [1,†], Androniki Papadopoulou [1,†], Maria Mermiri [2,*], Eleftherios Beltsios [3], Dimitrios Chatzis [4], Foteini Malli [5], Antonis Adamou [1], Konstantinos Gourgoulianis [5], Georgios Mavrovounis [1] and Ioannis Pantazopoulos [1]

1 Department of Emergency Medicine, Faculty of Medicine, University of Thessaly, Biopolis, 41110 Larissa, Greece
2 Department of Anaesthesiology, Faculty of Medicine, University of Thessaly, Biopolis, 41110 Larissa, Greece
3 Department of Thoracic and Cardiovascular Surgery, West Germany Heart Center, University Clinic Essen, 45147 Essen, Germany
4 School of Medicine, European University of Cyprus, 2404 Nicosia, Cyprus
5 Department of Respiratory Medicine, Faculty of Medicine, University of Thessaly, Biopolis, 41110 Larissa, Greece
* Correspondence: mmermiri@gmail.com; Tel.: +30-6988987175
† These authors contributed equally to this work.

Abstract: Pulmonary embolism (PE) is a rather common cardiovascular disorder constituting one of the major manifestations of venous thromboembolism (VTE). It is associated with high mortality and substantial recurrence rates, and its diagnosis may be challenging, especially in patients with respiratory comorbidities. Therefore, providing a prompt and accurate diagnosis for PE through developing highly sensitive and specific diagnostic algorithms would be of paramount importance. There is sound evidence supporting the use of biomarkers to enhance the diagnosis and predict the recurrence risk in patients with PE. Therefore, several novel biomarkers, such as factor VIII, Ischemia Modified Albumin, and fibrinogen, as well as several MicroRNAs and microparticles, have been investigated for the diagnosis of this clinical entity. The present review targets to comprehensively present the literature regarding the novel diagnostic biomarkers for PE, as well as to discuss the evidence for their use in daily routine.

Keywords: pulmonary embolism; diagnosis; D-dimers; biomarkers; ischemia modified albumin; microparticles; microRNAs; Factor VIII

Citation: Gkana, A.; Papadopoulou, A.; Mermiri, M.; Beltsios, E.; Chatzis, D.; Malli, F.; Adamou, A.; Gourgoulianis, K.; Mavrovounis, G.; Pantazopoulos, I. Contemporary Biomarkers in Pulmonary Embolism Diagnosis: Moving beyond D-Dimers. *J. Pers. Med.* **2022**, *12*, 1604. https://doi.org/10.3390/jpm12101604

Academic Editor: Eumorfia Kondili

Received: 13 August 2022
Accepted: 26 September 2022
Published: 29 September 2022

1. Introduction

Pulmonary embolism (PE) is a relatively common cardiovascular disorder that constitutes one of the two major manifestations of venous thromboembolism (VTE). PE may be associated with high mortality, especially in untreated cases; undiagnosed PE carries a 30% mortality rate, which falls to 8% when diagnosed [1]. PE diagnosis may be challenging, especially in patients with respiratory comorbidities [1]. Therefore, it is crucial to provide a prompt and accurate diagnosis for PE by developing highly sensitive and specific diagnostic algorithms.

The diagnosis of the disease is based on the individual patient's clinical probability for PE combined with laboratory and non-invasive imaging methods, mainly Computed Tomography Pulmonary Angiography (CTPA), which serves as the gold standard [2]. Since PE pathophysiology is rather complex, incorporating both thrombotic and inflammatory components, a plethora of "novel" biomarkers for PE diagnosis is currently under investigation with the ultimate goal to increase diagnostic accuracy, leading to the effective and appropriate management of this potentially lethal clinical entity.

The purpose of the present narrative review is to discuss some of the novel diagnostic biomarkers for PE and illustrate the evidence for their use in everyday clinical practice.

Furthermore, we provide an updated review of the contemporary approaches concerning D-dimer testing for the diagnosis of PE.

2. Methods

To identify relevant articles for the present literature review, we performed an electronic search of the PubMed (MEDLINE), Google Scholar, and Scopus databases. We used the following keywords combined with the Boolean operators "AND" and "OR", as appropriate: "Pulmonary Embolism", "Diagnosis", "D-dimers", "Biomarkers", "Ischemia Modified Albumin", "MicroRNAs", "Fibrinogen", "Factor VIII", and "Microparticles". The results were limited to those written in English. The last literature search was performed on 1 March 2022. Three independent investigators (A.G., A.P., M.M) screened the titles and abstracts to select potentially relevant articles for inclusion. The full text of the selected articles was thoroughly examined, and the studies presenting original data on PE diagnosis and different biomarkers were finally included.

3. Fibrinogen

Fibrinogen is a large, complex, fibrous glycoprotein, which is converted into fibrin during the coagulation cascade, yielding the fibrin clot for hemostasis [3,4]. Moreover, fibrinogen is produced as an acute phase reactant by the liver in response to inflammation or ischemia. The cleaving of fibrin by plasmin results in the production of D-dimers, which represent the expression of fibrin degradation occurring during the fibrinolytic activity of clot breakdown [5]. Due to its nature as an acute phase reactant, as well as a significant part of the coagulation cascade, the measurement of fibrinogen levels combined with D-dimer levels has been proposed as a valuable diagnostic tool for the diagnosis of PE.

A prospective study assessed the D-dimer and fibrinogen levels in 191 outpatients with suspected PE and observed that patients suffering from PE had a lower fibrinogen and higher D-dimer/fibrinogen (D/F) ratio versus those without PE [6]. The inverse relation of D-dimer and fibrinogen is indicative of activated coagulation leading to fibrinogen consumption and the simultaneous activation of endogenous fibrinolysis, resulting in D-dimer elevation. Moreover, low fibrinogen levels can be explained by the impaired fibrinogen synthesis due to liver congestion caused by right ventricular failure in patients with PE. At the cut-off point of 100% specificity, the true PPV of D/F ratio > 1.04 × 103 was approximately twice as high when compared with D-dimer > 7000 mg/L (57.6% vs. 29.4%). As such, the authors supported that a D/F ratio > 1000 is highly specific for acute PE and might be used as a "rule in" test. [6]. In the same context, Kara et al. [4] demonstrated that patients with PE had q significantly increased D/F ratio compared to controls. However, this change was attributed to increased D-dimer levels, since fibrinogen did not differ between groups. Importantly, the D/F ratio displayed greater specificity than D-dimer levels alone for PE diagnosis (37% vs. 27%, respectively) [4].

Interestingly, in a large Danish study of 77,608 individuals, high fibrinogen levels were observed in patients with PE in combination with DVT; fibrinogen levels $\geq$ 4.6 g/L were associated with a multivariate-adjusted odds ratio of 2.1 [7]. On the other hand, to make matters more complicated, in a prospective study of 40 PE patients, one-third of the patients had a fibrinogen level out of the normal range and the study did not reveal lower fibrinogen levels in patients with a positive D-dimer test [8].

Another argument that has been raised is whether the D/F ratio may be utilized for the diagnosis of PE in specific clinical settings, such as Intensive Care Unit (ICU) patients. Critically ill patients may have elevated D-dimer and low fibrinogen levels due to several factors, such as infections, malignancies, or severe cardiac or respiratory diseases, rendering them unreliable for the diagnosis of PE [9,10]. In these instances, the D/F ratio may be preferable instead. Indeed, Hajsadeghi et al. [10] suggested that the D/F ratio in ICU patients was significantly higher when PE was present, having almost the same AUC with D-dimer for diagnosing patients with PE (0.710 vs. 0.714 for D/F ratio and D-dimers, respectively), while in contrast, the fibrinogen levels did not differ significantly

(536.73 ± 186.32 vs. 586.33 ± 211.06, $p = 0.298$). More specifically, a D/F cut-off ratio of 0.233×10^{-3} had the highest accuracy in the diagnosis of PE in an ICU setting (sensitivity 70%, specificity 67.1%) [10].

In conclusion, the utility of the D-dimer/fibrinogen ratio as a diagnostic tool for the diagnosis of PE, although promising, remains controversial. The data found in the literature are not conclusive and are derived from small cohorts. One has to take into account that the aforementioned data lack external validation and cannot be safely applied in clinical practice before further larger randomized clinical trials confirm their findings [4,6,10]. Table 1 summarized the available data on the use of fibrinogen in the diagnosis of PE.

Table 1. Summary of the available studies on the use of fibrinogen in the diagnosis of PE [4,6,8,10].

Study/YOP	Number of Participants	Results
Kucher et al., 2003 [6]	191	A D/F ratio of >103 is highly specific for the presence of acute PE It doubles the diagnostic rate compared with D-dimer testing alone
Kara et al., 2014 [4]	200	D-dimer cutoff of 0.5 mg/mL vs. D/F ratio cutoff of 1.0: D/F ratio may have a better specificity than D-dimer level in PE diagnosis
Hajsadeghi et al., 2012 [10]	81	Significantly higher D/F ratio (0.913 ± 0.716 vs. $483 \pm 0.440 \times 10^{-3}$, $p = 0.003$) in PE patients than in non-PE patients. A D/F ratio of 0.417×10^{-3} (AUC = 0.710, $p = 0.004$) had 70.3% sensitivity and 61.6% specificity.
Calvo-Romero et al., 2004 [8]	40	Fibrinogen levels similar in patients with a negative vs. positive D-dimer test Fibrinogen levels not statistically different in patients with DVT and PE vs. patients with isolated DVT (trend observed, $p = 0.1$).

4. Ischemia-Modified Albumin (IMA)

Ischemia-Modified Albumin (IMA) is a molecule formed by the modification of albumin by reactive oxygen radicals [11]. Human serum albumins consist of 585 amino acids and the first 3 amino acids in the N-terminus, Asp-Ala-His, constitute a specific binding site for transition metals, which is susceptible to degradation. IMA is formed through the modification of this protein region due to the effect of reactive oxygen radicals produced by ischemia [12]. Serum IMA levels may increase in several acute conditions, namely, acute coronary syndrome, cardiac arrest, stroke, and mesenteric ischemia [11,13,14].

Published data from small cohort studies suggest that IMA levels are higher in PE patients vs. controls, and thus IMA has been proposed as a potential diagnostic biomarker for PE [15]. Turedi et al. [16] studied 30 PE patients and 30 healthy volunteers and demonstrated a statistically significant increase in serum IMA levels above 0.540 Absorbance Units in 97.7% of PE patients. In line with the aforementioned findings, a serum IMA above 0.4 had a sensitivity of 53.8% and specificity of 89.6% for PE, and the IMA levels were positively correlated with shock index and heart rate but failed to predict RV dysfunction in an experimental animal study [11]. A consequent study suggested that the IMA levels, in combination with clinical probability scores, had similar negative predictive value (NPV) and sensitivity to D-dimer testing [15]. However, IMA had a greater positive predictive value (PPV) compared to D-dimer (79.4% vs. 69.4%) but was not high enough to confirm the diagnosis of PE without additional investigation [15].

Despite that the aforementioned data favor a role of IMA in PE diagnosis, they should be interpreted with caution since they derive from small retrospective cohorts (i.e., patients were not followed-up for subsequent development of PE). The fact that there is no evidence about IMA's role in PE in the last 10 years highlights the need for more studies with greater sample sizes in order to conclude more reliable results. Furthermore, IMA may be elevated in many other conditions (e.g., exercise, congestive heart failure), thus performing multivariate analysis for possible confounders is crucial. Table 2 summarizes the available on the use of IMA in the diagnosis of PE.

Table 2. Summary of the available studies on the use of IMA in the diagnosis of PE [12,16].

Study/YOP	Number of Participants	Results
Turedi et al., 2006 [16]	60	Mean IMA levels in PE patients: 0.724 ± 0.122 ABSU Mean IMA levels in controls: 0.360 ± 0.090 ABSU Statistically significant difference ($p < 0.0005$)
Turedi et al., 2008 [12]	189	Cut-off point of 0.25 ABSU: Sensitivity = 93% Specificity = 75% PPV = 79.4% NPV = 78.6% For PE diagnosis

5. Factor VIII

Factor VIII (FVIII) is a glycoprotein produced in liver sinusoidal cells and endothelial cells which is essential in the coagulation cascade [17]. Activated Factor VIII (FVIIIa) is derived by limited proteolysis, catalyzed by thrombin or activated factor X. FVIIIa increases the catalytic efficiency of activated factor IX in the activation of factor X. FVIII accelerates, through Xa, the conversion of prothrombin to thrombin, which converts fibrinogen to fibrin. Additionally, high FVIII levels may increase the thrombotic risk by decreasing responsiveness to activated protein C (APC) [18]. Consequently, FVIII plays an important role in the amplification of the clotting cascade at sites of vascular injury [19]. Studies indicate a direct relationship between high plasma levels of FVIII and arterial or venous thrombosis and PE [20–30].

Several studies reported that elevated plasma FVIII levels may represent a significant, independent risk factor for PE in a quantitative dependent pattern [20,21,23,24,26–31]. In 1995, Koster et al. reported the independent quantitative response association between FVIII levels and DVT ($p < 0.001$). In patients with FVIII levels above 1500 IU/L, there was a dose–response relation of FVIII levels with the risk of thrombosis (OR = 4.8) [20]. Other investigators also confirmed this independent and quantitative relationship. Rietveld et al. in 2019 [31], performed a large case–control study that assessed the levels of coagulation factors in relation to the risk for VTE. Their results showed that FVIII levels, as well as Von Willebrand Factor levels, had the strongest association of all coagulation factors with VTE, and this association was found to be independent of BMI, major illness, or CRP levels. The relative risks were similar for patients with provoked and unprovoked (idiopathic) VTE. The relative risks were found to be 15.0 (95% CI 8.6–26.1) for PE, 27.8 (95% CI 16.9–45.8) for DVT, and 43.2 (95% CI 16.6–122.5) for PE with DVT, suggesting that FVIII levels play different roles in the DVT and PE etiology [31]. Payne et al. also supported the independent relationship between FVIII levels and VTE [30]. In addition, it has been shown that Von Willebrand Factor levels correlate with FVIII levels, and this combination elevates, even more, the risk for VTE [24,30,31]. Interestingly, O'Donnell J et al. reported that elevated FVIII:C levels following VTE are persistent and independent of the acute phase reaction [23]. This result was further supported by Sane et al. who measured FVIII levels during PE diagnosis in 63 patients and after a 7-month follow-up period. The levels of FVIII were higher during PE diagnosis compared with the follow-up levels (167.2% vs. 155.1%) but the difference was not statistically significant ($p = 0.07$) [32]. Moreover, Oger et al. demonstrated a quantitative relationship between FVIII levels and VTE, not only in young adults but elderly patients (>70 years old) as well [26].

Regarding PE, Erkekol et al. supported the existence of a quantitative correlation between factor VIII levels and thrombosis, since high plasma levels of FVIII (>168 U/dL) were found in 53.3% (OR 11.04; 95% CI 3.65–33.35) of isolated PE patients and 55.0% (OR 11.81; CI 3.49–39.92) of patients with a combined form of PE and DVT compared with

9.4% in control patients. The risk was not affected after adjustment for other possible risk factors [27]. Heerink et al. found that the levels of FVIII were higher in patients with PE when compared with healthy controls, but the population of PE patients in this study was small (n = 11) [33]. In contrast to the previous results pointing to the specificity of FVIII levels, Kamphuisen et al. found high FVIII levels (≥150 IU/dL) at the acute phase in both PE patients and subjects with various etiologic substrates (pneumonia, heart failure, or malignancy) [25].

While several studies have investigated the possible use of FVIII levels as a biomarker for the diagnosis of PE, their importance remains unclear. The aforementioned observations need further confirmation by studies focusing on the potential influence of comorbidities (such as cancer, heart disease, or lung disease) and the acute phase reactions at the FVIII plasma level.

6. MicroRNAs

MicroRNAs (miRNAs) are non-coding RNAs with a length of approximately 22 nucleotides that are involved in important cellular pathways such as development, proliferation, and apoptosis [34]. They are present in various body fluids, being remarkably stable due to carrier-protein binding [35] and consequently, in recent years, they have been studied as non-invasive biomarkers for various disorders such as cancer, cardiovascular, and cerebrovascular diseases [36,37]. Various miRNAs have been reported to regulate several hemostatic factors (fibrinogen, factor XI, etc.), modulate platelet activation and aggregation, and have been found to be dysregulated in venous thrombosis [38,39].

In 2011, Xiao et al. were the first group that investigated the possibility of identifying some miRNAs as potential biomarkers for the diagnosis of acute PE. Specifically, they reported that miRNA-134 was significantly elevated in patients with acute PE when compared with healthy individuals, reporting a sensitivity of 68.8% and specificity of 68.2% [40]. In 2016, Deng et al. [41] published a systematic review and meta-analysis based on three studies [40,42,43], concluding that, although more research is needed to validate their role as diagnostic biomarkers for acute PE, miRNAs seem to represent reliable novel biomarker candidates (pooled sensitivity: 83%, pooled specificity: 85%). Since then, more original studies have been published [44–46], reporting that various miRNAs are upregulated during acute PE episodes and can be an additional tool available to the physician. An interesting study reported that miRNA-1233 and miRNA-134 can be potentially used to identify patients with acute exacerbation of chronic obstructive pulmonary disease complicated by acute PE [46].

It is important to note that some groups have investigated the possibility of combining various miRNAs with each other and with other established biomarkers such as D-dimers to increase their diagnostic efficacy [45]. Combining miRNA-27a/b with D-dimers significantly increases the capacity for diagnosing acute PE [45]. In more detail, combining miRNA-27a or miRNA-27b with D-dimers resulted in a significant increase in the area under the receiver operating characteristic (ROC) curve, reaching 0.909 and 0.867, respectively.

Collectively, these findings support the hypothesis that miRNAs may serve as a novel biomarker for the diagnosis of acute PE; however, further research in this field has to be performed, as studies up to this date have limited statistical power and reproducibility. Table 3 summarizes the available data on the use of miRNAs in the diagnosis of PE.

Table 3. Summary of the available studies on the use of miRNAs in the diagnosis of PE [40,42–46].

Study/YOP	No Subjects/ Sample from	Cut-Off Value	Molecule	Results
Xiao J et al., 2011 [40]	54/plasma	0.003	miRNA-134	miRNA-134 levels were higher in patients with acute PE compared with healthy individuals, reporting a sensitivity of 68.8% and specificity of 68.2% Additionally, used miRNA-134 to differentiate between acute PE patients and non-PE patients that reported dyspnea, chest pain, or cough
Zhou X et al., 2016 [42]	74/plasma	1.66	miRNA-28-3p	MiRNA-28-3p was significantly elevated in the plasma of PE patients.
Kessler et al., 2016 [43]	42/plasma	0.53 0.63 0.51	miRNA-1233, miRNA-27a, miRNA-134	miRNA-1233, miRNA-27a, and miRNA-134 were significantly higher in the serum of acute PE patients in comparison to healthy controls The 1233-miRNA differentiated the acute PE patients and the NSTEMI, DVT, and chronic pulmonary hypertension patients
Liu T et al., 2018 [44]	110/plasma	NA	miRNA-221	The plasma levels of miRNA-221 were significantly increased in patients with acute PE when compared with healthy individuals. The levels in patients with acute PE were positively correlated with levels of BNP, troponin I, and D-dimer.
Wang Q et al., 2018 [45]	148/plasma	0.115, 0.059	miRNA-27a miRNA-27b	The plasma levels of miRNA-27a and miRNA-27b were significantly higher in APE patients ($p < 0.001$) compared with normal controls. Combining miRNA-27a/b with D-dimers significantly increased the capacity for diagnosing acute PE
Peng L et al., 2020 [46]	52/plasma	NA	miRNA-1233, miRNA-134	miRNA-1233 and miRNA-134 have high clinical value in the early diagnosis of patients of acute exacerbation of chronic obstructive pulmonary disease combined with PE These miRNAs could be used as potential biomarkers for clinical identification of acute exacerbation of chronic obstructive pulmonary disease with or without PE complications.

7. Microparticles

Microparticles (MPs) are small vesicles of <1 micron in size, derived from various cell types, including platelets, monocytes, endothelial, and cancer cells [5,47]. MPs are formed from membrane vesicles released from the cell surface by the proteolytic cleavage of the cytoskeleton. MPs provide procoagulant molecules, especially anionic phospholipids (particularly phosphatidylserine) and tissue factor (TF) protein, for the assembly of components of the coagulation cascade [47]. As a result, many studies aimed to investigate the role of MPs in inflammation, cancer, and other diseases [48]. Due to their involvement in the formation of thrombi, MPs have been proposed as potential biomarkers for the diagnosis of VTE and acute PE [48,49].

In a study by Rezania S et al. plasma MP levels were evaluated in PE patients and healthy volunteers using standard fluorescent polystyrene beads. A relative abundance of plasma MPs was noted in the PE patients [50]. Furthermore, there was a correlation between the PE and Platelet-Derived MPs (PDMPs) plasma levels; the PE patients exhibited higher levels of PDMPs as compared to their healthy counterparts [51]. The association between acute PE and procoagulant MPs levels was also highlighted by Bal et al. [52]. Specifically, circulating MPs and platelet MPs were significantly elevated in PE patients compared to healthy controls, but this correlation was not statistically significant when PE patients were compared with controls with cardiovascular risk factors such as hypertension and diabetes [52].

The correlation between MP levels and cardiovascular diseases, such as hypertension and coronary artery disease, has been previously reported [52,53]. These results highlight the importance of adjusting the measurement of MPs in patients with cardiac comorbidities when PE is suspected.

In conclusion, these studies provide evidence in favor of the clinical use of MPs for diagnosis, but potentially after adjustment for other comorbidities (cancer, cardiovascular diseases) which may also increase the levels of MPs in patients' serum.

8. Other Biomarkers and PE

There are several more novel biomarkers that have been proposed as potential biomarkers for the diagnosis of PE. Limited data on those biomarkers are available; thus, their use in clinical practice is still considered questionable.

Endothelial cell-specific molecule 1, or endocan, a soluble dermatan sulfate proteoglycan [54], has been associated with PE, predicting the severity of pulmonary artery occlusion [55,56]. Güzel et al. measured serum endocan levels in 46 PE patients and reported a significant difference in the serum endocan levels between PE patients and healthy controls 321.93 vs. 192.77 mg/L ($p < 0.03$) [55]. On the contrary, Mosevoll et al. dispute the diagnostic value of endocan in PE, showcasing that no difference in endocan levels between patients with PE and healthy controls was noted in their study [57]. Thus, the use of endocan as a PE biomarker has to be examined further before definite conclusions can be drawn.

The soluble urokinase-type plasminogen activator receptor (suPAR) is the soluble form of the urokinase-type plasminogen activator receptor, which is a glycosyl-phosphatidylinositol (GPI)-linked membrane protein [58] and an integral part of the fibrinolytic system. SuPAR has also been related to VTE. The incidence of VTE in 5203 subjects was higher in patients with high suPAR levels independently of several potential confounding factors (age, sex, BMI, smoking, systolic blood pressure, cholesterol, HDL, leukocyte count, diabetes, history of atrial fibrillation, history of cardiovascular disease) during a 15.7-year follow-up [58]. However, suPARs' role in PE is still unclear and needs further examination before definite conclusions can be drawn.

C-reactive protein (CRP) is a biomarker of systemic inflammation which has also been evaluated as a diagnostic marker in PE. CRP levels had a sensitivity of 95.7% [95% confidence interval (CI): 90–100] and an NPV of 98.4% (96–100). CRP < 5 mg/L with a clinical probability score indicating 'PE unlikely', had a sensitivity of 96.7% (90–100), specificity of 43.0% (37–49), and NPV 99.1% (97–100) [59]. Moreover, lower CRP levels have been shown to relate to unprovoked (idiopathic) PE [60], and changes in serum high-sensitivity CRP (Hs-CRP) levels could help in the severity categorization of PE (i.e., massive or minor PE) patients, as well as outcome prediction [61]. Thus, it has been proposed that CRP levels could be used to safely exclude PE, either alone or combined with clinical probability assessment [59,61].

A contemporary working hypothesis suggests that proteomic analysis could be used to identify potential biomarkers for PE. According to Granholm F et al. [62], the use of proteomic analysis showed that Complement component 9, Complement factor H, and Leucine-rich α-2-glycoprotein were increased in patients with PE, whereas Carboxylic ester hydrolase, Antithrombin-III, Procollagen C-endopeptidase enhancer, Serpin peptidase inhibitor, clade A, member 4, Afamin, and, *N*-acetylmuramoyl-L-alanine amidase, among others, were decreased. These findings consider proteins of general inflammation, atherosclerosis, and hemostasis as possible biomarkers in the diagnosis of PE while further research is needed to confirm it [62]. In the same context, data acquisition mass spectrometry and antibody microarray studies revealed that serum amyloid A1, calprotectin, and tenascin-C have promising value in PE diagnosis with acceptable sensitivity and specificity [63]. Few data support the use of haptoglobin (a hemoglobin-binding protein that serves as an acute-phase protein) as a biomarker of PE since its levels are increased in PE patients; the cut-off of 256.74 mg/L had a sensitivity of 62% and specificity of 83% for PE diagnosis [64].

9. Cost-Effectiveness Perspectives

Another significant parameter regarding the biomarkers in PE diagnosis is the evaluation of cost-effectiveness in health care systems worldwide. In fact, the use of an age-adjusted D-dimer cutoff of <500 ng/mL up to 50 years, then <age × 10 ng/mL, increases the cost savings by more than USD 80 million per year for the United States health care system [65]. Moreover, the D-dimer test and lower-limb compression ultrasonography are not only cost-effective in the diagnosis of PE but also easily available, thus allowing centers devoid of CTPAs to screen patients with suspected PE and avoid costly referrals [66]. On the other hand, novel biomarkers are usually expensive, and in an increasingly cost-conscious health care environment, regulatory approval will not be a guarantee of clinical adoption. Researchers must prove that a specific biomarker can change clinical practice and reduce costs by eliminating time-consuming, expensive, and sometimes ineffective diagnostic tests.

Table 4 summarizes the available data on the use of novel biomarkers in the diagnosis of PE, according to our literature search.

Table 4. Summary of the use of novel biomarkers in the diagnosis of PE.

Biomarker	Comments
Fibrinogen	• Fibrinogen as a biomarker itself seemed to be unreliable for PE diagnosis. • D-Dimer/Fibrinogen ratio had promising results, especially for critically ill patients, such as ICU patients. • Further larger randomized clinical trials have to confirm these findings.
Ischemia modified albumin	• IMA levels in combination with clinical probability scores (Geneva and Wells score) seem to play a role in the diagnosis of PE. • There is a lack of evidence in the last 10 years and a small number of available studies.
Factor VIII	• The correlation between FVIII and PE has been proven by a few studies over the last three decades. • Evidence in favor of specificity of FVIII in PE diagnosis. • Data supports that FVIII is independent of patients' comorbidities. • Other studies report that FVIII is high in various other disease processes. • Despite the promising evidence in favor of the FVIII in PE diagnosis, its specificity and accuracy are still questioned.
MicroRNAs	• Several miRNAs (miRNA-1233 and miRNA-134) are upregulated during acute PE episodes, making them potentially useful in PE diagnosis. • MiRNA-27a/b in combination with D-dimers significantly increases the capacity for diagnosing acute PE.
Microparticles	• MPs, especially platelet-derived, were found to be elevated in PE patients. However, MPs also increase in other cardiovascular diseases. • This points out the need for adjusting the measurement of MPs in patients with cardiac comorbidities

10. Conclusions

There is evidence supporting the use of biomarkers to enhance the diagnosis and predict the recurrence risk in patients with PE. There are several molecules related to both thrombotic and inflammatory PE-associated processes under investigation. So far, only D-dimer levels have been widely employed for the diagnosis of PE in daily clinical practice and have been implemented in international guidelines for PE diagnosis. This review was conducted in order to shed more light on non-D-dimer biomarkers, such as fibrinogen, IMA, factor VIII, microRNAs, and microparticles, which are present in the current bibliography, even though there are not yet randomized control trials to confirm and advance the existing evidence. Major caveats that should be addressed before the incorporation of biomarkers in clinical decision algorithms include the estimation of optimal cut-off values, the need for adjustment for cofounders (i.e., renal function), and the absence of studies that perform external validation. Further studies addressing the role of the aforementioned candidate biomarkers in PE should be designed to elucidate their importance in the diagnostic algorithm of the disease.

Author Contributions: Conceptualization, A.G., A.P., M.M., G.M. and I.P.; methodology E.B., A.A., A.G., A.P., M.M., G.M. and I.P.; writing—original draft preparation, A.G., A.P., M.M., E.B. and G.M.; writing—review and editing, E.B., A.A., D.C., F.M., K.G. and I.P.; supervision, K.G. and I.P.; project administration, I.P. All authors have read and agreed to the published version of the manuscript.

Funding: This research received no external funding.

Institutional Review Board Statement: No institutional Review acceptance was needed since this study is a narrative review.

Informed Consent Statement: Not applicable.

Data Availability Statement: Not applicable.

Conflicts of Interest: The authors declare no conflict of interest.

References

1. Bělohlávek, J.; Dytrych, V.; Linhart, A. Pulmonary Embolism, Part I: Epidemiology, Risk Factors and Risk Stratification, Pathophysiology, Clinical Presentation, Diagnosis and Nonthrombotic Pulmonary Embolism. *Exp. Clin. Cardiol.* **2013**, *18*, 129–138. [PubMed]
2. Konstantinides, S.V.; Meyer, G.; Becattini, C.; Bueno, H.; Geersing, G.-J.; Harjola, V.-P.; Huisman, M.V.; Humbert, M.; Jennings, C.S.; Jiménez, D.; et al. 2019 ESC Guidelines for the Diagnosis and Management of Acute Pulmonary Embolism Developed in Collaboration with the European Respiratory Society (ERS): The Task Force for the Diagnosis and Management of Acute Pulmonary Embolism of the European Society of Cardiology (ESC). *Eur. Respir. J.* **2019**, *54*, 1901647. [CrossRef] [PubMed]
3. Weisel, J.W. Fibrinogen and Fibrin. *Adv. Protein Chem.* **2005**, *70*, 247–299. [CrossRef] [PubMed]
4. Kara, H.; Bayir, A.; Degirmenci, S.; Kayis, S.A.; Akinci, M.; Ak, A.; Celik, B.; Dogru, A.; Ozturk, B. D-Dimer and D-Dimer/Fibrinogen Ratio in Predicting Pulmonary Embolism in Patients Evaluated in a Hospital Emergency Department. *Acta Clin. Belg.* **2014**, *69*, 240–245. [CrossRef]
5. Anghel, L.; Sascău, R.; Radu, R.; Stătescu, C. From Classical Laboratory Parameters to Novel Biomarkers for the Diagnosis of Venous Thrombosis. *Int. J. Mol. Sci.* **2020**, *21*, 1920. [CrossRef]
6. Kucher, N.; Kohler, H.-P.; Dornhöfer, T.; Wallmann, D.; Lämmle, B. Accuracy of D-Dimer/Fibrinogen Ratio to Predict Pulmonary Embolism: A Prospective Diagnostic Study. *J. Thromb. Haemost. JTH* **2003**, *1*, 708–713. [CrossRef]
7. Klovaite, J.; Nordestgaard, B.G.; Tybjærg-Hansen, A.; Benn, M. Elevated Fibrinogen Levels Are Associated with Risk of Pulmonary Embolism, but Not with Deep Venous Thrombosis. *Am. J. Respir. Crit. Care Med.* **2013**, *187*, 286–293. [CrossRef]
8. Calvo-Romero, J.M. Accuracy of D-Dimer/Fibrinogen Ratio to Predict Pulmonary Embolism: A Prospective Diagnostic Study - a Rebuttal. *J. Thromb. Haemost. JTH* **2004**, *2*, 1862–1863, author reply 1863–1864. [CrossRef]
9. Tataru, M.C.; Schulte, H.; von Eckardstein, A.; Heinrich, J.; Assmann, G.; Koehler, E. Plasma Fibrinogen in Relation to the Severity of Arteriosclerosis in Patients with Stable Angina Pectoris after Myocardial Infarction. *Coron. Artery Dis.* **2001**, *12*, 157–165. [CrossRef]
10. Hajsadeghi, S.; Kerman, S.R.; Khojandi, M.; Vaferi, H.; Ramezani, R.; Jourshari, N.M.; Mousavi, S.A.J.; Pouraliakbar, H. Accuracy of D-Dimer:Fibrinogen Ratio to Diagnose Pulmonary Thromboembolism in Patients Admitted to Intensive Care Units. *Cardiovasc. J. Afr.* **2012**, *23*, 446–456. [CrossRef]
11. Kaya, Z.; Kayrak, M.; Gul, E.E.; Altunbas, G.; Toker, A.; Kiyici, A.; Gunduz, M.; Alibaşiç, H.; Akilli, H.; Aribas, A. The Role of Ischemia Modified Albumin in Acute Pulmonary Embolism. *Heart Views Off. J. Gulf Heart Assoc.* **2014**, *15*, 106–110. [CrossRef] [PubMed]
12. Turedi, S.; Patan, T.; Gunduz, A.; Mentese, A.; Tekinbas, C.; Topbas, M.; Karahan, S.C.; Yulug, E.; Turkmen, S.; Ucar, U. Ischemia-Modified Albumin in the Diagnosis of Pulmonary Embolism: An Experimental Study. *Am. J. Emerg. Med.* **2009**, *27*, 635–640. [CrossRef] [PubMed]
13. Xanthos, T.; Iacovidou, N.; Pantazopoulos, I.; Vlachos, I.; Bassiakou, E.; Stroumpoulis, K.; Kouskouni, E.; Karabinis, A.; Papadimitriou, L. Ischaemia-Modified Albumin Predicts the Outcome of Cardiopulmonary Resuscitation: An Experimental Study. *Resuscitation* **2010**, *81*, 591–595. [CrossRef]
14. Pantazopoulos, I.; Papadimitriou, L.; Dontas, I.; Demestiha, T.; Iakovidou, N.; Xanthos, T. Ischaemia Modified Albumin in the Diagnosis of Acute Coronary Syndromes. *Resuscitation* **2009**, *80*, 306–310. [CrossRef] [PubMed]

15. Turedi, S.; Gunduz, A.; Mentese, A.; Topbas, M.; Karahan, S.C.; Yeniocak, S.; Turan, I.; Eroglu, O.; Ucar, U.; Karaca, Y.; et al. The Value of Ischemia-Modified Albumin Compared with d-Dimer in the Diagnosis of Pulmonary Embolism. *Respir. Res.* **2008**, *9*, 49. [CrossRef]
16. Turedi, S.; Gunduz, A.; Mentese, A.; Karahan, S.C.; Yilmaz, S.E.; Eroglu, O.; Nuhoglu, I.; Turan, I.; Topbas, M. Value of Ischemia-Modified Albumin in the Diagnosis of Pulmonary Embolism. *Am. J. Emerg. Med.* **2007**, *25*, 770–773. [CrossRef]
17. Turner, N.A.; Moake, J.L. Factor VIII Is Synthesized in Human Endothelial Cells, Packaged in Weibel-Palade Bodies and Secreted Bound to ULVWF Strings. *PLoS ONE* **2015**, *10*, e0140740. [CrossRef]
18. Kamphuisen, P.W.; Eikenboom, J.C.; Bertina, R.M. Elevated Factor Viii Levels and the Risk of Thrombosis. *Arterioscler. Thromb. Vasc. Biol.* **2001**, *21*, 731–738. [CrossRef]
19. Fang, H.; Wang, L.; Wang, H. The Protein Structure and Effect of Factor VIII. *Thromb. Res.* **2007**, *119*, 1–13. [CrossRef]
20. Koster, T.; Blann, A.D.; Briët, E.; Vandenbroucke, J.P.; Rosendaal, F.R. Role of Clotting Factor VIII in Effect of von Willebrand Factor on Occurrence of Deep-Vein Thrombosis. *Lancet Lond. Engl.* **1995**, *345*, 152–155. [CrossRef]
21. Kraaijenhagen, R.A.; in't Anker, P.S.; Koopman, M.M.; Reitsma, P.H.; Prins, M.H.; van den Ende, A.; Büller, H.R. High Plasma Concentration of Factor VIIIc Is a Major Risk Factor for Venous Thromboembolism. *Thromb. Haemost.* **2000**, *83*, 5–9. [PubMed]
22. Kyrle, P.A.; Minar, E.; Hirschl, M.; Bialonczyk, C.; Stain, M.; Schneider, B.; Weltermann, A.; Speiser, W.; Lechner, K.; Eichinger, S. High Plasma Levels of Factor VIII and the Risk of Recurrent Venous Thromboembolism. *N. Engl. J. Med.* **2000**, *343*, 457–462. [CrossRef] [PubMed]
23. O'Donnell, J.; Mumford, A.D.; Manning, R.A.; Laffan, M. Elevation of FVIII: C in Venous Thromboembolism Is Persistent and Independent of the Acute Phase Response. *Thromb. Haemost.* **2000**, *83*, 10–13.
24. Tsai, A.W.; Cushman, M.; Rosamond, W.D.; Heckbert, S.R.; Tracy, R.P.; Aleksic, N.; Folsom, A.R. Coagulation Factors, Inflammation Markers, and Venous Thromboembolism: The Longitudinal Investigation of Thromboembolism Etiology (LITE). *Am. J. Med.* **2002**, *113*, 636–642. [CrossRef]
25. Kamphuisen, P.W.; Ten Wolde, M.; Jacobs, E.M.G.; Ullmann, E.F.; Büller, H.R. Screening of High Factor VIII Levels Is Not Recommended in Patients with Recently Diagnosed Pulmonary Embolism. *J. Thromb. Haemost. JTH* **2003**, *1*, 2239–2240. [CrossRef] [PubMed]
26. Oger, E.; Lacut, K.; Van Dreden, P.; Bressollette, L.; Abgrall, J.-F.; Blouch, M.-T.; Scarabin, P.-Y.; Mottier, D. High Plasma Concentration of Factor VIII Coagulant Is Also a Risk Factor for Venous Thromboembolism in the Elderly. *Haematologica* **2003**, *88*, 465–469. [PubMed]
27. Erkekol, F.O.; Ulu, A.; Numanoglu, N.; Akar, N. High Plasma Levels of Factor VIII: An Important Risk Factor for Isolated Pulmonary Embolism. *Respirol. Carlton Vic* **2006**, *11*, 70–74. [CrossRef]
28. Vormittag, R.; Simanek, R.; Ay, C.; Dunkler, D.; Quehenberger, P.; Marosi, C.; Zielinski, C.; Pabinger, I. High Factor VIII Levels Independently Predict Venous Thromboembolism in Cancer Patients: The Cancer and Thrombosis Study. *Arterioscler. Thromb. Vasc. Biol.* **2009**, *29*, 2176–2181. [CrossRef]
29. Jenkins, P.V.; Rawley, O.; Smith, O.P.; O'Donnell, J.S. Elevated Factor VIII Levels and Risk of Venous Thrombosis. *Br. J. Haematol.* **2012**, *157*, 653–663. [CrossRef]
30. Payne, A.B.; Miller, C.H.; Hooper, W.C.; Lally, C.; Austin, H.D. High Factor VIII, von Willebrand Factor, and Fibrinogen Levels and Risk of Venous Thromboembolism in Blacks and Whites. *Ethn. Dis.* **2014**, *24*, 169–174.
31. Rietveld, I.M.; Lijfering, W.M.; le Cessie, S.; Bos, M.H.A.; Rosendaal, F.R.; Reitsma, P.H.; Cannegieter, S.C. High Levels of Coagulation Factors and Venous Thrombosis Risk: Strongest Association for Factor VIII and von Willebrand Factor. *J. Thromb. Haemost. JTH* **2019**, *17*, 99–109. [CrossRef]
32. Sane, M.; Granér, M.; Laukkanen, J.A.; Harjola, V.-P.; Mustonen, P. Plasma Levels of Haemostatic Factors in Patients with Pulmonary Embolism on Admission and Seven Months Later. *Int. J. Lab. Hematol.* **2018**, *40*, 66–71. [CrossRef] [PubMed]
33. Heerink, J.S.; Gemen, E.; Oudega, R.; Geersing, G.-J.; Hopstaken, R.; Kusters, R. Performance of C-Reactive Protein, Procalcitonin, TAT Complex, and Factor VIII in Addition to D-Dimer in the Exclusion of Venous Thromboembolism in Primary Care Patients. *J. Appl. Lab. Med.* **2022**, *7*, 444–455. [CrossRef]
34. Bartel, D.P. MicroRNAs: Genomics, Biogenesis, Mechanism, and Function. *Cell* **2004**, *116*, 281–297. [CrossRef]
35. Morelli, V.M.; Brækkan, S.K.; Hansen, J.-B. Role of MicroRNAs in Venous Thromboembolism. *Int. J. Mol. Sci.* **2020**, *21*, 2602. [CrossRef] [PubMed]
36. Li, M.; Zhang, J. Circulating MicroRNAs: Potential and Emerging Biomarkers for Diagnosis of Cardiovascular and Cerebrovascular Diseases. *BioMed Res. Int.* **2015**, *2015*, 730535. [CrossRef]
37. Harada, K.; Baba, Y.; Ishimoto, T.; Shigaki, H.; Kosumi, K.; Yoshida, N.; Watanabe, M.; Baba, H. The Role of MicroRNA in Esophageal Squamous Cell Carcinoma. *J. Gastroenterol.* **2016**, *51*, 520–530. [CrossRef]
38. Nourse, J.; Braun, J.; Lackner, K.; Hüttelmaier, S.; Danckwardt, S. Large-Scale Identification of Functional MicroRNA Targeting Reveals Cooperative Regulation of the Hemostatic System. *J. Thromb. Haemost. JTH* **2018**, *16*, 2233–2245. [CrossRef]
39. De Los Reyes-García, A.M.; Arroyo, A.B.; Teruel-Montoya, R.; Vicente, V.; Lozano, M.L.; González-Conejero, R.; Martínez, C. MicroRNAs as Potential Regulators of Platelet Function and Bleeding Diatheses. *Platelets* **2019**, *30*, 803–808. [CrossRef]
40. Xiao, J.; Jing, Z.-C.; Ellinor, P.T.; Liang, D.; Zhang, H.; Liu, Y.; Chen, X.; Pan, L.; Lyon, R.; Liu, Y.; et al. MicroRNA-134 as a Potential Plasma Biomarker for the Diagnosis of Acute Pulmonary Embolism. *J. Transl. Med.* **2011**, *9*, 159. [CrossRef]

41. Deng, H.-Y.; Li, G.; Luo, J.; Wang, Z.-Q.; Yang, X.-Y.; Lin, Y.-D.; Liu, L.-X. MicroRNAs Are Novel Non-Invasive Diagnostic Biomarkers for Pulmonary Embolism: A Meta-Analysis. *J. Thorac. Dis.* **2016**, *8*, 3580–3587. [CrossRef]
42. Zhou, X.; Wen, W.; Shan, X.; Qian, J.; Li, H.; Jiang, T.; Wang, W.; Cheng, W.; Wang, F.; Qi, L.; et al. MiR-28-3p as a Potential Plasma Marker in Diagnosis of Pulmonary Embolism. *Thromb. Res.* **2016**, *138*, 91–95. [CrossRef] [PubMed]
43. Kessler, T.; Erdmann, J.; Vilne, B.; Bruse, P.; Kurowski, V.; Diemert, P.; Schunkert, H.; Sager, H.B. Serum MicroRNA-1233 Is a Specific Biomarker for Diagnosing Acute Pulmonary Embolism. *J. Transl. Med.* **2016**, *14*, 120. [CrossRef] [PubMed]
44. Liu, T.; Kang, J.; Liu, F. Plasma Levels of MicroRNA-221 (MiR-221) Are Increased in Patients with Acute Pulmonary Embolism. *Med. Sci. Monit. Int. Med. J. Exp. Clin. Res.* **2018**, *24*, 8621–8626. [CrossRef] [PubMed]
45. Wang, Q.; Ma, J.; Jiang, Z.; Wu, F.; Ping, J.; Ming, L. Diagnostic Value of Circulating MicroRNA-27a/b in Patients with Acute Pulmonary Embolism. *Int. Angiol. J. Int. Union Angiol.* **2018**, *37*, 19–25. [CrossRef]
46. Peng, L.; Han, L.; Li, X.-N.; Miao, Y.-F.; Xue, F.; Zhou, C. The Predictive Value of MicroRNA-134 and MicroRNA-1233 for the Early Diagnosis of Acute Exacerbation of Chronic Obstructive Pulmonary Disease with Acute Pulmonary Embolism. *Int. J. Chron. Obstruct. Pulmon. Dis.* **2020**, *15*, 2495–2503. [CrossRef]
47. Owens, A.P.; Mackman, N. Microparticles in Hemostasis and Thrombosis. *Circ. Res.* **2011**, *108*, 1284–1297. [CrossRef]
48. Nieri, D.; Neri, T.; Petrini, S.; Vagaggini, B.; Paggiaro, P.; Celi, A. Cell-Derived Microparticles and the Lung. *Eur. Respir. Rev. Off. J. Eur. Respir. Soc.* **2016**, *25*, 266–277. [CrossRef]
49. Campello, E.; Spiezia, L.; Radu, C.M.; Simioni, P. Microparticles as Biomarkers of Venous Thromboembolic Events. *Biomark. Med.* **2016**, *10*, 743–755. [CrossRef]
50. Rezania, S.; Puskarich, M.A.; Petrusca, D.N.; Neto-Neves, E.M.; Rondina, M.T.; Kline, J.A. Platelet Hyperactivation, Apoptosis and Hypercoagulability in Patients with Acute Pulmonary Embolism. *Thromb. Res.* **2017**, *155*, 106–115. [CrossRef]
51. Inami, N.; Nomura, S.; Kikuchi, H.; Kajiura, T.; Yamada, K.; Nakamori, H.; Takahashi, N.; Tsuda, N.; Hikosaka, M.; Masaki, M.; et al. P-Selectin and Platelet-Derived Microparticles Associated with Monocyte Activation Markers in Patients with Pulmonary Embolism. *Clin. Appl. Thromb. Off. J. Int. Acad. Clin. Appl. Thromb.* **2003**, *9*, 309–316. [CrossRef]
52. Bal, L.; Ederhy, S.; Di Angelantonio, E.; Toti, F.; Zobairi, F.; Dufaitre, G.; Meuleman, C.; Mallat, Z.; Boccara, F.; Tedgui, A.; et al. Circulating Procoagulant Microparticles in Acute Pulmonary Embolism: A Case-Control Study. *Int. J. Cardiol.* **2010**, *145*, 321–322. [CrossRef] [PubMed]
53. Garcia Rodriguez, P.; Eikenboom, H.C.J.; Tesselaar, M.E.T.; Huisman, M.V.; Nijkeuter, M.; Osanto, S.; Bertina, R.M. Plasma Levels of Microparticle-Associated Tissue Factor Activity in Patients with Clinically Suspected Pulmonary Embolism. *Thromb. Res.* **2010**, *126*, 345–349. [CrossRef]
54. Kali, A.; Shetty, K.S.R. Endocan: A Novel Circulating Proteoglycan. *Indian J. Pharmacol.* **2014**, *46*, 579–583. [CrossRef] [PubMed]
55. Güzel, A.; Duran, L.; Köksal, N.; Torun, A.C.; Alaçam, H.; Ekiz, B.C.; Murat, N. Evaluation of Serum Endothelial Cell Specific Molecule-1 (Endocan) Levels as a Biomarker in Patients with Pulmonary Thromboembolism. *Blood Coagul. Fibrinolysis Int. J. Haemost. Thromb.* **2014**, *25*, 272–276. [CrossRef]
56. Kuluöztürk, M.; İn, E.; İlhan, N. Endocan as a Marker of Disease Severity in Pulmonary Thromboembolism. *Clin. Respir. J.* **2019**, *13*, 773–780. [CrossRef]
57. Mosevoll, K.A.; Lindås, R.; Wendelbo, O.; Bruserud, O.; Reikvam, H. Systemic Levels of the Endothelium-Derived Soluble Adhesion Molecules Endocan and E-Selectin in Patients with Suspected Deep Vein Thrombosis. *SpringerPlus* **2014**, *3*, 571. [CrossRef]
58. Engström, G.; Zöller, B.; Svensson, P.J.; Melander, O.; Persson, M. Soluble Urokinase Plasminogen Activator Receptor and Incidence of Venous Thromboembolism. *Thromb. Haemost.* **2016**, *115*, 657–662. [CrossRef]
59. Steeghs, N.; Goekoop, R.J.; Niessen, R.W.L.M.; Jonkers, G.J.P.M.; Dik, H.; Huisman, M.V. C-Reactive Protein and D-Dimer with Clinical Probability Score in the Exclusion of Pulmonary Embolism. *Br. J. Haematol.* **2005**, *130*, 614–619. [CrossRef]
60. Stoeva, N.; Kirova, G.; Staneva, M.; Lekova, D.; Penev, A.; Bakalova, R. Recognition of Unprovoked (Idiopathic) Pulmonary Embolism–Prospective Observational Study. *Respir. Med.* **2018**, *135*, 57–61. [CrossRef]
61. Araz, O.; Yilmazel Ucar, E.; Yalcin, A.; Kelercioglu, N.; Meral, M.; Gorguner, A.M.; Akgun, M. Predictive Value of Serum Hs-CRP Levels for Outcomes of Pulmonary Embolism: Pulmonary Embolism and Hs-CRP. *Clin. Respir. J.* **2016**, *10*, 163–167. [CrossRef] [PubMed]
62. Granholm, F.; Bylund, D.; Shevchenko, G.; Lind, S.B.; Henriksson, A.E. A Feasibility Study on the Identification of Potential Biomarkers in Pulmonary Embolism Using Proteomic Analysis. *Clin. Appl. Thromb. Off. J. Int. Acad. Clin. Appl. Thromb.* **2022**, *28*, 10760296221074348. [CrossRef]
63. Han, B.; Li, C.; Li, H.; Li, Y.; Luo, X.; Liu, Y.; Zhang, J.; Zhang, Z.; Yu, X.; Zhai, Z.; et al. Discovery of Plasma Biomarkers with Data-independent Acquisition Mass Spectrometry and Antibody Microarray for Diagnosis and Risk Stratification of Pulmonary Embolism. *J. Thromb. Haemost.* **2021**, *19*, 1738–1751. [CrossRef] [PubMed]
64. Zhang, Y.-X.; Li, J.-F.; Yang, Y.-H.; Huang, K.; Miao, R.; Zhai, Z.-G.; Wang, C. Identification of Haptoglobin as a Potential Diagnostic Biomarker of Acute Pulmonary Embolism. *Blood Coagul. Fibrinolysis* **2018**, *29*, 275–281. [CrossRef]

65. Blondon, M.; Le Gal, G.; Meyer, G.; Righini, M.; Robert-Ebadi, H. Age-Adjusted D-Dimer Cutoff for the Diagnosis of Pulmonary Embolism: A Cost-Effectiveness Analysis. *J. Thromb. Haemost. JTH* **2020**, *18*, 865–875. [CrossRef]
66. Perrier, A.; Buswell, L.; Bounameaux, H.; Didier, D.; Morabia, A.; de Moerloose, P.; Slosman, D.; Unger, P.F.; Junod, A. Cost-Effectiveness of Noninvasive Diagnostic Aids in Suspected Pulmonary Embolism. *Arch. Intern. Med.* **1997**, *157*, 2309–2316. [CrossRef]

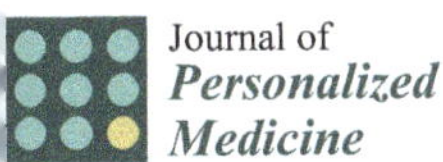
Journal of *Personalized Medicine*

MDPI

Article

C-Reactive Protein as a Predictor of Survival and Length of Hospital Stay in Community-Acquired Pneumonia

Apostolos Travlos, Agamemnon Bakakos, Konstantinos F. Vlachos, Nikoletta Rovina, Nikolaos Koulouris and Petros Bakakos *

1st University Department of Respiratory Medicine, National and Kapodistrian University of Athens, 11527 Athens, Greece
* Correspondence: petros44@hotmail.com

Abstract: Introduction: Community-acquired pneumonia (CAP) presents high mortality rates and high healthcare costs worldwide. C-reactive protein (CRP) has been widely used as a biomarker for the management of CAP. We evaluated the performance of CRP threshold values and ΔCRP as predictors of CAP survival and length of hospital stay. Methods: A total of 173 adult patients with CAP were followed for up to 30 days. We measured serum CRP levels on days 1, 4, and 7 (D1, D4, and D7) of hospitalization, and their variations between different days were calculated (ΔCRP). A multivariate logistic regression model was created with CAP 30-day survival and length of hospital stay as dependent variables, and absolute CRP values and ΔCRP, age, sex, smoking habit (pack-years), pO2/FiO2 ratio on D1, WBC on D1, and CURB-65 score as independent variables. Results: A total of six patients with CAP died (30-day mortality 3.47%). No difference was found in CRP levels and ΔCRP between survivors and non-survivors. Using a cut-off level of 9 mg/dL, the AUC (95% CI) for the prediction of survival of CRP on D4 and D7 were 0.765 (0.538–0.992) and 0.784 (0.580–0.989), respectively. A correlation between CRP values on any day and length of hospital stay was found, with it being stronger for CRPD4 and CRPD7 ($p < 0.0001$ and $p = 0.0024$, respectively). A reduction of CRP > 50% from D1 to D4 was associated with 4.11 fewer days of hospitalization ($p = 0.0308$). Conclusions: CRP levels on D4 and D7, but not ΔCRP, could fairly predict CAP survival. A reduction of CRP > 50% by the fourth day of hospitalization could predict a shorter hospital stay.

Keywords: C-reactive protein (CRP); community-acquired pneumonia (CAP); biomarkers; mortality; prognosis; length of stay

Citation: Travlos, A.; Bakakos, A.; Vlachos, K.F.; Rovina, N.; Koulouris, N.; Bakakos, P. C-Reactive Protein as a Predictor of Survival and Length of Hospital Stay in Community-Acquired Pneumonia. *J. Pers. Med.* **2022**, *12*, 1710. https://doi.org/10.3390/jpm12101710

Academic Editors: Ioannis Pantazopoulos and Ourania S. Kotsiou

Received: 14 August 2022
Accepted: 11 October 2022
Published: 13 October 2022

1. Introduction

Community-acquired pneumonia (CAP) is a major public health problem with a high mortality rate of approximately 5–15% and a considerable socio-economic burden worldwide [1,2]. It remains a main reason of hospitalization, death, and high healthcare costs in developed countries, especially among elderly people [3,4].

CRP is an acute-phase protein predominantly produced in the liver. Responding to infection or tissue inflammation, the production of CRP is rapidly stimulated by cytokines, particularly interleukin (IL)-6 [5]. Moreover, CRP is not only a marker, but also a driver of inflammation by human macrophages [6,7].

In patients with severe CAP, a decrease of less than 25% in CRP levels at the second day was significantly associated with 30-day all-cause mortality [8]. Additionally, a failure of CRP to fall by 50% or more at day 4 leads to an increased risk for 30-day mortality and a need for mechanical ventilation [9]. Conversely, a recent 5-year follow-up cohort study showed no higher admission levels of CRP in patients with CAP experiencing an adverse short-term outcome (intensive care unit admission and 30-day mortality) [10]. CRP levels have been shown to decrease after successful antibiotic treatment, and serial assessment of CRP aided in the early identification of CAP patients with poor outcomes [11,12].

The correlation of CRP values with the length of hospital stay has also been evaluated. In 823 adult patients hospitalized with CAP, a lack of a CRP decline within three days of hospitalization was associated with a high risk of complications and a prolonged hospital stay [13]. Similarly, in a study from Sweden, it was demonstrated that hospital-treated CAP patients with high IL-6 or CRP levels had a longer duration of fever and a longer hospital stay [14]. A reduced length of hospital stay can result in substantially lower costs [15].

The aim of the present study was to assess the predictive value of CRP levels in patients with CAP. We hypothesized that serum CRP levels on days 1 (D1), 4 (D4), and 7 (D7) could predict survival and hospital length of stay. We carried out a study in which we evaluated: (1) serum CRP levels on the first, fourth, and seventh day of CAP; and (2) ΔCRP, as a prognostic marker of CAP survival (up to D30) and length of hospital stay. We also evaluated whether CRP in any day measured was associated with the severity of respiratory failure.

2. Materials and Methods

2.1. Study Design and Population

The study was conducted at the 1st University Department of Respiratory Medicine, University of Athens, from January 2013 until September 2019. The local ethics committee approved the study.

Initially, 194 patients with CAP were screened. Patients with hospital-acquired pneumonia (HAP), immunocompromised patients (hematologic malignancies, HIV, neutropenia < 1000 cells/mL, and patients who had received chemotherapy or other immunosuppressive therapy over the past 2 months) were excluded from the study. Patients who died within the first 2 days of CAP diagnosis were also excluded from the study. Moreover, patients who had received antibiotic treatment at least 1 day prior to hospital admission were not included in the study. Finally, 173 patients with CAP comprised the study group. The day of CAP diagnosis was defined as D1 and was the day that empirical antibiotic treatment was started. The following days were termed as D2, D3, etc. CRP levels were measured on D1, D4, and D7 in all patients included in the study. Patients were followed until the 30th day after CAP diagnosis and then were considered survivors. Those who died before D30 were considered non-survivors. Antibiotic treatment was chosen by the treating physician and was modified according to the susceptibility pattern of the sputum and/or blood culture in case empirical treatment did not cover the isolated pathogen. Blood samples were collected on D1, D4, and D7. The samples were centrifuged at 2500 rpm for 15 min, and the plasma was aliquoted and stored at −80 °C until analyzed in a single batch. Circulating levels of CRP were measured using an immunoturbumetric method with a commercially available kit (Dade Behring). Normal values for CRP were <0.70 mg/dL.

2.2. Statistical Analysis

Values were expressed as mean (±SD) or median (interquartile range 25–75 percentile) in the case of a skewed distribution. Comparisons between patient groups were performed by using the Mann–Whitney U-test method. The difference Δ was calculated using the formula: Δ = D4-D1, D7-D4 and D7-D1, respectively. Therefore, ΔCRP4-1 = CRPD4-CRPD1, ΔCRP7-4 = CRPD7-CRPD4, and ΔCRP7-1 = CRPD7-CRPD1, where $\Delta > 0$ refers to increasing values and $\Delta \leq 0$ refers to reducing values. The ΔCRP values were classified as increasing or unchanging/decreasing. A univariate logistic regression analysis followed in order to define the risk factors for CAP survival and hospital length of stay. A multivariate logistic regression analysis model was created with CAP survival and hospital stay as dependent variables, whereas the absolute CRP values on D1, D4, and D7, as well as the changes in CRP values on days D1, D4, and D7 (ΔCRP4-1, ΔCRP7-1, and ΔCRP7-4), were set as the as independent variables. In order to deal with possible linearity, models were created that contained only absolute values or only changes, as well as models with absolute values and changes combined together. In order to control for potential confounding factors, age, gender, and CURB-65 score were included in the original model. Results were reported as ORs, adjusted at 95% CI.

Sensitivity and specificity were calculated. Threshold values that gave the best combination of sensitivity and specificity were judged by calculating the Youden's index, i.e., the maximum difference between sensitivity and specificity [16].

The SPSS statistical package was used. A p-value < 0.05 was considered significant.

3. Results

A total of 173 patients with CAP were eventually included in the study. All of them were hospitalized in the 1st University Department of Respiratory Medicine, University of Athens, Greece. A flowchart of the study population is shown in Figure 1. The demographic characteristics and the CRP values are shown in Table 1.

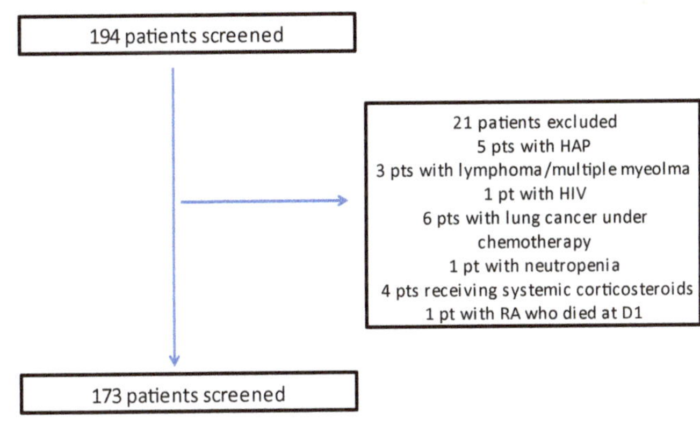

HAP: Hospital acquired pneumonia, HIV: Human Immunodeficiency Virus, RA: Rheumatoid arthritis

Figure 1. Flowchart of the study participants.

Table 1. Characteristics of patients with CAP.

Subjects (n = 173)	Survivors (n = 167)	Non-Survivors (n = 6)	p-Value
Age	62.6 ± 21.4	82.8 ± 13.7	0.011
Sex (M/F)	98/69	6/0	0.112
Smoking (C/Ex/N)	65/47/55	1/4/1	0.115
CRP D1	11.8 ± 9.1	17.8 ± 12.5	0.216
CRP D4	6.4 ± 6.2	16.9 ± 13.5	0.054
CRP D7	4.6 ± 5.8	12.8 ± 10.7	0.059
Length of stay (days)	14.4 ± 12.1	16.5 ± 9.2	0.397
pO2/FiO2	268.9 ± 76.2	210.5 ± 68.9	0.074
WBC	12,277 ± 4684	12,688 ± 5008	0.816
CURB-65 score			0.513
(0,1,2,3,4)	7/27/70/50/13	0/0/2/3/1	

Data are presented as n, mean ± SD. CRP: C-reactive protein, WBC: white blood cell count, CURB: confusion, urea, respiratory rate, and blood pressure.

In 11 patients, a positive sputum culture was found (Klebsiella Pneumoniae: 3, Staphylococcus Aureus: 1, Stenotrophomonas Maltophila: 1, MRSA: 1, Pseudomonas Aeruginosa: 3, other Gram (+) bacteria: 1, and other Gram (−) bacteria: 1). A total of 4 patients had a positive blood culture (Klebsiella Pneumoniae: 1, Streptococcus Pneumoniae: 1, Proteus Mirabilis: 1, and other Gram (+) bacteria: 1), while in 4 patients with CAP, a positive urine antigen for strep pneumonia (n = 3) and for Legionella (n = 1) was detected.

3.1. CAP Survival

CRP values exceeded normal levels in 172 out of 173 patients on D1.

During the study period, six patients with CAP died (3.47%). One death occurred on D3 of hospitalization, and five non-survivors died between D8 and D23. Non-survivors were older compared to survivors (p = 0.011). There was no difference in CRP levels between survivors and non-survivors on any day although non-survivors had higher CRP levels, especially on D4 and D7.

In the univariate analysis, CRPD4 and CRPD7 were able to predict survival of CAP. However, this predictive performance was lost in the multivariate analysis.

ΔCRP scores were not different between survivors and non-survivors either.

Using as cut-off level the value of 9 mg/dL, the AUC and 95% CI for the prediction of survival for CRP on D4 and D7 were 0.765 (0.538–0.992) and 0.784 (0.580–0.989), respectively (Figure 2A,B).

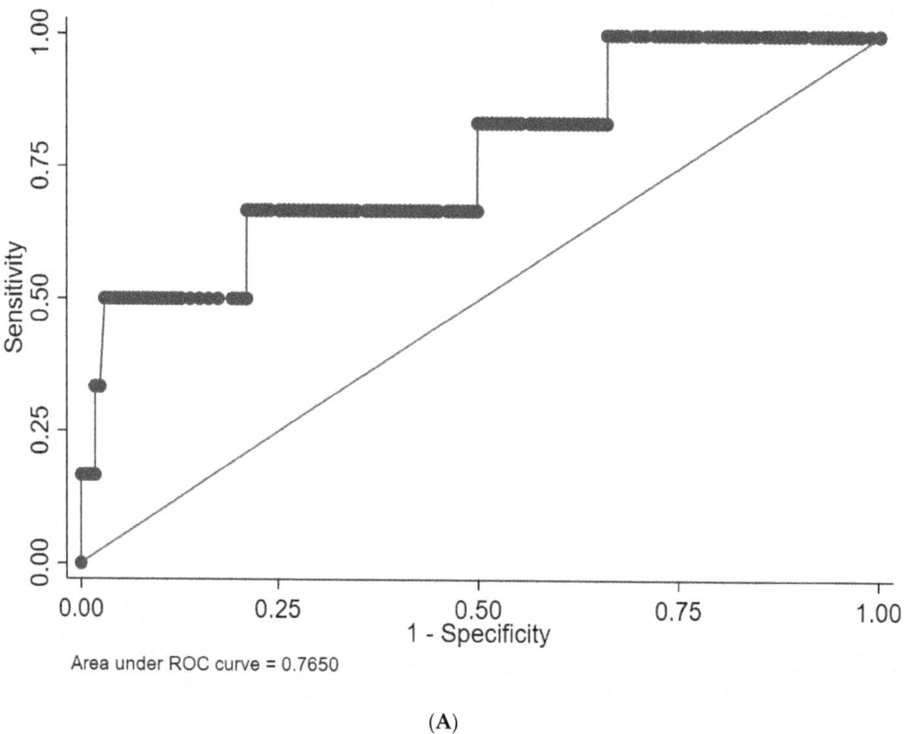

(A)

Figure 2. *Cont.*

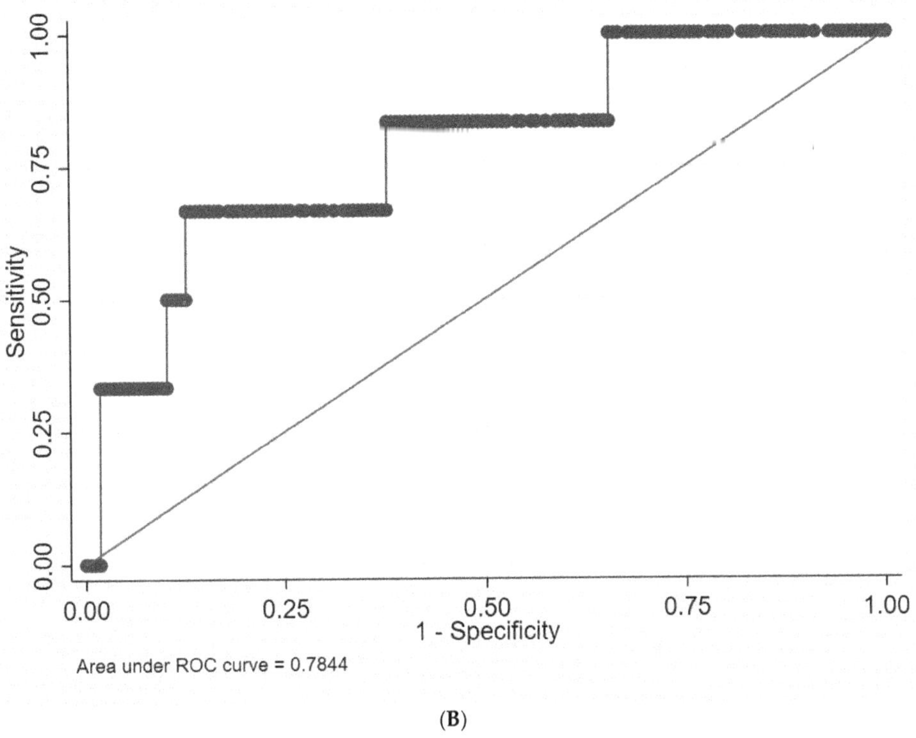

(**B**)

Figure 2. (**A**) ROC curve for CRP D4 in predicting CAP survival; (**B**) ROC curve for CRP D7 in predicting CAP survival.

Moreover, neither a reduction of CRP >50% from D1 to D4, nor a reduction >50% from D4 to D7 were associated with better survival ($p = 0.0688$ and 0.362, respectively).

CURB-65 was not associated with mortality ($p = 0.512$), and the addition of CURB-65 to absolute CRP values (D1, D4, and D7) did not improve its performance.

Using a cut-off value of 3 for CURB-65 (thus <3 and ≥3), the AUC and 95% CI for the prediction of survival was 0.702 (0.5245–0.8801).

One patient with a positive blood culture died, while no pathogen was isolated in the cultures of the other five non-survivors. Compared to those with a negative blood culture, patients with a positive blood culture had significantly higher CRP levels on D1 ($p = 0.016$), while levels on D4 and D7, although higher, did not reach significance ($p = 0.128$ and $p = 0.077$, respectively).

3.2. *CAP Hospital Length of Stay*

A correlation between CRP values on any day and length of hospital stay was found, being stronger for CRPD4 and CRPD7 ($p < 0.0001$ and $p = 0.0024$, respectively).

Furthermore, a reduction of CRP >50% from D1 to D4 was associated with a shorter hospital length of stay and corresponded to 4.11 fewer days of hospitalization ($p = 0.0308$). A reduction of CRP >50% from D4 to D7 corresponded to 1 fewer hospitalization days, which was not significant ($p = 0.5657$).

The CURB-65 score was not associated with hospital length of stay ($p = 0.2762$).

Additionally, a positive correlation was detected between PaO2/FiO2 and CRPD4 or CRPD7 ($p = 0.0008$ and $p = 0.0392$, respectively).

4. Discussion

Several biomarkers have been evaluated in an effort to assess the prognosis of patients with CAP, and these measurements are supplementary to traditional clinical tools.

CRP has been established as a widely used inflammatory biomarker in CAP and has been evaluated in several studies. It is included in the clinical protocols for CAP of several hospitals [17], and it is mentioned in the guidelines of lower respiratory tract infections (LRTIs) [18]. Currently, CRP and PCT are the best available tools to assess the severity of CAP [18]. When CRP levels remain unremarkable or low at follow-up measurements, a relevant severe infection is very unlikely [19].

In the present study, we aimed to evaluate the predictive performance of CRP in survival and hospital length of stay in hospitalized patients with CAP. The choice of D1, D4, and D7 was arbitrary and was based upon the clinical course of CAP, thus at admittance (D1), after three days of antibiotic treatment when re-evaluation usually occurs (D4), and towards the end of antibiotic treatment (D7). We did not find any association between absolute CRP values measured on D1, D4, and D7 and survival of patients hospitalized with CAP. Neither did we find any association between ΔCRP and CAP survival. However, a failure to reduce CRP levels <9 mg/dL on D4 and D7 after the initiation of antibiotic treatment could fairly predict CAP survival. Moreover, we found that a reduction of CRP of more than 50% from D1 to D4 could predict a shorter hospital length of stay. The findings of our study regarding mortality are in contrast to the findings of other studies. A retrospective study from Denmark, including 814 patients with CAP, showed that absolute CRP levels and relative decline on the third day of hospitalization were both predictors of 30-day mortality. Moreover, the highest mortality risk was found in CAP patients with a level of CRP > 75 mg/L who failed to decline 50% by day 3 [20]. Another study demonstrated that a failure to present a decline in CRP levels was associated with a poor prognosis, irrespective of the actual level of CRP [21]. Similarly, according to the German competence network CAPNETZ, in CAP patients without antimicrobial pre-treatment, survivors had lower values of CRP, as well as PCT and WBC, compared to non-survivors, and these biomarkers predicted 28-day mortality exclusively in these patients. However, in patients with antimicrobial pre-treatment, the values of PCT, WBC, and CRP did not differ significantly in survivors and non-survivors, indicating that there is an effect of antibiotic pre-treatment in the levels of inflammatory biomarkers [22]. This discrepancy may be attributed to the low number of deaths in our study population. Only 6 out of 173 patients died, and this corresponds to a percentage of 3.47%, which is lower in comparison to other studies. Moreover, the mean age of survivors was lower in comparison to other studies, possibly contributing to the low mortality since mortality has been shown to increase with age [23].

Patients with a positive blood culture had higher CRP levels on D1, indicating that they constituted a more severely ill population. However, this difference was not observed in D4 and D7 CRP levels, and most importantly, it did not influence the outcome (death or survival), demonstrating a less crucial effect after the initiation of antibiotic therapy.

The finding of an association of ΔCRP with hospital length of stay is important. CAP presents a varying spectrum of severity, and hospital stay increases its cost and morbidity significantly. We found that, of those patients with CAP in whom CRP decreased from D1 to D4, more than 50% stayed in the hospital for four fewer days. The decision of hospital discharge was based upon the clinician's decision and other factors, such as social factors and comorbidities. However, apart from being statistically significant, four fewer days of hospital stay are clinically important as they correspond to 30% less hospitalization time and a much lower cost. A relatively small decrease in the length of hospital stay in CAP can have a significant cost impact, and even a one-day reduction in length of stay has been shown to yield substantial cost savings [15,24]. Our findings are compatible with the results of a prospective observational cohort study in Israel which demonstrated that a greater decrease in CRP levels between the first and second day of hospitalization was associated with a shorter length of hospital stay [25]. Similarly, a failure of CRP to decline by day 3 of hospitalization has been associated with prolonged hospital stay [13].

There are limitations to this study. First, the decision to admit, as well as to discharge, the patient with CAP was made by the clinician and was not based on specific, pre-defined criteria. However, almost 80% of the admitted patients had a CURB-65 score ≥2 and fewer than 4% had a CURB-65 score of 0, indicating that the more severe patients were hospitalized. The lack of data regarding comorbidities and past vaccinations that are known to influence susceptibility to CAP is a major limitation of our study. Third, treating physicians—although in the same department—may have started antibiotic treatment with different regimens, as there was no specific protocol for guiding antibiotic therapy, and therefore, ΔCRP could not be strongly associated with successful treatment. However, the very low death rate demonstrates that, in the majority of CAP patients, the chosen antibiotic regimen was successful, but it may also be attributed to the lower mean age of our study group. Another limitation is the low number of patients with an established microbiological diagnosis. However, this is common in clinical practice. Moreover, since D1 was defined as the day of hospital admission and initiation of empirical antibiotic treatment, the time between the onset of patients' symptoms and hospital admission varied among patients and may have influenced the absolute CRP values at D1, and that is a limitation. Eventually, the study was conducted in a single center, and accordingly, this makes the generalizability of our findings ambiguous. A strength of this study is the relatively high number of patients, without any lost to follow-up, and the fact that it reflects common clinical practice, as in a real-life situation. None of the included patients had received antibiotic treatment prior to hospitalization, and thus, they constituted a homogenous population of in-patients with CAP.

Undoubtedly, there is need for further research on how to use the information provided by single biomarker measurements and to corroborate the additive value of these biomarkers in order to improve clinical decision-making regarding the management and prognosis of hospitalized patients with CAP in daily practice. In conclusion, we found that CRP levels on D4 and D7 could fairly predict CAP survival, and a reduction of CRP >50% by D4 of hospitalization corresponded to four fewer days of length of hospital stay.

Author Contributions: Conceptualization, A.T., A.B., K.F.V., N.R., N.K. and P.B.; methodology, A.T., A.B., K.F.V., N.R., N.K. and P.B.; software, A.T., A.B., K.F.V., N.R., N.K. and P.B.; validation, A.T., A.B., K.F.V., N.R., N.K. and P.B.; formal analysis, A.T., A.B., K.F.V., N.R., N.K. and P.B.; investigation, A.T., A.B., K.F.V., N.R., N.K. and P.B.; resources, A.T., A.B., K.F.V., N.R., N.K. and P.B.; data curation, A.T., A.B., K.F.V., N.R., N.K. and P.B.; writing—original draft preparation, A.T., A.B., K.F.V., N.R., N.K. and P.B.; writing—review and editing, A.T., A.B., K.F.V., N.R., N.K. and P.B.; visualization, A.T., A.B., K.F.V., N.R., N.K. and P.B.; supervision P.B.; project administration, P.B. All authors have read and agreed to the published version of the manuscript.

Funding: This research received no external funding.

Institutional Review Board Statement: The study was conducted in accordance with the Declaration of Helsinki, and approved by the Ethics Committee of "Sotiria" Chest Diseases Hospital (12271-13/5/13).

Informed Consent Statement: Informed consent was obtained from all subjects involved in the study.

Data Availability Statement: Not applicable.

Conflicts of Interest: The authors declare no conflict of interest.

References

1. Wunderink, R.; Waterer, G. Community-Acquired Pneumonia. *N. Engl. J. Med.* **2014**, *370*, 543–551. [CrossRef]
2. Yoon, H.K. Changes in the epidemiology and burden of community-acquired pneumonia in Korea. *Korean J. Intern. Med.* **2014**, *29*, 735–737. [CrossRef] [PubMed]

3. Torner, N.; Izquierdo, C.; Soldevila, N.; Toledo, D.; Chamorro, J.; Espejo, E.; Fernandez-Sierra, A.; Dominguez, A.; Project PI12/02079 Working Group. Factors associated with 30-day mortality in elderly inpatients with community acquired pneumonia during 2 influenza seasons. *Hum. Vaccin Immunother.* **2017**, *13*, 450–455. [CrossRef] [PubMed]
4. Blasi, F.; Mantero, M.; Santus, P.; Tarsia, P. Understanding the burden of pneumococcal disease in adults. *Clin. Microbiol. Infect.* **2012**, *18*, 7–14. [CrossRef]
5. Pepys, M.B.; Hirschfield, G.M. C-reactive protein: A critical update. *J. Clin. Investig.* **2003**, *111*, 1805–1812. [CrossRef]
6. Kaplan, M.H.; Volanakis, J.E. Interaction of C-reactive protein complexes with the complement system. I. Consumption of human complement associated with the reaction of C-reactive protein with pneumococcal C-polysaccharide and with the choline phosphatides, lecithin and sphingomyelin. *J. Immunol.* **1974**, *112*, 2135–2147.
7. Newling, M.; Sritharan, L.; van der Ham, A.J.; Hoepel, W.; Fiechter, R.H.; de Boer, L.; Zaat, S.A.J.; Bisoendial, R.J.; Baeten, D.L.P.; Everts, B.; et al. C-Reactive Protein Promotes Inflammation through FcγR-Induced Glycolytic Reprogramming of Human Macrophages. *J. Immunol.* **2019**, *203*, 225–235. [CrossRef]
8. Nseir, W.; Farah, R.; Mograbi, J.; Makhoul, N. Impact of serum C-reactive protein measurements in the first 2 days on the 30-day mortality in hospitalized patients with severe community-acquired pneumonia: A cohort study. *J. Crit. Care* **2013**, *28*, 291–295. [CrossRef]
9. Chalmers, J.D.; Singanayagam, A.; Hill, A.T. C-reactive protein is an independent predictor of severity in community-acquired pneumonia. *Am. J. Med.* **2008**, *121*, 219–225. [CrossRef]
10. Siljan, W.; Holter, J.; Michelsen, A.; Nymo, S.; Lauritzen, T.; Oppen, K.; Husebye, E.; Ueland, T.; Mollnes, T.E.; Aukrust, P.; et al. Inflammatory biomarkers are associated with aetiology and predict outcomes in community-acquired pneumonia: Results of a 5-year follow-up cohort study. *ERJ Open Res.* **2019**, *5*, 00014-2019. [CrossRef] [PubMed]
11. Coelho, L.; Salluh, J.; Soares, M.; Bozza, F.; Verdeal, J.C.; Povoa, P.; Lapa e Silva, J.R.; Bozza, P.T.; Póvoa, P. Patterns of c-reactive protein RATIO response in severe community-acquired pneumonia: A cohort study. *Crit. Care* **2012**, *16*, R53. [CrossRef] [PubMed]
12. Coelho, L.; Povoa, P.; Almeida, E.; Fernandes, A.; Mealha, R.; Moreira, P.; Sabino, H. Usefulness of C-reactive protein in monitoring the severe community-acquired pneumonia clinical course. *Crit. Care* **2007**, *11*, R92. [CrossRef]
13. Saldías, F.; Salinas, G.; Farcas, K.; Reyes, A.; Díaz, O. Immunocompetent adults hospitalized for a community-acquired pneumonia: Serum C-reactive protein as a prognostic marker. *Rev. Med. Chil.* **2019**, *147*, 983–992.
14. Örtqvist, A.; Hedlund, J.; Wretlind, B.; Carlström, A.; Kalin, M. Diagnostic and prognostic value of interleukin-6 and C-reactive protein in community-acquired pneumonia. *Scand J. Infect. Dis.* **1995**, *27*, 457–462. [CrossRef]
15. Fine, M.J.; Pratt, H.M.; Obrosky, D.S.; Lave, J.R.; McIntosh, L.J.; Singer, D.E.; Coley, C.M.; Kapoor, W.N. Relation between length of hospital stay and costs of care for patients with community-acquired pneumonia. *Am. J. Med.* **2000**, *109*, 378–385. [CrossRef]
16. Youden, W.J. Index for rating diagnostic tests. *Cancer* **1950**, *3*, 32–35. [CrossRef]
17. Seligman, R.; Ramos-Lima, L.F.; Oliveira, V.; Sanvicente, C.; Pacheco, E.F.; Dalla Rosa, K. Biomarkers in community-acquired pneumonia: A state-of-the-art review. *Clinics* **2012**, *67*, 1321–1325. [PubMed]
18. Woodhead, M.; Blasi, F.; Ewig, S.; Garau, J.; Huchon, G.; Ieven, M.; Ortqvist, A.; Schaberg, T.; Torres, A.; van der Heijden, G.; et al. Guidelines for the management of adult lower respiratory tract infections–full version. *Clin. Microbiol. Infect.* **2011**, *17*, E1–E59. [CrossRef] [PubMed]
19. Kruger, S.; Welte, T. Biomarkers in community-acquired pneumonia. *Expert Rev. Respir. Med.* **2012**, *6*, 203–214.
20. Andersen, S.B.; Baunbæk Egelund, G.; Jensen, A.V.; Peterson, P.T.; Rohde, G.; Ravn, P. Failure of CRP decline within three days of hospitalization is associated with poor prognosis of Community-acquired Pneumonia. *Infect. Dis.* **2017**, *49*, 251–260.
21. Andersen, S.; Baunbæk-Knudsen, G.L.; Jensen, A.V.; Petersen, P.T.; Ravn, P. The prognostic value of consecutive C-reactive protein measurements in community acquired pneumonia. *Eur. Respir. J.* **2015**, *46*, 2577.
22. Krüger, S.; Ewig, S.; Kunde, J.; Hartmann, O.; Marre, R.; Suttorp, N.; Welte, T. Assessment of inflammatory markers in patients with community-acquired pneumonia—Influence of antimicrobial pre-treatment: Results from the German competence network CAPNETZ. *Clin. Chim. Acta* **2010**, *411*, 1929–1934. [CrossRef] [PubMed]
23. Cillóniz, C.; Polverino, E.; Ewig, S.; Aliberti, S.; Gabarrús, A.; Menéndez, R.; Mensa, J.; Blasi, F.; Torres, A. Impact of Age and Comorbidity on Cause and Outcome in Community-Acquired Pneumonia. *Chest* **2013**, *144*, 999–1007. [CrossRef] [PubMed]
24. Raut, M.; Schein, J.; Mody, S.; Grant, R.; Benson, C.; Olson, W. Estimating the Economic Impact of a Half-Day Reduction in Length of Hospital Stay Among Patients with Community-Acquired Pneumonia in the US. *Curr. Med. Res. Opin.* **2009**, *25*, 2151–2157. [CrossRef] [PubMed]
25. Farah, R.; Khamisy-Farah, R.; Makhoul, N. Consecutive Measures of CRP Correlate with Length of Hospital Stay in Patients with Community-Acquired Pneumonia. *Isr. Med. Assoc. J.* **2018**, *20*, 345–348.

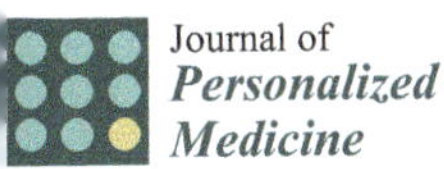
Journal of *Personalized Medicine*

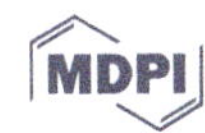

Review

Incorporating Biomarkers in COPD Management: The Research Keeps Going

Ioannis Pantazopoulos [1,*], Kalliopi Magounaki [2], Ourania Kotsiou [3], Erasmia Rouka [3], Fotis Perlikos [4], Sotirios Kakavas [5] and Konstantinos Gourgoulianis [3]

1 Department of Emergency Medicine, Faculty of Medicine, University of Thessaly, Biopolis, 41500 Larissa, Greece
2 Medical School, European University of Cyprus, Nicosia 2404, Cyprus; magounakikelly@gmail.com
3 Department of Respiratory Medicine, Faculty of Medicine, University of Thessaly, Biopolis, 41500 Larissa, Greece; raniakotsiou@gmail.com (O.K.); eri.rouka@gmail.com (E.R.); kgourg@uth.gr (K.G.)
4 ICU Department, Henry Dynant Hospital Center, 11526 Athens, Greece; perlykos@yahoo.com
5 Critical Care Department, "Sotiria" General Hospital of Chest Diseases, 11527 Athens, Greece; sotikaka@yahoo.com
* Correspondence: pantazopoulosioannis@yahoo.com; Tel.: +30-6945661525

Abstract: Globally, chronic obstructive pulmonary disease (COPD) remains a major cause of morbidity and mortality, having a significant socioeconomic effect. Several molecular mechanisms have been related to COPD including chronic inflammation, telomere shortening, and epigenetic modifications. Nowadays, there is an increasing need for novel therapeutic approaches for the management of COPD. These treatment strategies should be based on finding the source of acute exacerbation of COPD episodes and estimating the patient's own risk. The use of biomarkers and the measurement of their levels in conjunction with COPD exacerbation risk and disease prognosis is considered an encouraging approach. Many types of COPD biomarkers have been identified which include blood protein biomarkers, cellular biomarkers, and protease enzymes. They have been isolated from different sources including peripheral blood, sputum, bronchoalveolar fluid, exhaled air, and genetic material. However, there is still not an exclusive biomarker that is used for the evaluation of COPD but rather a combination of them, and this is attributed to disease complexity. In this review, we summarize the clinical significance of COPD-related biomarkers, their association with disease outcomes, and COPD patients' management. Finally, we depict the various samples that are used for identifying and measuring these biomarkers.

Keywords: biomarkers; chronic obstructive pulmonary disease; exacerbations; lung aging; oxidative stress

Citation: Pantazopoulos, I.; Magounaki, K.; Kotsiou, O.; Rouka, E.; Perlikos, F.; Kakavas, S.; Gourgoulianis, K. Incorporating Biomarkers in COPD Management: The Research Keeps Going. *J. Pers. Med.* **2022**, *12*, 379. https://doi.org/10.3390/jpm12030379

Academic Editor: Luisa Brussino

Received: 30 December 2021
Accepted: 28 February 2022
Published: 1 March 2022

1. Introduction

The pathogenesis of chronic obstructive pulmonary disease (COPD) involves a series of cellular and molecular processes driven by cytokines, chemokines, growth factors, oxidative stress, apoptosis, proteases-antiproteases imbalance, chronic tissue damage, and repair, and the relevant receptors and genetic signals [1]. It has become evident that COPD is not a single disease entity but comprises a set of distinct phenotypes with different underlying molecular and genetic pathways [2]. COPD-related research is increasingly focused on the search for biomarkers of the disease [3]. By definition, a biomarker is "objectively measured and evaluated as an indicator of normal biological processes, pathogenic processes, or pharmacologic responses to a therapeutic intervention" [4]. The multifactorial nature of the pathobiology of COPD implies that a large number of molecules could serve as biomarkers indicative of different aspects of the disease such as the presence or the extent of pulmonary damage, lung or systemic inflammation, and comorbidities. Moreover, there is a great interest in developing biomarkers that could enable the clear delineation and quantification of the distinct characteristics and outcomes associated with the various COPD phenotypes. The development of relevant biomarkers is also essential for the evaluation and discovery of individualized therapies that would combine improved clinical efficacy with minimal risk of adverse effects for patients in each of the COPD phenotypes.

Over the last years, a variety of biomarkers have been evaluated in COPD, derived from various sources including peripheral blood and genetic material [5]. Some of these tests have been reported to be useful to some degree for diagnostic or therapeutic purposes. However, in most cases, the value of the potential biomarkers in guiding COPD phenotyping and management is limited [6]. The Evaluation of COPD Longitudinally to Identify Predictive Surrogate End-points (ECLIPSE) study of 2.164 patients with COPD has provided valuable information concerning COPD phenotypes and relevant biomarkers and/or genetic parameters [7]. According to the ECLIPSE study, some potential biomarkers have been identified, but no single biomarker seems to fulfill all the necessary requirements. All these findings deserve further prospective validation in other COPD cohorts. Table 1 shows biomarkers currently being under investigation. This review aimed to present the most important recent findings on potential biomarkers derived from the peripheral blood and genetic material that can be used clinically to impact patient care in COPD.

Table 1. Biomarkers under investigation for COPD management.

Specimen Type	Readily Available and Currently Used Biomarkers	Extensively Investigated Biomarkers but Not Sufficiently Validated	Less Investigated Biomarkers
Peripheral Blood (plasma/ serum)	Eosinophils CRP	MDA GSH, GSH-Px, SOD IL-6, TNFα, MCP-1	Vitamins A, E, and C GGT vWF Extracellular vesicles (CD62E+, CD31+)
Exhaled air	FeNO		Ethane
Sputum		IL-6, IL-8, TNF-α MPO MMP-8, MMP-9, MMP-12, neutrophil elastase, Eosinophil peroxidase	8-isoprostane MDA SOD, GSH-Px Leptin
Exhaled breath condensate		8-isoprostane H_2O_2	MDA IL-8
Bronchoalveolar lavage fluid		Glutathione	EGFR, HSA, A1AT, TIMP1, IL-8 and Cal-protectin
Urine			8-isoprostane

MDA: Malondialdehyde, GSH: glutathione, GSH-Px: glutathione peroxidase, SOD: superoxide dismutase, GGT: γ-glutamyltransferase, CRP: C-reactive protein, IL: interleukin, TNF-α: tumor necrosis factor-alpha, MCP-1: monocyte chemoattractant protein-1, vWF: von Willebrand factor, FeNO: fraction of exhaled nitric oxide, MPO: myeloperoxidase, MMP: matrix metalloproteinase, EGFR: epidermal growth factor receptor, HSA: human serum albumin, A1AT: alpha-1-antitrypsin, TIMP1: tissue inhibitor matrix metalloproteinase 1.

2. Complete Blood Count-Based Biomarkers

The phenotype of frequent exacerbators (≥2 per year) is characterized by a persistent elevation of white blood cell (WBC) count, among other features [8,9]. These patients have a high risk of hospitalization and poorer prognosis, including increased mortality [10,11]. Additionally, peripheral eosinophil level from a complete blood count (CBC) has been evaluated as a surrogate marker for corticosteroid responsiveness, and eosinophilic bronchitis [12,13]. The analysis of the ECLIPSE cohort has shown that eosinophilic inflammation (eosinophil counts ≥2% at all visits) was present in 37.4% of patients and was associated with spirometrically and clinically less severe COPD [14]. More importantly, a higher blood eosinophil count appears to indicate a subgroup of COPD patients in which the use of inhaled corticosteroids (ICS) results in reduced exacerbation frequency [12,15,16]. Furthermore, significant elevations in peripheral eosinophil counts have been associated with a higher exacerbation rate when ICS is withdrawn [17–19]. In the setting of an acute exacerbation, peripheral eosinophil counts have been reported as an indicator of patients that would benefit from systemic corticosteroids [20]. This strategy could spare the use of corticosteroids in patients without eosinophilia avoiding possible adverse effects and poorer recovery rates [21,22]. The 2019 treatment guidelines from the Global Initiative for Chronic Obstructive Lung Disease (GOLD) have recommended blood eosinophil counts $\geq$300 cells$\cdot\mu L^{-1}$ in stable COPD as the diagnostic criterion for initiating therapy with ICS/long-acting β-agonist (LABA) [23]. However, further prospective validation is necessary to allow the widespread clinical implementation of peripheral blood eosinophils as a guide for the initiation of inhaled or systemic corticosteroids. The optimal cut-off value for the definition of significant eosinophilia has not been established yet [24]. Optimal cut-off values are fundamental for the clinical distinction of patients that would benefit from inhaled corticosteroid therapy. The realization that eosinophilic inflammation is significant in a subgroup of patients with COPD has been recently translated in the development of interleukin (IL)-5 receptor antagonists (benralizumab and mepolizumab) [25,26]. IL-5 expression is transduced through a cooperative signaling network that promotes eosinophil precursor maturation and prolongs the survival of eosinophils. Previously the inhibition of IL-5 has been proved efficacious in reducing severe exacerbations in patients with severe asthma [27]. In a recent phase III trial, mepolizumab at a dose of 100 mg was associated with a lower annual rate of moderate or severe exacerbations in patients with COPD and an eosinophilic phenotype documented by a blood eosinophil count of at least 150 per cubic millimeter at screening or at least 300 per cubic millimeter during the previous year [26]. Benralizumab is a human monoclonal antibody that enhances antibody-dependent cell-mediated cytotoxicity by the blockade of IL-5Rα expressed by eosinophils and basophils [28]. In COPD patients with higher baseline blood eosinophil counts the administration of benralizumab resulted in improved lung function and health status and a trend toward reduction in exacerbations [25]. Based on these encouraging findings phase III studies have been initiated.

Numerous serum biomarkers have been previously tested for their diagnostic, phenotyping, and prognostic ability in cohorts of COPD patients. Most of them are inflammatory markers, such as C-reactive protein (CRP) and IL-6, the circulating levels of which have been found elevated in patients with COPD [29–31]. These studies produced a series of associations most of which are summarized in Table 2. These findings should be taken into account as they may indicate clinical aspects useful for the integrative assessment of the COPD patient [32,33]. However, the reported associations are highly variable and sometimes poorly reproducible and seem inadequate to establish a clear relationship with relevant clinical outcomes of the disease. Thus, at present no single serum biomarker exhibits performance characteristics that allow a definite clinical translation and therapeutic guidance in COPD patients [34]. Therefore, the need for well-validated serum/plasma biomarkers in the COPD population remains.

Table 2. Summary table of biomarkers in COPD management.

Specimen Type	Biomarker	Main Findings	First Author [Ref]
Peripheral Blood (plasma/serum)	MDA	MDA levels were significantly higher in patients with AECOPD compared to stable COPD	Zinellu E. [35]
	Vitamins A, E, and C	Levels of vitamins A and E, but not C were significantly lower in patients with AECOPD than stable COPD	
	GSH, GSH-Px, SOD	Decreased levels of these antioxidant biomarkers were found in the plasma of patients with AECOPD compared to stable COPD	
	GGT	GGT levels were significantly higher in patients with AECOPD (adjusted for age, gender, smoking status) compared to stable COPD and a positive association was reported with CRP	Zinellu E. [36]
	IL-6, TNFα, MCP-1 vWF	Elevated serum levels of IL-6, TNFα and MCP-1, depict the systemic inflammation that occurs in COPD patients Increased concentration of vWF was reported in the serum of COPD smokers	Röpcke S. [37]
	CRP	Positive association of CRP with morbidity, mortality, and frequency of exacerbations Negative association with lung function parameters	Röpcke S. [37]
		CRP was used for the confirmation of AECOPD	Lacoma A. [38]
		CRP was used as a prognostic biomarker and as a marker of inflammatory response in COPD patients Increased CRP levels were found in both patients with AECOPD and stable COPD CRP had a sensitivity of 72.5% and a specificity of 100% for the diagnosis of patients with AECOPD	Heidari B. [31]
	Extracellular vesicles	CD31+ EVs, suggestive of endothelial cell apoptosis, were elevated in patients with emphysema CD62E+ EVs indicative of endothelial activation were elevated in severe COPD and hyperinflation	Thomashow M.A. [39]
		Higher baseline CD62E+ EVs may indicate COPD patients who are susceptible to exacerbation	Takahashi T [40]
	Blood eosinophilia	Peripheral blood eosinophilia (above 0.2×10^9/L) can be used for the detection of sputum eosinophilia mostly in stable COPD It is considered a sensitive biomarker for the detection of sputum eosinophilia in AECOPD (sensitivity 90%, specificity 60%)	Negewo N.A. [13]
Exhaled air	Ethane	Elevated levels of ethane are found in exhaled air of COPD patients and are associated with COPD severity	Barnes P.J. [41]
	FeNO	Smoking is considered a significant limitation of FeNO use because it negatively affects its concentration FeNO is elevated in patients with asthma-like component of COPD Potential biomarker for estimating treatment response in COPD patients	Angelis N. [42]
		FeNO levels increased at the onset of AECOPD and decreased with resolution FeNO had an inverse relationship with FEV1% Increase of FEV1% following a decrease in FeNO (sensitivity 74%, specificity 75%)	Koutsokera A. [43]
Sputum	MPO, 8-isoprostane	No significant elevation of MPO and 8-isoprostane was found in patients with AECOPD	Zinellu E. [35]
		Increased levels of 8-isoprostane were detected in COPD patients compared to non-smokers and smokers without COPD A positive association was observed between 8-isoprostane and pulmonary function parameters	Comandini A. [44]
	MDA, SOD, GSH-Px	Elevated levels of MDA, and reduced SOD and GSH-Px were observed in the sputum of patients with AECOPD compared to stable COPD A positive association was detected among these biomarkers in induced sputum	Zinellu E. [35]

Table 2. *Cont.*

Specimen Type	Biomarker	Main Findings	First Author [Ref]
Sputum	MMP-8, MMP-9, MMP-12, neutrophil elastase, Eosinophil peroxidase	Elevated levels of these biomarkers were found in COPD patients	Barnes P.J. [45]
			Comandini A. [44]
	IL-6, IL-8, TNF-α, Leptin	Elevated levels of IL-6, IL-8, TNF-a were observed in severe COPD cases compared to less severe COPD Increased levels of IL-8 were associated with COPD severity (predicted FEV1%) progression and AECOPD	Barnes P.J. [45]
	IL-6, IL-8, TNF-α	Elevated levels of IL-6, IL-8 and TNF-α are observed in patients with AECOPD compared to stable COPD	Koutsokera A. [43]
Exhaled breath condensate	MDA, H_2O_2	No difference was observed in the MDA levels in the EBC of patients with AECOPD and stable COPD H_2O_2 was highly elevated in both patients with AECOPD and stable COPD	Zinellu E. [35]
		MDA was elevated in the EBC of COPD patients and was even higher in patients with an AECOPD Elevated levels of H_2O_2 were found in both patients with AECOPD and stable COPD	Barnes P.J. [41]
	8-isoprostane	Increased levels of 8-isoprostane were observed in COPD patients	Chamitava L. [46]
			Koutsokera A. [43]
	8-isoprostaglandin F2a (8-isoprostane)	8-isoprostane was associated with disease severity Its concentration was found to be higher in COPD patients compared to smokers without COPD	Barnes P.J. [45]
	IL-8	There is an inverse relationship of IL-8 and PFTs at the onset of an AECOPD	Koutsokera A. [43]
Bronchoalveolar lavage fluid	Glutathione	Reduced glutathione levels were observed in severe AECOPD compared to stable COPD	Zinellu E. [35]
		Lower levels of glutathione were observed in frequent AECOPD compared to stable COPD.	Barnes P.J. [41]
	EGF-R, HSA, A1AT, TIMP1, IL-8 and Calprotectin	Low levels of EGF-R, HSA and A1AT were found in the BAL of COPD patients Increased concentrations of TIMP1, IL-8 and Calprotectin were detected in the BAL of COPD patients that were correlated with airway inflammation	Röpcke S. [37]
Urine	8-isoprostane	Increased levels of 8-isoprostane were observed in the urine of COPD patients	Chamitava L. [46]

MDA: Malondialdehyde, AECOPD: acute exacerbation of COPD, GSH: glutathione, GSH-Px: glutathione peroxidase, SOD: superoxide dismutase, GGT: γ-glutamyltransferase, CRP: C-reactive protein, IL: interleukin, TNF-α: tumor necrosis factor-alpha, MCP-1: monocyte chemoattractant protein-1, vWF: von Willebrand factor, FeNO: fraction of exhaled nitric oxide, FEV1: forced expiratory volume in one second, MPO: myeloperoxidase, MMP: matrix metalloproteinase, EBC: exhaled breath condensate, PFTs: pulmonary function tests, EGFR: epidermal growth factor receptor, HSA: human serum albumin, A1AT: alpha-1-antitrypsin, BAL: bronchoalveolar lavage, TIMP1: tissue inhibitor matrix metalloproteinase 1, EVs: extracellular vesicles.

COPD phenotype with persistent systemic inflammation has been proposed. This phenotype is associated with poor prognosis, including increased mortality [8,9]. The combination of a selective inflammatory panel with BODE index measured at baseline has been shown to improve the ability to predict 3-year and 8-year mortality [47]. This issue has been further addressed by the ECLIPSE study by analyzing the levels and the relationship of a panel of inflammatory markers [WBC count, CRP, IL-6, IL-8, fibrinogen, and tumor necrosis factor-alpha (TNF-α)] with clinical characteristics and relevant outcomes at 3 years follow-up [7,8]. According to this analysis, distinct inflammatory patterns seem to emerge. COPD patients show higher levels of some biomarkers (especially fibrinogen, and IL-6) in comparison with the control smokers and non-smokers. A subgroup of patients accounting for 16% of the sample had persistently high levels of inflammatory biomarkers and this was associated with a greater risk of exacerbations at 1 year regardless of the level of airflow limitation. Additionally, in smokers without COPD the levels of specific markers (IL-8,

TNF-α) are increased compared with both patients with COPD and non-smokers without COPD [7,8]. Finally, plasma CRP, fibrinogen, serum TNFα levels, and immunoglobulin E (IgE) levels are higher in patients with asthma and COPD overlap (ACO) compared to those with COPD alone [8,48]. Such findings represent another indication that patients with ACO may share a specific inflammatory pattern more responsive to corticosteroids and perhaps with a different prognosis. The data concerning therapeutic efficacy in this phenotype are limited since randomized controlled clinical trials exclude asthmatic smokers and patients with possible ACO.

3. Oxidative Stress Biomarkers

Oxidative stress has a significant role in the pathophysiology of COPD. The existence of an essential equilibrium among the cellular oxidant and antioxidant mechanisms plays a crucial role in the preservation of the physiological function of the respiratory system. This disequilibrium of the oxidant-antioxidant mechanism is attributed to the increased oxidants and decreased antioxidants production which subsequently contributes to COPD severity [35,46]. Thus, oxidative stress has significant adverse effects like DNA and protein damage, and lipid destruction. So far, numerous oxidative stress biomarkers including both oxidants and antioxidants have been examined in COPD cases [36]. Several both non-invasive [exhaled breath condensate (EBC), sputum] and invasive methods [bronchoalveolar lavage (BAL), bronchoscopy] have been used for the detection of biomarkers in the COPD [49]. The most commonly used biological samples for the identification of biomarkers include the blood, sputum, BAL, and exhaled air [50]. Malondialdehyde (MDA) and thiobarbituric acid reactive substances (TBARS) are the universal biomarkers used for the detection of oxidative stress mostly in blood samples [36]. Studies compared the MDA values in blood samples of stable COPD cases and acute exacerbation of COPD (AECOPD) cases. The results revealed high MDA values in those with AECOPD [35]. Additionally, the studies assessed the levels of antioxidant biomarkers like glutathione (GSH), glutathione peroxidase (GSH-Px), and superoxide dismutase (SOD) and found them at low levels in the AECOPD patients [35]. Moreover, many studies investigated the concentration of dietary antioxidants especially vitamin A, E, and C, and found a remarkable reduction of their levels in the AECOPD [35]. Various oxidative stress biomarkers such as ethane can be detected at high levels in the exhaled air of COPD individuals. Of interest, ethane is also associated with COPD intensity [41]. Furthermore, studies examined the levels of the hydrogen peroxide (H2O2) biomarker which was remarkably elevated in EBC samples of COPD individuals [35]. High levels of 4-hydroxynonenal (4HNE), MDA, and 8-isoprostane have been detected in patients with either stable or AECOPD [46]. Notably, 8-isoprostane has been investigated in several pulmonary samples like exhaled air and sputum. Many studies found increased 8-isoprostane concentration in the sputum of COPD individuals and even higher in AECOPD. However, a further increase of 8-isoprostane was observed in the sputum of smokers compared to that of non-smokers, concluding that smoking is a significant confounding factor. Publication data revealed that smokers had elevated 8-isoprostane for a period of at least three months following smoking cessation [49]. Thus, the elevated levels of this compound in ex-smokers indicate an endogenous source of oxidative stress and simultaneously an ongoing pulmonary inflammation [41]. Similarly, MDA was studied in both sputum and EBC samples. EBC MDA levels were higher in AECOPD individuals compared to stable cases, but sputum MDA levels were further elevated in AECOPD compared to stable COPD cases. Interestingly, only one study has examined biomarkers in BAL [35]. GSH, the main antioxidant in the respiratory system, was investigated in BAL of both stable and AECOPD cases and was found to be decreased in severe AECOPD patients [35]. However, the results regarding blood GSH levels are still controversial [49].

Moreover, increased γ-glutamyltransferase (GGT), an enzyme that is involved in the pathway of GSH production and the development of many conditions characterized by oxidative stress, was detected in the plasma of COPD patients [36]. A positive link between GGT and CRP levels, as well as COPD severity, has been reported [35].

4. Age-Related Biomarkers

COPD is a chronic disease that is characterized by accelerated lung aging [51]. Several pathological mechanisms of accelerated lung aging have been examined in COPD patients including telomere attrition, epigenetic changes, stem cell exhaustion, cellular senescence, epigenetic changes, oxidative stress, mitochondrial dysfunction, and genomic instability. Cellular senescence describes a process in which the presence of stressors such as reactive oxygen species (ROS) leads cells to a permanent cell arrest state which is correlated with phenotypic alterations [52]. Cellular senescence is an established lung aging process that is associated with both functional and structural impairment in COPD patients [53]. Moreover, cellular senescence occurs in patients with emphysematous lungs and is correlated with shorter telomeres and reduced anti-aging molecules, indicating accelerated lung aging [52]. Additionally, studies have found increased levels of cellular senescence biomarkers like p16, p19, and p21, which are tumor suppressors and cyclin kinase inhibitors, in COPD individuals [53,54]. Sirtuin-1 (SIRT1) is another cellular senescence biomarker that, in COPD patients is expressed in low concentrations in the respiratory epithelium of the small airways [53]. Furthermore, smoking contributes to the high levels of senescence biomarkers like protein p21 and b-galactosidase [53,54].

Stem cell exhaustion is another significant mechanism of aging that contributes to the COPD pathogenesis [54]. Stem cells can replace and regenerate diseased cells, a property which is lost with age leading to age-related disorders [52,54]. In COPD patients the stem cells which are responsible for the regeneration of respiratory epithelium possess a diminished capacity of cellular regeneration which subsequently affects the entire cellular repair process [52]. Concerning the relationship between COPD and other physiological parameters, it was found that PaO_2 has an important association with telomere length in COPD individuals because these patients have regular incidences of hypoxia, especially during COPD exacerbations, sleep, and physical activity which induces oxidative stress to the cells [54]. The length of telomeres has been used as a biomarker of aging and disease progression in COPD patients. Specifically, studies compared the length of the telomeres in leukocytes of COPD patients with both a control group and smokers without COPD. The results revealed shorter telomere length in white blood cells of COPD subjects even after matching for sex, age, and tobacco exposure [55,56]. However, shorter telomere length was observed in elderly patients with COPD and smokers without COPD. Moreover, a few large-scale studies have indicated a moderate association between telomere length and respiratory function related to forced expiratory volume in one second (FEV1) [57,58]. Recent studies in which many biomarkers of aging were examined in COPD patients, revealed that telomere length is the sole biomarker related to respiratory function. Additionally, a link between telomere length and other comorbidities like hypertension, cancer, diabetes mellitus in COPD subjects has not been established [56]. Systemic inflammation is another factor that affects the telomere length in COPD. High levels of inflammatory markers such as IL-6, IL-1β, IL-8, Transforming growth factor-beta (TGF-B) have been found in the respiratory tract and bloodstream of COPD subjects [56]. Specifically, IL-6 is considered a pro-inflammatory cytokine involved in aging and low-grade activation of chronic inflammation [54]. Interestingly, the telomeres length shortening was negatively associated with the levels of IL-6 in COPD individuals. Thus, inflammation influences the telomeres length [56]. Studies have also investigated the role of two main age-related hormonal biomarkers, dehydroepiandrosterone (DHEA) and growth hormone (GH) in the process of accelerated lung aging. The results revealed a remarkable decrease in DHEA and GH levels in COPD patients. Additionally, it was shown that a negative association exists among DHEA, GH, and age in COPD and non-COPD patients. Specifically, it was found that COPD patients present early biological aging, ranging from 13 to 23 years, compared to non-COPD patients depending on the variations of DHEA and GH levels. Moreover, both DHEA and GH showed an important association with many respiratory parameters like FEV1 and PaO2 [56]. To sum up, further studies are needed to elucidate the molecular mechanisms of aging in patients with aging-related diseases like COPD [56].

5. Bronchial Biomarkers

Several non-invasive techniques (exhaled air, induced sputum, EBC) and invasive diagnostic techniques (BAL, respiratory tissue biopsies) are currently used for the detection of bronchial biomarkers in COPD patients [42].

Regarding non-invasive methods, induced sputum is used for both the identification of inflammatory biomarkers and the presence of eosinophilia [42]. The sputum sampling is collected mostly from the large respiratory airways [45]. The main sputum inflammatory biomarkers that have been identified include cytokines especially IL-6, IL-8, and TNF-α. High levels of these cytokines were found in individuals with AECOPD. Moreover, it was noticed that in patients with COPD exacerbations the level of inflammatory biomarkers has an inverse relationship with FEV1 [43]. Additionally, high proteases levels, like matrix metalloproteinase (MMP)-8, MMP-9, MMP-12, and neutrophil elastase were found in sputum samples of COPD individuals. Also, elevated proportions of extracellular matrix (ECM) structural components were identified in the sputum of COPD patients [45]. Eosinophil peroxidase is used as an indicator of eosinophilia in the sputum samples of COPD patients and has been found elevated in COPD sputum samples [44]. In the exhaled air method, the fraction of exhaled nitric oxide (FeNO) was found as the predominant biomarker [42]. The measurement of FeNO concentration is considered difficult and can be influenced by factors like smoking and ICS. Remarkably, increased FeNO levels have been detected at the beginning of the AECOPD [43]. Moreover, FeNO has a positive association with FEV1 following COPD treatment, and specifically, the reduction of FeNO levels is associated with increased FEV1 [43].

BAL performed in COPD patients revealed the presence of numerous inflammatory biomarkers like myeloperoxidase, eosinophil cationic protein, and IL-8 at increased concentrations. Few studies showed increased levels of tryptase and histamine in COPD patients. Additionally, BAL sample results demonstrated high proteases and low anti-protease levels [41]. However, BAL has several limitations due to its invasive nature, sampling method, and other confounding factors like smoking and ICS [41]. Studies that have compared BAL samples of COPD patients versus healthy smokers, showed decreased concentrations of certain biomarkers including epidermal growth factor receptor (EGFR), human serum albumin (HSA), and alpha-1-antitrypsin (A1AT) in the BAL samples of COPD patients. In contrast, healthy smokers had elevated levels of HSA, A1AT, and MMP3. Simultaneously, BAL of COPD patients had high levels of IL-8, Tissue inhibitor matrix metalloproteinase 1 (TIMP1), and calprotectin indicative of respiratory tract neutrophilia. Interestingly, HSA and A1AT were the dominant biomarkers in BAL samples [37].

As mentioned above, oxidative stress has a dominant role in the pathogenesis of COPD, with adverse outcomes in the structural components of the cells. Inflammation of the respiratory system leads to ROS production by certain cells like macrophages, neutrophils, and epithelial cells. H2O2 and 8-isoprostaglandin F2a (8-isoprostane) are the two predominant biomarkers of oxidative stress that can be detected in an exhaled breath at a high concentration [42]. The use of EBC in COPD patients has shown high levels of both H2O2 and 8-isoprostaglandin F2a. Moreover, both biomarkers are associated with the intensity of the COPD [45]. The EBC pH is another potential biomarker, but it is still not well studied [43].

6. Mucine-Producing Pathways

The lining of the respiratory tract has an important mucociliary clearance mechanism which is involved in its protection by various environmental and infectious factors. Any impairment of this clearance mechanism can lead to mucus build-up and peripheral airways obstruction [59,60]. Increased mucin production is the main feature involved in

COPD pathogenesis and has been associated with a high risk of morbidity, mortality, as well as COPD exacerbations and disease severity [61,62]. Numerous mucin genes have been identified in the respiratory system of humans. The most abundant are the Mucin (MUC)5AC and MUC5B [61]. These two mucin genes are responsible for both the composition of mucus and its movement along the airways [62]. Specifically, in the airways of healthy individuals, MUC5B is the predominant mucin gene that is related to mucus clearance from the airways. Opposed to that, the MUC5AC gene is expressed at low rates in the airways of healthy patients. Remarkably, a significant increase in the expression of MUC5AC has been related to inflammatory states and muco-obstructive lung diseases compared to MUC5B [59,61]. Furthermore, several other factors are implicated in the increased production of mucins such as oxidative stress and smoking. Indeed, smoking augments mostly the MUC5AC expression and to a slighter degree the expression of MUC5B, in the respiratory epithelium of smokers compared to the non-smoker's [59,63]. The mechanism by which cigarette smoke enhances mucus production still needs further investigation, although oxidative stress is currently considered the main causative factor [63]. Moreover, studies showed a positive relationship between disease severity and high MUC5AC levels [59]. The results of pulmonary function tests revealed an inverse relationship among MUC5AC, and pulmonary function expressed as forced expiratory flow (FEF) 25–75%, which was not found for the MUC5B mucin gene [59,60]. Interestingly, a marked decrease in the pulmonary function (i.e., FEV1) with a parallel rise in MUC5AC levels was observed in smokers compared to ex-smokers with normal MUC5AC levels. Recent publications showed that ex-smokers with COPD had marginally increased MUC5AC levels which did not return to normal levels following smoking cessation. Similar reversibility rates were observed for the levels of MUC5B as well. However, early smoking cessation prior to airway obstruction was found to prevent pulmonary function decline and MUC5AC regulation. In conclusion, MUC5AC can be used as a potential biomarker for COPD detection, prognosis, and effectiveness of the treatment [59].

7. Extracellular Vesicles as Biomarkers in COPD

Recent studies have examined the use of extracellular vesicles (EVs) as both diagnostic and prognostic biomarkers in COPD and their potential role in distinguishing COPD exacerbations from the stable state as well as defining the COPD phenotype [64]. EVs are membrane particles that are released in systemic circulation by endothelial cells undergoing either apoptosis or activation [40]. Several body fluids have been used for the isolation of Evs including blood, urine, and BAL [64]. EVs express several endothelial cell markers which are specific to the stimuli that caused their release. More specifically, EVs that express CD31+ are related to apoptosis of endothelial cells whereas the expression of CD62E is related to activation of endothelial cells. Furthermore, the expression of CD51 is associated with the chronic injury [39]. Studies found that there is a link between CD31+ EVs and decreased diffusing capacity of carbon monoxide (DLCO). In addition, there is a negative association among EVs expressing CD31+ and FEV1. Increased levels of CD31+ EVs were found in COPD patients and were related to the severity of COPD. Additionally, CD31+ EVs were related to the emphysematous phenotype of COPD on imaging studies [39]. In contrast, EVs expressing CD62E+ were increased only in individuals with severe COPD and were related to lung hyperinflation [39]. Takahashi et al. showed that increased CD62E+ EVs (E-selectin) were observed in COPD individuals with regular episodes of AECOPD and those prone to exacerbations [40]. Concerning CD51+ EVs, elevated levels were detected in COPD individuals. However, no connection was observed between CD51+ or CD62E+ EVs and DLCO [39]. Overall, further research is needed upon the use of EVs as biomarkers for the diagnosis and management of COPD in the clinical practice [39].

8. Genetic Biomarkers

Mutations in the SERPINA1 gene leading to a1-antithrypsin deficiency represent at present the only established genetically based phenotype of COPD for which targeted therapy exists. Although this genetic condition accounts only for 1–2% of the total COPD population it may respond positively to replacement therapy with an alpha 1 proteinase inhibitor [65,66]. Increased susceptibility to smoking-induced emphysema has been associated with polymorphisms of the heme oxygenase (HO-1) promoter leading to reduced HO-1 expression [67,68]. Additionally, susceptibility to emphysema has been recently linked to a variant (single nucleotide polymorphisms; SNP) of the BICD1 gene [69]. Patients with ACO are characterized by an enhanced expression of several genes, such as toll-like receptor 10 (TLR10) which has been previously implicated in the pathogenesis of the asthma [48]. Other studies on genetic polymorphisms have identified several genes associated with the pathogenesis of different characteristics of COPD: cholinergic nicotine receptor alpha 3/5 (CHRNA3/5), iron regulatory binding protein 2 (IREB2), hedgehog-interacting protein (HHIP), family with sequence similarity 13, member A (FAM13A), and advanced glycosylation end product-specific receptor (AGER) [70–75]. Previously reported associations of these genetic variants include: airflow limitation (CHRNA3/5, IREB2, HHIP), [76] emphysema susceptibility and severity (CHRNA3/5, BICD1), [77] chronic bronchitis phenotype, [78] exacerbation rate (HHIP) [79] and pulmonary hypertension pathogenesis [80]. Nevertheless, the majority of these findings comprise suggestive liaisons and their clinical translation and applicability require replication in additional studies [81].

9. COPD Exacerbation-Related Biomarkers

AECOPD is related to poor health outcomes, increased morbidity, and mortality rates [82,83]. The diagnostic and therapeutic management of AECOPD is still considered insufficient due to its heterogeneity and complexity [84]. Currently, the diagnostic approach of AECOPD is mostly based on the patient's symptomatology [83,84]. Thus, biomarkers should be actively investigated to incorporate them in the clinical assessment [83].

Nowadays, inflammatory biomarkers serve as diagnostic and prognostic tools in patients with AECOPD. Such inflammatory biomarkers that are commonly used include CRP, procalcitonin (PCT), and fibrinogen. Additionally, biomarkers like serum amyloid A (SAA), serum surfactant protein-D (SP-D), vascular endothelial growth factor (VEGF), troponin-T (TNT), 4-HNE, β-thromboglobulin, platelet factor-4 (PF4), and copeptin were proven beneficial for the assessment of intensity and outcome of AECOPD. Recently, FeNO was identified as a promising upcoming biomarker [84].

The results of the ECLIPSE study indicated that AECOPD is associated with increased levels of inflammatory biomarkers including white blood cells, CRP, and fibrinogen during the first year of follow-up [10,85]. Interestingly, no link has been observed among elevated levels of IL-6 and acute COPD exacerbations [86]. However, three studies found an increased level of IL-6 in AECOPD, although the statistical significance was not reported in [87]. The TNF-α biomarker was also found to be elevated during AECOPD [87]. Recent studies found a positive interdependence between high levels of fibrinogen, CRP, and leukocytes in patients presenting with COPD exacerbations [38,85,88]. Remarkably, the ECLIPSE, COPDGene, and the Copenhagen Lung Study found that an increased number of eosinophils in the blood were associated with COPD exacerbations [83]. Moreover, the COPDGene cohort study demonstrated a significant association between serious AECOPD and five biomarkers, the plasminogen activator inhibitor-1 (PAI-1), soluble receptor for advanced glycation end products (sRAGE), A1AT, brain-derived neurotrophic factor (BDNF), and C-X-C Motif Chemokine Ligand 5 (CXCL5).

Other biomarkers that have been identified in prior studies include CRP, leukocytes, eosinophils, ILs, fibrinogen, extracellular adenosine triphosphate (eATP), and extracellular heat shock protein 70 (eHsp70) [89]. The extracellular ATP (eATP), a key molecule of the pro-inflammatory cascade pathway associated with respiratory airway diseases, was investigated in the plasma of COPD patients. High levels of eATP were associated with the frequency of COPD exacerbations, symptoms severity, and rate of airflow decline [90]. Similar results were reported for the heat shock protein 70, an important pro-inflammatory molecule having a crucial role in the regulation of immunological pathways [89,90].

Other studies have examined the connection between the AECOPD and respiratory tissue destruction. The results showed an increased number of circulating structural proteins of the respiratory extracellular matrix which can be used as diagnostic biomarkers [83,91,92]. In 2017, Noell et al. showed that the combined set of elevated CRP and neutrophil levels in conjunction with dyspnea can accurately diagnose AECOPD [84]. Additionally, studies have evaluated the measurement of volatile organic compounds during expiration in AECOPD cases and considered it as a useful, non-invasive diagnostic tool [83,93].

10. Combination of Biomarkers

Numerous protein biomarkers have been studied in the bloodstream of COPD individuals aiming to assess the disease outcomes [94]. Specifically, studies have found a link between biomarkers like the SP-D, CRP, fibrinogen, and high mortality rates in COPD patients. Nevertheless, no association has been found among SP-D, CRP, fibrinogen, soluble receptor of activated glycogen end-product (sRAGE), club cell protein 16 (CC-16), and the degree of FEV1 decline, hospitalizations, and COPD exacerbations [91].

The COPDGene cohort study showed that both the decrease of lung function and the progression of emphysema could be most reliably estimated by measuring the level of a specific panel of biomarkers (sRAGE, CC-16, and fibrinogen). Similarly, the ECLIPSE study used the same panel of biomarkers combined with SP-D and CRP strengthening, even more, the estimations [94]. Furthermore, elevated levels of the IL-1α, IL-1β, IL-6, IL-8, TNF-α cytokines have been found in the serum and sputum of COPD subjects. A positive association was found between CRP and IL-1β in the blood of COPD patients. Moreover, IL-1β and IL-6 were negatively associated with FEV1. Additionally, a positive correlation was observed between the cytokines IL-1β, IL-6, TNF-α, and COPD severity [89].

To sum up, more investigations are needed to find the association between the aforementioned panels of biomarkers and the COPD outcomes [91].

11. Conclusions

Age-related diseases like COPD are increasing in frequency due to population aging. In the last years, numerous biomarkers have been investigated in COPD patients, although their significance is not well established. The study of appropriate and ideal biomarkers is of high importance for the disease diagnosis, prognosis, and treatment effectiveness. Moreover, COPD prognosis and response to treatment could be assessed by evaluating the combination of biomarkers in COPD individuals. Many types of biological samples and diagnostic techniques are used for the detection of these numerous biomarkers in COPD patients, with each one having its sensitivity.

The recent therapeutic methods for COPD are mostly targeting the patients' COPD-related symptoms. For this reason, further research is warranted to develop novel therapies which could target the underlying pathways that lead to COPD pathogenesis. Furthermore, the disease heterogeneity among COPD individuals especially at the level of COPD severity, progression, and patients' comorbidities as well as clinical status, could set the foundations for more personalized management of these patients. Specifically, the measurement and evaluation of each patients' unique biomarker panel could be a quite convenient approach in the upcoming years. As a result of this, more effective, and targeted therapies could be followed.

Author Contributions: Conceptualization, I.P., and S.K.; investigation, K.M.; data curation, K.M.; writing—original draft preparation, K.M., O.K. and F.P.; writing—review and editing, I.P., E.R. and K.G.; supervision, K.G. All authors have read and agreed to the published version of the manuscript.

Funding: This research received no external funding.

Data Availability Statement: Not applicable.

Conflicts of Interest: The authors declare no conflict of interest.

References

1. Lange, P.; Celli, B.R.; Agustí, A.; Jensen, G.B.; Divo, M.; Faner, R.; Guerra, S.; Marott, J.L.; Martinez, F.D.; Martinez-Camblor, P.; et al. Lung-Function Trajectories Leading to Chronic Obstructive Pulmonary Disease. *N. Engl. J. Med.* **2015**, *373*, 111–122. [CrossRef] [PubMed]
2. Woodruff, P.G.; Agusti, A.; Roche, N.; Singh, D.; Martinez, F.J. Current concepts in targeting chronic obstructive pulmonary disease pharmacotherapy: Making progress towards personalised management. *Lancet* **2015**, *385*, 1789–1798. [CrossRef]
3. Stockley, R.A.; Halpin, D.M.G.; Celli, B.R.; Singh, D. Chronic Obstructive Pulmonary Disease Biomarkers and Their Interpretation. *Am. J. Respir. Crit. Care Med.* **2019**, *199*, 1195–1204. [CrossRef] [PubMed]
4. Biomarkers Definitions Working Group; Atkinson, A.J., Jr.; Colburn, W.A.; DeGruttola, V.G.; DeMets, D.L.; Downing, G.J.; Hoth, D.F.; Oates, J.A.; Peck, C.C.; Spilker, B.A. Biomarkers and surrogate endpoints: Preferred definitions and conceptual framework. *Clin. Pharmacol. Ther.* **2001**, *69*, 89–95. [CrossRef]
5. Ho, T.; Dasgupta, A.; Hargreave, F.E.; Nair, P. The use of cellular and molecular biomarkers to manage COPD exacerbations. *Expert Rev. Respir. Med.* **2017**, *11*, 403–411. [CrossRef]
6. Sin, D.D.; Hollander, Z.; Demarco, M.L.; McManus, B.M.; Ng, R.T. Biomarker Development for Chronic Obstructive Pulmonary Disease. From Discovery to Clinical Implementation. *Am. J. Respir. Crit. Care Med.* **2015**, *192*, 1162–1170. [CrossRef] [PubMed]
7. Faner, R.; Tal-Singer, R.; Riley, J.H.; Celli, B.; Vestbo, J.; MacNee, W.; Bakke, P.; Calverley, P.M.A.; Coxson, H.; Crim, C.; et al. Lessons from ECLIPSE: A review of COPD biomarkers. *Thorax* **2014**, *69*, 666–672. [CrossRef]
8. Agustí, A.; Edwards, L.D.; Rennard, S.I.; MacNee, W.; Tal-Singer, R.; Miller, B.E.; Vestbo, J.; Lomas, D.A.; Calverley, P.M.A.; Wouters, E.; et al. Persistent Systemic Inflammation is Associated with Poor Clinical Outcomes in COPD: A Novel Phenotype. *PLoS ONE* **2012**, *7*, e37483. [CrossRef]
9. Thomsen, M.; Dahl, M.; Lange, P.; Vestbo, J.; Nordestgaard, B.G. Inflammatory Biomarkers and Comorbidities in Chronic Obstructive Pulmonary Disease. *Am. J. Respir. Crit. Care Med.* **2012**, *186*, 982–988. [CrossRef]
10. Hurst, J.R.; Vestbo, J.; Anzueto, A.; Locantore, N.; Müllerová, H.; Tal-Singer, R.; Miller, B.; Lomas, D.A.; Agusti, A.; MacNee, W.; et al. Susceptibility to Exacerbation in Chronic Obstructive Pulmonary Disease. *N. Engl. J. Med.* **2010**, *363*, 1128–1138. [CrossRef]
11. Müllerová, H.; Maselli, D.J.; Locantore, N.; Vestbo, J.; Hurst, J.R.; Wedzicha, J.A.; Bakke, P.; Agusti, A.; Anzueto, A. Hospitalized Exacerbations of COPD: Risk Factors and Outcomes in the ECLIPSE Cohort. *Chest* **2015**, *147*, 999–1007. [CrossRef]
12. Pavord, I.; Lettis, S.; Locantore, N.; Pascoe, S.; Jones, P.W.; Wedzicha, J.A.; Barnes, N.C. Blood eosinophils and inhaled corticosteroid/long-acting β-2 agonist efficacy in COPD. *Thorax* **2015**, *71*, 118–125. [CrossRef] [PubMed]
13. Negewo, N.A.; McDonald, V.M.; Baines, K.; Wark, P.A.; Simpson, J.L.; Jones, P.W.; Gibson, P. Peripheral blood eosinophils: A surrogate marker for airway eosinophilia in stable COPD. *Int. J. Chronic Obstr. Pulm. Dis.* **2016**, *11*, 1495–1504. [CrossRef] [PubMed]
14. Singh, D.; Kolsum, U.; Brightling, C.; Locantore, N.; Agusti, A.; Tal-Singer, R. Eosinophilic inflammation in COPD: Prevalence and clinical characteristics. *Eur. Respir. J.* **2014**, *44*, 1697–1700. [CrossRef]
15. Pascoe, S.; Locantore, N.; Dransfield, M.T.; Barnes, N.C.; Pavord, I. Blood eosinophil counts, exacerbations, and response to the addition of inhaled fluticasone furoate to vilanterol in patients with chronic obstructive pulmonary disease: A secondary analysis of data from two parallel randomised controlled trials. *Lancet Respir. Med.* **2015**, *3*, 435–442. [CrossRef]
16. Siddiqui, S.; Guasconi, A.; Vestbo, J.; Jones, P.; Agusti, A.; Paggiaro, P.; Wedzicha, J.A.; Singh, D. Blood Eosinophils: A Biomarker of Response to Extrafine Beclomethasone/Formoterol in Chronic Obstructive Pulmonary Disease. *Am. J. Respir. Crit. Care Med.* **2015**, *192*, 523–525. [CrossRef]
17. Magnussen, H.; Disse, B.; Rodriguez-Roisin, R.; Kirsten, A.; Watz, H.; Tetzlaff, K.; Towse, L.; Finnigan, H.; Dahl, R.; Decramer, M.; et al. Withdrawal of Inhaled Glucocorticoids and Exacerbations of COPD. *N. Engl. J. Med.* **2014**, *371*, 1285–1294. [CrossRef]
18. Cosio, M.; Baraldo, S.; Saetta, M.; Singanayagam, A.; Johnston, S.L.; Mallia, P.; Magnussen, H.; Tetzlaff, K.; Calverley, P.M.A.; Brightling, C.E.; et al. Inhaled Glucocorticoids and COPD Exacerbations. *N. Engl. J. Med.* **2015**, *372*, 93–94. [CrossRef]
19. Watz, H.; Tetzlaff, K.; Wouters, E.F.M.; Kirsten, A.; Magnussen, H.; Rodriguez-Roisin, R.; Vogelmeier, C.; Fabbri, L.; Chanez, P.; Dahl, R.; et al. Blood eosinophil count and exacerbations in severe chronic obstructive pulmonary disease after withdrawal of inhaled corticosteroids: A post-hoc analysis of the WISDOM trial. *Lancet Respir. Med.* **2016**, *4*, 390–398. [CrossRef]
20. Aaron, S.D.; Vandemheen, K.L.; Maltais, F.; Field, S.; Sin, D.D.; Bourbeau, J.; Marciniuk, D.D.; FitzGerald, J.M.; Nair, P.; Mallick, R. TNFα antagonists for acute exacerbations of COPD: A randomised double-blind controlled trial. *Thorax* **2012**, *68*, 142–148. [CrossRef]
21. Bafadhel, M.; Greening, N.; Harvey-Dunstan, T.C.; Williams, J.E.; Morgan, M.D.; Brightling, C.; Hussain, S.F.; Pavord, I.; Singh, S.J.; Steiner, M. Blood Eosinophils and Outcomes in Severe Hospitalized Exacerbations of COPD. *Chest* **2016**, *150*, 320–328. [CrossRef] [PubMed]
22. Bafadhel, M.; Davies, L.; Calverley, P.M.; Aaron, S.; Brightling, C.; Pavord, I. Blood eosinophil guided prednisolone therapy for exacerbations of COPD: A further analysis. *Eur. Respir. J.* **2014**, *44*, 789–791. [CrossRef] [PubMed]
23. Singh, D.; Agusti, A.; Anzueto, A.; Barnes, P.J.; Bourbeau, J.; Celli, B.R.; Criner, G.J.; Frith, P.; Halpin, D.M.G.; Han, M.; et al. Global Strategy for the Diagnosis, Management, and Prevention of Chronic Obstructive Lung Disease: The GOLD science committee report 2019. *Eur. Respir. J.* **2019**, *53*, 1900164. [CrossRef] [PubMed]

24. Barnes, N.C.; Sharma, R.; Lettis, S.; Calverley, P.M. Blood eosinophils as a marker of response to inhaled corticosteroids in COPD. *Eur. Respir. J.* **2016**, *47*, 1374–1382. [CrossRef]
25. Brightling, C.E.; Bleecker, E.R.; Panettieri, R.A.; Bafadhel, M.; She, D.; Ward, C.K.; Xu, X.; Birrell, C.; van der Merwe, R. Benralizumab for chronic obstructive pulmonary disease and sputum eosinophilia: A randomised, double-blind, placebo-controlled, phase 2a study. *Lancet Respir. Med.* **2014**, *2*, 891–901. [CrossRef]
26. Pavord, I.D.; Chanez, P.; Criner, G.J.; Kerstjens, H.; Korn, S.; Lugogo, N.; Martinot, J.-B.; Sagara, H.; Albers, F.C.; Bradford, E.S.; et al. Mepolizumab for Eosinophilic Chronic Obstructive Pulmonary Disease. *N. Engl. J. Med.* **2017**, *377*, 1613–1629. [CrossRef]
27. Garcia, G.; Taille, C.; Laveneziana, P.; Bourdin, A.; Chanez, P.; Humbert, M. Anti-interleukin-5 therapy in severe asthma. *Eur. Respir. Rev. Off. J. Eur. Respir. Soc.* **2013**, *22*, 251–257. [CrossRef]
28. Ghazi, A.; Trikha, A.; Calhoun, W.J. Benralizumab—A humanized mAb to IL-5Rα with enhanced antibody-dependent cell-mediated cytotoxicity—A novel approach for the treatment of asthma. *Expert Opin. Biol. Ther.* **2011**, *12*, 113–118. [CrossRef]
29. Fabbri, L.; Rabe, K.F. From COPD to chronic systemic inflammatory syndrome? *Lancet* **2007**, *370*, 797–799. [CrossRef]
30. Gan, W.Q.; Man, S.F.P.; Senthilselvan, A.; Sin, D.D. Association between chronic obstructive pulmonary disease and systemic inflammation: A systematic review and a meta-analysis. *Thorax* **2004**, *59*, 574–580. [CrossRef]
31. Heidari, B. The importance of C-reactive protein and other inflammatory markers in patients with chronic obstructive pulmonary disease. *Casp. J. Intern. Med.* **2012**, *3*, 428–435.
32. Hurst, J.R.; Donaldson, G.C.; Perera, W.R.; Wilkinson, T.M.A.; Bilello, J.A.; Hagan, G.W.; Vessey, R.S.; Wedzicha, J.A. Use of Plasma Biomarkers at Exacerbation of Chronic Obstructive Pulmonary Disease. *Am. J. Respir. Crit. Care Med.* **2006**, *174*, 867–874. [CrossRef] [PubMed]
33. Asiimwe, A.C.; Brims, F.J.H.; Andrews, N.P.; Prytherch, D.R.; Higgins, B.R.; Kilburn, S.A.; Chauhan, A.J. Routine Laboratory Tests Can Predict In-hospital Mortality in Acute Exacerbations of COPD. *Lung* **2011**, *189*, 225–232. [CrossRef]
34. Hollander, Z.; DeMarco, M.L.; Sadatsafavi, M.; McManus, B.M.; Ng, R.T.; Sin, D.D. Biomarker Development in COPD: Moving From P Values to Products to Impact Patient Care. *Chest* **2017**, *151*, 455–467. [CrossRef] [PubMed]
35. Zinellu, E.; Zinellu, A.; Fois, A.; Pau, M.; Scano, V.; Piras, B.; Carru, C.; Pirina, P. Oxidative Stress Biomarkers in Chronic Obstructive Pulmonary Disease Exacerbations: A Systematic Review. *Antioxidants* **2021**, *10*, 710. [CrossRef]
36. Zinellu, E.; Zinellu, A.; Fois, A.G.; Carru, C.; Pirina, P. Circulating biomarkers of oxidative stress in chronic obstructive pulmonary disease: A systematic review. *Respir. Res.* **2016**, *17*, 150. [CrossRef]
37. Röpcke, S.; Holz, O.; Lauer, G.; Muller, M.; Rittinghausen, S.; Ernst, P.; Lahu, G.; Elmlinger, M.; Krug, N.; Hohlfeld, J.M. Repeatability of and Relationship between Potential COPD Biomarkers in Bronchoalveolar Lavage, Bronchial Biopsies, Serum, and Induced Sputum. *PLoS ONE* **2012**, *7*, e46207. [CrossRef]
38. Domínguez, J.; Lacoma, A.; Prat, C.; Andreo, F.; Lores, L.; Ruiz-Manzano, J.; Ausina, V. Value of procalcitonin, C-reactive protein, and neopterin in exacerbations of chronic obstructive pulmonary disease. *Int. J. Chronic Obstr. Pulm. Dis.* **2011**, *6*, 157–169. [CrossRef]
39. Thomashow, M.A.; Shimbo, D.; Parikh, M.A.; Hoffman, E.A.; Vogel-Claussen, J.; Hueper, K.; Fu, J.; Liu, C.-Y.; Bluemke, D.A.; Ventetuolo, C.E.; et al. Endothelial Microparticles in Mild Chronic Obstructive Pulmonary Disease and Emphysema. The Multi-Ethnic Study of Atherosclerosis Chronic Obstructive Pulmonary Disease Study. *Am. J. Respir. Crit. Care Med.* **2013**, *188*, 60–68. [CrossRef]
40. Takahashi, T.; Kobayashi, S.; Fujino, N.; Suzuki, T.; Ota, C.; He, M.; Yamada, M.; Suzuki, S.; Yanai, M.; Kurosawa, S.; et al. Increased circulating endothelial microparticles in COPD patients: A potential biomarker for COPD exacerbation susceptibility. *Thorax* **2012**, *67*, 1067–1074. [CrossRef] [PubMed]
41. Barnes, P.J. Oxidative stress-based therapeutics in COPD. *Redox Biol.* **2020**, *33*, 101544. [CrossRef] [PubMed]
42. Angelis, N.; Porpodis, K.; Zarogoulidis, P.; Spyratos, D.; Kioumis, I.; Papaiwannou, A.; Pitsiou, G.; Tsakiridis, K.; Mpakas, A.; Arikas, S.; et al. Airway inflammation in chronic obstructive pulmonary disease. *J. Thorac. Dis.* **2014**, *6*, S167–S172. [CrossRef] [PubMed]
43. Koutsokera, A.; Kostikas, K.; Nicod, L.P.; Fitting, J.-W. Pulmonary biomarkers in COPD exacerbations: A systematic review. *Respir. Res.* **2013**, *14*, 111. [CrossRef]
44. Comandini, A.; Rogliani, P.; Nunziata, A.; Cazzola, M.; Curradi, G.; Saltini, C. Biomarkers of lung damage associated with tobacco smoke in induced sputum. *Respir. Med.* **2009**, *103*, 1592–1613. [CrossRef] [PubMed]
45. Barnes, P.J.; Chowdhury, B.; Kharitonov, S.A.; Magnussen, H.; Page, C.P.; Postma, D.; Saetta, M. Pulmonary Biomarkers in Chronic Obstructive Pulmonary Disease. *Am. J. Respir. Crit. Care Med.* **2006**, *174*, 6–14. [CrossRef] [PubMed]
46. Chamitava, L.; Cazzoletti, L.; Ferrari, M.; Garcia-Larsen, V.; Jalil, A.; Degan, P.; Fois, A.G.; Zinellu, E.; Fois, S.S.; Pasini, A.M.F.; et al. Biomarkers of Oxidative Stress and Inflammation in Chronic Airway Diseases. *Int. J. Mol. Sci.* **2020**, *21*, E4339. [CrossRef]
47. Cote, C.G. Surrogates of Mortality in Chronic Obstructive Pulmonary Disease. *Am. J. Med.* **2006**, *119*, 54–62. [CrossRef]
48. Wurst, K.E.; Rheault, T.R.; Edwards, L.; Tal-Singer, R.; Agustí, A.; Vestbo, J. A comparison of COPD patients with and without ACOS in the ECLIPSE study. *Eur. Respir. J.* **2016**, *47*, 1559–1562. [CrossRef]
49. Antus, B. Oxidative Stress Markers in Sputum. *Oxidative Med. Cell. Longev.* **2016**, *2016*, 1–12. [CrossRef]

50. Kant, S.; Bajpai, J.; Prakash, V.; Verma, A.K.; Srivastava, A.; Bajaj, D.K.; Ahmad, M.; Agarwal, A. Study of oxidative stress biomarkers in chronic obstructive pulmonary disease and their correlation with disease severity in north Indian population cohort. *Lung India Off. Organ Indian Chest Soc.* **2017**, *34*, 324–329. [CrossRef]
51. Albrecht, E.; Sillanpää, E.; Karrasch, S.; Alves, A.C.; Codd, V.; Hovatta, I.; Buxton, J.L.; Nelson, C.P.; Broer, L.; Hägg, S.; et al. Telomere length in circulating leukocytes is associated with lung function and disease. *Eur. Respir. J.* **2013**, *43*, 983–992. [CrossRef] [PubMed]
52. MacNee, W. Is Chronic Obstructive Pulmonary Disease an Accelerated Aging Disease? *Ann. Am. Thorac. Soc.* **2016**, *13*, S429–S437. [CrossRef]
53. Birch, J.; Anderson, R.K.; Correia-Melo, C.; Jurk, D.; Hewitt, G.; Marques, F.M.; Green, N.J.; Moisey, E.; Birrell, M.A.; Belvisi, M.G.; et al. DNA damage response at telomeres contributes to lung aging and chronic obstructive pulmonary disease. *Am. J. Physiol. Cell. Mol. Physiol.* **2015**, *309*, L1124–L1137. [CrossRef] [PubMed]
54. Easter, M.; Bollenbecker, S.; Barnes, J.W.; Krick, S. Targeting Aging Pathways in Chronic Obstructive Pulmonary Disease. *Int. J. Mol. Sci.* **2020**, *21*, E6924. [CrossRef] [PubMed]
55. Córdoba-Lanús, E.; Cazorla-Rivero, S.; Espinoza-Jiménez, A.; De-Torres, J.P.; Pajares, M.J.; Aguirre-Jaime, A.; Celli, B.; Casanova, C. Telomere shortening and accelerated aging in COPD: Findings from the BODE cohort. *Respir. Res.* **2017**, *18*, 59. [CrossRef]
56. Savale, L.; Chaouat, A.; Bastuji-Garin, S.; Marcos, E.; Boyer, L.; Maitre, B.; Sarni, M.; Housset, B.; Weitzenblum, E.; Matrat, M.; et al. Shortened Telomeres in Circulating Leukocytes of Patients with Chronic Obstructive Pulmonary Disease. *Am. J. Respir. Crit. Care Med.* **2009**, *179*, 566–571. [CrossRef]
57. Moon, D.H.; Kim, J.; Lim, M.N.; Bak, S.H.; Kim, W.J. Correlation between Telomere Length and Chronic Obstructive Pulmonary Disease—Related Phenotypes: Results from the Chronic Obstructive Pulmonary Disease in Dusty Areas (CODA) Cohort. *Tuberc. Respir. Dis.* **2021**, *84*, 188–199. [CrossRef]
58. Rode, L.; Bojesen, S.E.; Weischer, M.; Vestbo, J.; Nordestgaard, B.G. Short telomere length, lung function and chronic obstructive pulmonary disease in 46 396 individuals. *Thorax* **2012**, *68*, 429–435. [CrossRef]
59. Radicioni, G.; Ceppe, A.; Ford, A.A.; Alexis, N.E.; Barr, R.G.; Bleecker, E.R.; Christenson, S.A.; Cooper, C.B.; Han, M.K.; Hansel, N.N.; et al. Airway mucin MUC5AC and MUC5B concentrations and the initiation and progression of chronic obstructive pulmonary disease: An analysis of the SPIROMICS cohort. *Lancet Respir. Med.* **2021**, *9*, 1241–1254. [CrossRef]
60. Kesimer, M.; Smith, B.M.; Ceppe, A.; Ford, A.A.; Anderson, W.H.; Barr, R.G.; O'Neal, W.K.; Boucher, R.C.; Woodruff, P.G.; Han, M.K.; et al. Mucin Concentrations and Peripheral Airway Obstruction in Chronic Obstructive Pulmonary Disease. *Am. J. Respir. Crit. Care Med.* **2018**, *198*, 1453–1456. [CrossRef]
61. Fujisawa, T.; Velichko, S.; Thai, P.; Hung, L.-Y.; Huang, F.; Wu, R. Regulation of AirwayMUC5ACExpression by IL-1β and IL-17A; the NF-κB Paradigm. *J. Immunol.* **2009**, *183*, 6236–6243. [CrossRef]
62. Kesimer, M.; Ford, A.A.; Ceppe, A.; Radicioni, G.; Cao, R.; Davis, C.W.; Doerschuk, C.M.; Alexis, N.E.; Anderson, W.H.; Henderson, A.G.; et al. Airway Mucin Concentration as a Marker of Chronic Bronchitis. *N. Engl. J. Med.* **2017**, *377*, 911–922. [CrossRef]
63. Kanai, K.; Koarai, A.; Shishikura, Y.; Sugiura, H.; Ichikawa, T.; Kikuchi, T.; Akamatsu, K.; Hirano, T.; Nakanishi, M.; Matsunaga, K.; et al. Cigarette smoke augments MUC5AC production via the TLR3-EGFR pathway in airway epithelial cells. *Respir. Investig.* **2015**, *53*, 137–148. [CrossRef]
64. Reid, L.V.; Spalluto, C.M.; Watson, A.; Staples, K.J.; Wilkinson, T.M.A. The Role of Extracellular Vesicles as a Shared Disease Mechanism Contributing to Multimorbidity in Patients with COPD. *Front. Immunol.* **2021**, *12*. [CrossRef] [PubMed]
65. Chapman, K.R.; Burdon, J.G.W.; Piitulainen, E.; Sandhaus, R.A.; Seersholm, N.; Stocks, J.M.; Stoel, B.C.; Huang, L.; Yao, Z.; Edelman, J.M.; et al. Intravenous augmentation treatment and lung density in severe α1 antitrypsin deficiency (RAPID): A randomised, double-blind, placebo-controlled trial. *Lancet* **2015**, *386*, 360–368. [CrossRef]
66. Silverman, E.K.; Sandhaus, R.A. Alpha1-Antitrypsin Deficiency. *N. Engl. J. Med.* **2009**, *360*, 2749–2757. [CrossRef] [PubMed]
67. Guenegou, A.; Leynaert, B.; Bénessiano, J.; Pin, I.; Demoly, P.; Neukirch, F.; Boczkowski, J.; Aubier, M. Association of lung function decline with the heme oxygenase-1 gene promoter microsatellite polymorphism in a general population sample. Results from the European Community Respiratory Health Survey (ECRHS), France. *J. Med. Genet.* **2006**, *43*, e43. [CrossRef]
68. Yamada, N.; Yamaya, M.; Okinaga, S.; Nakayama, K.; Sekizawa, K.; Shibahara, S.; Sasaki, H. Microsatellite Polymorphism in the Heme Oxygenase-1 Gene Promoter Is Associated with Susceptibility to Emphysema. *Am. J. Hum. Genet.* **2000**, *66*, 187–195. [CrossRef] [PubMed]
69. Kong, X.; Cho, M.H.; Anderson, W.; Coxson, H.O.; Müller, N.; Washko, G.; Hoffman, E.A.; Bakke, P.; Gulsvik, A.; Lomas, D.A.; et al. Genome-wide Association Study IdentifiesBICD1as a Susceptibility Gene for Emphysema. *Am. J. Respir. Crit. Care Med.* **2011**, *183*, 43–49. [CrossRef]
70. Faner, R.; Rojas, M.; MacNee, W.; Agustí, A. Abnormal Lung Aging in Chronic Obstructive Pulmonary Disease and Idiopathic Pulmonary Fibrosis. *Am. J. Respir. Crit. Care Med.* **2012**, *186*, 306–313. [CrossRef]
71. Kim, D.K.; Cho, M.H.; Hersh, C.P.; Lomas, D.A.; Miller, B.E.; Kong, X.; Bakke, P.; Gulsvik, A.; Agustí, A.; Wouters, E.; et al. Genome-Wide Association Analysis of Blood Biomarkers in Chronic Obstructive Pulmonary Disease. *Am. J. Respir. Crit. Care Med.* **2012**, *186*, 1238–1247. [CrossRef] [PubMed]

72. Pillai, S.G.; Ge, D.; Zhu, G.; Kong, X.; Shianna, K.V.; Need, A.; Feng, S.; Hersh, C.P.; Bakke, P.; Gulsvick, A.; et al. A Genome-Wide Association Study in Chronic Obstructive Pulmonary Disease (COPD): Identification of Two Major Susceptibility Loci. *PLoS Genet.* **2009**, *5*, e1000421. [CrossRef] [PubMed]
73. Cho, M.H.; Castaldi, P.J.; Wan, E.S.; Siedlinski, M.; Hersh, C.P.; Demeo, D.L.; Himes, B.E.; Sylvia, J.S.; Klanderman, B.J.; Ziniti, J.P.; et al. A genome-wide association study of COPD identifies a susceptibility locus on chromosome 19q13. *Hum. Mol. Genet.* **2012**, *21*, 947–957. [CrossRef] [PubMed]
74. Cho, M.H.; Boutaoui, N.; Klanderman, B.J.; Sylvia, J.S.; Ziniti, J.P.; Hersh, C.P.; DeMeo, D.L.; Hunninghake, G.M.; Litonjua, A.; Sparrow, D.; et al. Variants in FAM13A are associated with chronic obstructive pulmonary disease. *Nat. Genet.* **2010**, *42*, 200–202. [CrossRef]
75. Artigas, M.S.; Wain, L.V.; Repapi, E.; Obeidat, M.; Sayers, I.; Burton, P.R.; Johnson, T.; Zhao, J.H.; Albrecht, E.; Dominiczak, A.F.; et al. Effect of Five Genetic Variants Associated with Lung Function on the Risk of Chronic Obstructive Lung Disease, and Their Joint Effects on Lung Function. *Am. J. Respir. Crit. Care Med.* **2011**, *184*, 786–795. [CrossRef]
76. Hancock, D.; Eijgelsheim, M.; Wilk, J.B.; Gharib, S.A.; Loehr, L.; Marciante, K.D.; Franceschini, N.; Van Durme, Y.M.T.A.; Chen, T.-H.; Barr, R.G.; et al. Meta-analyses of genome-wide association studies identify multiple loci associated with pulmonary function. *Nat. Genet.* **2010**, *42*, 45–52. [CrossRef]
77. Castaldi, P.J.; Cho, M.H.; Estepar, R.S.J.; McDonald, M.-L.N.; Laird, N.; Beaty, T.H.; Washko, G.; Crapo, J.D.; Silverman, E.K. Genome-Wide Association Identifies Regulatory Loci Associated with Distinct Local Histogram Emphysema Patterns. *Am. J. Respir. Crit. Care Med.* **2014**, *190*, 399–409. [CrossRef]
78. Lee, J.H.; Cho, M.H.; Hersh, C.P.; McDonald, M.-L.N.; Crapo, J.D.; Bakke, P.S.; Gulsvik, A.; Comellas, A.P.; Wendt, C.H.; Lomas, D.A.; et al. Genetic susceptibility for chronic bronchitis in chronic obstructive pulmonary disease. *Respir. Res.* **2014**, *15*, 113. [CrossRef]
79. Pillai, S.G.; Kong, X.; Edwards, L.D.; Cho, M.H.; Anderson, W.H.; Coxson, H.O.; Lomas, D.A.; Silverman, E.K. Loci Identified by Genome-wide Association Studies Influence Different Disease-related Phenotypes in Chronic Obstructive Pulmonary Disease. *Am. J. Respir. Crit. Care Med.* **2010**, *182*, 1498–1505. [CrossRef]
80. Bleecker, E.R.; Cho, M.H.; Hersh, C.P.; McDonald, M.-L.N.; Wells, J.M.; Dransfield, M.T.; Bowler, R.P.; Lynch, D.A.; Lomas, D.A.; Crapo, J.D.; et al. IREB2andGALCAre Associated with Pulmonary Artery Enlargement in Chronic Obstructive Pulmonary Disease. *Am. J. Respir. Cell Mol. Biol.* **2015**, *52*, 365–376. [CrossRef]
81. Li, X.; Zhou, G.; Tian, X.; Chen, F.; Li, G.; Ding, Y. The polymorphisms of FGFR2 and MGAT5 affect the susceptibility to COPD in the Chinese people. *BMC Pulm. Med.* **2021**, *21*, 129. [CrossRef] [PubMed]
82. Li, D.; Wu, Y.; Guo, S.; Qin, J.; Feng, M.; An, Y.; Zhang, J.; Li, Y.; Xiong, S.; Zhou, H.; et al. Circulating syndecan-1 as a novel biomarker relates to lung function, systemic inflammation, and exacerbation in COPD. *Int. J. Chronic Obstr. Pulm. Dis.* **2019**, *14*, 1933–1941. [CrossRef] [PubMed]
83. Mathioudakis, A.G.; Janssens, W.; Sivapalan, P.; Singanayagam, A.; Dransfield, M.T.; Jensen, J.-U.S.; Vestbo, J. Acute exacerbations of chronic obstructive pulmonary disease: In search of diagnostic biomarkers and treatable traits. *Thorax* **2020**, *75*, 520–527. [CrossRef]
84. Noell, G.; Cosío, B.G.; Faner, R.; Monsó, E.; Peces-Barba, G.; De Diego, A.; Esteban, C.; Gea, J.; Rodriguez-Roisin, R.; Garcia-Nuñez, M.; et al. Multi-level differential network analysis of COPD exacerbations. *Eur. Respir. J.* **2017**, *50*, 1700075. [CrossRef]
85. Thomsen, M.; Ingebrigtsen, T.S.; Marott, J.L.; Dahl, M.; Lange, P.; Vestbo, J.; Nordestgaard, B.G. Inflammatory Biomarkers and Exacerbations in Chronic Obstructive Pulmonary Disease. *JAMA* **2013**, *309*, 2353–2361. [CrossRef] [PubMed]
86. Fermont, J.M.; Masconi, K.L.; Jensen, M.T.; Ferrari, R.; Di Lorenzo, V.A.P.; Marott, J.M.; Schuetz, P.; Watz, H.; Waschki, B.; Müllerova, H.; et al. Biomarkers and clinical outcomes in COPD: A systematic review and meta-analysis. *Thorax* **2019**, *74*, 439–446. [CrossRef]
87. Chen, Y.-W.R.; Leung, J.M.; Sin, D.D. A Systematic Review of Diagnostic Biomarkers of COPD Exacerbation. *PLoS ONE* **2016**, *11*, e0158843. [CrossRef]
88. Celli, B.R.; Locantore, N.; Yates, J.; Tal-Singer, R.; Miller, B.E.; Bakke, P.; Calverley, P.; Coxson, H.; Crim, C.; Edwards, L.; et al. Inflammatory Biomarkers Improve Clinical Prediction of Mortality in Chronic Obstructive Pulmonary Disease. *Am. J. Respir. Crit. Care Med.* **2012**, *185*, 1065–1072. [CrossRef]
89. Hlapčić, I.; Belamarić, D.; Bosnar, M.; Kifer, D.; Dugac, A.V.; Rumora, L. Combination of Systemic Inflammatory Biomarkers in Assessment of Chronic Obstructive Pulmonary Disease: Diagnostic Performance and Identification of Networks and Clusters. *Diagnostics* **2020**, *10*, 1029. [CrossRef]
90. Hlapčić, I.; Hulina-Tomašković, A.; Rajković, M.G.; Popović-Grle, S.; Dugac, A.V.; Rumora, L. Association of Plasma Heat Shock Protein 70 with Disease Severity, Smoking and Lung Function of Patients with Chronic Obstructive Pulmonary Disease. *J. Clin. Med.* **2020**, *9*, 3097. [CrossRef]
91. Celli, B.R.; Anderson, J.A.; Brook, R.; Calverley, P.; Cowans, N.J.; Crim, C.; Dixon, I.; Kim, V.; Martinez, F.J.; Morris, A.; et al. Serum biomarkers and outcomes in patients with moderate COPD: A substudy of the randomised SUMMIT trial. *BMJ Open Respir. Res.* **2019**, *6*, e000431. [CrossRef]

92. Schumann, D.M.; Leeming, D.; Papakonstantinou, E.; Blasi, F.; Kostikas, K.; Boersma, W.; Louis, R.; Milenkovic, B.; Aerts, J.; Sand, J.M.; et al. Collagen Degradation and Formation Are Elevated in Exacerbated COPD Compared with Stable Disease. *Chest* **2018**, *154*, 798–807. [CrossRef]
93. Pizzini, A.; Filipiak, W.; Wille, J.; Ager, C.; Wiesenhofer, H.; Kubinec, R.; Blaško, J.; Tschurtschenthaler, C.; Mayhew, C.A.; Weiss, G.; et al. Analysis of volatile organic compounds in the breath of patients with stable or acute exacerbation of chronic obstructive pulmonary disease. *J. Breath Res.* **2018**, *12*, 036002. [CrossRef]
94. Zemans, R.L.; Jacobson, S.; Keene, J.; Kechris, K.; Miller, B.E.; Tal-Singer, R.; Bowler, R.P. Multiple biomarkers predict disease severity, progression and mortality in COPD. *Respir. Res.* **2017**, *18*, 117. [CrossRef]

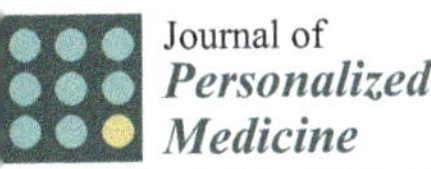

Journal of *Personalized Medicine*

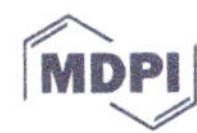

Article

Interferon-Inducible Protein-10 as a Marker to Detect Latent Tuberculosis Infection in Patients with Inflammatory Rheumatic Diseases

Mediha Gonenc Ortakoylu [1,*], Ayse Bahadir [1], Sinem Iliaz [2], Derya Soy Bugdayci [3], Mehmet Atilla Uysal [1], Nurdan PAKER [3] and Seda Tural Onur [1]

1 Department of Pulmonary Disease, University of Health Sciences Turkey, Yedikule Chest Diseases and Thoracic Surgery Training and Research Hospital, Istanbul 34020, Turkey; aysebahadir@yahoo.com (A.B.); dratilla@yahoo.com (M.A.U.); sedatural@yahoo.com (S.T.O.)

2 Department of Pulmonary Disease, Koc University Hospital, Istanbul 34010, Turkey; snmkaraosman@gmail.com

3 Department of Physical Medicine and Rehabilitation, Istanbul Physical Medicine and Rehabilitation Training Hospital, Istanbul 34186, Turkey; deryabugdayci@yahoo.com (D.S.B.); nurdanpaker@hotmail.com (N.P.)

* Correspondence: gonencorta@yahoo.com; Tel.: +90-535-219-81-49

Abstract: It is important to identify cases of latent tuberculosis infection (LTBI) who are at risk for tuberculosis (TB) reactivation. We aimed to evaluate the performance of interferon (IFN)-gamma-inducible protein 10 (IP-10) as a marker to detect LTBI in patients with inflammatory rheumatic diseases (IRD). This study comprised 76 consecutive subjects with IRD. Patients with a history of TB or having active TB were excluded. In all patients, IP-10 level was measured and tuberculin skin test (TST) and QuantiFERON-TB Gold In-Tube test (QFT-GIT) were performed. Seventy patients with complete test results were analyzed. Twenty-one (30%) QFT-GIT-positive patients were defined as having LTBI. IP-10 yielded 2197 pg/mL cut-off point. At this cut-off point, IP-10 showed 89% specificity with a sensitivity of 91% (AUC: 0.950, 95% CI 0.906–0.994). TST, QFT-GIT, and IP-10 were positive in 77.1%, 30%, and 44.3% of the patients, respectively. Concordance among the results of TST, QFT-GIT, and IP-10 tests was evaluated. Agreement was poor between IP-10 and TST (58.6%, $\kappa = 0.19$), whereas it was good between QFT-GIT and IP-10 (84.3%, $\kappa = 0.65$). The results of the present study demonstrated that sensitivity and specificity of released IP-10 were as high as those of QFT-GIT in indicating LTBI in IRD patient group.

Keywords: latent tuberculosis; inflammatory rheumatoid disease; interferon-inducible protein-10

Citation: Ortakoylu, M.G.; Bahadir, A.; Iliaz, S.; Soy Bugdayci, D.; Uysal, M.A.; PAKER, N.; Tural Onur, S. Interferon-Inducible Protein-10 as a Marker to Detect Latent Tuberculosis Infection in Patients with Inflammatory Rheumatic Diseases. *J. Pers. Med.* **2022**, *12*, 1027. https://doi.org/10.3390/jpm12071027

Academic Editors: Ioannis Pantazopoulos and Ourania S. Kotsiou

Received: 31 May 2022
Accepted: 20 June 2022
Published: 23 June 2022

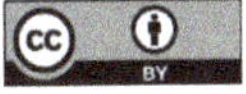

1. Introduction

Tuberculosis (TB) remains as an important problem all over the world. For a TB-free world, it is essential to reduce the prevalence of latent *Mycobacterium tuberculosis* infection and transition from latent infection to active disease [1]. Increase in immunosuppressive conditions highlight the need for additional strategies to maintain and improve TB control.

After the introduction of tumor necrosis factor (TNF)-α inhibitors (anti-TNFs) into inflammatory rheumatic diseases (IRD) treatment, we experienced more severe and more common TB infections in this group of patients [2,3]. Therefore, it has become obligatory to identify cases of latent tuberculosis infection (LTBI) prior to anti-TNFs [4].

Tuberculin skin test (TST), which is widely used in the diagnosis of LTBI, has some drawbacks, including variability in test application and low specificity due to purified protein derivative (PPD) presenting in non-tuberculous mycobacteria as well as in Bacille Calmette-Guérin (BCG) strains [5]. Moreover, TST use in IRD patients presents a major complicating factor: there is a decreased responsiveness of peripheral mononuclear cells, leading to a loss in delayed hypersensitivity, which is fundamental for the recognition of antigens, such as PPD [6].

Interferon (IFN)-gamma release assays (IGRAs) measure in-vitro T cell response to Mycobacterium TB-specific antigens [7]. Its results are more specific than those of TST, since mycobacterium TB-specific antigens [Early Secretory Antigenic Target-6 (ESAT-6) and Culture Filtrate Protein-10 (CFP-10)] that are not present in BCG and most of non-tuberculous mycobacteria are used during IGRA test on the contrary to PPD [8–10].

There are several unresolved issues on the potential clinical use of IGRAs. One area of controversy is whether they can be used in immunocompromised patients, in addition or as an alternative to the TST. The lack of a gold standard for LTBI diagnosis has complicated the assessment of diagnostic accuracy of IGRAs and the comparison of these tests with the TST [11]. Other Potential biomarkers to detect LTBI more accurately in IRD patients are needed. IFN-gamma-inducible protein-10 kDa (IP-10, CXCL10 [C-X-C motif chemokine 10]) is a pro-inflammatory chemokine involved in trafficking monocytes and T-cells to inflamed foci. In the studies, IP-10 level have been found to be much higher in the QuantiFERON-TB Gold in-Tube test (QFT-GIT) supernatants of TB patients as compared to the healthy individuals and it was thought that TB-specific antigen-stimulated IP-10 could be a potential biomarker for TB infection [12]. We aimed to evaluate the performance of IP-10 as a marker to detect LTBI and the agreement among TST or QFT-GIT in patients with IRD from moderate prevalence setting.

2. Materials and Methods

2.1. Study Population

This cross-sectional study comprised all consecutive subjects with IRD [rheumatoid arthritis (RA) and ankylosing spondylitis (AS)], who were being treated and followed in the Istanbul Physical Medicine and Rehabilitation Training and Research Hospital and referred to our pulmonology clinic to be evaluated in terms of pulmonary diseases during a six-month period of time. All patients' BCG status and medications used for IRD were reviewed and their chest graphs were evaluated. Patients with a history of TB in the past and the patients considered to have active TB were excluded. All patients were Human immunodeficiency virus (HIV) (−). This study was approved by Yedikule Chest Diseases and Thoracic Surgery Training and Research Hospital Ethics Committee (ID:2017/ 73) and all patients read and signed the informed consent.

Of the patients, 28 were on TNF-α treatment, 12 were on steroid treatment, and 21 were on disease-modifying antirheumatic drugs (DMARD). We assessed BCG vaccination status based on interviewing past vaccinations and scar inspection. All subjects underwent a chest radiograph, they were questioned about history of previous TB, and results of previous TST.

2.2. Performing and Assessing TST

Immediately after blood was drawn, TST was performed by intradermal injection of 0.1 mL (5TU) of PPD (RT-23-tween80). The transverse diameter of induration was measured in millimeters 72 h later using the ballpoint pen method by only one examiner in all patients [13]. In IRD group, TST induration was interpreted according to published guideline as follows: 0 to 4 mm as negative and $\geq$5 mm as positive [14]. To maximize the detection rate for LTBI, two-step TST was performed, with a second TST administered 7–10 days after a negative initial test.

2.3. Whole Blood Stimulation

For the test, 1 mL of whole blood was drawn in each of three vacutainer tubes provided as part of the QFG-GIT system (Cellestis, Carnegie, Australia), a new generation of QFT test. These tubes are already pre-coated with saline (negative control), peptides of ESAT-6, CFP10, and antigen TB 7.7 (antigen stimulated), and PHA (positive mitogen control). The tubes were mixed and incubated for 20–24 h at 37 °C and they were frozen until further analysis. This plasma provided the unstimulated, antigen stimulated and mitogen stimulated supernatant samples.

2.4. IFN-Gamma Level Quantification

IFN-gamma measurement was performed by enzyme-linked immunosorbent assay (ELISA) using QFG-GIT test according to the manufacturer's instructions [15]. A result of ≥0.35 IU/mL of IFN-gamma in the TB antigen tube minus the negative control (or nil) tube was considered a positive result. If the level was less than this and the mitogen control was positive (≥0.5 IU/mL), a negative result was recorded. If the level in both the TB antigen and mitogen tube was less than the threshold for positive, or the level in the nil tube was >8.0 IU/mL, then an indeterminate result was recorded. As there is no gold standard for the diagnosis of LTBI, and BCG being a routine in our vaccination programme, IRD patients with a positive QFT-GIT were defined as having LTBI.

2.5. IP-10 Level Quantification

For the quantification of IP-10 level, the RayBio Human IP-10 ELISA kit is used (RayBiotech, Inc., Norcross, GA, USA). The kit has a microplate with 96 wells pre-coated with a specific monoclonal antibody for human IP-10. IP-10 supernatant levels were measured using a sandwich ELISA according to the manufacturer's instructions [16].

Samples were diluted 1:2. Fifty μL samples from each three QFG-GIT test tubes were taken and put in the wells. Wells were covered and incubated for 2.5 h at room temperature. After washing four times, 50 μL prepared biotin antibody was added to each well and incubated 1 h at room temperature. Washing procedure was repeated. A hundred μL streptavidin was added to the wells and incubated 45 min at room temperature. After the washing procedure, 50 μL of TMB One-Step Substrate Reagent was added to each well and incubate for 30 min at room temperature in the dark. Finally, 100 μL of Stop Solution was added to each well and read at 450 nm ELISA reader immediately.

2.6. Statistical Analysis

Qualitative measurements were defined in numbers and percentages. Descriptive analyses were expressed as means and standard deviation (SD) for normally distributed variables or median values and minimum-maximum for the non-normal distributed variables. Chi-square or Fisher's exact test was used to compare frequencies or values of variables within the TST positive, QFT-GIT and IP-10 groups. We used receiver operating characteristic (ROC) analysis to examine discriminant validity. The concordance between TST, QFT-GIT and IP-10 was assessed by computing the Kappa statistics. Statistical analyses were performed using XLSTAT 2015.2.03 for Windows by Addinsoft. Statistical significance was at $p < 0.05$, two-tailed.

3. Results

A total of 70 subjects (51.4% males) with IRD were enrolled in the study. Out of 70 patients, 45 had AS and 25 had RA. The present population was characterized by a mean age of 47 ± 14 years; the prevalence of BCG was 77.1%. In IRD group, 54 (77.1%) patients had positive TST, 21 (30%) had positive QFT-GIT. Characteristics of the patients are demonstrated in Table 1.

3.1. Level of IP-10

TB antigen-stimulated plasma IP-10 level was found to be higher in QFT-GIT(+) patients (median: 26,060.3 ± 18,626.5 pg/mL, min–max: 165–60,000 pg/mL) as compared to QFT-GIT(−) patient group (median:1982.7 ± 3607.6 pg/mL, min–max: 0–20,982 pg/mL) ($p < 0.0001$). The released plasma IP-10 level was significantly higher in QFT-GIT(+) patients (median: 3680.5 ± 1954.0 pg/mL, min–max: 110–8899 pg/mL) as compared to QFT-GIT(−) patient group (median:789.5 ± 1543.7 pg/mL, min–max: 0–8115 pg/mL) ($p < 0.0001$).

Table 1. Characteristics of the patients (n = 70).

Type of IRD [1]	(n/%)
Ankylosing spondylitis, n/%	45/64.3%
Rheumotoid arthritis, n/%	25/35.7%
Mean age, years ± SD	47 ± 14
Male, n/%	36/51.4%
BCG positivity, n/%	54/77.1%
TST positivity, n/%	54/77.1%
QFT-GIT positivity, n/%	21/30%

[1] IRD, inflammatory rheumatic diseases; BCG, Bacillus Calmette–Guérin, TST, tuberculin skin test; QFT-GIT, QuantiFERON-TB Gold in-Tube test.

3.2. Cut-Off Point Determination for IP-10

IP-10 value in nil tube was extracted from the plasma IP-10 value which was stimulated by TB antigen. Thus, we calculated the amount of IP-10 produced after stimulation with TB antigen. This value was called as released IP-10. To determine the diagnostic performance of TB antigen dependent IP-10, receiver-operator characteristic (ROC) curve analysis was performed in QFT-GIT(−) and QFT-GIT(+) IRD patients. It yielded 2197 pg/mL cut-off point. At this cut-off point, IP-10 showed 89% of specificity with a sensitivity of 91% (AUC: 0.950, 95% CI:0.906–0.994) (Figure 1).

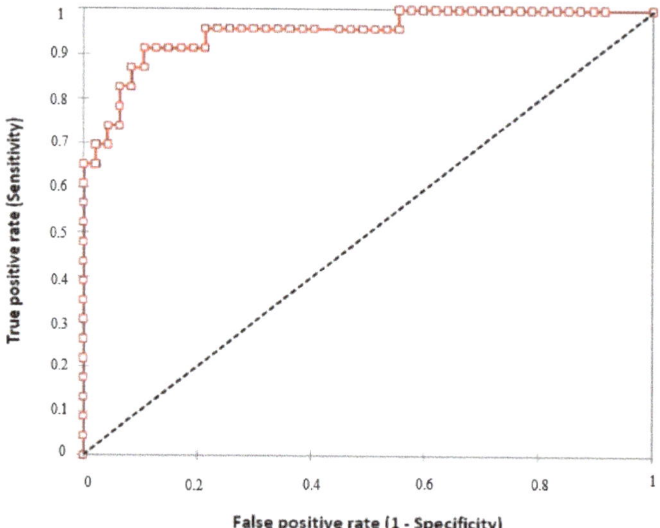

Figure 1. ROC curve analysis for the released plasma inducible protein-10. The cut-off values were determined using QFT-GIT(+) and QFT-GIT(−) patients with inflammatory rheumatic diseases. The area under curve was 0.950 (95% CI 0.906–0.994). (Red line: stimulated IP-10 levels; Black line: reference).

Using the released IP-10, the results obtained with the cut-off value of ≥2197 pg/mL were considered positive. According to this cut-off value, IP-10 test was positive in 31 (44.3%) patients with IRD. Demographic and clinical features of the patients are demonstrated in Table 2.

Table 2. Associations of demographic, epidemiological and clinical characteristics and therapy with QuantiFERON-TB Gold intube (QFT-GIT) and tuberculin skin test (TST) and Interferon-Inducible Protein-10 (IP-10) positive results in subjects with IRD patients.

	n	TST (+) [1] (*n* = 54)	*p*	QFT-GIT (+) (*n* = 21)	*p*	IP-10 (+) (*n* = 31)	*p*
Gender, *n* (%)							
Female	34	23 (67.6)	0.660	8 (23.5)	>0.05	9 (26.5)	0.004
Male	36	31 (86.1)		13 (36.1)	data	22 (61.1)	
Age, years, *n* (%)			0.03		>0.05		0.66
<29	8	7 (87.5)	-	1 (12.5)		2 (25.0)	-
30–49	35	31 (88.6)		10 (28.6)		16 (45.7)	
50–69	22	15 (68.2)		10 (45.5)	data	11 (50.0)	
>70	5	1 (20.0)		0 (0.0)	data	2 (40.0)	
BCG vaccinated, *n* (%)							
Yes	54	44 (82.4)	0.230	15 (42.9)	0.190	22 (43.1)	0.160
No	16	10 (64.3)		6 (29.4)	data	9 (64.3)	
Diagnosis, *n* (%)							
RA	25	14 (56.0)	0.020	6 (24.0)	0.410	9 (12.9)	0.290
AS	45	40 (88.8)		15 (33.3)		22 (31.4)	
Treatment TNF-α inhibitors, *n* (%)							
Yes	28	20 (71.4)	0.350	5 (25.0)	0.700	9 (12.9)	0.090
No	42	34 (80.9)		16 (38.0)		22 (52.3)	
Steroid, *n* (%)							
Yes	12	8 (75)	0.45	5 (62.5)	0.25	6 (50)	0.52
No	58	46 (85.2)		16 (27.6)		25(43.1)	

[1] TST assessment limit according to ≥5 mm. TST, tuberculin skin test; QFT-GIT, QuantiFERON-TB Gold In-Tube test; IP-10, interferon-gamma-inducible protein 10; BCG, Bacillus Calmette–Guérin; RA, rheumatoid arthritis; AS, ankylosing spondylitis; TNF, tumor necrosis factor.

Tuberculin skin test positivity was significantly higher in AS patients versus RA patients and IP-10 positivity was significantly higher in male versus female patients. No difference was determined between the patients with and without BCG vaccination, as well as the patients received and not received TNF-α inhibitor therapy, in terms of positivity of the tests (TST, QFT-GIT, IP-10). Likewise, it was observed that steroid use has no statistically significant effect on test results. TST positivity decreased with older age (p = 0.03). Contrary to TST, QFT-GIT and IP-10 positivity increased with age, but this increment was not statistically significant.

Concordance between the results of TST, QFT-GIT and IP-10 tests is demonstrated in Table 3. According to the TST threshold taken as ≥5 mm, agreement between QFT-GIT and TST was poor (55.7%, κ = 0.24), and it was also poor between IP-10 and TST (58.6%, κ = 0.19). The agreement was good between QFT-GIT and IP-10 (84.3%, κ = 0.65).

Table 3. Concordance among latent tuberculosis infection tests.

Tests	Test Results				Kappa Value
	−/−	+/−	−/+	+/+	
TST/QFT-GIT	16	33	0	21	0.24
TST/IP-10	12	27	4	27	0.19
QFT-GIT/IP-10	38	1	11	20	0.65

TST: Tuberculin skin test, QFT-GIT: QuantiFERON-TB Gold In-Tube test, IP-10: Interferon-gamma-inducible protein 10. TST assessment limit according to ≥5 mm.

TST induration was observed in IRD patients with TST(+)/QFT-GIT(+) results (16.09 ± 4.35 mm); and with TST(+)/QFT-GIT(−) results (14.09 ± 4.20 mm) (*p* = 0.123). Likewise, the diameter of TST induration was found to be 16.11 ± 4.37 mm in TST(+)/IP-10(+) IRD patients and 13.18 ± 4.53 mm in TST(+)/IP-10(−) patients (*p* = 0.06).

4. Discussion

We aimed to evaluate the performance of IP-10 as a marker to detect LTBI and the concordance among TST or QFT-GIT in patients with IRD. The results revealed good agreement between QFT-GIT and IP-10 but poor agreement between TST and either QFT-GIT or IP-10.

It has been demonstrated that TST had poor performance and gave false negative results in the diagnosis of LTBI in immunocompromised patient group including those with IRD [6]. In a study that evaluated TST response between RA patients and healthy controls, TST was found to be negative independent from duration and activity of disease in 76.6% of the patients with RA, whereas it was negative in 26% of the control group [17]. In the present study, TST positivity was found to be 77% in IRD patient group (86.1% in males, 67.6% in females). BCG scar was present in 82.4% of the patients. In a large-scale study performed in normal population living in a tuberculosis endemic country, TST positivity (TST $\geq$ 10 mm) was found to be 69.3%. At least one BCG scar was detected in 91.2% of the cases and it was demonstrated that TST positivity is higher in male gender (70% vs. 55%) [18]. Similarity of these results with the results of present study suggests that TST responsiveness is not poor at all in our study group. Since there is no gold standard in the diagnosis of LTBI, all studies on IRD patient group in the literature are based on evaluating and comparing TST and new-generation IGRA tests and investigating agreement between these tests. In the IRD patient group, IGRA positivity was reported to be 13–44%, whereas TST positivity was reported to be 1–61%. Different inflammatory diseases of the patients in the study populations and different immunosuppressive medications that they have been receiving and also different BCG vaccination status in their own populations make the interpretation of outcomes difficult [19]. In a large meta-analysis, the sensitivity and specificity of IGRA tests were found to be 76% and 98%, respectively. It has been stated that IGRA tests have excellent specificity that is not influenced by BCG vaccination but that data from pediatric and immunocompromised patients are limited [8]. In the studies conducted in IRD patient group, the agreement between TST and IGRA was found to be good in the countries where the rate of BCG vaccination is low, whereas it was found to be poor in the countries where the rate of vaccination is high [10,20]. In the present study, the agreement between TST and QFT-GIT was poor (kappa = 0.24).

An important IGRA-related disadvantage is high indeterminate test results in immunocompromised patients. It was reported as 13–38.2% depending on the patient group and it was emphasized that this was accompanied by immunosuppressive therapy and particularly peripheral lymphocytopenia [21,22]. This is different in the IRD patient group; it was reported that indeterminate IGRA results were not prevalent in IRD patients and were seen by less than 5% [19]. The prevalence of indeterminate test results was reported to be 1.2% in an IRD patient group consisted of 398 patients [11]. Among 70 patients in our study, there was no patient with indeterminate IGRA result.

In 2006, QFT-GIT supernatants were screened for cytokines and chemokines that could be the markers of *M. tuberculosis* antigen-specific cell-mediated immune response. It was demonstrated that IP-10 was overexpressed in the patients with active tuberculosis but there was no expression in unexposed controls. This suggested that IP-10 might be an alternative marker to IFN-γ and may lead to development of IGRA tests [23]. Studies were performed to investigate diagnostic performance of IP-10 in tuberculosis and they have been frequently compared with IGRA tests. Studies that compared the results of IP-10 and QFT-GIT one-to-one in indicating active TB reported comparable rates of positivity (74–91% vs. 79–100%) [12,24,25]. Consistency between the two tests was investigated in only two of these studies and was found good. Specificity was found to be 98% for IP-10 and 100% for QFT-GIT in unexposed healthy controls in Italy and Denmark and no cross-reaction was observed with BCG [26]. IP-10 was found to be 55% positive and QFT-GIT was found to be 48% positive in an Indian population without symptom or contact with tuberculosis and it was interpreted in the way that the test could reflect the prevalence of LTBI [27]. In a multicenter study conducted in Europe in the patients with non-tuberculosis disease, IP-10 was 35% positive and QFT-GIT test was 27% positive and increase in the positivity of IP-10 was interpreted in the way that IP-10 might have superior sensitivity or impaired specificity as compared to QFT-GIT [25]. Obtaining similar results in the present study (IP-10 31% positive, QFT-GIT 21% positive) suggested that sensitivity of IP-10 might be considered to be superior. Also, a few recent studies showed that IP-10 might help to differentiate healthy controls, LTBI, and active TB from each other, but it did not reach sufficient sensitivity and specificity [28,29].

Making accurate diagnosis of LTBI is important for the treatment and follow-up in immunocompromised patients, who have high risk of progression to active TB. In a novel randomized controlled study, the occurrence of tuberculosis was evaluated in patients receiving TNF-α inhibitors and exposure to TNF-α inhibitors was associated with a statistically significant threefold increase in the risk of TB. These findings confirm that appropriate screening with TST/IGRA test should be performed before starting treatment with TNF-α inhibitors [30]. Murdaca et al. also pointed to the negative TST should be interpreted with caution in any patient who is under treatment with an immunosuppressive agent as they ae more likely to have false-negative TST results, IGRAs for the LTBI have recently been proven to be more spesifiic for LTBI than the TST in immunocomponent subjects as an expert opinion [31].

Unfortunately, both TST and IGRA tests may give false negative outcomes in such patients. In a study conducted with IP-10 in HIV(+) patient group, it was reported that IP-10 is slightly better than QFT-GIT in demonstrating active TB and is influenced less by CD4 cell count [25]. In another study by Villar-Hernandez et al., using IP-10 and IFN-γ together led to higher detection rate of LTBI in patients with inflammatory rheumatic diseases without being affected by immunosuppressive treatment [32].

A study, which evaluated IP-10 in the diagnosis of LTBI in RA patients receiving immunosuppressive therapy, reported significantly higher IP-10 level in TST(+) patients; similar results were obtained in the present study. In the same study, it was demonstrated that baseline unstimulated IP-10 level was high but decreased after treatment in the patient that developed active TB [33]. Serum IP-10 measurement appears to be one of the most promising tests that might contribute to the diagnosis of LTBI.

The most striking problem in the comparison of studies that are conducted with IP-10 as a new diagnostic marker is associated with technical aspects of the measures used to detect IP-10. The use of different brand kits in the studies, measuring the samples at different dilutions, wide range of measures, and taking different cut-off values in the studies have been specified as the main problems [34]. Detecting cut-off value using released IP-10 narrowed the range of measure in our study. Limitations of the present study, as in the similar studies, include the facts that study population is small, since it is a specific patient group, and patients have been receiving different therapies. However, the limited number of studies investigating IP-10 in a specific patient group makes the present study critical.

In conclusion, the results of the present study demonstrated that IP-10 is as comparable as QFT-GIT in the diagnosis of LTBI in IRD patient group. It suggests that IP-10 assay could be an alternative biomarker for diagnosis of LTBI in countries where the BCG vaccine is routinely administered.

Author Contributions: Conceptualization, M.G.O.; methodology, M.G.O.; software, M.A.U. and A.B.; investigation, M.G.O. and A.B.; resources, S.I. and S.T.O.; data curation, M.G.O. and D.S.B.; writing—original draft preparation, M.G.O. and N.P.; writing—review and editing, M.G.O., S.I. and S.T.O.; All authors have read and agreed to the published version of the manuscript.

Funding: This research received no external funding.

Institutional Review Board Statement: The study was conducted in accordance with the Declaration of Helsinki, and approved by the or Ethics Committee of Istanbul Yedikule Chest Diseases and Thoracic Surgery Training and Research Hospital (protocol code 2017/73 and March 2017).

Informed Consent Statement: Informed consent was obtained from all subjects involved in the study.

Data Availability Statement: The data presented in this study are available on request from the corresponding author. The data are not publicly available due to privacy reasons.

Acknowledgments: Authors thank to Gungor Ates, Ekrem Cengiz Seyhan, Kaya Koksalan and Emel Caglar for their valuable contributions.

Conflicts of Interest: The authors declare no conflict of interest.

References

1. Chiang, C.-Y.; Van Weezenbeek, C.; Mori, T.; Enarson, D.A. Challenges to the Global Control of Tuberculosis: Global Control of TB. *Respirology* **2013**, *18*, 596–604. [CrossRef] [PubMed]
2. Cantini, F.; Nannini, C.; Niccoli, L.; Petrone, L.; Ippolito, G.; Goletti, D. Risk of Tuberculosis Reactivation in Patients with Rheumatoid Arthritis, Ankylosing Spondylitis, and Psoriatic Arthritis Receiving Non-Anti-TNF-Targeted Biologics. *Mediat. Inflamm.* **2017**, *2017*, 8909834. [CrossRef] [PubMed]
3. Saidenberg-Kermanac'h, N.; Semerano, L.; Naccache, J.M.; Brauner, M.; Falgarone, G.; Dumont-Fischer, D.; Guillot, X.; Valeyre, D.; Boissier, M.-C. Screening for Latent Tuberculosis in Anti-TNF-α Candidate Patients in a High Tuberculosis Incidence Setting. *Int. J. Tuberc. Lung Dis.* **2012**, *16*, 1307–1314. [CrossRef] [PubMed]
4. Cantini, F.; Nannini, C.; Niccoli, L.; Iannone, F.; Delogu, G.; Garlaschi, G.; Sanduzzi, A.; Matucci, A.; Prignano, F.; Conversano, M.; et al. Guidance for the Management of Patients with Latent Tuberculosis Infection Requiring Biologic Therapy in Rheumatology and Dermatology Clinical Practice. *Autoimmun. Rev.* **2015**, *14*, 503–509. [CrossRef] [PubMed]
5. Brock, I.; Weldingh, K.; Lillebaek, T.; Follmann, F.; Andersen, P. Comparison of Tuberculin Skin Test and New Specific Blood Test in Tuberculosis Contacts. *Am. J. Respir. Crit. Care Med.* **2004**, *170*, 65–69. [CrossRef]
6. Martins, M.V.B.S.; Lima, M.C.B.S.; Duppre, N.C.; Matos, H.J.; Spencer, J.S.; Brennan, P.J.; Sarno, E.N.; Fonseca, L.; Pereira, G.M.B.; Pessolani, M.C.V. The Level of PPD-Specific IFN-γ-Producing CD4+ T Cells in the Blood Predicts the in Vivo Response to PPD. *Tuberculosis* **2007**, *87*, 202–211. [CrossRef]
7. Andersen, P.; Munk, M.E.; Pollock, J.M.; Doherty, T.M. Specific Immune-Based Diagnosis of Tuberculosis. *Lancet* **2000**, *356*, 1099–1104. [CrossRef]
8. Pai, M.; Zwerling, A.; Menzies, D. Systematic Review: T-Cell–Based Assays for the Diagnosis of Latent Tuberculosis Infection: An Update. *Ann. Intern. Med.* **2008**, *149*, 177. [CrossRef]
9. Jeong, D.H.; Kang, J.; Jung, Y.J.; Yoo, B.; Lee, C.-K.; Kim, Y.-G.; Hong, S.; Shim, T.S.; Jo, K.-W. Comparison of Latent Tuberculosis Infection Screening Strategies before Tumor Necrosis Factor Inhibitor Treatment in Inflammatory Arthritis: IGRA-Alone versus Combination of TST and IGRA. *PLoS ONE* **2018**, *13*, e0198756. [CrossRef]
10. Diel, R.; Goletti, D.; Ferrara, G.; Bothamley, G.; Cirillo, D.; Kampmann, B.; Lange, C.; Losi, M.; Markova, R.; Migliori, G.B.; et al. Interferon- Release Assays for the Diagnosis of Latent Mycobacterium Tuberculosis Infection: A Systematic Review and Meta-Analysis. *Eur. Respir. J.* **2011**, *37*, 88–99. [CrossRef]
11. Bartalesi, F.; Vicidomini, S.; Goletti, D.; Fiorelli, C.; Fiori, G.; Melchiorre, D.; Tortoli, E.; Mantella, A.; Benucci, M.; Girardi, E.; et al. QuantiFERON-TB Gold and the TST Are Both Useful for Latent Tuberculosis Infection Screening in Autoimmune Diseases. *Eur. Respir. J.* **2009**, *33*, 586–593. [CrossRef] [PubMed]
12. Ruhwald, M.; Bodmer, T.; Maier, C.; Jepsen, M.; Haaland, M.B.; Eugen-Olsen, J.; Ravn, P.; on behalf of TBNET. Evaluating the Potential of IP-10 and MCP-2 as Biomarkers for the Diagnosis of Tuberculosis. *Eur. Respir. J.* **2008**, *32*, 1607–1615. [CrossRef] [PubMed]
13. Sokal, J.E. Measurement of Delayed Skin-Test Responses. *N. Engl. J. Med.* **1975**, *293*, 501–502. [CrossRef]
14. Republic of Turkey Ministry of Health. Directorate General of the Public Health, Tuberculosis Diagnosis and Treatment Guide, Tuberculosis Guideline in Patients Receiving Anti-TNF Treatment, Ankara, May 2019. Available online: https://hsgm.saglik.gov.tr/depo/birimler/tuberkuloz_db/haberler/Tuberkuloz_Tani_Ve_Tedavi_Rehberi_/Tuberkuloz_Tani_ve_Tedavi_Rehberi.pdf (accessed on 16 June 2022).
15. Cellestis. QuantiFERON s-TB Gold Package Insert. Available online: https://www.quantiferon.com/products/quantiferon-tb-gold/package-inserts/ (accessed on 16 June 2022).
16. RayBiotech. RayBio Human IP-10 ELISA Kit User Manual. Available online: https://www.raybiotech.com/human-ip-10-elisa/ (accessed on 16 June 2022).
17. Ponce de Leon, D. Attenuated Response to Purified Protein Derivative in Patients with Rheumatoid Arthritis: Study in a Population with a High Prevalence of Tuberculosis. *Ann. Rheum. Dis.* **2005**, *64*, 1360–1361. [CrossRef] [PubMed]
18. Ucan, E.; Sevinc, C.; Abadoglu, O.; Arpaz, S.; Ellidokuz, H. Interpretation of tuberculin test results standards of our country and new needs. *J. Toraks* **2000**, *1*, 25–29. Available online: https://turkthoracj.org/en/interpretation-of-tuberculin-test-results-standards-of-our-country-and-new-needs-1317/ (accessed on 16 June 2022).
19. Smith, R.; Cattamanchi, A.; Steingart, K.R.; Denkinger, C.; Dheda, K.; Winthrop, K.L.; Pai, M. Interferon-Gamma Release Assays for Diagnosis of Latent Tuberculosis Infection: Evidence in Immune-Mediated Inflammatory Disorders. *Curr. Opin. Rheumatol.* **2011**, *23*, 377–384. [CrossRef]

20. Cobanoglu, N.; Ozcelik, U.; Kalyoncu, U.; Ozen, S.; Kiraz, S.; Gurcan, N.; Kaplan, M.; Dogru, D.; Yalcin, E.; Pekcan, S.; et al. Interferon-Gamma Assays for the Diagnosis of Tuberculosis Infection before Using Tumour Necrosis Factor-Alpha Blockers. *Int. J. Tuberc. Lung Dis.* **2007**, *11*, 1177–1182.
21. Ferrara, G.; Losi, M.; Meacci, M.; Meccugni, B.; Piro, R.; Roversi, P.; Bergamini, B.M.; D'Amico, R.; Marchegiano, P.; Rumpianesi, F.; et al. Routine Hospital Use of a New Commercial Whole Blood Interferon-Gamma Assay for the Diagnosis of Tuberculosis Infection. *Am. J. Respir. Crit. Care Med.* **2005**, *172*, 631–635. [CrossRef]
22. Kobashi, Y.; Mouri, K.; Obase, Y.; Fukuda, M.; Miyashita, N.; Oka, M. Clinical Evaluation of QuantiFERON TB-2G Test for Immunocompromised Patients. *Eur. Respir. J.* **2007**, *30*, 945–950. [CrossRef]
23. Ruhwald, M.; Bjerregaard-Andersen, M.; Rabna, P.; Kofoed, K.; Eugen-Olsen, J.; Ravn, P. CXCL10/IP-10 Release Is Induced by Incubation of Whole Blood from Tuberculosis Patients with ESAT-6, CFP10 and TB7.7. *Microbes Infect.* **2007**, *9*, 806–812. [CrossRef]
24. Kabeer, B.S.A.; Raja, A.; Raman, B.; Thangaraj, S.; Leportier, M.; Ippolito, G.; Girardi, E.; Lagrange, P.H.; Goletti, D. IP-10 Response to RD1 Antigens Might Be a Useful Biomarker for Monitoring Tuberculosis Therapy. *BMC Infect. Dis.* **2011**, *11*, 135. [CrossRef] [PubMed]
25. Aabye, M.G.; Ruhwald, M.; PrayGod, G.; Jeremiah, K.; Faurholt-Jepsen, M.; Faurholt-Jepsen, D.; Range, N.; Friis, H.; Changalucha, J.; Andersen, A.B.; et al. Potential of Interferon-γ-Inducible Protein 10 in Improving Tuberculosis Diagnosis in HIV-Infected Patients. *Eur. Respir. J.* **2010**, *36*, 1488–1490. [CrossRef] [PubMed]
26. Ruhwald, M.; Dominguez, J.; Latorre, I.; Losi, M.; Richeldi, L.; Pasticci, M.B.; Mazzolla, R.; Goletti, D.; Butera, O.; Bruchfeld, J.; et al. A Multicentre Evaluation of the Accuracy and Performance of IP-10 for the Diagnosis of Infection with *M. tuberculosis*. *Tuberculosis* **2011**, *91*, 260–267. [CrossRef]
27. Syed Ahamed Kabeer, B.; Raman, B.; Thomas, A.; Perumal, V.; Raja, A. Role of QuantiFERON-TB Gold, Interferon Gamma Inducible Protein-10 and Tuberculin Skin Test in Active Tuberculosis Diagnosis. *PLoS ONE* **2010**, *5*, e9051. [CrossRef] [PubMed]
28. Mamishi, S.; Mahmoudi, S.; Banar, M.; Hosseinpour Sadeghi, R.; Marjani, M.; Pourakbari, B. Diagnostic Accuracy of Interferon (IFN)-γ Inducible Protein 10 (IP-10) as a Biomarker for the Discrimination of Active and Latent Tuberculosis. *Mol. Biol. Rep.* **2019**, *46*, 6263–6269. [CrossRef]
29. Ghanaie, R.M.; Karimi, A.; Azimi, L.; James, S.; Nasehi, M.; Mishkar, A.P.; Sheikhi, M.; Fallah, F.; Tabatabaei, S.R.; Hoseini-Alfatemi, S.M. Diagnosis of Latent Tuberculosis Infection among Pediatric Household Contacts of Iranian Tuberculosis Cases Using Tuberculin Skin Test, IFN- γ Release Assay and IFN-γ-Induced Protein-10. *BMC Pediatr.* **2021**, *21*, 76. [CrossRef]
30. Murdaca, G.; Negrini, S.; Pellecchio, M.; Greco, M.; Schiavi, C.; Giusti, F.; Puppo, F. Update upon the Infection Risk in Patients Receiving TNF Alpha Inhibitors. *Expert Opin. Drug Saf.* **2019**, *18*, 219–229. [CrossRef]
31. Murdaca, G.; Spanò, F.; Contatore, M.; Guastalla, A.; Penza, E.; Magnani, O.; Puppo, F. Infection Risk Associated with Anti-TNF-α Agents: A Review. *Expert Opin. Drug Saf.* **2015**, *14*, 571–582. [CrossRef]
32. Villar-Hernández, R.; Latorre, I.; Mínguez, S.; Díaz, J.; García-García, E.; Muriel-Moreno, B.; Lacoma, A.; Prat, C.; Olivé, A.; Ruhwald, M.; et al. Use of IFN-γ and IP-10 Detection in the Diagnosis of Latent Tuberculosis Infection in Patients with Inflammatory Rheumatic Diseases. *J. Infect.* **2017**, *75*, 315–325. [CrossRef]
33. Chen, D.-Y.; Shen, G.-H.; Chen, Y.-M.; Chen, H.-H.; Lin, C.-C.; Hsieh, C.-W.; Lan, J.-L. Interferon-Inducible Protein-10 as a Marker to Detect Latent and Active Tuberculosis in Rheumatoid Arthritis. *Int. J. Tuberc. Lung Dis.* **2011**, *15*, 192–200.
34. Ruhwald, M.; Aabye, M.G.; Ravn, P. IP-10 Release Assays in the Diagnosis of Tuberculosis Infection: Current Status and Future Directions. *Expert Rev. Mol. Diagn* **2012**, *12*, 175–187. [CrossRef] [PubMed]

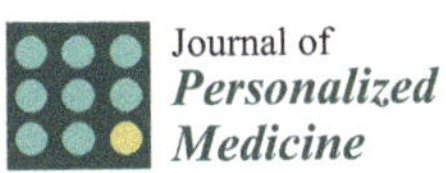

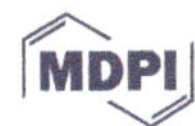

Article

High-Sensitivity Troponin T: A Potential Safety Predictive Biomarker for Discharge from the Emergency Department of Patients with Confirmed Influenza

Manuel Antonio Tazón-Varela [1,2], Jon Ortiz de Salido-Menchaca [1], Pedro Muñoz-Cacho [2,3,*], Enara Iriondo-Bernabeu [1], María Josefa Martos-Almagro [1], Emma Lavín-López [1], Ander Vega-Zubiaur [1], Edgar José Escalona-Canal [1], Iratxe Alcalde-Díez [1], Carmen Gómez-Vildosola [1], Ainhoa Belzunegui-Gárate [1], Fabiola Espinoza-Cuba [1], José Antonio López-Cejuela [1], Alba García-García [1], Alejandro Torrejón-Cereceda [1], Elena Sabina Nisa-Martínez [1], Diana Moreira Nieto [1], Cintia Hellín-Mercadal [1], Ander García-Caballero [1] and Héctor Alonso-Valle [2,4]

1 Servicio de Urgencias, Hospital de Laredo, 39770 Laredo, Spain; tazovare@yahoo.es (M.A.T.-V.); jonortiz1989@gmail.com (J.O.d.S.-M.); enarairiondo1@gmail.com (E.I.-B.); majos1709@hotmail.com (M.J.M.-A.); emmuca@hotmail.com (E.L.-L.); andervz@hotmail.com (A.V.-Z.); edgar.escalona.canal@gmail.com (E.J.E.-C.); iratxealkalde@gmail.com (I.A.-D.); cgomezvildo@hotmail.com (C.G.-V.); ainhobelzu@gmail.com (A.B.-G.); fecuba@hotmail.com (F.E.-C.); joselc7@hotmail.es (J.A.L.-C.); albagg95@hotmail.com (A.G.-G.); alextorcer@gmail.com (A.T.-C.); hnmhelen@gmail.com (E.S.N.-M.); dayana_m_n@yahoo.es (D.M.N.); cintiahellin@gmail.com (C.H.-M.); ander.garcia38@gmail.com (A.G.-C.)

2 Grupo Salud Comunitaria, Instituto de Investigación Sanitaria Valdecilla (IDIVAL), 39011 Santander, Spain

3 Unidad Docente Gerencia de Atención Primaria, Servicio Cántabro de Salud, 39011 Santander, Spain

4 Servicio de Urgencias, Hospital Universitario Marqués de Valdecilla, Santander, 39008 Santander, Spain; jefaturaestudios.humv@scsalud.es

* Correspondence: pedro.munoz@scsalud.es

Citation: Tazón-Varela, M.A.; Ortiz de Salido-Menchaca, J.; Muñoz-Cacho, P.; Iriondo-Bernabeu, E.; Martos-Almagro, M.J.; Lavín-López, E.; Vega-Zubiaur, A.; Escalona-Canal, E.J.; Alcalde-Díez, I.; Gómez-Vildosola, C.; et al. High-Sensitivity Troponin T: A Potential Safety Predictive Biomarker for Discharge from the Emergency Department of Patients with Confirmed Influenza. *J. Pers. Med.* **2022**, *12*, 520. https://doi.org/10.3390/jpm12040520

Academic Editors: Ioannis Pantazopoulos and Ourania S. Kotsiou

Received: 24 February 2022
Accepted: 20 March 2022
Published: 23 March 2022

Abstract: The purpose of the study was to analyze the relationship between the high-sensitivity troponin T levels in patients with confirmed influenza virus infection and its severity determined by mortality during the care process. In addition, a high-sensitivity troponin T cut-off value was sought to allow us to a safe discharge from the emergency department. An analytical retrospective observational study was designed in which high-sensitivity troponin T is determined as an exposure factor, patients are followed until the resolution of the clinical picture, and the frequency of mortality is analyzed. We included patients $\geq$ 16 years old with confirmed influenza virus infection and determination of high-sensitivity troponin T. One hundred twenty-eight patients were included (96.9% survivors, 3.1% deceased). Mean and median blood levels of high-sensitivity troponin T of survivors were 26.2 $\pm$ 58.3 ng/L and 14.5 ng/L (IQR 16 ng/L), respectively, and were statistically different when compared with those of the deceased patients, 120.5 $\pm$ 170.1 ng/L and 40.5 ng/L (IQR 266.5 ng/L), respectively, $p = 0.012$. The Youden index using mortality as the reference method was 0.76, and the cut-off value associated with this index was 24 ng/L (sensitivity 100%, specificity 76%, NPV 100%, PPV 4%) with AUC of 88,8% (95% CI: 79.8–92.2%), $p < 0.001$. We conclude that high-sensitivity troponin T levels in confirmed virus influenza infection are a good predictor of mortality in our population, and this predictor is useful for safely discharging patients from the emergency department.

Keywords: influenza; human; troponin; biomarkers; SARS-CoV-2; cardiovascular infections; virus diseases; usTnT

1. Introduction

Influenza virus infection (IVI) is a substantial global public health problem that causes significant morbidity and mortality. Annual epidemics are estimated to infect 5–10% of the world's population, causing 3–5 million severe cases and more than 650,000 deaths [1,2]. In the 2019–2020 season, the impact of the flu epidemic in Spain caused 27,700 hospitalizations with confirmed influenza infection, 1800 patients in the intensive care unit (ICU) services, and 3900 deaths [3].

Although IVI is a usually self-limited pathology that normally infects only the upper respiratory tract, sometimes in relation to its aggressiveness and the characteristics of the host, it can have a complexity and severity that make it difficult for us to predict the evolution upon arrival at health services. In addition, the appearance of the SARS-CoV-2 virus has produced a significant distortion, with a drastic decrease in the incidence of IVI. In the 2020–2021 season by the date of 2 May 2021, 15 IVIs had been reported in Spain, 2 from sentinel samples and 13 nonsentinel samples [4]. We do not know if in the future the influenza virus will disappear in its fight with other viruses in the same ecological niche or will rebound and be a promoter of other infections, but the European Center for Disease Prevention and Control and the World Health Organization (WHO) propose establishing sentinel surveillance systems for influenza, COVID-19 and any other respiratory virus or emerging etiological agent in the future [5].

A growing body of evidence says that infectious diseases cause cardiovascular complications in the short and medium term. There is increasing evidence of the relationship between bacterial pneumonia or COVID-19 infection and important cardiovascular complications with increased biomarkers [6–8]. IVI is not an exception, increasing deaths from cardiovascular problems during influenza epidemics and triggering or aggravating episodes of arrhythmias, acute coronary syndrome, acute myocarditis, or acute heart failure [9]. During the last century, the healthcare community has observed cardiovascular complications in patients with IVI. The first reference to the increase in cardiovascular morbidity and mortality during IVI epidemics was described in 1932 by Dr. Selwyn D. Collins [10].

Several large epidemiological studies in Russia, the United States, the United Kingdom, and Hong Kong have revealed a temporal association between influenza virus circulation and increased deaths from ischemic heart disease [11]. In 2015 a meta-analysis determined that a recent diagnosis of IVI doubled the risk of developing an acute coronary syndrome [12], and this risk was found to be able to increase up to 6 times in the seven days after IVI confirmation [13]. There is increasing evidence that a recent flu infection is associated with an increased risk of developing acute coronary syndrome, heart failure, myocarditis, and arrhythmias, increasing hospital admissions and mortality [12–14]. In a study of 600 patients with confirmed IVI, 86% of the events associated with acute cardiac injury occurred during the three days after flu laboratory ratification [15]. In short, IVI can predispose to suffering a coronary event in the following days. IVI can also cause other cardiovascular complications, multiplying 3–5 times the risk of heart failure, acute lung edema, and arrhythmias, especially in the first three days of infection [16].

A recent systematic review that analyzed 14 articles that evaluated the elevation of any type of troponin (conventional T and I; ultrasensitive T and I) in patients with IVI concluded that troponin elevation is a rare phenomenon but that when it occurs it increases the risk of death [10].

Searching for a safe cut-off point would decant the patients who could potentially be discharged from the emergency department, with the potential financial savings for the health system in a disease with a large absolute number of seasonal infections.

Therefore, we propose a study whose objective is to determine the prognostic capacity of hsTnT to detect mortality in patients with confirmed IVI, searching for a cut-off point that optimizes the sensitivity and negative predictive value (NPV) of the diagnostic test.

2. Materials and Methods

2.1. Enrolled Patients' Characteristics

An analytical retrospective observational study was designed in a 145-bed hospital in northern Spain, covering a population of 104,800 people. Subjects $\geq$ 16 years of age with confirmed IVI and determination of usTnT in the emergency room were included and were followed up until resolution of the condition. The patient inclusion period was from 1 January 2009 to 31 December 2020.

Demographic variables; comorbidity; clinical characteristics; and laboratory values including biomarkers, radiological data, and evolution data were collected.

2.2. Diagnostic

The outcome predictor variable was the blood determination of hsTnT (measured in ng/L) and mortality during the care process as a dependent variable.

For the diagnosis of IVI, oropharyngeal samples were collected with swabs, which were analyzed by a rapid diagnostic test that uses an immunochromatographic analysis for the qualitative detection of influenza nucleoprotein antigens and/or molecular biological diagnosis by genomic amplification techniques by polymerase chain reaction (RT-PCR) methods. We consider IVI confirmed by the positivity of either of the two methods due to their high specificity.

hsTnT measurement was performed within the first hour of the patient's arrival at the emergency department. Electrochemiluminescent immunoassay technique was used to determine hsTnT (Roche Elecsys Diagnostics GMBH autoanalyzer, Sandhofer Strasse 116, D-68305 Mannheim, Germany). For the rest of the biomarkers, immunoturbidimetric tests for C-reactive protein and electrochemiluminescent immunoassay for NT-proBNP were used.

2.3. Statistical Analysis

For the statistical analysis, the categorical variables were described as absolute value and percentage, and the continuous variables were described by their mean, standard deviations, medians, and interquartile ranges. To assess the differences between the levels of hsTnT and the rest of the quantitative variables in patients with IVI, an analysis was performed between the surviving and nonsurviving groups for each of the variables using the Mann–Whitney U test. To evaluate differences between groups for qualitative variables, the chi-square test or Fisher's test was used.

For the analysis of hsTnT as a predictor of mortality, the ideal cut-off point was calculated by optimizing the product of sensitivity by specificity, maximizing the Youden index, and using mortality as the reference method, representing the receiver operating characteristic (ROC) curve and area under the curve (AUC).

Values of $p < 0.05$ were considered statistically significant. The analysis was performed with SPSS for Windows, version 25 (IBM Corp. Released 2017. IBM SPSS Statistics for Windows, Version 25.0. Armonk, NY, USA: IBM Corp.), and MedCalc for the diagnostic utility (MedCalc Statistical Software version 19.6 (MedCalc Software bv, Ostend, Belgium; https://www.medcalc.org; accessed on 22 February 2022)

2.4. Bioethical Statement

This study was designed following the ethical principles of the Declaration of Helsinki. It was positively evaluated and certified by the Cantabria Clinical Research Ethics Committee (CEIm 2020.082 certificate) and by the Laredo Hospital Teaching Commission.

3. Results

During the study period, 489,825 patients were assisted in the emergency department. Of these patients, 1411 patients were diagnosed with flu syndrome. In 920 patients, IVI was confirmed by immunochromatographic analysis and/or genomic amplification techniques. One hundred twenty-eight patients $\geq$16 years with confirmed IVI and determination of hsTnT were included in the study (Figure 1).

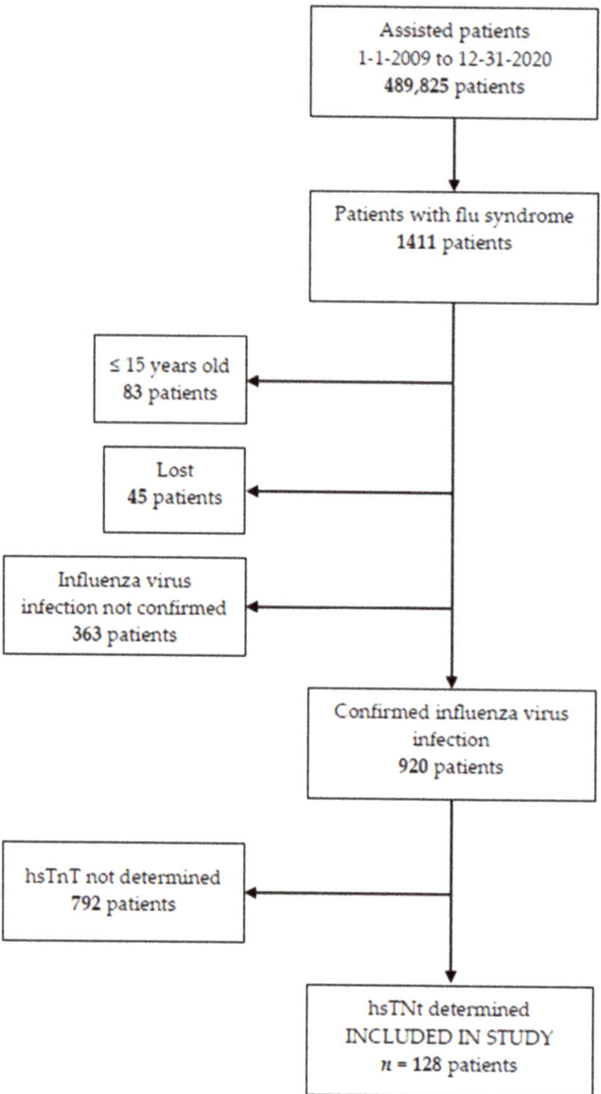

Figure 1. Patients included in the study.

The mean age was 68.8 ± 15.7 years, and 37.1% were women. In the study population, 19.5% had a history of ischemic heart disease, 11.7% had a history of heart failure, 20.3% had chronic obstructive pulmonary disease, and 19.4% had chronic renal failure. The proportion of patients admitted was 67.2%, 65.6% in the conventional ward and 1.6% in the ICU. Of the patients, 3.1% died, with a mean survival of 5.5 days (SD 4.5). The general characteristics of the sample are shown in the Table 1

Table 1. General characteristics of the sample.

Chart. General Characteristics of the Sample.					
	SURVIVORS (n = 124)		DECEASED (n = 4)		p-Value
	n	%	n	%	
SOCIODEMOGRAPHIC VARIABLES					
Age (years) [mean (SD)]	68.2	15.7	85.8	4.9	0.008
Female sex	46	37.1	3	75	0.156
ASSOCIATED COMORBIDITY					
Active smoker (n = 19)	19	15.3	0	0	0.822
Essential hypertension (n = 79)	76	61.3	3	75	0.504
DM-1 (n = 2)	2	1.6	0	0	0.936
DM-2 (n = 28)	28	22.6	0	0	0.546
Dyslipidemia (n = 57)	56	45.2	1	25	0.396
Heart failure (n = 15)	14	11.3	1	25	0.396
Ischemic heart disease (n = 25)	25	20.2	0	0	0.414
Cardiac arrhythmia (n = 22)	21	16.9	1	25	0.534
Asthma (n = 14)	12	9.7	2	50	0.059
COPD (n = 26)	25	20.2	1	25	0.813
Chronic Kidney Disease (n = 12)	11	8.9	1	25	0.329
Chronic liver disease (n = 12)	11	8.9	1	25	0.546
Cognitive dysfunction (n = 7)	5	4	2	50	0.015
Neoplasia (n = 11)	10	8.1	1	25	0.305
CLINICAL PRESENTING VARIABLES					
Dyspneic feeling (n = 65)	61	49.2	4	100	0.062
Body temperature (°C) [mean (SD)] (n = 125)	37.1	0.9	36.8	0.4	0.487
HR (bpm) [median (IQR)] (n = 124)	88	28.3	71	7.3	0.035
RF (rpm) [median (IQR)] (n = 67)	15	6	14.5	2.5	0.716
TAS (mmHg) [median (IQR)] (n = 126)	136	37.3	140	37.3	0.765
DBP (mmHg) [median (IQR)] (n = 126)	75	17.3	78.5	22.3	0.440
Pulse oximetry (n = 119)	96	4	86.5	4	0.002
ANALYTICAL VARIABLES					
Leukocytes x103/µL [median (IQR)] (n = 127)	8000	4100	7250	4575	0.310
Neutrophils x103/µL [median (IQR)] (n = 125)	5450	3825	5400	1800	0.904
Lymphocytes x103/µL [median (IQR)] (n = 125)	900	900	800	700	0.784
Hematocrit % [median (IQR)] (n = 127)	41	6.2	41.3	11.3	0.836
Hemoglobin g/dL [median (IQR)] (n = 127)	13.6	1.9	13.7	4	0.820
Platelets x103/µL [median (IQR)] (n = 126)	176	74	140	99	0.300
Glucose mg/dL [median (IQR)] (n = 127)	126	73	144.5	64	0.945
Urea mg/dL [median (IQR)] (n = 127)	41	26	38.5	17.8	0.709
Creatinine mg/dL [median (IQR)] (n = 126)	0.91	0.33	1.17	0.78	0.337
Sodium mEq/L [median (IQR)] (n = 124)	136	4	139	3	0.214
Potassium mEq/L [median (IQR)] (n = 120)	4.2	0.7	4.2	0.8	0.372
Bilirubin mg/dL [median (IQR)] (n = 56)	0.4	0.4	0.5	0.2	0.941
Prothrombin time % [median (IQR)] (n = 119)	88	30	64	75	0.272

Table 1. *Cont.*

Chart. General Characteristics of the Sample.					
	SURVIVORS (*n* = 124)		DECEASED (*n* = 4)		*p*-Value
	n	%	*n*	%	
Arterial pH [median (IQR)] (*n* = 100)	7.45	0.06	7.41	0.07	0.085
pO2 mmHg [median (IQR)] (*n* = 99)	62	16	53.5	8.5	0.052
pCO2 mmHg [median (IQR)] (*n* = 100)	36.5	9	40.5	8	0.149
BIOMARKERS					
CRP mg/dL [median (IQR)] (n = 124)	3.8	8.4	1.9	1.1	0.095
Lactate mg/dL [median (IQR)] (*n* = 22)	14	10	13	0	0.909
NT-proBNP ng/L [median (IQR)] (*n* = 71)	575	2186	3481	4408	0.077
hsTnT ng/L [median (IQR)] (*n* = 128)	14.5	16	40.5	266.5	0.012
RADIOLOGICAL CHARACTERISTICS					
Chest X-ray performed (*n* = 124)	120	96.8	4	100	0.936
Parenchymal condensation/infiltrate (*n* = 27)	27	21.8	0	0	0.383
Pleural effusion (*n* = 3)	2	1.6	1	25	0.009
EVOLUTION VARIABLES					
Entrance to conventional ward (*n* = 88)	84	67.7	4	100	0.391
Admission to intensive care unit (*n* = 2)	2	1.6	0	0	0.936
Days of survival in deceased [mean (SD)]	-	-	7.3	5.6	-

bpm: beats per minute; brpm: breaths per minute; COPD: chronic obstructive pulmonary disease; CRP: C-reactive protein; DBP: diastolic blood pressure; DM: diabetes mellitus; hsTnT: high-sensitivity troponin T; IQR: interquartile range; NT-proBNP: Amino-terminal fragment of brain natriuretic peptide; Rx: X-rays; SD: standard deviation; TAS: systolic blood pressure.

The mean value of hsTnT in the surviving patients was 26.2 ± 58.3 ng/L, and the median was 14.5 ng/L (IQR 16). In the deceased, the mean was 120.5 ± 170.1 ng/L and median was 40.5 ng/L (IQR 266.5), $p = 0.012$ (Figure 2).

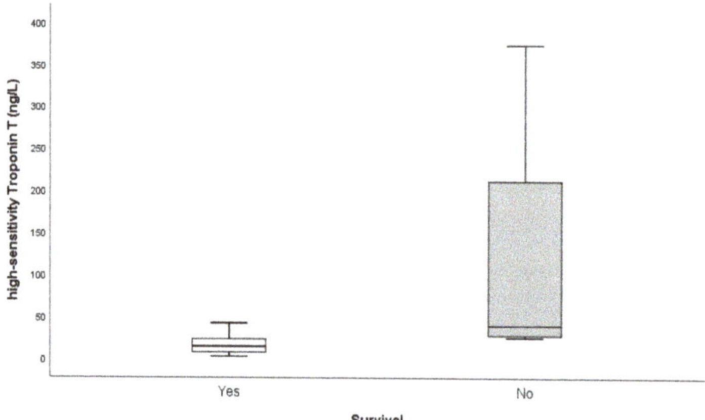

Figure 2. Box plot showing high-sensitivity troponin T values (ng/L) of survivors (*n* = 124) and nonsurvivors (*n* = 4) due to influenza virus infection confirmed by rapid immunochromatographic diagnosis and/or molecular biological diagnosis by techniques. of genomic amplification by polymerase chain reaction methods. Data are presented as medians with 25th and 75th percentiles (boxes) and 95th and 5th percentiles (whiskers).

The Youden index was 0.76, and the cut-off point associated with this index was 24 ng/L (sensitivity 100%, specificity 76%, NPV 100%, positive predictive value (PPV) 4%) with area under the ROC curve (AUC) of 88.8% (95% CI: 79.8–92.2%), $p < 0.001$ (Figure 3).

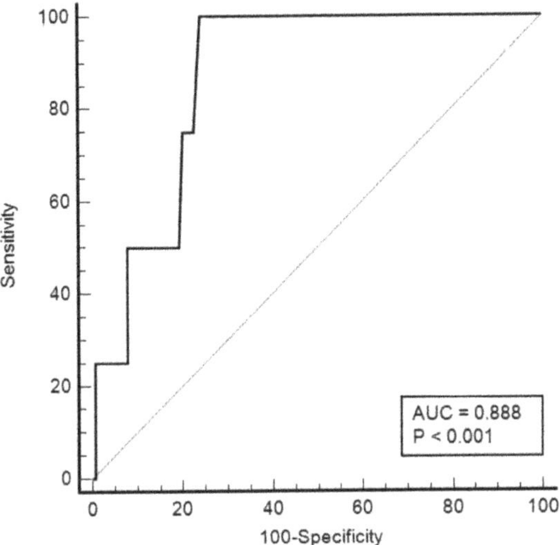

Figure 3. ROC curve plot for ultrasensitive troponin T as a function of mortality. AUC: area under the curve. ROC: receiver operating characteristic.

4. Discussion

The main complications of IVI are respiratory (primary influenza pneumonia or viral pneumonia superinfected by bacteria), but when it comes to extrapulmonary complications, a systematic review of 218 articles found that acute myocarditis and acute coronary syndrome were among the most frequent clinical entities [11,17].

On the other hand, troponin is a globular protein widely used for the early detection of acute coronary syndrome when its values are higher than the 99th percentile of the normal reference population, but it also increases in situations of heart failure, myocarditis, and arrhythmias [18,19].

At this point, we have to consider the reasons why a clinician requests the determination of a cardiac biomarker in a patient with influenza syndrome. Possibly it is because we assume that the patient is seriously ill and therefore we suspect that the patient is developing silent acute myocardial damage or some complication secondary to infection, such as myocarditis due to direct myocardial injury or due to substances that decrease contractility, myocardial ischemia due to an imbalance between demands and oxygen supply, ischemia due to plaque instability due to transient loss of anticoagulant properties of the endothelium when infiltrated by components of the mononuclear phagocyte system, arrhythmias due to increased sympathetic–adrenal activity, catecholaminergic coronary spasm, etc. We could also conjecture that troponin is requested in polypathological patients due to suspicion of atypical presentation of coronary syndrome or suspicion of pathology where troponin is useful as a prognostic tool, such as in pulmonary thromboembolic disease. Whatever the etiopathogenic mechanism, any of these fatal complications of IVI cause an increase in hsTnT in peripheral blood.

The elevation of troponin in IVI is not described as frequent, but when it occurs, it worsens the prognosis, increasing the risk of death [20].

The body of evidence in this regard is increasing. A study of 1131 patients with IVI found an increase in TnI by 2.9%, with 26.6% of this subgroup dying [21]. A recent retrospective study on 264 patients with IVI confirmed by RT-PCR that stratified patients with IVI according to normality of hsTnT found that hsTnT values were significantly higher in patients who died within 30 days of diagnosis compared to those who survived ($p < 0.01$) [22]. Lippi et al. determined that troponin elevation as an indicator of complicated IVI is a relatively rare phenomenon in patients with IVI, being more likely in elderly patients with significant comorbidities [20]. These results go in the same direction as our study, where we found statistically significant differences in the blood levels of hsTnT between deceased and survivors with IVI ($p = 0.012$).

Therefore, in this context in which acute cardiovascular symptoms are a potential wake-up call to indicate a complication due to severe IVI, hsTnT is postulated as a valuable prognostic tool to detect bad evolution. However, one aspect that has not been studied much is the ability of hsTnT to detect patients with confirmed IVI who can be safely discharged from the emergency department. Pizzini et al., with a mortality of 3.8% and using hsTnT with a cut-off point of 46.4 ng/L, achieved an NPV of 89% to rule out acute cardiac events (acute coronary syndrome, acute heart failure, or arrhythmia) in patients with confirmed IVI [22].

In our sample, whose mortality is 3.1%, using the proposed cut-off point of 24 ng/L to safely discharge patients with confirmed IVI (NPV of 100% with AUC of 88.8% to detect mortality), we would have been able to avoid 52 admissions, that is, 60.5% of them (52/86), reducing the therapeutic effort in the emergency department and the pressure on hospitalization wards. Furthermore, no patient below the cut-off point died or required intensive care unit assistance.

If we take into account the RAE-CMBD (Specialized Health Care Activity Register) data from the annual report of the National Health System, the average cost per admission in Spain is EUR 4,741.94. During the 10 years of the study, 558 patients were admitted (545 in a conventional ward and 13 in an intensive care unit). Therefore, if we apply our model, 338 patients would not have been admitted, with the potential saving in direct costs being EUR 1,602,775.7 [23].

Elevated baseline troponin levels are detected in the elderly, heart disease, diabetics, or patients with chronic renal failure, which may act as a confounder. In our sample, the group of patients who died were significantly older. However, we do not think that these baseline differences invalidate our results, because we did not find statistically significant differences in other comorbidities. Furthermore, the main objective of our study was to detect patients with potentially severe IVI upon arrival at the hospital, regardless of the etiology being that the troponin increased acutely or that the elevation was in a patient who already had chronically high troponin levels. This idea is supported by studies that confirm that hospital mortality in patients with IVI is significantly higher in both acutely and chronically elevated hsTnT patients [24].

The limitations of the study are fundamentally those derived from a retrospective single-center study that requires the clinician's request for hsTnT as an inclusion criterion, which could lead to a selection bias. Due to the type of study, it was not possible to carry out further determinations of hsTnT or cardiological evaluation. Nor was the time elapsed from the onset of flu-like symptoms to attendance at the emergency department recorded.

We are also aware that age and chronic heart and kidney disease history are potential confounders that may require different cut-off points to avoid interference. Given the small number of ominous events, future studies aimed at consolidating these results will be useful.

Near the end of World War, I an unknown disease ravaged the world's population, especially the elderly, diabetics, and pregnant and lactating women [25]. The autopsies detected pneumonia and myocarditis. It was the Influenza A virus. We are currently facing another pandemic situation with COVID-19. Both SARS-CoV-2 and influenza are similar in clinical presentation, transmission mechanisms, and vulnerable risk groups and generate similar pulmonary and extrapulmonary complications. In addition, patients with coinfection with IVI and SARS-CoV-2 are more likely to suffer cardiac lesions and earlier cytokine storm [26,27].

The European Center for Disease Prevention and Control and the WHO propose establishing sentinel surveillance systems for influenza and COVID-19 because we do not know what will happen in the near future. A possible scenario would be the coexistence of both viruses, one being a facilitator of the other and both being facilitators of pneumotropic bacteria.

So, in this turbulent period from the microbiological point of view of fighting viruses in health systems, as important as preventive measures with vaccination campaigns aimed at vulnerable groups are, it will also be important to find tools that, once the disease is acquired, allow clinicians to discriminate between stable patients who will have a good evolution and will be able to leave the care area quickly, especially at times of pressure on the health system.

5. Conclusions

Therefore, we conclude, first of all, that in our sample the elevation of hsTnT at the time of IVI diagnosis in the emergency department is significantly associated with increased mortality during the care process.

Secondly, in our sample, the proposed cut-off point of 24 ng/L would allow the safe discharge of patients with IVI confirmed by immunochromatographic analysis and/or genomic amplification techniques, helping to reduce the therapeutic effort and stress on the system.

Thirdly, the retrospective application of our model suggests important economic savings for the health system in the direct cost of care, due to the high percentage of admissions avoided (60.5%), while allowing safe discharge planning from the emergency service for patients with IVI.

hsTnT could be one more block on the retaining wall that we will be forced to develop against viral infections. Paraphrasing Miguel de Cervantes, we can say that in this unpredictable time in which we are living, "being prepared will be half a victory".

Author Contributions: Conceptualization, M.A.T.-V., J.O.d.S.-M., P.M.-C. and H.A.-V.; Methodology, M.A.T.-V. and P.M.-C.; Software, M.A.T.-V., J.O.d.S.-M., P.M.-C. and H.A.-V.; Validation, M.A.T.-V., J.O.d.S.-M., P.M.-C. and H.A.-V.; Formal Analysis, M.A.T.-V. and P.M.-C.; Investigation, M.A.T.-V., J.O.d.S.-M., E.I.-B., M.J.M.-A., E.L.-L., A.V.-Z., I.A.-D., F.E.-C., A.G.-G., A.T.-C., E.J.E.-C., A.B.-G., C.G.-V., E.S.N.-M., D.M.N., C.H.-M., A.G.-C. and J.A.L.-C.; Resources, P.M.-C.; Data Curation, M.A.T.-V. and P.M.-C.; Writing—Original Draft Preparation, M.A.T.-V., J.O.d.S.-M., P.M.-C. and H.A.-V.; Writing—Review and Editing, M.A.T.-V., J.O.d.S.-M., P.M.-C. and H.A.-V.; Visualization, M.A.T.-V., J.O.d.S.-M., P.M.-C. and H.A.-V.; Supervision, M.A.T.-V., J.O.d.S.-M., P.M.-C. and H.A.-V.; Project Administration, M.A.T.-V., J.O.d.S.-M., P.M.-C. and H.A.-V. All authors have read and agreed to the published version of the manuscript.

Funding: This research received no external funding.

Institutional Review Board Statement: The study was conducted in accordance with the Declaration of Helsinki, and the protocol was approved by the Ethics Committee of Cantabria (CEIm 2020.082).

Informed Consent Statement: Patient consent was waived because it was a retrospective study.

Data Availability Statement: The data presented in this study are available on request from the corresponding author.

Conflicts of Interest: The authors declare no conflict of interest.

References

1. WHO. Available online: https://www.who.int/mediacentre/infographic/influenza/en/ (accessed on 11 May 2021).
2. Iuliano, A.D.; Roguski, K.M.; Chang, H.H.; Muscatello, D.J.; Palekar, R.; Tempia, S.; Cohen, C.; Gran, J.M.; Schanzer, D.; Cowling, B.J.; et al. Global Seasonal Influenza-associated Mor-tality Collaborator Network. Estimates of global seasonal influenza-associated respiratory mortality: A modelling study. *Lancet* **2018**, *391*, 1285–1300. [CrossRef]
3. Ministerio de Sanidad, Consumo y Bienestar Social. Available online: https://www.mscbs.gob.es/profesionales/saludPublica/prevPromocion/vacunaciones/programasDeVacunacion/gripe/faq/home.htm#:~{}:text=En%20la%20temporada%202019%2

D2020%20se%20produjeron%2027.700%20hospitalizaciones%2C%201.800,factor%20de%20riesgo%20de%20complicaciones (accessed on 11 May 2021).
4. Instituto de Salud Carlos III. Sistema de Vigilancia de la Gripe y otros virus respiratorios en España (SVGE). Available online: https://vgripe.isciii.es/documentos/20202021/boletines/Informe%20semanal%20SVGE%20y%20otros%20virus%20respiratorios_2020-2021_172021.pdf (accessed on 11 May 2021).
5. Instituto de Salud Carlos III. Sistema de Vigilancia de la Gripe y Otros Virus Respiratorios en España (SVGE). Available online: https://vgripe.isciii.es/inicio.do;jsessionid=71A23A4BFD707E40C4C9E68F89829CB9 (accessed on 11 May 2021).
6. Kunutsor, S.K.; Laukkanen, J.A. Cardiovascular complications in COVID-19: A systematic review and meta-analysis. *J. Infect.* **2020**, *81*, e139–e141. [CrossRef] [PubMed]
7. Tazón Varela, M.A.; Alonso Valle, H.; Muñoz Cacho, P.; Colomo Mármol, L.F.; Gallo Terán, J.; Hernández Herrero, M. N-terminal fragment of pro-brain natriuretic peptide plasma concentration: A new predictive biomarker for community acquired pneumonia? *Emergencias* **2014**, *26*, 94–100.
8. Tazón-Varela, M.A.; Muñoz-Cacho, P.; Alonso-Valle, H.; Gallo-Terán, J.; Pérez-Mier, L.A.; Colomo-Mármol, L.F. The Amino-Terminal Fragment of Pro-Brain Natriuretic Peptide in Plasma as a Biological Marker for Predicting Mortality in Community-Acquired Pneumonia: A Cohort Study. *Eurasian J. Emerg. Med.* **2016**, *15*, 30–38. [CrossRef]
9. Warren-Gash, C.; Smeeth, L.; Hayward, A. Influenza as a trigger for acute myocardial infarction or death from cardiovascular disease: A systematic review. *Lancet Infect. Dis.* **2009**, *9*, 601–610. [CrossRef]
10. Lippi, G.; Sanchis-Gomar, F. Cardiac troponin elevation in patients with influenza virus infections. *Biomed. J.* **2020**, *44*, 183–189. [CrossRef]
11. Collins, S.D. Excess Mortality from Causes Other than Influenza and Pneumonia during Influenza Epidemics. *Public Health Rep.* **1932**, *47*, 2159. [CrossRef]
12. Kwong, J.C.; Schwartz, K.L.; Campitelli, M.A.; Chung, H.; Crowcroft, N.S.; Karnauchow, T.; Katz, K.; Ko, D.; McGeer, A.J.; McNally, D.; et al. Acute Myocardial Infarction after Laboratory-Confirmed Influenza Infection. *New Engl. J. Med.* **2018**, *378*, 345–353. [CrossRef]
13. Sellers, S.A.; Hagan, R.S.; Hayden, F.G.; Fischer, W.A. The hidden burden of influenza: A review of the extra-pulmonary complications of influenza infection. *Influ. Other Respir. Viruses* **2017**, *11*, 372–393. [CrossRef] [PubMed]
14. López-Fernández, L.; López-Messa, J.; Llano, J.A.-D.; Garmendia-Leiza, J.R.; García-Cruces, J.; García-Crespo, J. Relación entre las tasas de gripe estacional y las tasas de hospitalización y mortalidad hospitalaria por enfermedades cardiovasculares agudas en una región española. *Med. Clin.* **2019**, *153*, 133–140. [CrossRef]
15. Barnes, M.; E Heywood, A.; Mahimbo, A.; Rahman, B.; Newall, A.; MacIntyre, C.R. Acute myocardial infarction and influenza: A meta-analysis of case–control studies. *Heart* **2015**, *101*, 1738–1747. [CrossRef]
16. Ludwig, A.; Lucero-Obusan, C.; Schirmer, P.; Winston, C.; Holodniy, M. Acute cardiac injury events $\leq$ 30 days after laboratory-confirmed influenza virus infection among U.S.veterans, 2010–2012. *BMC Cardiovasc. Disord.* **2015**, *15*, 109. [CrossRef] [PubMed]
17. Tazón-Varela, M.; Alonso-Valle, H.; Muñoz-Cacho, P.; Gallo-Terán, J.; Piris-García, X.; Pérez-Mier, L. Aumento de microorganismos no habituales en la neumonía adquirida en la comunidad. *SEMERGEN-Med. Fam.* **2017**, *43*, 437–444. [CrossRef] [PubMed]
18. Thygesen, K.; Alpert, J.S.; Jaffe, A.S.; Chaitman, B.R.; Bax, J.J.; Morrow, D.A.; White, H.D. Executive Group on behalf of the Joint European Society of Cardiology (ESC)/American College of Cardiology (ACC)/American Heart Association (AHA)/World Heart Federation (WHF) Task Force for the Universal Definition of Myocardial Infarction Fourth Universal Definition of Myocardial Infarction (2018). *J. Am. Coll. Cardiol.* **2018**, *72*, 2231–2264. [CrossRef]
19. Azar, R.R.; Sarkis, A.; Giannitsis, E. A Practical Approach for the Use of High-Sensitivity Cardiac Troponin Assays in the Evaluation of Patients With Chest Pain. *Am. J. Cardiol.* **2020**, *139*, 1–7. [CrossRef]
20. Lee, N.; Ison, M.G. Diagnosis, management and outcomes of adults hospitalized with influenza. *Antivir. Ther.* **2012**, *17*, 143–157. [CrossRef] [PubMed]
21. Harris, J.; Shah, P.J.; Korimilli, V.; Win, H. Frequency of troponin elevations in patients with influenza infection during the 2017–2018 influenza season. *IJC Hear. Vasc.* **2019**, *22*, 145–147. [CrossRef]
22. Pizzini, A.; Burkert, F.; Theurl, I.; Weiss, G.; Bellmann-Weiler, R. Prognostic impact of high sensitive Troponin T in patients with influenza virus infection: A retrospective analysis. *Hear. Lung* **2020**, *49*, 105–109. [CrossRef]
23. Gobierno de España. Ministerio de Sanidad. Sistema de Información de Atención Especializada (SIAE). Registro de Actividad de Atención Especializada. RAE-CMBD. Available online: https://www.sanidad.gob.es/estadEstudios/estadisticas/cmbdhome.htm (accessed on 11 May 2021).
24. Sharma, Y.; Horwood, C.; Chua, A.; Hakendorf, P.; Thompson, C. Prognostic impact of high sensitive troponin in predicting 30-day mortality among patients admitted to hospital with influenza. *IJC Hear. Vasc.* **2020**, *32*, 100682. [CrossRef]
25. Rezkalla, S.H.; Kloner, R.A. Viral myocarditis: 1917–2020: From the Influenza A to the COVID-19 pandemics. *Trends Cardiovasc. Med.* **2020**, *31*, 163–169. [CrossRef]
26. Cuadrado-Payán, E.; Montagud-Marrahi, E.; Torres-Elorza, M.; Bodro, M.; Blasco, M.; Poch, E.; Soriano, A.; Piñeiro, G.J. SARS-CoV-2 and influenza virus co-infection. *Lancet* **2020**, *395*, e84. [CrossRef]
27. Ma, S.; Lai, X.; Chen, Z.; Tu, S.; Qin, K. Clinical characteristics of critically ill patients co-infected with SARS-CoV-2 and the influenza virus in Wuhan, China. *Int. J. Infect. Dis.* **2020**, *96*, 683–687. [CrossRef] [PubMed]

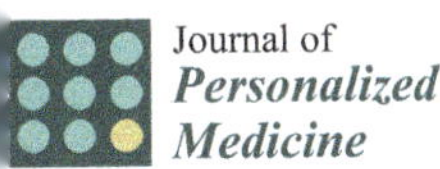
Journal of *Personalized Medicine*

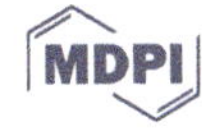

Article

Assessment of Dynamic Changes in Stressed Volume and Venous Return during Hyperdynamic Septic Shock

Athanasios Chalkias [1,2,3,*], Eleni Laou [1], Nikolaos Papagiannakis [4], Vaios Spyropoulos [5], Evaggelia Kouskouni [6], Kassiani Theodoraki [7,†] and Theodoros Xanthos [8,†]

1 Department of Anesthesiology, Faculty of Medicine, University of Thessaly, 41500 Larisa, Greece; elenilaou1@gmail.com
2 Outcomes Research Consortium, Cleveland, OH 44195, USA
3 Hellenic Society of Cardiopulmonary Resuscitation, 11528 Athens, Greece
4 First Department of Neurology, Eginition University Hospital, Medical School, National and Kapodistrian University of Athens, 11528 Athens, Greece; nikolas.papagia@gmail.com
5 Medical Supervision S.A., 10680 Athens, Greece; sp.vaios@gmail.com
6 Department of Biopathology, Aretaieion University Hospital, Medical School, National and Kapodistrian University of Athens, 11528 Athens, Greece; ekouskouni@yahoo.com
7 Department of Anesthesiology, Aretaieion University Hospital, National and Kapodistrian University of Athens, 15772 Athens, Greece; ktheodoraki@hotmail.com
8 School of Medicine, European University Cyprus, Nicosia 2404, Cyprus; theodorosxanthos@yahoo.com
* Correspondence: thanoschalkias@yahoo.gr
† These authors contributed equally to this work.

Citation: Chalkias, A.; Laou, E.; Papagiannakis, N.; Spyropoulos, V.; Kouskouni, E.; Theodoraki, K.; Xanthos, T. Assessment of Dynamic Changes in Stressed Volume and Venous Return during Hyperdynamic Septic Shock. *J. Pers. Med.* **2022**, *12*, 724. https://doi.org/10.3390/jpm12050724

Academic Editor: Bruno Mégarbané

Received: 1 April 2022
Accepted: 28 April 2022
Published: 29 April 2022

Abstract: The present work investigated the dynamic changes in stressed volume (*Vs*) and other determinants of venous return using a porcine model of hyperdynamic septic shock. Septicemia was induced in 10 anesthetized swine, and fluid challenges were started after the diagnosis of sepsis-induced arterial hypotension and/or tissue hypoperfusion. Norepinephrine infusion targeting a mean arterial pressure (MAP) of 65 mmHg was started after three consecutive fluid challenges. After septic shock was confirmed, norepinephrine infusion was discontinued, and the animals were left untreated until cardiac arrest occurred. Baseline *Vs* decreased by 7% for each mmHg decrease in MAP during progression of septic shock. Mean circulatory filling pressure (Pmcf) analogue (Pmca), right atrial pressure, resistance to venous return, and efficiency of the heart decreased with time ($p < 0.001$ for all). Fluid challenges did not improve hemodynamics, but noradrenaline increased *Vs* from 107 mL to 257 mL (140%) and MAP from 45 mmHg to 66 mmHg (47%). Baseline Pmca and post-cardiac arrest Pmcf did not differ significantly (14.3 ± 1.23 mmHg vs. 14.75 ± 1.5 mmHg, $p = 0.24$), but the difference between pre-arrest Pmca and post-cardiac arrest Pmcf was statistically significant (9.5 ± 0.57 mmHg vs. 14.75 ± 1.5 mmHg, $p < 0.001$). In conclusion, the baseline *Vs* decreased by 7% for each mmHg decrease in MAP during progression of hyperdynamic septic shock. Significant changes were also observed in other determinants of venous return. A new physiological intravascular volume existing at zero transmural distending pressure was identified, termed as the rest volume (*Vr*).

Keywords: septic shock; venous return; mean circulatory filling pressure; stressed volume; unstressed volume; rest volume; cardiovascular dynamics; hemodynamics; anesthesiology; intensive care medicine

1. Introduction

The traditional management of shock focuses on the regulation of left ventricular cardiac output (CO). However, it is the venous return theory that provides an understanding of the circulation, emphasizing that CO is associated with, and regulated by, the amount of blood returning to the heart. In general, venous return occurs because of a pressure gradient between the periphery and the right atrium. As a matter of fact, not all the blood leaving the venous system returns to the heart at the same time because the largest quantity remains within the veins to regulate venous return [1]; therefore, approximately 30% of the total blood volume (TBV) represents stressed volume (*Vs*, i.e., the volume in blood vessels when transmural distending pressure (Ptm) is above zero), while the remaining 70% is unstressed volume (*Vu*), i.e., the volume in blood vessels when Ptm equals zero.

The modification of the venous system that occurs in sepsis is poorly understood. Experimental studies have indicated a diverse pathophysiology with biphasic hemodynamic responses and/or hyperdynamic hypotensive circulatory states [2–4], suggesting a disproportionate impairment in peripheral vasoregulation [5]. Sepsis increases venous capacitance and decreases systemic vascular resistance (SVR), leading to cardiovascular compromise and tissue hypoperfusion. In septic shock, the TBV status is unchanged, but the progressive vasodilation shifts a portion of the *Vs* to *Vu*, which decreases mean circulatory filling pressure (Pmcf) and venous return [6].

The use of the *Vs*:*Vu* ratio introduced novel strategies for fluid resuscitation and vasopressor administration. Nevertheless, the current recommendations on sepsis and septic shock have failed to reach hemodynamic goals [7]. After decades of research, it seems that the optimal management requires a basic understanding of the underlying evolving pathophysiology and an individualized, physiology-guided strategy [8]. An important asset to this would be the comprehension of *Vs*:*Vu* ratio changes during progression of the condition. In the present study, we aimed to elucidate this topic in greater detail. To this end, we investigated the dynamic changes in *Vs* and other determinants of venous return during progression and resuscitation of hyperdynamic septic shock in an experimental swine model.

2. Materials and Methods

2.1. Extrapolation Model of Calculation of Stressed Volume

An extrapolation model was created to assess circulatory volumes in steady-state and pathophysiological conditions using 20-kg Landrace–Large White swine. As the animals' baseline hemodynamics closely resemble human hemodynamics [9,10], we accepted that 30% of their TBV represents *Vs* and the remaining 70% is *Vu* [11–14]. The TBV of the Landrace–Large White swine is 7% of the total body weight, i.e., 1400 mL for a 20 kg animal, and therefore, their baseline *Vs* is 420 mL.

We have recently shown that the blood volume that has to be removed from the 20-kg swine to induce cardiac arrest is ≈860 mL [15]. This volume includes the *Vs* and the *Vu* that converts to *Vs* during hemorrhage [14,16]. Considering that the *Vs* is 420 mL, the blood volume mobilized from the splanchnic and other compliant veins to maintain Ptm > 0, and thus *Vs* and venous return, in the 20-kg swine during hemorrhage is 440 mL [15]. Although in severe hypovolemia the homeostatic mechanisms involved in hemodynamics and CO regulation may empty the splanchnic reservoir [17], the remaining 540 mL of the 1400 mL of blood in our animals was volume that was not mobilized from the venous pool, probably due to depletion of sympathoadrenal system reserves or splanchnic sequestration, or mobilization could have occurred only with the use of exogenous vasopressor. This volume can be characterized as the "rest volume" (*Vr*), i.e., the volume that cannot be mobilized without the use of an external vasopressor or without decreasing arterial and/or venous resistance. The *Vs* and the *Vu* (i.e., the volume that can be converted to *Vs* or *Vr*) constitute the potential total circulating blood volume (*Vc*). In our model, the following apply:

$$\text{Total blood volume (mL)} = Vc + Vr = (Vs + Vu) + Vr \quad (1)$$

and

Steady state: *Vs* = 420 mL, *Vu* = 440 mL, *Vr* = 540 mL (TBV = 1400 mL).
During hemorrhage: *Vs* = 420 mL + 440 mL from *Vu* (to maintain Ptm > 0), *Vr* = 540 mL.
Hypovolemic cardiac arrest: 860 mL removed and *Vr* = 540 mL (Ptm ≈ 0).

In summary, in the hemorrhagic model, the *Vs* (420 mL in the 20-kg swine with TBV 1400 mL) was related to a MAP of 88.4 mmHg, while the *Vr* (540 mL) was the blood volume at MAP 30 mmHg (cardiac arrest) [15]. The *Vs*, *Vu*, and *Vr* during hemorrhage are depicted in Figure S1. The extrapolation of the aforementioned baseline data from the hemorrhagic model to animals of the same age, weight, TBV, and baseline hemodynamics [9,15] allows the study of circulatory volumes in other experimental conditions using linear regression analysis.

2.2. *Experimental Model*

2.2.1. Ethics Approval

Taking into consideration the principles of 3R, i.e., Replacement, Reduction, and Refinement, which represent a responsible approach for performing more humane animal research [18], we conducted a post hoc analysis of high-quality hemodynamic data derived from a previous study investigating resuscitation in hyperdynamic septic shock [9]. The original protocol was approved by the General Directorate of Veterinary Services (license No. 26, 10 January 2012) according to the national legislation regarding ethical and experimental procedures. These procedures conformed to the guidelines from Directive 2010/63/EU of the European Parliament on the protection of animals used for scientific purposes or the current National Institutes of Health guidelines. The manuscript adheres to the applicable ARRIVE 2.0 and Minimum Quality Threshold in Pre-Clinical Sepsis Studies (MQTiPSS) guidelines [19,20].

2.2.2. Study Objectives

The primary objective was to assess the dynamic changes in *Vs* and other determinants of venous return during progression and resuscitation of hyperdynamic septic shock. Secondary objective was to measure Pmcf after sepsis-induced cardiac arrest.

2.2.3. Origin and Source of the Animals

This analysis included 10 healthy female Landrace–Large White piglets aged 19–21 weeks with average weight of 20 $\pm$ 1 kg, all purchased from the same breeder (Validakis, Koropi, Greece). One week prior to the experiments, the animals were transported to the research facility (Experimental-Research Center Elpen, European Ref Number EL 09 BIO 03) and were acclimatized to laboratory conditions, as previously described [10]. The day before the experimentation, the animals were fasted, but access to water was ad libitum. All animals received anesthetic and surgical procedures in compliance with the Guide for the Care and Use of Laboratory Animals [21].

2.2.4. Animal Preparation

The animals were premedicated with intramuscular ketamine hydrochloride (Merial, Lyon, France), 10 $mg{\cdot}kg^{-1}$, midazolam (Roche, Athens, Greece), 0.5 $mg{\cdot}kg^{-1}$, and atropine sulphate (Demo, Athens, Greece), 0.05 $mg{\cdot}kg^{-1}$, and were subsequently transported to the operation research facility. Intravascular access was obtained through the auricular veins, and induction of anesthesia was achieved with an intravenous bolus dose of propofol (Diprivan 1% w/v; AstraZeneca, Luton, United Kingdom), 2 $mg{\cdot}kg^{-1}$, and fentanyl (Janssen Pharmaceutica, Beerse, Belgium), 2 $\mu g{\cdot}kg^{-1}$. While breathing spontaneously, the animals were intubated with a size 6.0 mm cuffed endotracheal tube, which was secured on the lower jaw. Successful intubation was ascertained by auscultation of both lungs while ventilated with a self-inflating bag.

The animals were then immobilized in the supine position on the operating table and were volume-controlled ventilated (tidal volume 10 $mg{\cdot}kg^{-1}$, inspiratory-to-expiratory time ratio 1:2, positive end-expiratory pressure 0 cm H_20, fraction of inspired oxygen 0.21; Siare Alpha-Delta Lung Ventilator; Siare s.r.l. Hospital Supplies, Bologna, Italy) [22]. Additional amounts of 1 $mg{\cdot}kg^{-1}$ propofol, 0.15 $mg{\cdot}kg^{-1}$ cis-atracurium, and 4 $\mu g{\cdot}kg^{-1}$ fentanyl were administered intravenously to ascertain synchrony with the ventilator. Amounts of propofol 0.1 $mg{\cdot}kg^{-1}{\cdot}min^{-1}$, cis-atracurium 20 $\mu g{\cdot}kg^{-1}{\cdot}min^{-1}$, and fentanyl 0.6 $\mu g{\cdot}kg^{-1}{\cdot}min^{-1}$ were administered to maintain adequate anesthetic depth, assessed by the jaw tone, throughout the study [9,10,22]. Normocapnia was achieved using continuous monitoring of end-tidal carbon dioxide ($ETCO_2$, Tonocap TC-200-22-01; Engstrom Division, Instrumentarium Corp, Helsinki, Finland), and the respiratory rate was adjusted to maintain $ETCO_2$ 35–40 mmHg. Pulse oximetry was monitored throughout the experiment. Body temperature was monitored by a rectal temperature probe and was maintained between 38.5 °C and 39.5 °C with a heating blanket [22].

Electrocardiographic monitoring was used using leads I, II, III, aVR, aVL, and aVF, which were connected to a monitor (Mennen Medical, Envoy; Papapostolou, Athens, Greece) that electronically calculated the heart rate. For measurement of the aortic pressures, an arterial catheter (model 6523, USCI CR, Bart; Papapostolou, Athens, Greece) was inserted and moved forward into the descending aorta after surgical preparation of the right internal carotid artery. A FloTrac sensor kit was connected to the arterial line and coupled to a Vigileo monitor (FloTrac/Vigileo; Edwards Lifescience, Irvine, CA, USA). Then, the internal jugular vein was cannulated, and a Swan–Ganz catheter (Opticath 5.5F, 75 cm; Abbott, Ladakis, Athens, Greece) was inserted into the right atrium. Intravascular catheters were zeroed to ambient pressure at the phlebostatic axis, and measurements initiated after the systems' dynamic response was confirmed with fast-flush tests. These allowed the recording of systolic (SAP), diastolic (DAP), and mean (MAP) arterial pressure, and CO, SVR, and right atrial pressure (P_{RA}). Arterial blood gases were measured on a blood gas analyzer (IRMA SL Blood Analysis System, Part 436301; Diametrics Medical Inc., Roseville, MN, USA). Baseline data were collected after allowing each animal to stabilize for 30 min.

2.2.5. Preparation of Bacterial Suspensions

We used bacterial suspensions in normal saline with a concentration of approximately 1×10^8 cfu·mL^{-1} and therefore 0.5 McFarland turbidity [9]. The strains (lipopolysaccharide *Escherichia coli* (*E. coli*) ATCC 25922) were derived from the Microbiology Laboratory of the Aretaieion University Hospital in Athens, Greece, and stored at −70 °C in 50% glycerol solution. Each vial contained 5×10^8 cfu·mL^{-1} bacteria in logarithmic phase. Two days prior to the experimental procedure, the vials were allowed to defrost at room temperature and then cultured in blood agar plates. They were incubated at 37 °C for 14 h and then recultured every 14 h. At the middle of the logarithmic phase, the colonies were skimmed from the surface and suspended in 12.5 mL of sterile normal saline that was equally divided into four tubes (3.125 mL each). The 12.5 mL were removed from a sterile normal saline bottle of 100 mL. In each tube, we created a bacterial suspension with a turbidity of 4 McFarland. Then, the suspensions were reinfused back in the 100 mL bottle of normal saline. After vigorous shaking (vortex) we removed 3 mL from the 100 mL and counted the turbidity. If it was 0.5 McFarland, the suspension was accepted. The turbidity was measured with a spectrophotometer at a wavelength of 580 nm (Densicheck Plus Biomerieux). The suspensions were stored at 4 °C for 6–8 h and were left at room temperature 30 min prior to the infusion.

2.2.6. Experimental Procedure

After baseline data were collected, septicemia was induced by an intravenous infusion of a bolus of 20 mL of bacterial suspension over two minutes, followed by a continuous infusion (1 mL·kg^{-1}·h^{-1}; 1 mL = 10^8 cfu) during the rest of the experiment (Figure 1) [9]. Hemodynamic measurements were obtained every one hour after inoculation and sepsis was documented by the presence of systemic manifestations. The definitions of sepsis and septic shock were based on the 2012 Surviving Sepsis Campaign Guidelines, and septic shock was defined as sepsis-induced hypotension persisting despite adequate fluid resuscitation [23].

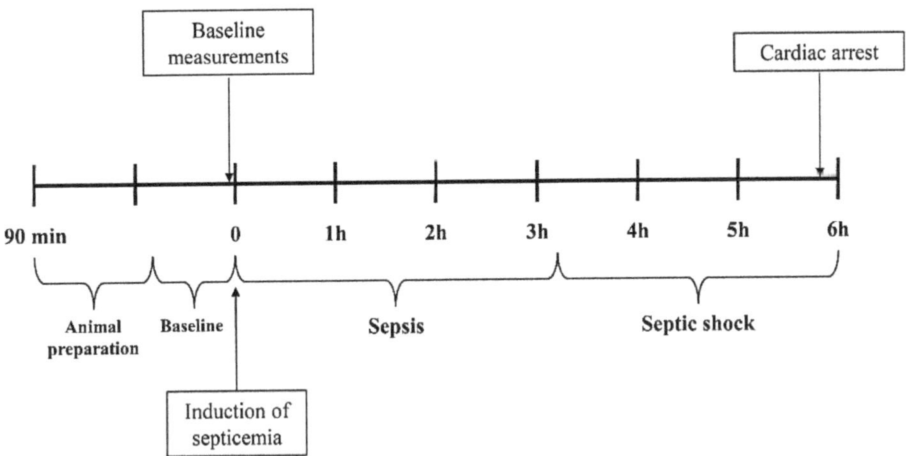

Figure 1. Experimental protocol outline.

Fluid challenges of 10 mL·kg^{-1} isotonic sodium chloride were started with the diagnosis of sepsis-induced arterial hypotension and/or tissue hypoperfusion (lactate > 1 mmol·L^{-1}) [23]. Particular attention was paid to infuse the fluid challenges over 20–30 min and not faster in order to prevent an artificial stress response [9]. Norepinephrine infusion of 0.01–3 µg·kg^{-1}·min^{-1} targeting a MAP of 65 mmHg was started after three consecutive fluid challenges without improvement in MAP. When MAP ≥ 65 mmHg, septic shock was confirmed and norepinephrine infusion was discontinued [9,23]. No other fluids, vasopressors, or inotropes were used, and no other adjustments were performed despite further deterioration, and all animals were left untreated until cardiac arrest occurred.

2.2.7. Calculation of Baseline Mean Circulatory Filling Pressure Analogue and Related Variables

Mean circulatory filling pressure analog (Pmca) was calculated from running hemodynamic data to assess the effective circulating volume and the driving pressure for venous return. The methods of the Pmca algorithm have been described in detail before [24–28]. Briefly, based on a Guytonian model of the systemic circulation [CO = VR = (Pmcf − P_{RA})/R_{VR}], an analogue of Pmcf can be derived using the mathematical model Pmca = ($a \times P_{RA}$) + ($b \times$ MAP) + ($c \times$ CO), where P_{RA} is right atrial pressure and R_{VR} is resistance to venous return [29,30]. In this formula, a and b are dimensionless constants ($a + b = 1$). Assuming a veno-arterial compliance ratio of 24:1, $a = 0.96$ and $b = 0.04$, reflecting the contribution of venous and arterial compartments, and c resembles arteriovenous resistance and is based on a formula including age, height, and weight [27,30,31]:

$$c = \frac{0.038\ (94.17 + 0.193 \times \text{age})}{4.5\ \left(0.99^{\text{age}-15}\right)\ 0.007184 \cdot \left(\text{height}^{0.725}\right)\ \left(\text{weight}^{0.425}\right)} \quad (2)$$

In addition, the following variables were determined: (1) pressure gradient for venous return (PG_{VR}) was defined as the pressure difference between Pmca and P_{RA} [PG_{VR} = Pmca − P_{RA}]; (2) resistance to venous return was defined as the ratio of the pressure difference between Pmca and P_{RA} and CO [R_{VR} = (Pmca − P_{RA})/CO], a formula that is used to describe venous return during transient states of imbalances (Pmca is the average pressure in the systemic circulation, and R_{VR} is the resistance encountered by the heart) [32,33]; and (3) efficiency of the heart (Eh) was defined as the ratio of the pressure difference between Pmca and P_{RA} and Pmca [Eh = (Pmca − P_{RA})/Pmca]. This equation was proposed for the measurement of heart performance. During the cardiac stop ejection, P_{RA} is equal to the Pmca, and Eh approaches zero [27,34].

2.2.8. Analysis of the Dynamic Changes in Stressed Volume during Progression of Septic Shock

So as to assess *Vs* during septic shock, we used our extrapolation model in swine of the same age, weight, TBV, and baseline hemodynamics. The baseline *Vs* value and the hourly MAP values during progression of hyperdynamic septic shock were separately determined on a line plot. Using extrapolation lines and linear regression of MAP − *Vs* relationship, we estimated the hourly decrease in *Vs* considering that the total volume status was unchanged.

2.2.9. Calculation of Mean Circulatory Filling Pressure during Cardiac Arrest

Significant changes in vasomotor tone occur after the onset of cardiac arrest. The arterial pressure falls and the venous pressure rises until they almost reach equilibrium [35,36]. Thus, the measurement of Pmcf must be made within the first few seconds after arrest [35,37]. However, the hypotension-induced baroreflex withdrawal maintains an antegrade and pulmonary blood flow that may continue for more than 30–60 s [37]. As Pmcf may vary among individuals, the maximum flow could be better assessed if the time of arrest is more than 20 s [14,38]. Therefore, we initially measured Pmcf using the equilibrium mean P_{RA} between 5 and 7.5 s after the onset of cardiac arrest, before the reflex response had significantly altered the measured plateau pressure [36,39,40]. Then, we continued measuring Pmcf every 10 s until 1 min post-cardiac arrest, provided that the measured plateau pressure was not significantly altered. In this study, Pmcf was measured at six time points (5–7.5 s, 15–17.5 s, 25–27.5 s, 35–37.5 s, 45–47.5 s, and 55–57.5 s post-cardiac arrest).

As arteries are much less compliant than veins, transfer of the remaining arterial volume sufficient to equalize pressures throughout the vasculature could not significantly increase Pmcf or affect measurements in our study [39]. In this context, a plateau was considered adequate to allow accurate measurement if mean P_{RA} rose by less than one mmHg over the period from 5 to 7.5 s after the onset of cardiac arrest [39]. In the present study, all animals had adequate plateau and were included for further analysis.

2.2.10. Statistical Analysis

Statistical analysis was performed using R v4.1. Pearson's method was used to correlate hemodynamic measurements with Pmca at baseline. Repeated-measures ANOVA was used to assess differences between groups. Linear mixed effects (LME) models were used when needed to assess coefficients additionally to p-values. The different subjects (swine) were included as random factor. p-values less than 0.05 were deemed significant.

3. Results

3.1. *Progression of Sepsis and Septic Shock*

Sepsis progressively evolved with time, and hyperdynamic septic shock was evident after the second hour from induction of septicemia. The progression of sepsis had a significant effect on hemodynamic (Table 1) and metabolic variables (Table S1).

Table 1. Hemodynamic changes in animals during progression of sepsis and septic shock.

	Baseline	**1 h**	**2 h**	**3 h**	**4 h**	**5 h**	**6 h**	***p*-Value**
Heart rate (beat·min^{-1})	127.2 (14.23)	137.4 (12.19)	137 (19.09)	134.6 (18.63)	142.7 (18.03)	123.5 (14.94)	129.1 (15.56)	0.135
MAP (mmHg)	88.4 (20.94)	78.8 (20.35)	59.6 (13.50)	48.6 (13.81)	48.6 (15.94)	42.7 (12.26)	33.2 (3.36)	<0.001
CO (L·min^{-1})	6.4 (0.34)	6.9 (0.22)	7.1 (0.25)	8 (0.11)	8.6 (0.19)	8.7 (0.41)	10.1 (0.53)	<0.001
SVR (dynes·sec·cm^{-5})	1012.7 (61.24)	827.5 (42.79)	585.3 (18.06)	443.4 (11.99)	416.2 (14.16)	346.2 (16.98)	241.6 (17.78)	<0.001
P_{RA} (mmHg)	7.3 (1.16)	6.6 (0.84)	5.5 (0.71)	4.1 (0.74)	4 (0.67)	4.9 (0.32)	2.4 (0.52)	<0.001
Pmca (mmHg)	14.3 (1.23)	13.5 (0.85)	11.9 (0.74)	10.5 (0.71)	10.8 (0.64)	11.5 (0.38)	9.5 (0.57)	<0.001
PG_{VR} (mmHg)	6.9 (0.16)	6.9 (0.11)	6.4 (0.18)	6.4 (0.08)	6.8 (0.12)	6.6 (0.24)	7.1 (0.3)	0.934
R_{VR} (mmHg·min·L^{-1})	1.1 (0.03)	1 (0.02)	0.87 (0.01)	0.8 (0.01)	0.79 (0.01)	0.75 (0.01)	0.7 (0.01)	<0.001
Eh	0.49 (0.04)	0.52 (0.03)	0.54 (0.03)	0.61 (0.04)	0.63 (0.04)	0.57 (0.02)	0.75 (0.04)	<0.001
Vs (mL)	420	350	214	136	136	93	≈0	<0.001

Values are expressed as mean (SD). MAP, mean arterial pressure; CO, cardiac output; SVR, systemic vascular resistance; P_{RA}, right atrial pressure; Pmca, mean circulatory filling pressure analog; PG_{VR}, pressure gradient for venous return; R_{VR}, resistance to venous return; Eh, efficiency of the heart.

3.2. Dynamic Changes in Stressed Volume during Progression of Septic Shock

The dynamic changes in *Vs* during progression of septic shock are depicted in Figure 2. A 7% decrease in *Vs* was observed for each mmHg decrease in MAP during progression of sepsis and septic shock (Figure 3).

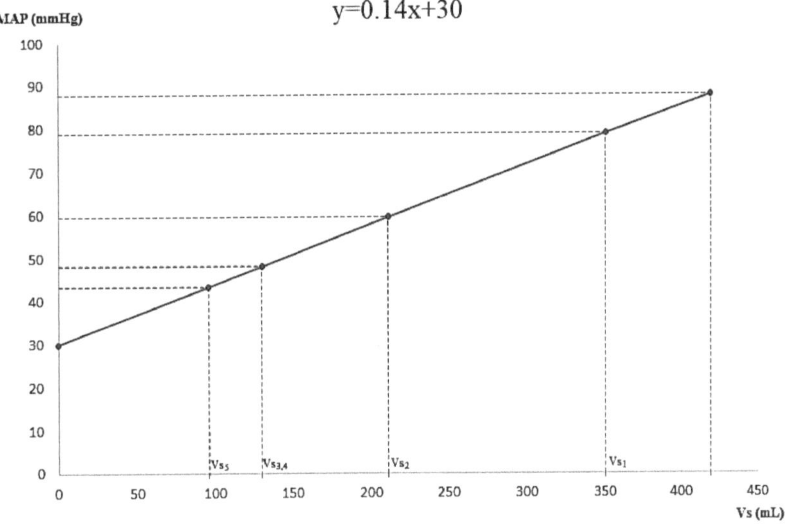

Figure 2. Changes in stressed volume during progression of hyperdynamic septic shock. Cardiac arrest (MAP = 30 mmHg) occurs when Vs = 0. MAP, mean arterial pressure; Vs, stressed volume.

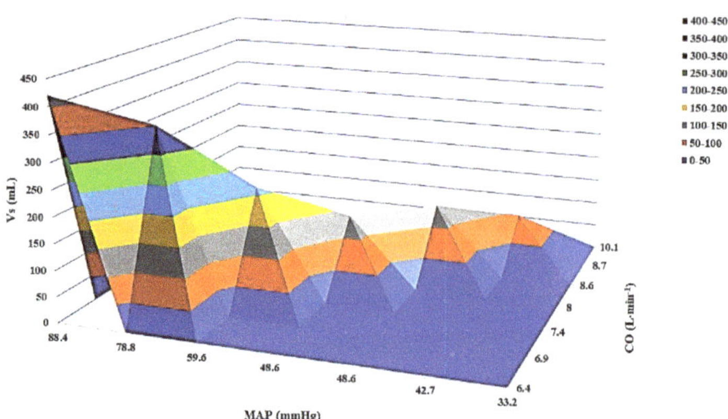

Figure 3. Three-dimensional surface plot showing the functional relationship between stressed volume, mean arterial pressure, and cardiac output during progression of hyperdynamic septic shock. The decrease in stressed volume was the result of progressive vasodilation and was not affected by changes in cardiac output, which increased in an effort to maintain tissue perfusion during progression of shock. Vs, stressed volume; MAP, mean arterial pressure; CO, cardiac output.

3.3. *Changes in Mean Circulatory Filling Pressure Analogue and Other Determinants of Venous Return during Septic Shock*

Mean circulatory filling pressure analogue decreased with time ($p < 0.001$), along with P_{RA} ($p < 0.001$) and R_{VR} ($p < 0.001$). The PG_{VR} also decreased, but the difference between time points was not statistically significant ($p = 0.934$). In addition, a statistically significant decrease in Eh was observed with time ($p < 0.001$).

3.4. *Effects of Fluid Challenges and Noradrenaline on Determinants of Venous Return*

In total, 30 mL·kg^{-1} were administered within the first three hours from diagnosis of septic shock. The infusion of the first 50 mL of isotonic sodium chloride increased MAP from 61 mmHg to 64 mmHg (5%) and *Vs* from 221 mL to 243 mL (10%). However, neither this nor the subsequent amount of isotonic sodium chloride significantly affected hemodynamics, implying an increase in *Vu* and *Vr* (Table 2, Figure 4).

Table 2. Effect of fluid challenges on hemodynamic variables.

	2 h (100 mL)		3 h (300 mL)		4 h (200 mL)		
	Before	After	Before	After	Before	After	*p*-Value
Heart rate (beat·min^{-1})	140 (15)	126 (7)	138 (4)	137 (6)	148 (12)	148 (9)	1
MAP (mmHg)	61 (11)	64 (6)	46 (5)	46 (6)	45 (7)	45 (4)	1
CO (L·min^{-1})	7.1 (2)	7.3 (2)	7.9 (2)	8 (2)	8.5 (2)	8.6 (2)	0.79
SVR (dynes·sec·cm^{-5})	629 (14)	642 (8)	424 (16)	420 (11)	386 (24)	381 (17)	0.98
P_{RA} (mmHg)	5.2 (0.2)	5.4 (0.5)	4.1 (0.3)	4 (0.2)	4 (0.4)	4 (0.5)	1
Pmca (mmHg)	11.6 (0.4)	12 (0.3)	10.4 (0.8)	10.3 (0.2)	10.6 (0.3)	10.6 (0.3)	1
PG_{VR} (mmHg)	6.4 (0.5)	6.6 (0.2)	6.3 (0.2)	6.3 (0.3)	6.6 (0.3)	6.6 (0.1)	1
R_{VR} (mmHg·min·L^{-1})	0.9 (0.1)	0.9 (0.2)	0.8 (0.2)	0.8 (0.3)	0.8 (0.2)	0.8 (0.2)	1
Eh	0.55 (0.02)	0.55 (0.03)	0.61 (0.01)	0.61 (0.01)	0.62 (0.01)	0.62 (0.01)	1
Vs (mL)	221	243	119	119	119	119	0.962

Values are expressed as mean (SD). MAP, mean arterial pressure; CO, cardiac output; SVR, systemic vascular resistance; P_{RA}, right atrial pressure; Pmca, mean circulatory filling pressure analog; PG_{VR}, pressure gradient for venous return; R_{VR}, resistance to venous return; Eh, efficiency of the heart.

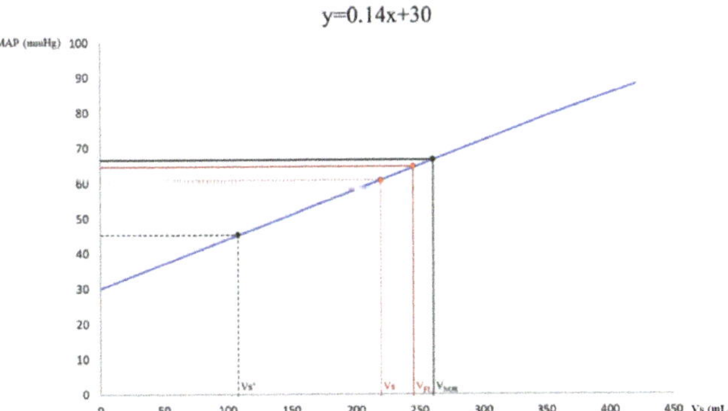

Figure 4. Effect of fluid challenge and noradrenaline on stressed volume. After infusion of 50 mL of isotonic sodium chloride, MAP increased from 61 mmHg to 64 mmHg and Vs increased from 221 mL to 243 mL (V_{FL}). After noradrenaline infusion, MAP increased from 45 mmHg to 66 mmHg and Vs increased from 107 mL (Vs') to 257 mL (V_{NOR}). MAP, mean arterial pressure; Vs, stressed volume before fluid infusion; V_{FL}, stressed volume after fluid infusion; Vs', stressed volume before noradrenaline infusion; V_{NOR}, stressed volume after noradrenaline infusion.

On the contrary, noradrenaline increased *Vs* from 107 mL to 257 mL (140%) and MAP from 45 mmHg to 66 mmHg (47%). In addition, most systemic hemodynamic variables and determinants of venous return significantly improved after the onset of noradrenaline infusion (Table 3, Figure 4).

Table 3. Effect of noradrenaline on hemodynamic variables.

	Before	After	*p*-Value
Heart rate (beat·min^{-1})	147 (8)	119 (9)	<0.001
MAP (mmHg)	45 (5)	66 (1)	<0.001
CO (L·min^{-1})	8 (2)	8.6 (2)	0.510
SVR (dynes·sec·cm^{-5})	410 (11)	572 (9)	<0.001
P_{RA} (mmHg)	4 (0.2)	4.5 (0.1)	<0.001
Pmca (mmHg)	10.3 (0.3)	11.9 (0.2)	<0.001
PG_{VR} (mmHg)	6.3 (0.1)	7.4 (0.1)	<0.001
R_{VR} (mmHg·min·L^{-1})	0.8 (0.2)	0.9 (0.1)	0.174
Eh	0.61 (0.01)	0.62 (0.01)	0.826
Vs (mL)	107	257	<0.001

Values are expressed as mean (SD). MAP, mean arterial pressure; CO, cardiac output; SVR, systemic vascular resistance; P_{RA}, right atrial pressure; Pmca, mean circulatory filling pressure analog; PG_{VR}, pressure gradient for venous return; R_{VR}, resistance to venous return; Eh, efficiency of the heart.

3.5. Measurement of Mean Circulatory Filling Pressure after Cardiac Arrest

Post-cardiac arrest Pmcf was 14.75 ± 1.5 mmHg. The change in Pmcf during the first minute after cardiac arrest is depicted in Table S2. Baseline Pmca and post-cardiac arrest Pmcf did not differ significantly (14.3 ± 1.23 mmHg vs. 14.75 ± 1.5 mmHg, $p = 0.24$), but the difference between pre-arrest Pmca and post-cardiac arrest Pmcf was statistically significant (9.5 ± 0.57 mmHg vs. 14.75 ± 1.5 mmHg, $p < 0.001$).

4. Discussion

The aim of this experimental study was to investigate the dynamic changes in *Vs* and other determinants of venous return during progression and resuscitation of hyperdynamic septic shock in a swine model that closely resembles human hemodynamics. The main findings of the present analysis are: (1) the baseline *Vs* was estimated at 420 mL and decreased by 7% for each mmHg decrease in MAP during progression of septic shock; (2) we revealed a new physiological volume existing at Ptm ≈ 0, the *Vr*, which has important physiological significance and cannot be mobilized without the use of an external vasopressor or without decreasing arterial and/or venous resistance; (3) during septic shock, Pmca, P_{RA}, R_{VR}, and Eh significantly decreased with time, while PG_{VR} also decreased but did not reach statistical significance; (4) fluid challenges (in total 30 mL·kg^{-1}) did not improve systemic parameters or determinants of venous return, while the infusion of noradrenaline significantly improved hemodynamics except for CO, Eh, and R_{VR}; and (5) post-cardiac arrest Pmcf did not differ significantly from baseline Pmca, but the difference between pre-arrest Pmca and post-cardiac arrest Pmcf was statistically significant. The present study investigated for the first time the dynamic changes in intravascular volumes and venous return during progression of sepsis to hyperdynamic septic shock and cardiac arrest, providing novel insights into the evolution of cardiovascular dynamics during the condition.

4.1. Estimation and Dynamic Changes in Stressed Volume

The evidence on *Vs* estimation in healthy state and sepsis is limited. Ogilvie et al. reported mean *Vs* values of 812 mL (43% of TBV), 952 mL (50% of TBV), and 1148 mL (60% of TBV) for three different ways of inducing circulatory arrest [37]. A model-based computation method of *Vs* from a preload reduction maneuver reported an average *Vs* of 486 mL (22.4% of TBV) in swine [41]. Studies in dogs using the capacity vessel pressure–volume relationship demonstrated *Vs* ranging between 322–653 mL (15–45% of TBV) [42–44]. In humans, *Vs* was determined by extrapolating the mean systemic filling pressure (Pmsf, i.e., Pmcf excluding the cardiopulmonary compartment)–volume curve to zero pressure intercept after inspiratory holds and arm stop-flow maneuvers and was estimated to be 1265 mL (≈30% of the predicted TBV) [45]. In another study with postoperative cardiac surgery patients, *Vs* was estimated with inspiratory hold maneuvers at 1677 mL (26% of TBV) [46]. The differences in *Vs* can be explained by the physiological characteristics of species and the method used for its estimation.

In the present experimental study, *Vs* was estimated at 420 mL and had decreased by 17% after 60 min from the onset of sepsis (no fluid challenges up to this time point), and by 50% after 120 min from the onset of sepsis (100 mL of isotonic sodium chloride had been infused but did not affect *Vs*). Murphy et al. used a three-chambered cardiovascular system model to identify *Vs* in swine and reported that it decreased by 29% after 30–40 min from the infusion of *E. coli* endotoxin [47]. However, 500 mL of saline solution had been administered before endotoxin infusion. Additionally, in a canine model of *E. coli* endotoxin shock, Uemura et al. reported a decrease in *Vs* of 50% after the end of 60 min endotoxin infusion [48]. In either case, it is important to remember that *Vs* and *Vu* are virtual values, not separated, and they change their names and function depending on Ptm at every moment [11]. Nevertheless, the aforementioned data suggest that research on the dynamic changes in *Vs* may lead to distinct shock phenotypes requiring distinct hemodynamic management. Considering the close resemblance between the Landrace–Large White swine and human hemodynamics, this species seems suitable for studying venous return and its determinants in steady and shock states [9,15,49,50].

4.2. Conceptual Approach and Characteristics of Rest Volume

One of the most significant findings to emerge from this study is the identification of *Vr* as the volume that cannot be mobilized/converted without the use of an external vasopressor or without decreasing arterial and/or venous resistance, e.g., by decreasing the dose of pure α-adrenergic agonists, such as phenylephrine. The utilization of *Vr* in research and clinical practice is extremely intriguing and helpful. Brengelmann has proposed the same term for the volume (*Vu*) beyond which further addition (in volume) would result in stretching of the vessel walls (distending volume or *Vs*) [51]. However, our analyses show that *Vr* is different from *Vu*, although they both exist at Ptm ≈ 0. In normal conditions, *Vu* can be mobilized, if required, but *Vr* cannot be without external intervention. In particular, *Vr* seems to have dual main functions at the steady state, i.e., to prevent an increase in venous resistance and maintain critical closing pressure, which is the pressure below which small vessels collapse and effective capillary blood flow ceases. As critical closing pressure is related to vascular tone, the *Vr* exerts the peripheral venous pressure required to sustain a vasomotor reflex, resulting in the maintenance of critical closing pressure [52,53]. Indeed, there is evidence showing that profound arterial hypotension during prolonged septic shock may be associated with a drastic increase in venous resistance, especially within the distal part of the splanchnic vasculature [11,54,55]. The aforementioned characteristics of *Vr* mandate that it should not be iatrogenically deranged or should be only minimally affected, even in patients with shock. A severe derangement of *Vr* could explain the devastating effects of exogenous adrenergic agonists, especially when administered in hypovolemic individuals and/or at high doses.

In our animals, the evolving vasoplegia decreased *Vs* until cardiac arrest occurred (*Vs* = 0 mL, *Vu* = 860 mL, *Vr* = 540 mL). In severe septic shock with low *Vs*, the use of exogenous vasopressors may not be sufficient to completely convert the increased amount of *Vu* (baseline *Vu* plus the converted part of *Vs*) to *Vs*, implying an increase in *Vr* (baseline *Vr* plus part of *Vu* that is not converted to *Vs*) and thus a lower *Vc*. In such a case, increasing vasopressor doses will result in arterial vasoconstriction, increased exit resistance from the arterial compartment, and decreased capillary perfusion [11,56]. In clinical practice, this may be the appropriate time along the pathophysiologic continuum of sepsis/septic shock at which fluid infusion will improve *Vs*, CO, and tissue perfusion.

Based on the aforementioned characteristics of *Vr*, a drug that stimulates both the α- and β-adrenergic receptors is expected to more effectively maintain systemic hemodynamics than one that activates either α- or β-adrenergic receptors [17]. Indeed, administration of norepinephrine causes arterial and venous constriction and dilatation of the splanchnic vasculature (decreasing splanchnic sequestration at low to moderate doses), which enhance the conversion of *Vu* to *Vs* and facilitate flow through the splanchnic system [11,57], and therefore can improve venous return in patients with septic shock [58].

4.3. Dynamic Changes in Mean Circulatory Filling Pressure and Other Determinants of Venous Return

Accurate data on Pmcf in septic patients are also scarce. A meta-analysis investigating the effects of vasopressor-induced hemodynamic changes in adults with shock reported that vasopressor infusion increased Pmsf analogue (Pmsa) from 16 $\pm$ 3.3 mmHg to 18 $\pm$ 3.4 mmHg, but had variable effects on central venous pressure, Eh, and CO [59]. Guarracino et al. estimated Pmsa in septic shock patients at admission and after resuscitation with fluid and norepinephrine at 13.0 $\pm$ 1.4 mmHg and 15.2 $\pm$ 1.8 mmHg, respectively, with a PG_{VR} of 6.2 $\pm$ 0.8 mmHg [60]. In both Guarracino's study and our own, fluid resuscitation probably caused hemodilution that decreased and/or prevented an increase in R_{VR} [61–65]. In another study using inspiratory hold maneuvers in septic patients, Pmsf was found to be 26–33 mmHg, depending on the rate of norepinephrine infusion [57]. In the latter study, however, inspiratory holds may have overestimated zero-flow measurements [33]. Of note, Lee et al. investigated the hemodynamic changes in splenectomized dogs after *E. coli* endotoxin infusion and reported an increase in CO concomitantly with a decrease in MAP and Pmsa; however, volume loading (20 mL·kg^{-1}) significantly increased Pmsa above baseline values [31]. The improvement in Pmsa can be explained by the pre-endotoxin splenectomy, which prevents volume loss in canine models [65,66]. In the present study, only the first 50 mL of isotonic sodium chloride had a slight effect on MAP, CO, Pmca, and PG_{VR} (R_{VR} and Eh did not change), but neither these nor the total amount of administered fluids (30 mL·kg^{-1}) significantly improved hemodynamics. In addition, post-cardiac arrest Pmcf was 14.75 $\pm$ 1.5 mmHg in our animals, which was similar to their baseline Pmca, but significantly higher than the Pmca value before the onset of cardiac arrest, implying an increase in *Vu* and *Vr*. In humans, Pmcf measured one minute after death from septic shock was 12.7 $\pm$ 5.7 mmHg [67], which is similar to our post-cardiac arrest value. Despite the reported inadequacies in calculating Pmca [37], our findings support its use as a functional hemodynamic monitoring variable to track changes in Pmcf over time, coupling it with other functional hemodynamic parameters in the normal state and septic shock [31,68]. Most especially, the difference between the pre-arrest Pmca and post-cardiac arrest (equilibrium) Pmcf in the present study further strengthens the importance of *Vr* and its characteristics in the healthy state and disease state, as previously discussed in this section.

4.4. Clinical Implications

Although the clinical and pathophysiological understanding of septic shock has progressed in the previous decades, many questions still exist. Fluid resuscitation in septic shock is an effective intervention to increase venous return; however, timely fluid resuscitation is critical, and many patients do not respond to treatment [69–71]. Administration of fluids is based on the available static and dynamic methods, yet it may also result in overtreatment and organ injury. On the other hand, vasopressor administration can improve systemic hemodynamics, but may not always improve tissue perfusion and may result in adverse effects as well.

The present study revealed the hourly decrease in *Vs* during hyperdynamic septic shock, which increases our understanding of sepsis-induced vasoplegia. As the currently available methods for assessing fluid responsiveness have limitations [72–75], the use of *Vs* may further support the assessment of the procedure in patients with septic shock. Moreover, our findings can aid in the decision to start vasopressor support according to the decrease in vasomotor tone, a common characteristic of sepsis-related hypotension. Assessment of *Vs* can be also helpful in starting vasopressors simultaneously with fluids or following a very limited fluid resuscitation, which can improve Pmcf/Pmca, venous return, and CO, and decrease net fluid balance, incidence of complications, and mortality [76–80].

In addition, our analysis identified a new circulatory volume, the *Vr*. This volume cannot be mobilized/converted without the use of an external vasopressor or without decreasing arterial and/or venous resistance. The *Vr* seems to have a dual function, i.e., to prevent an increase in venous resistance and maintain critical closing pressure. These findings suggest that fluid management and administration of vasopressors in patients with shock should be considered only if they do not affect or minimally affect the *Vr*. The *Vr* seems extremely important for maintaining hemodynamic homeostasis both in the steady state and disease state.

The present study provides a deeper physiological understanding of hyperdynamic septic shock and new information on how to optimize fluid administration and the use of vasoactive drugs within an individualized treatment strategy. Furthermore, our findings may help in identifying novel phenotypes of septic shock patients.

4.5. Strengths and Limitations

The major strength of this experimental study was the resemblance of the hemodynamic and biochemical/metabolic changes during hyperdynamic septic shock between Landrace–Large White swine and humans [9,81]. We acknowledge that this experiment was performed on 10 healthy normovolemic swine and that the use of anesthetics may have affected their response to stress. Nevertheless, the hemodynamic changes during the progression of septic shock were robust. In addition, the present post hoc analysis included only female Landrace–Large White piglets. Furthermore, we did not address the effect of pulsatility on Pmca. However, the oscillations in P_{RA} during the cardiac cycle and vascular buffering minimize this effect [32,33].

5. Conclusions

The baseline *Vs* was estimated at 420 mL and decreased by 7% for each mmHg decrease in MAP during progression of hyperdynamic septic shock. Significant changes were also observed in other determinants of venous return. A new physiological intravascular volume existing at Ptm ≈ 0 was identified, termed as *Vr*, which cannot be mobilized/converted without vasopressor support or without decreasing arterial and/or venous resistance.

Supplementary Materials: The following supporting information can be downloaded at: https://www.mdpi.com/xxx/s1. Figure S1: Total blood volume in a 20-kg swine; Table S1: Metabolic changes in animals during progression of sepsis and septic shock; Table S2: Mean circulatory filling pressure after cardiac arrest.

Author Contributions: Conceptualization, A.C.; methodology, A.C.; software, A.C., E.L. and N.P.; validation, A.C., E.L., N.P., V.S., E.K., K.T. and T.X.; formal analysis, A.C., E.L. and N.P.; investigation, A.C., V.S. and T.X.; resources, A.C., E.K. and T.X.; data curation, A.C., E.L., N.P., V.S., E.K., K.T. and T.X.; writing—original draft preparation, A.C.; writing—review and editing, A.C., E.L., N.P., V.S., E.K., K.T. and T.X.; visualization, A.C. and N.P.; supervision, A.C.; project administration, A.C. and T.X.; funding acquisition, T.X. All authors have read and agreed to the published version of the manuscript.

Funding: This research received no external funding.

Institutional Review Board Statement: This was a post hoc analysis. The original protocol was approved by the General Directorate of Veterinary Services (license No. 26, 10 January 2012) according to the national legislation regarding ethical and experimental procedures. These procedures conformed to the guidelines from Directive 2010/63/EU of the European Parliament on the protection of animals used for scientific purposes or the current National Institutes of Health guidelines. The manuscript adheres to the applicable ARRIVE 2.0 and Minimum Quality Threshold in Pre-Clinical Sepsis Studies (MQTiPSS) guidelines.

Informed Consent Statement: Not applicable.

Data Availability Statement: Data can be made available upon request after publication through a collaborative process. Researchers should provide a methodically sound proposal with specific objectives in an approval proposal. Please contact the corresponding author for additional information.

Acknowledgments: We would like to thank A. Zacharioudaki, E. Karampela, K. Tsarea, M. Karamperi, N. Psychalakis, A. Karaiskos, S. Gerakis and E. Gerakis, staff members of the E.R.C.E., for their assistance during the experiments. Athanasios Chalkias would also like to thank Simon Gelman, Vandam/Covino of Anaesthesia, Brigham and additionally Women's Hospital, Harvard Medical School, Boston, USA, for his outstanding contribution and significant impact on the specialty of anesthesia and cardiovascular physiology.

Conflicts of Interest: The authors declare no conflict of interest.

Short Biography of Authors

Athanasios Chalkias is an asst. professor of anesthesiology at the Faculty of Medicine of the University of Thessaly, Greece. His clinical activity and research are dedicated to anesthesiology, intensive care, cardiovascular dynamics, translational physiology, and resuscitation. His main areas of interest include hemodynamic management of high-risk patients having surgery and of critically ill patients, venous return, heart–lung interactions, hemodynamic coherence, microcirculation, oxygen transport to tissue, shock, and advanced hemodynamic support. Prof. Chalkias is the Co-Chair of the Scientific Writing & Task Forces Subcommittee and a member of the Committee on Research of the Society of Critical Care Anesthesiologists, a member of the Guidelines Committee and the Critical Emergency Medicine-Trauma and Resuscitation Subcommittee of the European Society of Anaesthesiology and Intensive Care, an active member of the Outcomes Research Consortium, USA, a member of the Council on Basic Cardiovascular Science of the European Society of Cardiology, and the Treasurer and Chair of the Committee on Shock of the Hellenic Society of Cardiopulmonary Resuscitation. LinkedIn profile: https://www.linkedin.com/in/athanasios-chalkias-835b7845/

References

1. Gelman, S.; Bigatello, L. The physiologic basis for goal-directed hemodynamic and fluid therapy: The pivotal role of the venous circulation. *Can. J. Anaesth.* **2018**, *65*, 294–308. [CrossRef] [PubMed]
2. Chien, S.; Chang, C.; Dellenback, R.J.; Usami, S.; Gregersen, M.I. Hemodynamic changes in endotoxin shock. *Am. J. Physiol.* **1966**, *210*, 1401–1410. [CrossRef] [PubMed]
3. Pinsky, M.R.; Matuschak, G.M. Cardiovascular determinants of the hemodynamic response to acute endotoxemia in the dog. *J. Crit. Care* **1986**, *1*, 18–31. [CrossRef]

4. Teule, G.J.; den Hollander, W.; Bronsveld, W.; Koopman, P.A.; Bezemer, P.D.; Heidendal, G.A.; Thijs, L.G. Effect of volume loading and dopamine on hemodynamics and red-cell redistribution in canine endotoxin shock. *Circ. Shock.* **1983**, *10*, 41–50. [PubMed]
5. Stephan, F.; Novara, A.; Tournier, B.; Maillet, J.M.; London, G.M.; Safar, M.E.; Fagon, J.Y. Determination of total effective vascular compliance in patients with sepsis syndrome. *Am. J. Respir. Crit. Care Med.* **1998**, *157*, 50–56. [CrossRef]
6. Funk, D.J.; Jacobsohn, E.; Kumar, A. Role of the venous return in critical illness and shock: Part II-shock and mechanical ventilation. *Crit. Care Med.* **2013**, *41*, 573–579. [CrossRef]
7. Marik, P.E.; Weinmann, M. Optimizing fluid therapy in shock. *Curr. Opin. Crit. Care* **2019**, *25*, 246–251. [CrossRef]
8. Marik, P.E.; Farkas, J.D. The Changing Paradigm of Sepsis: Early Diagnosis, Early Antibiotics, Early Pressors, and Early Adjuvant Treatment. *Crit. Care Med.* **2018**, *46*, 1690–1692. [CrossRef]
9. Chalkias, A.; Spyropoulos, V.; Koutsovasilis, A.; Papalois, A.; Kouskouni, E.; Xanthos, T. Cardiopulmonary Arrest and Resuscitation in Severe Sepsis and Septic Shock: A Research Model. *Shock* **2015**, *43*, 285–291. [CrossRef]
10. Xanthos, T.; Lelovas, P.; Vlachos, I.; Tsirikos-Karapanos, N.; Kouskouni, E.; Perrea, D.; Dontas, I. Cardiopulmonary arrest and resuscitation in Landrace/Large White swine: A research model. *Lab. Anim.* **2007**, *41*, 353–362. [CrossRef]
11. Gelman, S. Venous Circulation: A Few Challenging Concepts in Goal-Directed Hemodynamic Therapy (GDHT). In *Perioperative Fluid Management*; Farag, E., Kurz, A., Troianos, C., Eds.; Springer Nature: Cham, Switzerland, 2020; pp. 365–385.
12. Rothe, C.F. Mean circulatory filling pressure: Its meaning and measurement. *J. Appl. Physiol.* **1985**, *1993*, 499–509. [CrossRef] [PubMed]
13. Gelman, S. Venous function and central venous pressure: A physiologic story. *Anesthesiology* **2008**, *108*, 735–748. [CrossRef] [PubMed]
14. Magder, S. Volume and its relationship to cardiac output and venous return. *Crit. Care* **2016**, *20*, 271. [CrossRef] [PubMed]
15. Chalkias, A.; Koutsovasilis, A.; Laou, E.; Papalois, A.; Xanthos, T. Measurement of mean systemic filling pressure after severe hemorrhagic shock in swine anesthetized with propofol-based total intravenous anesthesia: Implications for vasopressor-free resuscitation. *Acute. Crit. Care* **2020**, *35*, 93–101. [CrossRef] [PubMed]
16. Magder, S.; De Varennes, B. Clinical death and the measurement of stressed vascular volume. *Crit. Care Med.* **1998**, *26*, 1061–1064. [CrossRef] [PubMed]
17. Gelman, S.; Mushlin, P.S. Catecholamine-induced changes in the splanchnic circulation affecting systemic hemodynamics. *Anesthesiology* **2004**, *100*, 434–439. [CrossRef] [PubMed]
18. National Centre for the Replacement, Refinement & Reduction of Animals in Research. The 3Rs. Available online: https://www.nc3rs.org.uk/the-3rs (accessed on 10 February 2022).
19. Percie du Sert, N.; Ahluwalia, A.; Alam, S.; Avey, M.T.; Baker, M.; Browne, W.J.; Clark, A.; Cuthill, I.C.; Dirnagl, U.; Emerson, M.; et al. Reporting animal research: Explanation and elaboration for the ARRIVE guidelines 2.0. *PLoS Biol.* **2020**, *18*, e3000411. [CrossRef]
20. Osuchowski, M.F.; Ayala, A.; Bahrami, S.; Bauer, M.; Boros, M.; Cavaillon, J.M.; Chaudry, I.H.; Coopersmith, C.M.; Deutschman, C.; Drechsler, S.; et al. Minimum quality threshold in pre-clinical sepsis studies (MQTiPSS): An international expert consensus initiative for improvement of animal modeling in sepsis. *Intensive Care Med. Exp.* **2018**, *6*, 26. [CrossRef]
21. National Research Council. *Guide for the Care and Use of Laboratory Animals*, 8th ed.; The National Academies Press: Washington, DC, USA, 2011.
22. Swindle, M.M.; Vogler, G.A.; Fulton, L.K.; Marini, R.P.; Popilskis, S. Preanaesthesia, anesthesia, analgesia and euthanasia. In *Laboratory Animal Medicine*, 2nd ed.; Fox, J.G., Anderson, L.C., Loew, F.M., Quimby, F.W., Eds.; Academic Press: New York, NY, USA, 2002; pp. 955–1003.
23. Dellinger, R.P.; Levy, M.M.; Rhodes, A.; Annane, D.; Gerlach, H.; Opal, S.M.; Sevransky, J.E.; Sprung, C.L.; Douglas, I.S.; Jaeschke, R.; et al. Surviving sepsis campaign: International guidelines for management of severe sepsis and septic shock: 2012. *Crit. Care Med.* **2013**, *41*, 580–637. [CrossRef]
24. Wodack, K.H.; Graessler, M.F.; Nishimoto, S.A.; Behem, C.R.; Pinnschmidt, H.O.; Punke, M.A.; Monge-García, M.I.; Trepte, C.J.C.; Reuter, D.A. Assessment of central hemodynamic effects of phenylephrine: An animal experiment. *J. Clin. Monit. Comput.* **2019**, *33*, 377–384. [CrossRef]
25. Parkin, G.; Wright, C.; Bellomo, R.; Boyce, N. Use of a mean systemic filling pressure analogue during the closed-loop control of fluid replacement in continuous hemodiafiltration. *J. Crit. Care* **1994**, *9*, 124–133. [CrossRef]
26. Parkin, W.G. Volume state control—A new approach. *Crit. Care Resusc.* **1999**, *1*, 311–321. [PubMed]
27. Parkin, W.G.; Leaning, M.S. Therapeutic control of the circulation. *J. Clin. Monit. Comput.* **2008**, *22*, 391–400. [CrossRef] [PubMed]
28. Pellegrino, V.A.; Mudaliar, Y.; Gopalakrishnan, M.; Horton, M.D.; Killick, C.J.; Parkin, W.G.; Playford, H.R.; Raper, R.F. Computer based haemodynamic guidance system is effective and safe in management of postoperative cardiac surgery patients. *Anaesth. Intensive. Care* **2011**, *39*, 191–201. [CrossRef] [PubMed]
29. Meijs, L.P.B.; van Houte, J.; Conjaerts, B.C.M.; Bindels, A.J.G.H.; Bouwman, A.; Houterman, S.; Bakker, J. Clinical validation of a computerized algorithm to determine mean systemic filling pressure. *J. Clin. Monit. Comput.* **2022**, *36*, 191–198. [CrossRef] [PubMed]
30. Wijnberge, M.; Sindhunata, D.P.; Pinsky, M.R.; Vlaar, A.P.; Ouweneel, E.; Jansen, J.R.; Veelo, D.P.; Geerts, B.F. Estimating mean circulatory filling pressure in clinical practice: A systematic review comparing three bedside methods in the critically ill. *Ann. Intensive. Care* **2018**, *8*, 73. [CrossRef]

31. Lee, J.M.; Ogundele, O.; Pike, F.; Pinsky, M.R. Effect of acute endotoxemia on analog estimates of mean systemic pressure. *J. Crit. Care* **2013**, *28*, 880.e9–880.e15. [CrossRef] [PubMed]
32. Berger, D.; Moller, P.W.; Takala, J. Reply to "Letter to the editor: Why persist in the fallacy that mean systemic pressure drives venous return?". *Am. J. Physiol. Heart. Circ. Physiol.* **2016**, *311*, H1336–H1337. [CrossRef]
33. Berger, D.; Moller, P.W.; Weber, A.; Bloch, A.; Bloechlinger, S.; Haenggi, M.; Sondergaard, S.; Jakob, S.M.; Magder, S.; Takala, J. Effect of PEEP, blood volume, and inspiratory hold maneuvers on venous return. *Am. J. Physiol. Heart. Circ. Physiol.* **2016**, *311*, H794–H806. [CrossRef]
34. He, H.; Yuan, S.; Long, Y.; Liu, D.; Zhou, X.; Ince, C. Effect of norepinephrine challenge on cardiovascular determinants assessed using a mathematical model in septic shock: A physiological study. *Ann. Transl. Med.* **2021**, *9*, 561. [CrossRef]
35. Guyton, A.C.; Polizo, D.; Armstrong, G.G. Mean circulatory filling pressure measured immediately after cessation of heart pumping. *Am. J. Physiol.* **1954**, *179*, 261–267. [CrossRef] [PubMed]
36. Chalkias, A.; Xanthos, T. Pathophysiology and pathogenesis of post-resuscitation myocardial stunning. *Heart. Fail. Rev.* **2012**, *17*, 117–128. [CrossRef] [PubMed]
37. Ogilvie, R.I.; Zborowska-Sluis, D.; Tenaschuk, B. Measurement of mean circulatory filling pressure and vascular compliance in domestic pigs. *Am. J. Physiol.* **1990**, *258*, H1925–H1932. [CrossRef] [PubMed]
38. Schipke, J.D.; Heusch, G.; Sanii, A.P.; Gams, E.; Winter, J. Static filling pressure in patients during induced ventricular fibrillation. *Am. J. Physiol. Heart. Circ. Physiol.* **2003**, *285*, H2510–H2515. [CrossRef] [PubMed]
39. Fessler, H.E.; Brower, R.G.; Wise, R.A.; Permutt, S. Effects of positive end-expiratory pressure on the gradient for venous return. *Am. Rev. Respir. Dis.* **1991**, *143*, 19–24. [CrossRef]
40. Jellinek, H.; Krenn, H.; Oczenski, W.; Veit, F.; Schwarz, S.; Fitzgerald, R.D. Influence of positive airway pressure on the pressure gradient for venous return in humans. *J. Appl. Physiol.* **2000**, *88*, 926–932. [CrossRef]
41. Pironet, A.; Desaive, T.; Geoffrey Chase, J.; Morimont, P.; Dauby, P.C. Model-based computation of total stressed blood volume from a preload reduction manoeuvre. *Math. Biosci.* **2015**, *265*, 28–39. [CrossRef]
42. Drees, J.A.; Rothe, C.F. Reflex venoconstriction and capacity vessel pressure-volume relationships in dogs. *Circ. Res.* **1974**, *34*, 360–373. [CrossRef]
43. Rothe, C.F.; Drees, J.A. Vascular capacitance and fluid shifts in dogs during prolonged hemorrhagic hypotension. *Circ. Res.* **1976**, *38*, 347–356. [CrossRef]
44. Ogilvie, R.I.; Zborowska-Sluis, D. Effect of chronic rapid ventricular pacing on total vascular capacitance. *Circulation* **1992**, *85*, 1524–1530. [CrossRef]
45. Maas, J.J.; Pinsky, M.R.; Aarts, L.P.; Jansen, J.R. Bedside assessment of total systemic vascular compliance, stressed volume, and cardiac function curves in intensive care unit patients. *Anesth. Analg.* **2012**, *115*, 880–887. [CrossRef] [PubMed]
46. Maas, J.J.; Geerts, B.F.; van den Berg, P.C.; Pinsky, M.R.; Jansen, J.R. Assessment of venous return curve and mean systemic filling pressure in postoperative cardiac surgery patients. *Crit. Care Med.* **2009**, *37*, 912–918. [CrossRef] [PubMed]
47. Murphy, L.; Davidson, S.; Chase, J.G.; Knopp, J.L.; Zhou, T.; Desaive, T. Patient-Specific Monitoring and Trend Analysis of Model-Based Markers of Fluid Responsiveness in Sepsis: A Proof-of-Concept Animal Study. *Ann. Biomed. Eng.* **2020**, *48*, 682–694. [CrossRef] [PubMed]
48. Uemura, K.; Kawada, T.; Zheng, C.; Li, M.; Sugimachi, M. Computer-controlled closed-loop drug infusion system for automated hemodynamic resuscitation in endotoxin-induced shock. *BMC Anesthesiol.* **2017**, *17*, 145. [CrossRef]
49. Kontouli, Z.; Staikou, C.; Iacovidou, N.; Mamais, I.; Kouskouni, E.; Papalois, A.; Papapanagiotou, P.; Gulati, A.; Chalkias, A.; Xanthos, T. Resuscitation with centhaquin and 6% hydroxyethyl starch 130/0.4 improves survival in a swine model of hemorrhagic shock: A randomized experimental study. *Eur. J. Trauma. Emerg. Surg.* **2019**, *45*, 1077–1085. [CrossRef]
50. Chalkias, A.; Spyropoulos, V.; Georgiou, G.; Laou, E.; Koutsovasilis, A.; Pantazopoulos, I.; Kolonia, K.; Vrakas, S.; Papalois, A.; Demeridou, S.; et al. Baseline Values and Kinetics of IL-6, Procalcitonin, and TNF-α in Landrace-Large White Swine Anesthetized with Propofol-Based Total Intravenous Anesthesia. *BioMed Res. Int.* **2021**, *2021*, 6672573. [CrossRef]
51. Brengelmann, G.L. Venous return and the physical connection between distribution of segmental pressures and volumes. *Am. J. Physiol. Heart. Circ. Physiol.* **2019**, *317*, H939–H953. [CrossRef]
52. Girling, F. Critical closing pressure and venous pressure. *Am. J. Physiol.* **1952**, *171*, 204–207. [CrossRef]
53. Thiele, R.H.; Nemergut, E.C.; Lynch, C., 3rd. The physiologic implications of isolated alpha(1) adrenergic stimulation. *Anesth. Analg.* **2011**, *113*, 284–296. [CrossRef]
54. Bressack, M.A.; Morton, N.S.; Hortop, J. Group B streptococcal sepsis in the piglet: Effects of fluid therapy on venous return, organ edema, and organ blood flow. *Circ. Res.* **1987**, *61*, 659–669. [CrossRef]
55. Ayuse, T.; Brienza, N.; Revelly, J.P.; O'Donnell, C.P.; Boitnott, J.K.; Robotham, J.L. Alternations in liver hemodynamics in an intact porcine model of endotoxin shock. *Am. J. Physiol.* **1995**, *268*, H1106–H1114. [CrossRef]
56. Thiele, R.H.; Nemergut, E.C.; Lynch, C., 3rd. The clinical implications of isolated alpha1 adrenergic stimulation. *Anesth. Analg.* **2011**, *113*, 297–304. [CrossRef] [PubMed]
57. Persichini, R.; Silva, S.; Teboul, J.L.; Jozwiak, M.; Chemla, D.; Richard, C.; Monnet, X. Effects of norepinephrine on mean systemic pressure and venous return in human septic shock. *Crit. Care Med.* **2012**, *40*, 3146–3153. [CrossRef] [PubMed]

58. Evans, L.; Rhodes, A.; Alhazzani, W.; Antonelli, M.; Coopersmith, C.M.; French, C.; Machado, F.R.; Mcintyre, L.; Ostermann, M.; Prescott, H.C.; et al. Surviving Sepsis Campaign: International Guidelines for Management of Sepsis and Septic Shock 2021. *Crit. Care Med.* **2021**, *49*, e1063–e1143. [CrossRef]
59. Åneman, A.; Wilander, P.; Zoerner, F.; Lipcsey, M.; Chew, M.S. Vasopressor Responsiveness Beyond Arterial Pressure: A Conceptual Systematic Review Using Venous Return Physiology. *Shock.* **2021**, *56*, 352–359.
60. Guarracino, F.; Bertini, P.; Pinsky, M.R. Cardiovascular determinants of resuscitation from sepsis and septic shock. *Crit. Care* **2019**, *23*, 118. [CrossRef] [PubMed]
61. Blain, C.M.; Anderson, T.O.; Pietras, R.J.; Gunnar, R.M. Immediate hemodynamic effects of gram-negative vs gram-positive bacteremia in man. *Arch. Intern. Med.* **1970**, *126*, 260–265. [CrossRef] [PubMed]
62. Kumar, A.; Haery, C.; Parrillo, J.E. Myocardial dysfunction in septic shock: Part I. Clinical manifestation of cardiovascular dysfunction. *J. Cardiothorac. Vasc. Anesth.* **2001**, *15*, 364–376. [CrossRef]
63. MacLean, L.D.; Mulligan, W.G.; McLean, A.P.; Duff, J.H. Patterns of septic shock in man—A detailed study of 56 patients. *Ann. Surg.* **1967**, *166*, 543–562. [CrossRef]
64. Weil, M.H.; Nishjima, H. Cardiac output in bacterial shock. *Am. J. Med.* **1978**, *64*, 920–922. [CrossRef]
65. Chien, S.; Dellenback, R.J.; Usami, S.; Treitel, K.; Chang, C.; Gregersen, M.I. Blood volume and its distribution in endotoxin shock. *Am. J. Physiol.* **1966**, *210*, 1411–1418. [CrossRef] [PubMed]
66. Teule, G.J.; Kester, A.D.; Bezemer, P.D.; Thijs, L.J.; Heidendal, G.A. Hepatic trapping of red cells in canine endotoxin shock: A variable phenomenon after splenectomy. *Cardiovasc. Res.* **1985**, *19*, 201–205. [CrossRef] [PubMed]
67. Repessé, X.; Charron, C.; Fink, J.; Beauchet, A.; Deleu, F.; Slama, M.; Belliard, G.; Vieillard-Baron, A. Value and determinants of the mean systemic filling pressure in critically ill patients. *Am. J. Physiol. Heart. Circ. Physiol.* **2015**, *309*, H1003–H1007. [CrossRef] [PubMed]
68. Pinsky, M.R.; Payen, D. Functional hemodynamic monitoring. *Crit. Care* **2005**, *9*, 566–572. [CrossRef]
69. Toscani, L.; Aya, H.D.; Antonakaki, D.; Bastoni, D.; Watson, X.; Arulkumaran, N.; Rhodes, A.; Cecconi, M. What is the impact of the fluid challenge technique on diagnosis of fluid responsiveness? A systematic review and meta-analysis. *Crit. Care* **2017**, *21*, 207. [CrossRef]
70. Guarracino, F.; Bertini, P.; Pinsky, M.R. Heterogeneity of cardiovascular response to standardized sepsis resuscitation. *Crit. Care* **2020**, *24*, 99. [CrossRef] [PubMed]
71. Hernandez, G.; Ospina-Tascon, G.A.; Damiani, L.P.; Estenssoro, E.; Dubin, A.; Hurtado, J.; Friedman, G.; Castro, R.; Alegria, L.; Teboul, J.L.; et al. Effect of a Resuscitation Strategy Targeting Peripheral Perfusion Status vs Serum Lactate Levels on 28-Day Mortality among Patients with Septic Shock: The ANDROMEDA-SHOCK Randomized Clinical Trial. *JAMA.* **2019**, *321*, 654–664. [CrossRef]
72. Monnet, X.; Marik, P.E.; Teboul, J.L. Prediction of fluid responsiveness: An update. *Ann. Intensive. Care* **2016**, *6*, 111. [CrossRef]
73. Vincent, J.L.; Cecconi, M.; De Backer, D. The fluid challenge. *Crit. Care* **2020**, *24*, 703. [CrossRef]
74. Shi, R.; Monnet, X.; Teboul, J.L. Parameters of fluid responsiveness. *Curr. Opin. Crit. Care* **2020**, *26*, 319–326. [CrossRef]
75. Vignon, P.; Repesse, X.; Begot, E.; Leger, J.; Jacob, C.; Bouferrache, K.; Slama, M.; Prat, G.; Vieillard-Baron, A. Comparison of echocardiographic indices used to predict fluid responsiveness in ventilated patients. *Am. J. Respir. Crit. Care Med.* **2017**, *195*, 1022–1032. [CrossRef] [PubMed]
76. Ospina-Tascon, G.A.; Teboul, J.L.; Hernandez, G.; Alvarez, I.; Sanchez-Ortiz, A.I.; Calderon-Tapia, L.E.; Manzano-Nunez, R.; Quinones, E.; Madrinan-Navia, H.J.; Ruiz, J.E.; et al. Diastolic shock index and clinical outcomes in patients with septic shock. *Ann. Intensive. Care* **2020**, *10*, 41. [CrossRef] [PubMed]
77. Colon Hidalgo, D.; Patel, J.; Masic, D.; Park, D.; Rech, M.A. Delayed vasopressor initiation is associated with increased mortality in patients with septic shock. *J. Crit. Care* **2020**, *55*, 145–148. [CrossRef] [PubMed]
78. Ospina-Tascon, G.A.; Hernandez, G.; Alvarez, I.; Calderon-Tapia, L.E.; Manzano-Nunez, R.; Sanchez-Ortiz, A.I.; Quinones, E.; Ruiz-Yucuma, J.E.; Aldana, J.L.; Teboul, J.L.; et al. Effects of very early start of norepinephrine in patients with septic shock: A propensity score-based analysis. *Crit. Care* **2020**, *24*, 52. [CrossRef] [PubMed]
79. Permpikul, C.; Tongyoo, S.; Viarasilpa, T.; Trainarongsakul, T.; Chakorn, T.; Udompanturak, S. Early use of norepinephrine in septic shock resuscitation (CENSER): A randomized trial. *Am. J. Respir. Crit. Care Med.* **2019**, *199*, 1097–1105. [CrossRef] [PubMed]
80. Li, Y.; Li, H.; Zhang, D. Timing of norepinephrine initiation in patients with septic shock: A systematic review and meta-analysis. *Crit. Care* **2020**, *24*, 488. [CrossRef]
81. Pecchiari, M.; Pontikis, K.; Alevrakis, E.; Vasileiadis, I.; Kompoti, M.; Koutsoukou, A. Cardiovascular Responses During Sepsis. *Compr. Physiol.* **2021**, *11*, 1605–1652.

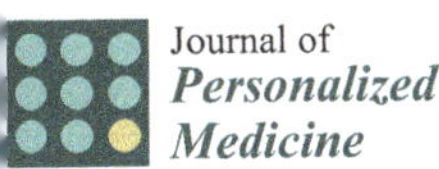
Journal of
Personalized
Medicine

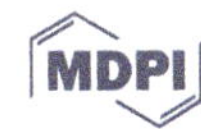

Article

Effects of Iloprost on Arterial Oxygenation and Lung Mechanics during One-Lung Ventilation in Supine-Positioned Patients: A Randomized Controlled Study

Kyuho Lee [1,2], Mina Kim [3], Namo Kim [1,2], Su Jeong Kang [1] and Young Jun Oh [1,2,*]

1 Department of Anesthesiology and Pain Medicine, Yonsei University College of Medicine, Seoul 03722, Korea; theoneimlee@yuhs.ac (K.L.); namo@yuhs.ac (N.K.); kangsuda@yuhs.ac (S.J.K.)
2 Anesthesia and Pain Research Institute, Yonsei University College of Medicine, Seoul 03722, Korea
3 Department of Anesthesiology and Pain Medicine, Dongguk University Ilsan Hospital, Goyang-si 10326, Gyeonggi-do, Korea; exrexr20@gmail.com
* Correspondence: yjoh@yuhs.ac; Tel.: +82-2-2228-2428

Abstract: Patients undergoing one-lung ventilation (OLV) in the supine position face an increased risk of intraoperative hypoxia compared with those in the lateral decubitus position. We hypothesized that iloprost (ILO) inhalation improves arterial oxygenation and lung mechanics. Sixty-four patients were enrolled and allocated to either the ILO or control group ($n = 32$ each), to whom ILO or normal saline was administered. The partial pressure of the arterial oxygen/fraction of inspired oxygen (PaO_2/FiO_2) ratio, dynamic compliance, alveolar dead space, and hemodynamic variables were assessed 20 min after anesthesia induction with both lungs ventilated (T1) and 20 min after drug nebulization in OLV (T2). A linear mixed model adjusted for group and time was used to analyze repeated variables. While the alveolar dead space remained unchanged in the ILO group, it increased at T2 in the control group ($n = 30$ each) ($p = 0.002$). No significant differences were observed in the heart rate, mean blood pressure, PaO_2/FiO_2 ratio, or dynamic compliance in either group. Selective ILO nebulization was inadequate to enhance oxygenation parameters during OLV in the supine position. However, it favorably affected alveolar ventilation during OLV in supine-positioned patients without adverse hemodynamic effects.

Keywords: one-lung ventilation; supine position; iloprost; oxygenation; lung mechanics

Citation: Lee, K.; Kim, M.; Kim, N.; Kang, S.J.; Oh, Y.J. Effects of Iloprost on Arterial Oxygenation and Lung Mechanics during One-Lung Ventilation in Supine-Positioned Patients: A Randomized Controlled Study. *J. Pers. Med.* **2022**, *12*, 1054. https://doi.org/10.3390/jpm12071054

Academic Editors: Ioannis Pantazopoulos and Ourania S. Kotsiou

Received: 15 June 2022
Accepted: 26 June 2022
Published: 27 June 2022

Publisher's Note: MDPI stays neutral with regard to jurisdictional claims in published maps and institutional affiliations.

1. Introduction

One-lung ventilation (OLV) is an essential part of thoracic anesthesia which allows access to the surgical field [1]. However, inevitable development of intrapulmonary shunt during OLV makes the maintenance of adequate oxygenation a major issue for this ventilation technique [2]. Arterial oxygenation during OLV is affected by the distribution of pulmonary perfusion to the ventilated and non-ventilated lungs [3]. Hypoxemia induced by collapse of one lung activates hypoxic pulmonary vasoconstriction, which reduces intrapulmonary shunt by redirecting pulmonary perfusion to the well-ventilated lung [4].

Along with hypoxic pulmonary vasoconstriction, body position may further affect the distribution of pulmonary perfusion [3]. Most thoracic surgeries are performed in the lateral decubitus position, and gravity induces better perfusion of the lower, ventilated lung than that of the upper, non-ventilated lung [3]. However, surgeries involving the anterior mediastinum often require OLV in the supine position, in which favorable gravitational modulation of pulmonary perfusion cannot be anticipated [5]. Hence, patients scheduled for these surgeries face an increased risk of hypoxemia during OLV [6].

Iloprost (ILO) is a prostacyclin analogue, and inhalation of the drug induces vasodilation in the well-ventilated areas of the lung with little effect on systemic circulation [7]. Hence, recent studies have investigated the capability of ILO as a potential rescue drug for hypoxia during OLV, and demonstrated that selective ILO nebulization to the ventilated lung improved arterial oxygenation and lung mechanics in pulmonary resections [8–10]. However, whether ILO would provide similar effects during OLV in the supine position is not known. Hence, we hypothesized that ILO would improve arterial oxygenation and lung mechanics in patients scheduled for anterior mediastinal mass excision and investigated the effects of ILO in this cohort.

2. Materials and Methods

2.1. Study Population

This prospective, randomized, controlled study included patients scheduled for video-assisted thoracoscopic anterior mediastinal mass excision between July 2021 and March 2022 and adhered to the Consolidated Standards of Reporting Trials (CONSORT) guidelines. The study was approved by the Institutional Review Board of Severance Hospital, Yonsei University Health System, Seoul, Korea (IRB, no. 4-2021-0694) and was registered at Clinicaltrials.gov (NCT 04927039). After IRB approval, written informed consent was obtained from all participants involved in the study, and the study methods were performed in accordance with the relevant guidelines and regulations. The inclusion criteria were as follows: (1) scheduled for video-assisted thoracoscopic mediastinal mass excision requiring OLV, (2) aged between 20 and 80 years, and (3) American Society of Anesthesiologists physical status class between II and III. The exclusion criteria included morbid obesity, heart failure (New York Heart Association class III or IV), arrhythmia, and severe hepatic, renal or pulmonary diseases.

2.2. Anesthetic Management

Anesthesia was induced using propofol (1.0–2.0 mg/kg), remifentanil (0.5–1.0 μg/kg), and rocuronium (0.8–1.0 mg/kg). Patients were intubated with left-sided double-lumen endobronchial tubes (DLT) (VentiBronc^{TM} Anchor; Flexicare Medical Ltd., Mountain Ash, UK). A fiberoptic bronchoscope was used to confirm the correct position of the DLT before the OLV was provided. The radial artery was cannulated for continuous pressure monitoring and arterial blood gas analysis. Mechanical ventilation was provided using autoflow pressure-controlled ventilation mode (Primus®; Dräger Medical, Lubeck, Germany). The fraction of inspired oxygen (FiO_2) was set at 0.6. The tidal volume was adjusted to 6 mL/kg, and a positive end-expiratory pressure (PEEP) of 5 mm Hg was applied. The respiratory rate was adjusted to maintain the end-tidal carbon dioxide ($etCO_2$) at the range of 35–40 mmHg. Anesthesia was maintained with 1.0–2.0 vol% sevoflurane and 0.1–0.3 μg/kg/min remifentanil, and the depth of anesthesia was assessed using a Sedline® brain function monitor (Masimo, Irvine, CA, USA). The rate of intravenous fluid administration was set at a rate of 3 mL/kg/h, and additional fluid was administered to compensate for intraoperative blood loss.

After anesthesia induction, OLV was initiated. Carbon dioxide (CO_2) insufflation was initiated on the operating side of the thorax by the surgeon with a pressure limit of 10 mmHg and a flow rate of 4 L/min. Vasoactive drugs, such as phenylephrine, were administered if systolic blood pressure (SBP) fell below 80 mmHg. In cases of desaturation (saturation of percutaneous oxygen [SpO_2] < 95%), the FiO_2 level increased by 0.2 up to 1.0.

2.3. Study Design and Outcome Measurements

All enrolled patients were randomly allocated to either the ILO or the control group using a randomized sequence, and surgeons and anesthesiologists were blinded to the group allocation. After the initiation of OLV, ILO (20 μg (2 mL, Ventavis®; Bayer AG, Leverkusen, Germany) was administered to the ILO group. ILO was mixed with normal saline (3 mL) and aerosolized using an ultrasonic nebulizer (Aerogen® Pro; Aerogen Ltd., Galway, Ireland), which was connected to the inspiratory limb of the ventilator system. A comparable volume (5 mL) of normal saline was nebulized to the control group in the same manner. The medications were nebulized for 20 min.

The study time points were as follows: (1) 20 min after anaesthesiainduction with both lungs ventilated (T1) and (2) 20 min after ILO or normal saline nebulization in OLV (T2). Respiratory and hemodynamic parameters were recorded and arterial blood samples were collected during each study period. Respiratory parameters included FiO_2, $etCO_2$, partial pressure of arterial oxygen (PaO_2), the ratio of PaO_2 to FiO_2 (PaO_2/FiO_2), alveolar dead space, and dynamic compliance. A blood gas analyzer (GEM® Premier 4000; Instrumentation Laboratory, Lexington, MA, USA) was used to obtain PaO_2 and the partial pressure of arterial carbon dioxide ($PaCO_2$). Dead space ventilation was calculated according to the Hardman and Aitkenhead equation as follows: ($1.135 \times (PaCO_2 - etCO_2)/PaCO_2 - 0.005$) [11]. Dynamic compliance was calculated using the following equation: (tidal volume/(plateau airway pressure-PEEP)). Hemodynamic parameters included the heart rate and arterial blood pressure. The incidence of intraoperative hypotension (SBP < 80 mmHg) and hypoxia (SpO_2 < 90%) after the initiation of drug administration was recorded.

2.4. Statistical Analysis

The primary outcome was the change in PaO_2/FiO_2 at 20 min at T2, and the secondary outcome was the change in other respiratory mechanics such as alveolar dead space and dynamic compliance. Considering the results of a previous study in which the difference in PaO_2/FiO_2 ratio was 30 mmHg with a standard deviation of 30 mmHg between patients who inhaled ILO and those who did not [9], a sample size of 27 participants per group was needed to achieve a power of 0.95 and an alpha level of 0.05. Assuming a 20% dropout rate, 32 patients were enrolled in each group.

The student's t-test was used to analyze continuous variables, and the Wilcoxon signed-rank test was used to analyze variables which did not meet normality. To compare categorical variables between the groups, chi-square test or Fisher's exact test was used. Repeated variables were analyzed using a linear mixed model with group and time and the interaction between groups and time as a fixed effect. Post hoc analysis with Bonferroni correction for within-group comparisons versus T1 and between-group comparisons versus T2 was performed for multiple comparisons. The results are expressed as mean ± standard deviation, median (interquartile range), or number (percentage). SPSS 25.0 software (IBM Corp., Armonk, NY, USA) was used for the statistical analyses, and $p < 0.05$ was considered statistically significant.

3. Results

Sixty-four patients scheduled for video-assisted thoracoscopic mediastinal mass excision were enrolled in this study (Figure 1). Two patients in the ILO group were excluded because of patient refusal, and two in the control group were excluded as the measurement protocol could not be properly executed owing to the short operation time. Hence, the data of 30 patients in each group were analyzed.

Intergroup comparisons of the preoperative variables between the two groups are shown in Table 1. Age, sex, height, weight, body mass index, and ASA classification were similar between groups. The incidence of hypertension and diabetes mellitus, history of cigarette smoking, incidence of pulmonary abnormalities according to preoperative computed tomography, and variables derived from preoperative spirometry were also comparable between the groups, except for FEV_1.

Intraoperative data are presented in Table 2. All variables, including the side of the operation, anesthesia time, operation time, OLV time, incidence of intraoperative hypotension, hypoxia, fluid intake, urine output, and estimated blood loss during surgery, were comparable between the two groups, with the exception of the incidence of FiO_2 elevation, which was more frequent in the control group ($p = 0.006$).

Data regarding hemodynamics and lung mechanics are presented in Table 3. No clinically relevant differences were observed between the two groups at T1. At T2, PaO_2, PaO_2/FiO_2 ratio, and dynamic compliance of the two groups were significantly decreased compared to those at T1; however, no statistical significance was observed in the linear mixed-model analysis adjusted for group and time. Changes in heart rate, mean blood pressure, and $etCO_2$ were insignificant in both groups. While $PaCO_2$ and alveolar dead space remained unchanged in the ILO group, those of the control group were significantly increased at T2 ($p = 0.04$ and 0.002, respectively).

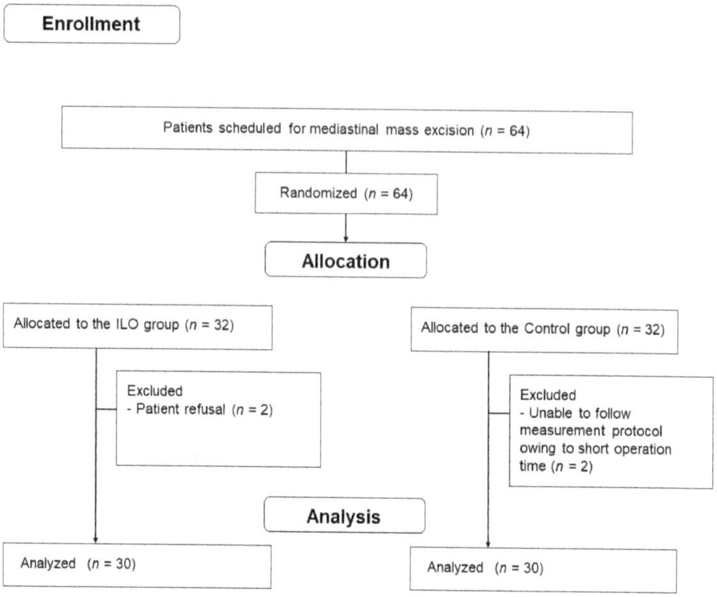

Enrollment

Patients scheduled for mediastinal mass excision ($n = 64$)

Randomized ($n = 64$)

Allocation

Allocated to the ILO group ($n = 32$)

Excluded
- Patient refusal ($n = 2$)

Allocated to the Control group ($n = 32$)

Excluded
- Unable to follow measurement protocol owing to short operation time ($n = 2$)

Analysis

Analyzed ($n = 30$)

Analyzed ($n = 30$)

Figure 1. Patient enrollment.

Table 1. Preoperative data.

	Control Group ($n = 30$)	ILO Group ($n = 30$)	p-Value
Age (yrs)	50 ± 12	53 ± 14	0.374
Women (n)	15 (50)	16 (53)	0.796
Height (cm)	164.4 ± 9.2	164.2 ± 11.1	0.923
Weight (kg)	67.9 ± 12.3	66.6 ± 13.9	0.705
Body mass index (kg/m^2)	24.9 ± 3.0	24.5 ± 3.4	0.622
ASA classification 2/3 (n)	28 (93)/2 (7)	26 (87)/4 (13)	0.389
Hypertension (n)	10 (33)	12 (40)	0.592
Diabetes mellitus (n)	2 (7)	5 (17)	0.228
Smoking history			
Ex-smoker or current smoker (n)	9 (30)	14 (47)	0.184
Smoking index (pack × years)	0 [0–11]	0 [0–10]	0.412
Preoperative chest CT			
Atelectasis (n)	1 (3)	4 (13)	0.161
Bronchiectasis (n)	1 (3)	3 (10)	0.301
Emphysema (n)	0 (0)	2 (7)	0.150
Bronchitis (n)	3 (10)	1 (3)	0.301
Preoperative spirometry			
FEV_1 (L)	2.9 ± 0.8	2.6 ± 1.1 *	0.037
FEV_1 (% predicted)	92 [85–96]	83 [75–94]	0.368
FVC (L)	3.6 ± 1.0	3.4 ± 1.2	0.569
FVC (% predicted)	89 [83–98]	88 [77–97]	0.276
FEV_1/FVC (%)	81 [76–84]	77 [72–81]	0.069

Data presented as mean ± standard deviation, number (%), or median [interquartile range]. ASA, American Society of Anesthesiologists; CT, computed tomography; FEV_1, forced expiratory volume in 1 s; FVC, forced vital capacity. * $p < 0.05$ vs. control group.

Table 2. Intraoperative data.

	Control Group (n = 30)	ILO Group (n = 30)	p-Value
Approach direction (right/left) (n)	16 (53)/14 (47)	15 (50)/15 (50)	0.796
Anesthesia time (min)	109 ± 32	116 ± 38	0.480
Operation time (min)	70 ± 29	76 ± 35	0.481
OLV time (min)	51 [42–66]	49 [40–61]	0.812
FiO_2 elevation (n)	9 (30)	1 (3) *	0.006
Hypoxia (n)	1 (3)	1 (3)	1.000
Hypotension (n)	14 (47)	13 (43)	0.795
Intake fluid (mL)	702 ± 259	700 ± 302	0.982
Urine output (mL)	25 ± 45	43 ± 71	0.254
Estimated blood loss (mL)	35 ± 20	34 ± 18	0.738

Data are presented as the mean ± standard deviation, number (%), or median (interquartile range). ILO, iloprost; OLV, one-lung ventilation; FiO_2, fraction of inspired oxygen; SpO_2, oxygen saturation (pulse oximetry); hypotensive event defined as the incidence of systolic blood pressure < 80 mmHg; hypoxic event defined as the incidence of SpO_2 < 90% requiring anesthetic intervention. * $p < 0.05$ vs. control group.

Table 3. Effects of iloprost on hemodynamics and lung mechanics.

	Control Group (n = 30)	ILO Group (n = 30)	p-Value
Heart rate (beat/min)			0.83
T1	72 ± 10	78 ± 14	
T2	74 ± 14	81 ± 12	
Mean blood pressure (mmHg)			0.95
T1	77 ± 11	80 ± 11	
T2	81 ± 12	85 ± 13	
PaO_2 (mmHg)			0.77
T1	253 ± 66	255 ± 68	
T2	108 ± 37 *	115 ± 45 *	
PaO_2/FiO_2 ratio (mmHg)			0.29
T1	422 ± 111	425 ± 113	
T2	156 ± 42 *	190 ± 75 *	
$EtCO_2$ (mmHg)			0.49
T1	39 ± 5	40 ± 4	
T2	40 ± 3	42 ± 5	
$PaCO_2$ (mmHg)			0.04
T1	43 ± 5	45 ± 5	
T2	48 ± 5 *	47 ± 6	
Alveolar dead space			0.002
T1	12 ± 12	12 ± 9	
T2	19 ± 6 *	11 ± 5	
Dynamic compliance (mL/cmH_2O)			0.41
T1	28 ± 5	27 ± 6	
T2	16 ± 3 *	16 ± 5 *	

Data are presented as the mean ± standard deviation. ILO, iloprost; T1, 20 min after initiation of two-lung ventilation; T2, 20 min after iloprost or saline administration; PaO_2, partial pressure of arterial oxygen; PaO_2/FiO_2 ratio, ratio of PaO_2 to fraction of inspired oxygen; $EtCO_2$, end-tidal carbon dioxide; $PaCO_2$, partial pressure of arterial carbon dioxide. p values in the rightmost column represent p group × time. * $p < 0.05$ vs. T1.

4. Discussion

In this study, we demonstrated that selective nebulization of ILO favorably affected alveolar ventilation in patients who underwent OLV in the supine position, with a significant difference in alveolar dead space observed between the ILO and control groups. However, ILO nebulization did not lead to a significant improvement in arterial oxygenation.

Inhaled ILO selectively dilates pulmonary terminal capillaries surrounded by alveoli, resulting in increased pulmonary blood flow in the well-ventilated areas of the lung [12]. Hence, the effects of ILO were recently investigated by anesthesiologists as a potential rescue drug for hypoxia during OLV in thoracic surgery [8–10]. Indeed, previous studies indicated that the selective ILO administration to the ventilated lung during OLV induced a decrease in ventilation/perfusion (V/Q) mismatch and improved oxygenation [8–10]. Yet these results were confined to patients who underwent pulmonary resection, which is performed in the lateral decubitus position. As the lateral position itself improves the V/Q match in OLV owing to gravitational forces reducing the shunt of the upper non-ventilated lung [3], it is reasonable to assume that patient positioning significantly contributed to enhanced lung mechanics and arterial oxygenation in these studies. However, it is not yet clear whether ILO would still demonstrate similar favorable effects in the OLV of supine-positioned patients, in whom favorable modulation of perfusion by gravity cannot be anticipated [5].

Our results indicate that ILO positively affected alveolar ventilation in the supine position, which is consistent with the results of previous studies [9,10]. While the $etCO_2$ of the two groups remained unchanged since we adjusted the respiratory rate to maintain the parameter at its target range throughout the measurement periods, significant increases were observed in $PaCO_2$ of the control group, leading to an increase in the alveolar dead space. In contrast, no significant change in the alveolar dead space was observed within the ILO group, indicating ameliorated alveolar ventilation induced by ILO.

Nonetheless, we did not observe a significant improvement in PaO_2 or the PaO_2/FiO_2 ratio in the ILO group. Indeed, some studies reported that ILO inhalation produced similar results in patients with pulmonary hypertension secondary to chronic obstructive pulmonary disease [13,14]. However, we speculate that in those studies, non-selective administration of ILO to patients with severe cardiopulmonary diseases may have induced vasodilation not only in well-ventilated areas but also in poorly ventilated areas of the lung, which would have aggravated the V/Q mismatch. However, most of our patients were classified as ASA II without severe cardiopulmonary diseases, and since we selectively administered ILO to the ventilated lung with the aid of a double-lumen endobronchial tube, unintended vasodilation of poorly ventilated areas of the lung seems unlikely. Rather, with gravity affecting both lungs equally in the supine position, we presume that the pharmacological vasodilation confined to the ventilated lung was inadequate to decrease the shunt induced in the non-ventilated lung. Nonetheless, it is notable that the number of patients who required FiO_2 elevation, which was triggered when SpO_2 fell below 95%, significantly differed between the two groups (one in the ILO group and nine in the control group), implying that ILO may have contributed to oxygenation. Given that the majority of our patients exhibited normal pulmonary function and successfully endured OLV without experiencing severe hypoxia, studies involving morbid patients with pulmonary diseases undergoing OLV in the supine position are warranted to further elucidate the impact of ILO on arterial oxygenation.

Evidence indicates that ILO administration may be associated with systemic vasodilation and inhibition of platelet aggregation [15]. Indeed, we frequently observed hypotension during OLV in both groups. However, the incidence was comparable between the groups, indicating that short-term ILO nebulization was not significantly associated with intraoperative hypotension. Considering that CO_2 was routinely insufflated in all cases to achieve a clear surgical view, we presume that induction of capnothorax may have contributed to the comparably high incidence of hypotension [16,17]. With regard to platelet function, the estimated blood loss was minor, and no significant difference was observed between the two groups, implying platelet inhibition induced by ILO to be negligible. Comprehensively, a short-term ILO nebulization seems less likely to be associated with intraoperative adverse events.

The limitations of the study are as follows: owing to the short operative time, the baseline measurement (T1) was inevitably performed during two-lung ventilation. The effects of ILO on arterial oxygenation may have been more clearly elucidated if all parameters could be measured during the OLV. However, pursuing such a measurement protocol would otherwise have compelled undesirable elongation of anesthesia time since mediastinal mass excision in our institution generally requires less than 50 min of OLV. In addition, we could not measure pulmonary shunts because pulmonary artery catheterization is not routinely performed during mediastinal mass excision.

5. Conclusions

In conclusion, selective ILO nebulization was inadequate to enhance the PaO_2/FiO_2 ratio in healthy, supine-positioned patients. Nonetheless, it positively affected alveolar ventilation without adverse hemodynamic effects and decreased the requirement for FiO_2 elevation during OLV. Whether ILO ameliorates arterial oxygenation in morbid patients remains to be proven in future studies.

Author Contributions: Conceptualization, K.L. and Y.J.O.; methodology, Y.J.O. and N.K.; software, K.L.; validation, Y.J.O. and M.K.; formal analysis, M.K. and S.J.K.; writing—original draft, K.L.; writing—review and editing, K.L., Y.J.O., M.K., S.J.K. and N.K.; visualization, S.J.K. and N.K.; supervision, Y.J.O.; project administration, N.K. All authors have read and agreed to the published version of the manuscript.

Funding: This research received no external funding.

Institutional Review Board Statement: The study was conducted in accordance with the Declaration of Helsinki, and approved by the Institutional Review Board of Severance Hospital, Yonsei University Health System, Seoul, Republic of Korea (IRB, no. 4-2021-0694), and was registered at Clinicaltrials.gov (NCT 04927039).

Informed Consent Statement: Written informed consent has been obtained from all participants involved in the study.

Data Availability Statement: Data are available from the corresponding author upon reasonable requests.

Conflicts of Interest: The authors declare no conflict of interest.

References

1. Campos, J.H. Current techniques for perioperative lung isolation in adults. *Anesthesiology* **2002**, *97*, 1295–1301. [CrossRef] [PubMed]
2. Campos, J.H.; Feider, A. Hypoxia During One-Lung Ventilation-A Review and Update. *J. Cardiothorac. Vasc. Anesth.* **2018**, *32*, 2330–2338. [CrossRef] [PubMed]
3. Wittenstein, J.; Scharffenberg, M.; Ran, X.; Zhang, Y.; Keller, D.; Tauer, S.; Theilen, R.; Chai, Y.; Ferreira, J.; Muller, S.; et al. Effects of Body Position and Hypovolemia on the Regional Distribution of Pulmonary Perfusion During One-Lung Ventilation in Endotoxemic Pigs. *Front. Physiol.* **2021**, *12*, 717269. [CrossRef] [PubMed]
4. Lumb, A.B.; Slinger, P. Hypoxic pulmonary vasoconstriction: Physiology and anesthetic implications. *Anesthesiology* **2015**, *122*, 932–946. [CrossRef] [PubMed]
5. Szegedi, L.L.; D'Hollander, A.A.; Vermassen, F.E.; Deryck, F.; Wouters, P.F. Gravity is an important determinant of oxygenation during one-lung ventilation. *Acta Anaesthesiol. Scand.* **2010**, *54*, 744–750. [CrossRef] [PubMed]
6. Rollin, A.; Mandel, F.; Grunenwald, E.; Mondoly, P.; Monteil, B.; Marcheix, B.; Maury, P. Hybrid surgical ablation for persistent or long standing persistent atrial fibrillation: A French single centre experience. *Ann. Cardiol. Angeiol.* **2020**, *69*, 86–92. [CrossRef] [PubMed]
7. Sawheny, E.; Ellis, A.L.; Kinasewitz, G.T. Iloprost improves gas exchange in patients with pulmonary hypertension and ARDS. *Chest* **2013**, *144*, 55–62. [CrossRef] [PubMed]
8. Choi, H.; Jeon, J.; Huh, J.; Koo, J.; Yang, S.; Hwang, W. The Effects of Iloprost on Oxygenation During One-Lung Ventilation for Lung Surgery: A Randomized Controlled Trial. *J. Clin. Med.* **2019**, *8*, 982. [CrossRef] [PubMed]
9. Kim, N.; Lee, S.H.; Joe, Y.; Kim, T.; Shin, H.; Oh, Y.J. Effects of Inhaled Iloprost on Lung Mechanics and Myocardial Function During One-Lung Ventilation in Chronic Obstructive Pulmonary Disease Patients Combined with Poor Lung Oxygenation. *Anesth. Analg.* **2020**, *130*, 1407–1414. [CrossRef]
10. Lee, K.; Oh, Y.J.; Kim, M.; Song, S.H.; Kim, N. Effects of Iloprost on Oxygenation during One-Lung Ventilation in Patients with Low Diffusing Capacity for Carbon Monoxide: A Randomized Controlled Study. *J. Clin. Med.* **2022**, *11*, 1542. [CrossRef]
11. Hardman, J.G.; Aitkenhead, A.R. Estimation of alveolar deadspace fraction using arterial and end-tidal CO_2: A factor analysis using a physiological simulation. *Anaesth. Intensive Care* **1999**, *27*, 452–458. [CrossRef] [PubMed]
12. Olschewski, H.; Simonneau, G.; Galie, N.; Higenbottam, T.; Naeije, R.; Rubin, L.J.; Nikkho, S.; Speich, R.; Hoeper, M.M.; Behr, J.; et al. Inhaled iloprost for severe pulmonary hypertension. *N. Engl. J. Med.* **2002**, *347*, 322–329. [CrossRef] [PubMed]
13. Boeck, L.; Tamm, M.; Grendelmeier, P.; Stolz, D. Acute effects of aerosolized iloprost in COPD related pulmonary hypertension—A randomized controlled crossover trial. *PLoS ONE* **2012**, *7*, e52248. [CrossRef]
14. Wang, L.; Jin, Y.Z.; Zhao, Q.H.; Jiang, R.; Wu, W.H.; Gong, S.G.; He, J.; Liu, J.M.; Jing, Z.C. Hemodynamic and gas exchange effects of inhaled iloprost in patients with COPD and pulmonary hypertension. *Int. J. Chronic Obstr. Pulm. Dis.* **2017**, *12*, 3353–3360. [CrossRef] [PubMed]

15. Liu, K.; Wang, H.; Yu, S.J.; Tu, G.W.; Luo, Z. Inhaled pulmonary vasodilators: A narrative review. *Ann. Transl. Med.* **2021**, *9*, 597. [CrossRef] [PubMed]
16. Jones, D.R.; Graeber, G.M.; Tanguilig, G.G.; Hobbs, G.; Murray, G.F. Effects of insufflation on hemodynamics during thoracoscopy. *Ann. Thorac. Surg.* **1993**, *55*, 1379–1382. [CrossRef]
17. Brock, H.; Rieger, R.; Gabriel, C.; Polz, W.; Moosbauer, W.; Necek, S. Haemodynamic changes during thoracoscopic surgery the effects of one-lung ventilation compared with carbon dioxide insufflation. *Anaesthesia* **2000**, *55*, 10–16. [CrossRef]

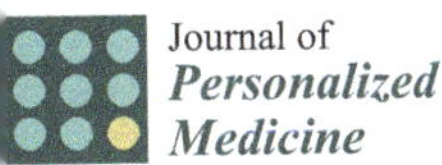
Journal of *Personalized Medicine*

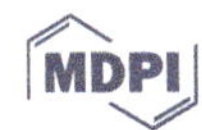

Article

Effect of General Anesthesia Maintenance with Propofol or Sevoflurane on Fractional Exhaled Nitric Oxide and Eosinophil Blood Count: A Prospective, Single Blind, Randomized, Clinical Study on Patients Undergoing Thyroidectomy

Artemis Vekrakou [1], Panagiota Papacharalampous [1], Helena Logotheti [2], Serena Valsami [3], Eriphyli Argyra [1], Ioannis Vassileiou [4] and Kassiani Theodoraki [1,*]

1 Department of Anaesthesiology, Aretaieion University Hospital, National and Kapodistrian University of Athens, 11528 Athens, Greece
2 Department of Anaesthesiology, Achillopouleion General Hospital of Volos, 38222 Magnesia, Greece
3 Hematology Laboratory—Blood Bank, Aretaieion University Hospital, National and Kapodistrian University of Athens, 11528 Athens, Greece
4 Second Department of Surgery, Aretaieion University Hospital, National and Kapodistrian University of Athens, 11528 Athens, Greece
* Correspondence: ktheod@med.uoa.gr

Citation: Vekrakou, A.; Papacharalampous, P.; Logotheti, H.; Valsami, S.; Argyra, E.; Vassileiou, I.; Theodoraki, K. Effect of General Anesthesia Maintenance with Propofol or Sevoflurane on Fractional Exhaled Nitric Oxide and Eosinophil Blood Count: A Prospective, Single Blind, Randomized, Clinical Study on Patients Undergoing Thyroidectomy. *J. Pers. Med.* **2022**, *12*, 1455. https://doi.org/10.3390/jpm12091455

Academic Editors: Ioannis Pantazopoulos and Ourania S. Kotsiou

Received: 11 August 2022
Accepted: 1 September 2022
Published: 5 September 2022

Abstract: Background: Nitric oxide (NO) is considered a means of detecting airway hyperresponsiveness, since even non-asthmatic patients experiencing bronchospasm intraoperatively or postoperatively display higher levels of exhaled NO. It can also be used as a non-invasive biomarker of lung inflammation and injury. This prospective, single-blind, randomized study aimed to evaluate the impact of two different anesthesia maintenance techniques on fractional exhaled nitric oxide (FeNO) in patients without respiratory disease undergoing total thyroidectomy under general anesthesia. **Methods:** Sixty patients without respiratory disease, atopy or known allergies undergoing total thyroidectomy were randomly allocated to receive either inhalational anesthesia maintenance with sevoflurane at a concentration that maintained Bispectral Index (BIS) values between 40 and 50 intraoperatively or intravenous anesthesia maintenance with propofol 1% targeting the same BIS values. FeNO was measured immediately preoperatively (baseline), postoperatively in the Postanesthesia Care Unit and at 24 h post-extubation with a portable device. Other variables measured were eosinophil blood count preoperatively and postoperatively and respiratory parameters intraoperatively. **Results:** Patients in both groups presented lower than baseline values of FeNO measurements postoperatively, which returned to baseline measurements at 24 h post-extubation. In the peripheral blood, a decrease in the percentage of eosinophils was demonstrated, which was significant only in the propofol group. Respiratory lung mechanics were better maintained in the propofol group as compared to the sevoflurane group. None of the patients suffered intraoperative bronchospasm. **Conclusions:** Both propofol and sevoflurane lead to the temporary inhibition of NO exhalation. They also seem to attenuate systemic hypersensitivity response by reducing the eosinophil count in the peripheral blood, with propofol displaying a more pronounced effect and ensuring a more favorable mechanical ventilation profile as compared to sevoflurane. The attenuation of NO exhalation by both agents may be one of the underlying mechanisms in the reduction in airway hyperreactivity. The clinical significance of this fluctuation remains to be studied in patients with respiratory disease.

Keywords: fractional exhaled NO; sevoflurane; propofol; eosinophil blood count; thyroidectomy

1. Introduction

Nitric oxide (NO) is a free radical in gas state, which plays an important role in a variety of processes relevant to respiratory physiology. The generation of NO follows both enzymatic and non-enzymatic pathways [1]. NO enzymatic production is catalyzed by three distinct isoforms of NO synthase: (i) neuronal NOS-1 (nNOS), mainly expressed in central and peripheral neurons, (ii) inducible NOS-2 (iNOS), expressed by many cell types as response to cytokines and other agents, and (iii) endothelial NOS-3 (eNOS), mostly expressed by endothelial cells. Non-enzymatic pathways, which are not clearly understood, produce NO through the reduction of NO_3 (nitrate) to NO_2 (nitrite) [2]. An imbalance between iNOS and its constitutive isoforms (nNOS and eNOS) has been implicated in the pathophysiology of many cardiopulmonary diseases, since it can lead to excessive NO synthesis [3]. While physiological levels of NO possess anti-inflammatory properties, when increased due to the aforementioned upregulation of iNOS, NO becomes a pro-inflammatory mediator [2,4]. In fact, high concentrations of NO can be transformed into peroxynitrite radicals in the presence of oxygen-derived free radicals and play a significant role in the cellular damage associated with overproduction of NO [5].

Airways of patients with bronchial hyperreactivity may respond in an exaggerated way to a variety of stimuli, while airway instrumentation in such patients may lead to life-threatening bronchospasm, adding to the burden of morbidity this population may suffer in case they undergo general anesthesia for a surgical or diagnostic procedure [6]. Fractional exhaled NO (FeNO) has been used in the diagnosis of asthma, especially of the eosinophilic phenotype, and has also proved useful in guiding treatment of asthmatic individuals [7,8]. Additionally, non-asthmatic patients experiencing bronchospasm intra-operatively or postoperatively display higher levels of exhaled NO, a fact suggesting that the upregulation of the production of NO may play a role in airway hyperreactivity [9]. Increased levels of FeNO have also been found to correlate with sputum eosinophilia and eosinophilia in bronchoalveolar lavage fluid [10,11]. Furthermore, an increase in exhaled NO concentration has been used as an early marker of lung inflammation and injury in models of sepsis or acute lung injury induced by toxins [12,13]. Therefore, exhaled NO can be considered an efficient method for the prediction of airway hyperresponsiveness perioperatively, even in patients without known respiratory disease [14]. Additionally, it may be considered as an invaluable non-invasive biomarker reflecting early airway injury and inflammation.

Propofol, an intravenous anesthetic agent, can modify NO production by inhibiting the inducible production of NO in lipopolysaccharide-stimulated macrophages [15,16]. It has also been shown to exert protective effects in acute lung injury in experimental models [17,18]. There is also evidence that some intravenous anesthetics can influence chemotaxis of eosinophils in vitro [19]. Similarly, volatile anesthetics have been shown to attenuate the expression of inflammatory mediators and to alleviate bronchial hyperresponsiveness [20]. Sevoflurane-borne protection could also be mediated via the suppression of the iNOS/NO pathway, as decreased levels of NO metabolites have been demonstrated in plasma or lung perfusate of sevoflurane-pretreated rat models [20,21].

The variation of exhaled NO and eosinophils in surgical patients undergoing anesthesia has not been studied before. We hypothesized that there is a different effect of intravenous and inhalational techniques on the potential for airway hyperresponsiveness perioperatively, as this can be assessed by the measurement of exhaled NO and eosinophil blood count. If this is the case, it could also affect the selection of anesthetic maintenance techniques for patients with known hyperreactive airways. Therefore, the aim of the present study was to investigate the differential impact of two general anesthesia maintenance techniques on the exhaled NO and eosinophil blood count of patients without respiratory disease or airway hyperreactivity.

2. Materials and Methods

2.1. Study Population

This is a prospective, single-blind, randomized, pragmatic trial, conducted between May 2014 and April 2018 in Aretaieion University Hospital, Athens, Greece. The protocol of the study was registered on www.clinicaltrials.gov (NCT02065635) (accessed on 30 April 2022). The study took place in compliance with the Helsinki Declaration, and its design was in accordance with the Consolidated Standards of Reporting Clinical Trials [22]. The study protocol was approved by the Ethics Committee of Aretaieion University Hospital, Aretaieion Hospital, National and Kapodistrian University of Athens, Chairperson Professor Ioannis Vasileiou on 19 December 2013 (B-19/19-12-2013).

After evaluating all eligible patients that were scheduled for thyroidectomy during this period, 60 patients were enrolled. Inclusion criteria were: age 18–75 years, all sexes, American Society of Anesthesiologists (ASA) physical status I-III, total thyroidectomy. Indications for thyroidectomy were: thyroid nodules, hyperthyroidism, substernal goiter, differentiated (papillary or follicular) thyroid cancer and medullary thyroid cancer. None of the patients presented with either clinical or radiological evidence for tracheomalacia. All patients were operated on by the same experienced surgeon and managed by the same anesthesiologist to avoid confounding. Exclusion criteria were: refusal or inability to consent due to language barriers or cognitive dysfunction, smoking, history of atopy, allergy, airway hyperresponsiveness or other respiratory disease, such as asthma and chronic obstructive pulmonary disease, contraindication to the administration of paracetamol, parecoxib or tramadol and treatment with nitrate medication. Informed consent for participation in the study was obtained at the preanesthetic visit.

Patients were randomized by a computer-generated list of random numbers (www.randomizer.org (accessed on 30 April 2022)) into two groups of different maintenance techniques: either inhalational anesthesia with sevoflurane (sevoflurane group) or continuous intravenous infusion of propofol 1% (propofol group).

2.2. Study Design and Anesthetic Management

On the operation day, patients undertook a fractional exhaled NO measurement using a portable analyzer of Nitric Oxide (NObreath®, Bedfont® Scientific Ltd., Maidstone, UK) during the preanesthetic visit (T_0). Patients had avoided the use of coffee during the last 12 h [23]. The NO measurement had to be performed at expiratory rates of 50 mL/s for 12 s and was expressed at parts per billion (ppb). If the patient exhaled outside the exhalation guidelines, the test failed. We complied with the American Thoracic Society suggestion for performance of two sequential measurements and calculation of their mean value for each patient [24]. Measurements with this portable analyzer have proven to be reliable in comparison to measurements performed with stationary analyzers [25].

On arrival to the operating room, standard monitoring (consisting of five-lead electrocardiography, pulse oximetry and non-invasive blood pressure measurement), peripheral nerve stimulator and Bispectral Index monitor (BIS) were applied. Additionally, intravenous access was secured and the first blood sample for eosinophil and polymorphonuclear leukocyte count was collected. All patients were premedicated with midazolam 0.02 mg/kg IV and received metoclopramide 10 mg and ranitidine 50 mg IV before induction. Anesthesia was induced with the same regimen in both groups: fentanyl 2 mcg/kg, propofol 2.5 mg/kg and rocuronium 0.8 mg/kg. When the BIS value was below 50 and the train of four (TOF) ratio was 0, direct laryngoscopy was performed, and the airway was secured with a flexible cuffed endotracheal tube of the appropriate size. Subsequently, capnography was applied, and the sevoflurane group was also monitored for minimum alveolar concentration (MAC). All patients were ventilated with protective lung ventilation with FiO_2: 0.4 on air mixture, a tidal volume of 6–8 mL/kg of the ideal body weight and a positive end-expiratory pressure (PEEP) of 5 cm H_2O. Partial pressure of end tidal CO_2 ($ETCO_2$) was maintained between 35–45 mmHg, while peak inspiratory pressure (Ppeak), plateau pressure (Ppl) and compliance were monitored.

Anesthesia maintenance was achieved either with a continuous infusion of propofol 1% (propofol group) or with sevoflurane (sevoflurane group) aiming at maintaining BIS values between 40 and 50. Muscle relaxation was maintained with bolus doses of rocuronium 0.3 mg/kg in order to maintain a TOF ratio < 3. The analgesic regimen consisted of fentanyl 3–5 mcg/kg/h, paracetamol 1 g, parecoxib 40 mg and tramadol 1 mg/kg intravenously. Intravenous ondansetron 4 mg was administered for postoperative nausea and vomiting prophylaxis approximately 30 min before recovery. Maintenance fluids were infused at a rate of 1 mL/kg/h.

During the operation, all parameters, such as heart rate (HR), systolic blood pressure (SBP), diastolic blood pressure (DBP), mean blood pressure (MAP), O_2 saturation (SpO_2), $ETCO_2$, Ppeak, Ppl, PEEP, compliance, MAC and BIS, were recorded every 10 min.

On surgery completion, propofol infusion or sevoflurane inhalation were discontinued, residual muscle blockade was reversed with sugammadex 2 mg/kg and patients were extubated when spontaneous breathing was resumed, the TOF ratio was >90%, and there was response to verbal commands.

Patients were transferred to the Post Anesthesia Care Unit (PACU), where the second blood sample for eosinophil and polymorphonuclear leukocyte count was collected. When patients scored >8 on the modified Aldrete score, the second measurement of exhaled NO was performed (T_1). As soon as patients scored >9 on the modified Aldrete score, with no postoperative nausea and vomiting, and a score < 3 on the pain Numeric Rating Scale (graded from 0: no pain to 10: worst pain imaginable), they were discharged from the PACU.

While on the ward, patients received paracetamol 1 g every 8 h, one dose of parecoxib (40 mg) and 1 mg/kg tramadol as rescue analgesia for acute pain.

At 24 h after the patients' extubation, a third measurement of exhaled NO was performed (T_2).

2.3. Study Endpoints

The primary endpoint of the study was to assess the alteration, if any, from the preoperative FeNO measurement (T_0) to the immediate postoperative FeNO measurement (T_1) in each group. Secondary outcomes of the study were the measurement of FeNO at 24 h after extubation (T_2) in each group, the variation of eosinophil and polymorphonuclear leukocyte blood count immediately postoperatively in each group and the variation of Ppeak, Ppl and compliance in each group.

2.4. Statistical Analysis

Prior to this study, we conducted a pilot study on 10 patients per group in order to estimate the needed sample size for the detection of a significant fluctuation in the measurements of exhaled NO from the preoperative to the postoperative status. We demonstrated a mean drop of 5.5 ppb in the exhaled NO in the 10 patients of the propofol group and a mean drop of 5.3 ppb in the 10 patients of the sevoflurane group from the preoperative to the postoperative period. Therefore, by considering an average change of 5.4 ppb from the preoperative to the postoperative period to be clinically meaningful, and by hypothesizing a standard deviation (SD) of change of 10 ppb, we calculated that 29 patients should be included in each group in order to detect such a change with a power of 0.80 and an alpha error of 0.05. We enrolled 30 patients in each group to allow for drop-outs. The Kolmogorov–Smirnoff test was used to test the normality of distributions of the investigated parameters. Comparisons of numeric data between the two groups were performed with the unpaired *t*-test or the Mann–Whitney U-test for independent samples, depending on whether the variables followed a normal or non-normal distribution. The chi-square test or Fisher's exact test, as appropriate, was used for comparisons of categorical data. Exhaled NO fluctuation in the two groups was analyzed by ANOVA for repeated measures and eosinophil and polymorphonuclear leukocyte variation within groups with the Wilcoxon signed rank test. Serial data (HR, SBP, DBP, MAP, SpO_2, $ETCO_2$, Ppeak, Ppl and compliance) were analyzed and compared between the two groups with a two-step summary measures technique [26]. Since there was variation in surgical times among patients, it was not deemed appropriate to compare mean values at every particular timepoint. In contrast, the area under the curve for values plotted against time was calculated for each patient, which was then divided by the number of recording points to provide one standardized value. Standardized data were then compared by intergroup analysis using unpaired *t*-test or Mann–Whitney U-test, as appropriate.

Data were expressed in terms of mean ± standard deviation (SD) or as median (25th–75th percentiles), depending on the normality of distributions for numeric variables and as number for categorical variables. For all statistical procedures, a value of $p < 0.05$ was considered statistically significant. Data were analyzed with IBM SPSS® V21.0 for Windows (IBM Corp. Released 2012. IBM SPSS Statistics for Windows, Version 21.0. Armonk, NY, USA: IBM Corp.).

3. Results

Seventy-one patients were scheduled for total thyroidectomy with the same surgeon between May 2014 and April 2018. Sixty-two of them met the inclusion criteria, and two of them declined participation in the study. Therefore, 60 patients were enrolled. One patient in the propofol group was complicated by recurrent laryngeal nerve damage and was unable to perform the FeNO measurement at T_1 and T_2. Two patients in the sevoflurane group were unable to cooperate in order to perform the FeNO measurement at T_1 (both of them) and at T_2 (one of them). Central, lateral or bilateral lymph node dissection was not indicated in any of the patients with malignant conditions. The flowchart of the study including patient enrollment, allocation and analysis is presented in Figure 1. Patients' demographics, surgery and anesthesia duration as well as baseline hemodynamic parameters were similar in the two groups (Table 1).

Table 1. Demographic and baseline hemodynamic characteristics of the two groups.

Variables	Propofol Group (n = 30)	Sevoflurane Group (n = 30)	p Value, Group Comparison
Sex (M/F)	5/25	4/26	1.000
ASA (I/II/III)	28/2/0	25/5/0	0.424
Age (years), mean ± SD	48.8 ± 12.0	49.3 ± 12.2	0.88
Weight (kg), mean ± SD	70.2 ± 13.9	76.1 ± 13.1	0.097
Height (cm), mean ± SD	164.7 ± 5.4	164.8 ± 5.9	0.910
Smoking status (non-smoker/ex-smoker/smoker)	30/0/0	26/4/0	0.117
Indication for surgery; Thyroid nodule/Hyperthyroidism/Substernal goiter/Thyroid cancer	8/6/11/5	12/1/9/8	0.153
Duration of surgery (min), median [IQR]	95.0 [75.0–105.0]	90.0 [75.0–105.0]	0.542
Duration of anesthesia, (min), median [IQR]	110.0 [90.0–130.0]	110.0 [100.0–120.0]	0.591
Baseline SBP (mmHg), mean ± SD	135.2 ± 21.1	137.1 ± 19.5	0.714
Baseline DBP (mmHg), mean ± SD	77.6 ± 8.1	74.2 ± 8.1	0.111
Baseline MAP (mmHg), mean ± SD	96.2 ± 11.3	93.7 ± 12.1	0.413
Baseline HR (bpm), mean ± SD	76.0 ± 8.7	78.6 ± 9.7	0.268

Abbreviations: SD, standard deviation; IQR, interquartile range; n, number; SBP, systolic arterial pressure; DBP, diastolic arterial pressure; MAP, mean arterial pressure; HR, heart rate.

Both propofol and sevoflurane groups displayed decreased NO exhalation postoperatively (T_1) in comparison to baseline values (T_0) (7.93 ± 0.70 vs. 12.86 ± 1.19 ppb, $p < 0.001$ for the propofol group and 9.39 ± 2.45 vs. 14.13 ± 3.31 ppb, $p < 0.001$ for the sevoflurane group). Twenty-four hours postoperatively (T_2), exhaled NO was no longer different from baseline in both the propofol and sevoflurane groups (12.83 ± 1.20 vs. 12.86 ± 1.19 ppb, $p = 0.964$ for the propofol group and 13.85 ± 2.85 vs. 14.13 ± 3.31 ppb, $p = 0.535$ for the sevoflurane group) (Figure 2).

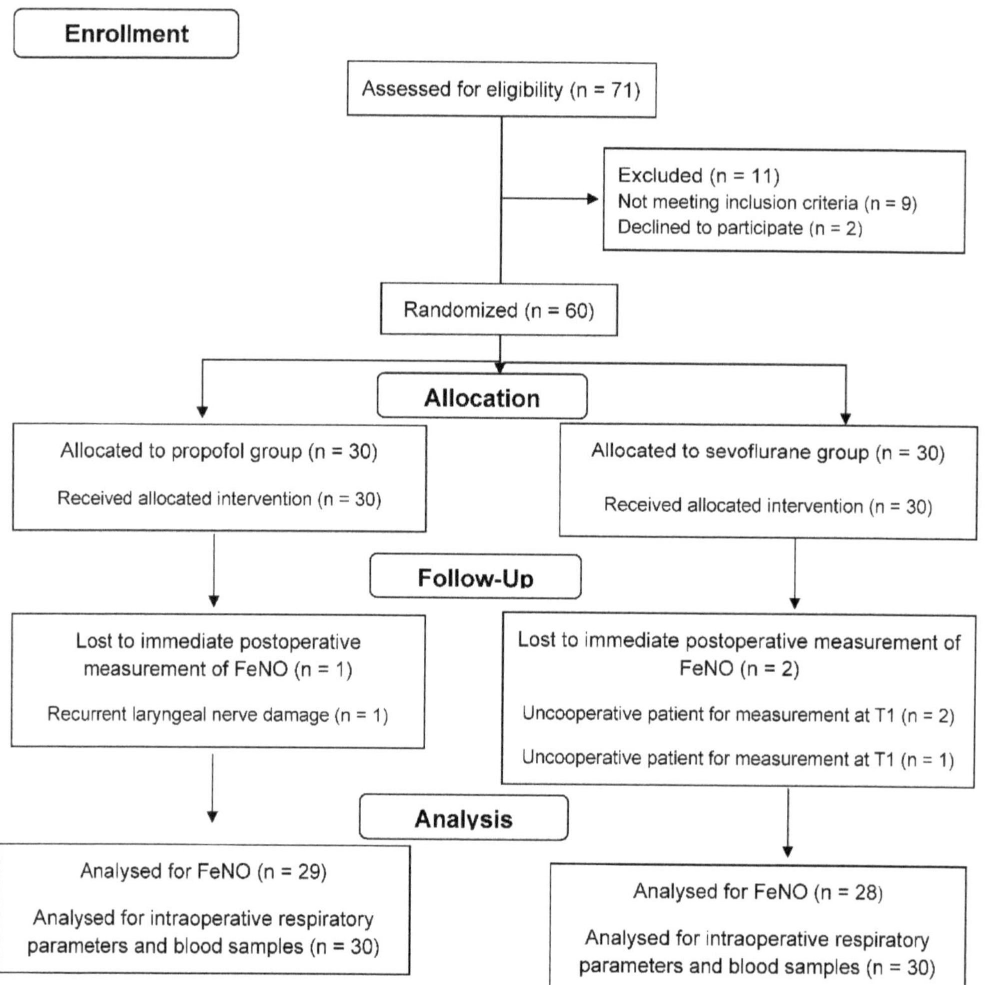

Figure 1. Study Flow Diagram.

In the peripheral blood, a significant decrease in the eosinophil count was demonstrated in the propofol group postoperatively in comparison to baseline values (93.0 [63.7–129.7] vs. 128.0 [76.7–179.7] $10^3/\mu L$, $p < 0.001$). There was no significant difference in the eosinophil blood count postoperatively in comparison to baseline values in the sevoflurane group (136.0 [75.0–267.0] vs. 157.0 [62.0–267.0] $10^3/\mu L$, $p = 0.746$) (Figure 3).

Additionally, there was a significant increase in the polymorphonuclear blood count postoperatively in comparison to baseline in both the propofol and sevoflurane groups (5023.0 [3740.2–6465.2] vs. 3743.0 [2940.2–4707.2] $10^3/\mu L$, $p < 0.001$ for the propofol group and 6863.0 [4665.5–10314.5] vs. 3705.0 [2842.0–5656.0] $10^3/\mu L$, $p < 0.001$ for the sevoflurane group) (Figure 4).

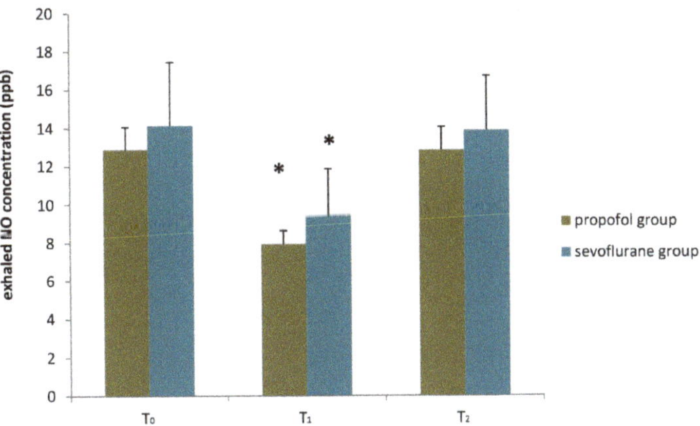

Figure 2. Exhaled NO fluctuation in the propofol and sevoflurane maintenance groups; * $p < 0.05$ in comparison to baseline (T_0).

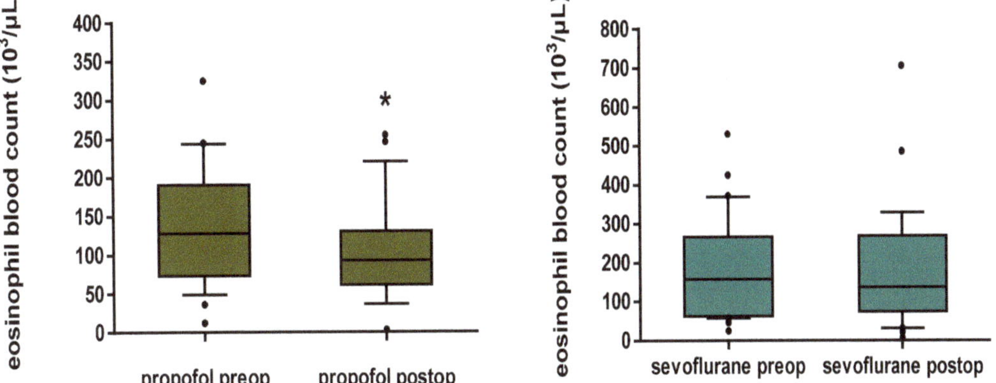

Figure 3. Box plots of eosinophil blood count in peripheral blood in the propofol and sevoflurane group preoperatively and postoperatively. Propofol maintenance caused a significant decrease in the eosinophil blood count ($p < 0.001$), while sevoflurane maintenance did not have a statistically significant effect ($p = 0.746$). The box plots depict the median and the interquartile range and the whiskers depict the 10th and 90th percentiles; * $p < 0.05$ in comparison to the preoperative status.

The propofol group presented with lower standardized Ppeak and Ppl over time versus the sevoflurane group (16.6 ± 4.3 vs. 18.8 ± 3.4 cm H_2O, $p = 0.032$ and 14.6 ± 4.2 vs. 16.6 ± 3.4 cm H_2O, $p = 0.054$, respectively) and higher standardized compliance over time (42.4 [35.0–52.9] vs. 33.0 [30.0–41.5] mL/cm H_2O, $p = 0.027$) (Table 2). Additionally, the propofol group had lower standardized heart rate over time versus the sevoflurane group (71.6 ± 7.7 vs. 76.6 ± 8.3 bpm, $p = 0.019$) and higher standardized DBP and MAP over time versus the sevoflurane group (76.8 ± 8.9 vs. 68.4 ± 8.8 mmHg, $p < 0.001$ and 93.2 ± 10.1 vs. 86.2 ± 9.2 mmHg, $p = 0.007$, respectively). Finally, the propofol group had lower standardized BIS values over time versus the sevoflurane group (45.2 ± 3.8 vs. 47.2 ± 2.6, $p = 0.019$). No differences between the two groups for standardized values of SBP, $ETCO_2$ and SpO_2 were demonstrated (Table 2).

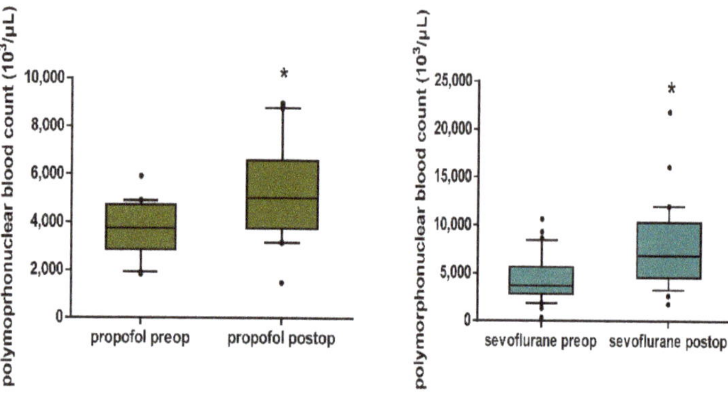

Figure 4. Box plots of polymorphonuclear blood count in peripheral blood in the propofol and sevoflurane group, preoperatively and postoperatively. Both propofol and sevoflurane maintenance caused a significant increase in the polymorphonuclear blood count ($p < 0.001$, respectively). The box plots depict the median and the interquartile range, and the whiskers depict the 10th and 90th percentiles; * $p < 0.05$ in comparison to the preoperative status.

Table 2. Standardized values for serial variables and comparisons between the two groups. * significant difference between groups.

Variables	Propofol Group (n = 30)	Sevoflurane Group (n = 30)	p Value, Group Comparison
Standardized SBP over time (mmHg), mean ± SD	123.4 ± 14.3	119.6 ± 11.2	0.260
Standardized DBP over time (mmHg), mean ± SD	76.8 ± 8.9	68.4 ± 8.8 *	**0.001**
Standardized MAP over time (mmHg), mean ± SD	93.2 ± 10.1	86.2 ± 9.2 *	**0.007**
Standardized HR over time (bpm), mean ± SD	71.6 ± 7.7	76.6 ± 8.3 *	**0.019**
Standardized BIS over time, mean ± SD	45.2 ± 3.8	47.2 ± 2.6 *	**0.019**
Standardized SaO_2 over time (%), mean ± SD	98.7 ± 0.5	98.6 ± 0.6	0.301
Standardized $ETCO_2$ over time (mmHg), mean ± SD	36.4 ± 2.9	36.5 ± 3.8	0.925
Standardized Ppeak over time (cm H_2O), mean ± SD	16.6 ± 4.3	18.8 ± 3.4 *	**0.032**
Standardized Ppl over time (cm H_2O), mean ± SD	14.6 ± 4.2	16.6 ± 3.4	0.054
Standardized compliance over time (mL/cm H_2O), median [IQR]	42.4 [35.0–52.9]	33.0 [30.0–41.5] *	**0.027**

abbreviations: SD, standard deviation; IQR, interquartile range; SBP, systolic arterial pressure; DBP, diastolic arterial pressure; MAP, mean arterial pressure; HR, heart rate; Ppl, plateau pressure; bold is for significant differences.

None of the patients suffered allergic or anaphylactic reaction or bronchospasm, nor was any patient treated with exogenous nitric donors, such as nitroglycerin.

4. Discussion

According to the main results of this randomized controlled trial, anesthesia maintenance with either propofol or sevoflurane caused a significant reduction in immediate postoperative FeNO levels in adult patients subjected to thyroidectomy. This decrease was accompanied by a decrease in the postoperative eosinophil blood count as compared to the preoperative status, which, however, was significant only in the propofol group. Finally, respiratory lung mechanics seem to be better maintained in the propofol group as compared to the sevoflurane group, with the preservation of higher lung compliance and lower Ppeak and Pplateau over time in the former group.

We are not aware of other studies in the literature comparing the two modes of anesthetic maintenance as to NO exhalation in humans, which prompted us to undertake the current protocol. We selected only thyroidectomy patients in our study, where the operation was performed by the same experienced surgeon, mainly so that there would be consistency in both the surgeon and type of surgery and, as a result, manipulations and surgical stress would be similar for all patients, and secondly, because abdominal walls are not manipulated at all during thyroidectomy, and therefore, the postoperative measurement of exhaled NO would be literally painless for patients.

Since the early 1990s, when NO was first detected in exhaled breathing of all humans, its actions in the airway and the lungs have been constantly studied, as they reflect its versatile role as a bronchodilator, vasodilator, neurotransmitter and inflammatory response mediator [27]. In the early years, chemiluminescent analyzers were used in order to detect exhaled NO [27]. It was already at that time that FeNO was noted to be higher in asthmatic patients and to decrease in response to treatment with corticosteroids [28,29]. Currently, chemiluminescent analyzers are used mostly for laboratory analyses due to their greater size and weight, and electrochemical sensors have replaced them in clinical practice for the detection and reliable measurement of exhaled NO [30]. NObreath (Bedfont® Scientific Ltd., Maidstone, UK), which we used in our study, is a portable, low-weight (≈400 g) analyzer with an electrochemical sensor, with FeNO measurement ranges from 5 to 500 ppb [31].

Even if FeNO does not seem to have the strength to confirm or rule out a diagnosis of asthma, as it can be elevated in non-asthma conditions or not elevated in some asthma phenotypes, it remains a useful tool for monitoring airway hyperresponsiveness and inflammation [24,32,33]. Particularly, when the FeNO level is co-evaluated with blood eosinophil count measurement, it has important specificity and sensitivity in predicting airway eosinophilia in asthma [34]. In addition, the measurement of FeNO, in combination with other risk assessment tools during the preanesthetic evaluation of patients with respiratory disease, might make the risk of perioperative and postoperative complications more predictable [35].

The significant reduction in NO exhalation in the propofol group in our study is in accordance with other studies reported in the literature, with, however, the vast majority of them dealing with NO measurement in the systemic circulation. Propofol, a safe and effective intravenous anesthetic routinely used for the induction and maintenance of anesthesia, also has a number of non-anesthetic effects related to NO activity. It displays an antioxidant potential by being able to directly scavenge hydroxyl chloride, superoxide, hydrogen peroxide and hydroxyl radicals and protect a variety of tissues from oxidant-related injury [36]. The antioxidant properties of propofol could be due to the fact that its chemical structure contains a phenolic hydroxyl group, which chemically resembles the antioxidant α-tocopherol [37]. Propofol can also protect macrophages from NO-induced cell death [38]. It has been shown that propofol enhances the activity of constitutive NO synthase (cNOS), but on the other hand, it inhibits the inducible production of NO both in vitro in experiments using whole blood from healthy volunteers and in surgical patients [39]. Propofol has also been found to have a direct inhibitory effect on iNOS expression in lipopolysaccharide-activated macrophages, thus downregulating the levels of NO production in macrophages [15,16]. Consequently, propofol may modify the excess production of NO and decrease the production of free radicals. These antioxidant and immunomodulating effects of propofol could contribute to the reduction in oxidative-related stress and inflammation in surgical patients [39].

Therefore, the reduction in FeNO levels in the propofol group in our study could be attributed to the direct action of propofol on the synthesis of iNOS isoform or to the inhibition of the release of inflammatory mediators from lung parenchyma, in accordance with the aforementioned findings. In fact, a reduction in the levels of such mediators by propofol has been demonstrated in in vivo experimental models, which have also demonstrated the protective effects of propofol on endotoxin-induced acute lung injury [17,18]. In fact, in a study by Chu et al., the attenuation by propofol of an endotoxin-induced increase in pro-inflammatory cytokines abrogated the microvascular leakage of protein and water in the lungs, thus preserving endothelial integrity [17]. In the same study, propofol significantly decreased exhaled NO and protein concentration in the bronchoalveolar lavage fluid, with its effects more evident in high doses. It was postulated by the authors that the protective action of propofol on endotoxin-induced acute lung injury could be mediated by the reduction in NO production. In a study by Gao et al., the early administration of propofol in rats subjected to endotoxin-induced acute lung injury resulted in reduced concentrations of nitrite/nitrate in the bronchoalveolar lavage fluid and attenuated iNOS expression in lung tissue [18]. In another study, propofol was able to reverse the oleic-acid-induced endothelial damage and subsequent inflammation and injury of lung parenchyma in conscious rats [40]. The authors suggested that NO production was involved in the oleic-acid-induced acute lung injury, since, in their study, an increase in exhaled NO and iNOS upregulation was noted in rats not treated with propofol, and these changes were reversed in propofol-treated animals. It could therefore be postulated that a similar pathophysiological mechanism of the suppression of the iNOS-NO-dependent pathway in the human lung parenchyma may underlie the decrease in FeNO levels by propofol, thus reducing the potential for inflammatory perturbation of the airway.

In our study, we also demonstrated a significant reduction in FeNO in the sevoflurane group. This is compatible with previous experimental studies investigating the effect of sevoflurane in several models of acute lung injury. In an experimental rat model of sepsis, pretreatment with sevoflurane attenuated sepsis-induced inflammatory response through a reduction in chemotactic cytokine levels and mitigated lipid peroxidation and oxidative stress [20]. It has already been shown that the induction of the expression of iNOS and, subsequently, overproduction of NO is implicated in the pathogenesis of acute lung injury in animals with endotoxemia [13,41,42]. In the Bedirli study, plasma NO levels were significantly reduced in comparison to the control group, prompting the authors to attribute decreased expression of inflammatory mediators in the sevoflurane group to the inhibition of intracellular NO-related signal transmission pathway [20]. Additionally, in an isolated buffer-perfused rat lung model, pretreatment with sevoflurane protected the lung against ischemia-reperfusion-induced injury, decreasing vascular permeability and reducing the production of NO metabolites in the perfusate [21]. This reduction indicates that the protective effects of sevoflurane against ischemia-reperfusion lung injury may be mediated through the inhibition of NO release. Both sevoflurane and isoflurane might share common pathways involving NO in the alleviation of acute lung injury, since, in an endotoxin-induced acute lung injury in rats, the proadministration of isoflurane resulted in the decreased pulmonary accumulation of proinflammatory cytokines, pulmonary nitrite/nitrate levels and significantly reduced iNOS gene expression in lung tissue [43]. It seems, therefore, that lung anti-inflammatory protection afforded by volatile anesthetics could be partially mediated through the inhibition of iNOS/NO pathway activation. Consequently, according to our results, sevoflurane seems to suppress the iNOS-dependent NO production in the human lung in a way similar to propofol, reducing the potential for inflammation.

In our study, polymorphonuclear blood count was increased in both groups. We consider that this response might be due to the effect of the surgical procedure. It is already known that immune responses after anesthesia and surgery are characterized by neutrophilia and that the surgical procedure plays a more important role than anesthesia per se in this response [44]. However, we demonstrated a significant decrease in eosinophil blood count postoperatively only in the propofol group. Eosinophils, after their release into the circulation, translocate into submucosal tissues, thus forming part of the immunological response at body surfaces, producing cytokines that influence acute and chronic inflammatory responses. The significant decrease in eosinophils in the propofol group is compatible with previous studies. Specifically, in a study examining the effect of various anesthetic agents on the chemotaxis of eosinophils in vitro, although the inhibition of eosinophilic chemotaxis was demonstrated only for thiopental and etomidate, the authors concluded that a similar effect for propofol could not be ruled out but could not be demonstrated due to the small power of the study [19]. Actually, in another study investigating a mouse model of allergic asthma, propofol significantly decreased the eosinophil count and the levels of proinflammatory mediators in the bronchoalveolar lavage fluid, attenuating infiltrating inflammatory cells and mucus production in histological samples [45]. The different response of eosinophils between propofol and sevoflurane anesthesia could be due to the different effect propofol and sevoflurane have on interleukin 10 (IL-10), whose role in the inflammatory response of the airway is a great significance. Il-10 has been found to be a strong inhibitor of eosinophil recruitment in mucosal tissue, contributing to the protection or resolution of airway inflammation in conditions such as asthma and chronic obstructive pulmonary disease [46–48]. In fact, the administration of propofol has been associated with reduced proinflammatory IL-6 levels and enhanced anti-inflammatory IL-10 generation as compared to sevoflurane, suggesting a more favorable anti-inflammatory effect of intravenous anesthesia in comparison to an inhalational technique [49]. This is obvious even in operations that require one-lung ventilation, which is a well-known factor to exert great stress on pulmonary function and homeostasis via the upregulation of proinflammatory cytokine expression either in systemic circulation or in the epithelial lining fluid [50,51]. In fact, there are several studies demonstrating that propofol anesthesia can more effectively suppress the perioperative inflammatory response as compared to inhalational techniques in operations involving one-lung ventilation [50–52].

An additional finding of our study was the more favorable respiratory profile and better preservation of lung mechanics in the propofol group, with demonstration of better compliance maintenance and favorable Ppeak and Ppl over time in comparison to the sevoflurane group. Sevoflurane has long been perceived as the preferable inhalational agent for anesthesia maintenance in patients suffering from asthma due to its favorable bronchodilatory effect [6]. However, when its use was studied in asthmatic children, the results were controversial [53], while on the other hand, propofol is also considered safe for asthmatic patients and has been shown to decrease airway resistance in patients with already hyperreactive airways [54,55]. It appears, therefore, that the expected increase in lung compliance due to bronchodilation caused by volatile anesthetics has perhaps been overestimated. In fact, animal experiments have shown that inhaled anesthetics inhibit the generation of lung surfactant by type II endothelial cells or reduce the efficacy of surfactant activity, thereby decreasing lung compliance [56]. Our finding of better respiratory mechanics over time with propofol maintenance are in accordance with an experimental study where sevoflurane maintenance resulted in significantly higher airway pressures than propofol during laparoscopy in a porcine model [57]. The protective effect of propofol against bronchoconstriction and increased respiratory resistance is perhaps mediated via the initiation of an anticholinergic mechanism during mechanical ventilation and resulting direct airway smooth muscle relaxant action, a fact that has been demonstrated in in vitro, experimental and human studies [58–60]. In fact, propofol anesthesia has been shown to decrease airway resistance even when no previous bronchoconstriction was present and was also associated with central airway dilatation observed at lung histology in a rat study [59]. The mechanism of the bronchodilatory effect of propofol remains to be elucidated, being perhaps associated with the inhibition of voltage-dependent calcium channels [61]. Propofol has also been shown to provide a dose-dependent relaxing effect in the chest wall muscles, affording an additional favorable effect on chest wall resistance [62–64]. A more potent muscle-relaxing effect of propofol versus sevoflurane at the same depth of anesthesia and a stronger relaxant action on airway muscles might account for its favorable effect on peak inspiratory pressures in our study.

Our study has a few limitations. First, we measured eosinophil blood count and not sputum eosinophil in our set of patients. Sputum eosinophil count has been long regarded as the most reliable indicator of eosinophilic airway inflammation. However, evolving evidence shows that eosinophil blood count seems to be equally reliable in predicting both eosinophilic airway inflammation and sputum eosinophil count [65]. It is important to note that the measurement of blood eosinophil count provides an easy sampling technique compared to the induction of sputum, particularly in the immediate postoperative period, because the latter would not only pose a risk of postoperative hemorrhage due to induced coughing but also create discomfort to the patient. Secondly, we can only make speculations about the aforementioned differential release of proinflammatory and anti-inflammatory cytokines between the two modes of anesthesia maintenance and the impact that these might have had on airway inflammation, because these were not measured in the current study. A further limitation is the fact that we did not evaluate the postoperative respiratory function of our patients via spirometry to confirm whether the aforementioned effects of the two anesthetic regimes on respiratory mechanics were sustained into the postoperative period. In addition, we did not correlate the preoperative volume of the thyroid gland with postoperative measurements of FeNO. Finally, we only enrolled patients without respiratory disease or airway hyperresponsiveness in our study, so it remains to be determined if our findings can be applied in those populations.

5. Conclusions

In conclusion, under the current study design, both propofol and sevoflurane maintenance techniques during thyroidectomy seem to decrease postoperative FeNO levels, with propofol additionally exerting a significant decrease in postoperative eosinophil blood count and providing a more favorable respiratory profile for the whole duration of the operation as compared to sevoflurane. The ease of measurement of FeNO by a portable device such as NObreath both for the anesthesiologist and the patient even in busy settings combined with its low cost could make it a useful tool in perianesthetic patient evaluation. According to our results, it appears that intravenous techniques may offer advantages in terms of the suppression of perioperative inflammatory perturbation in the local milieu of the airway as compared to inhalational techniques. Whether these findings can be extrapolated to patients with respiratory comorbidities or patients suffering from asthma or other forms of airway inflammation and hyperresponsiveness remains to be elucidated in future studies encompassing such patient populations.

Author Contributions: Conceptualization, A.V. and K.T.; data curation, P.P., H.L., S.V., E.A. and I.V.; formal analysis, A.V. and K.T.; investigation, P.P., H.L., S.V., E.A. and I.V.; methodology, A.V. and K.T.; project administration, A.V. and K.T.; software, K.T.; supervision, K.T.; writing—original draft, A.V.; writing—review and editing, K.T. All authors have read and agreed to the published version of the manuscript.

Funding: This research did not receive any specific grant from funding agencies in the public, commercial, or not-for-profit sectors.

Institutional Review Board Statement: This study was approved by the Ethics Committee of Aretaieion University Hospital, Aretaieion Hospital, National and Kapodistrian University of Athens, Chairperson Professor Ioannis Vassileiou on 19 December 2013 (B-19/19-12-2013).

Informed Consent Statement: All patients gave their informed consent for publication.

Data Availability Statement: The datasets generated during and/or analyzed during the current study are available from the corresponding author on reasonable request.

Conflicts of Interest: The authors declare that they have no potential conflict of interest.

References

1. Maniscalco, M.; Sofia, M.; Pelaia, G. Nitric oxide in upper airways inflammatory diseases. *Inflamm. Res.* **2007**, *56*, 58–69. [CrossRef] [PubMed]
2. Levine, A.B.; Punihaole, D.; Levine, T.B. Characterization of the Role of Nitric Oxide and Its Clinical Applications. *Cardiology* **2012**, *122*, 55–68. [CrossRef] [PubMed]
3. Panduri, V.; Weitzman, S.A.; Chandel, N.S.; Kamp, D.W. Mitochondrial-derived free radicals mediate asbestos-induced alveolar epithelial cell apoptosis. *Am. J. Physiol. Cell. Mol. Physiol.* **2004**, *286*, L1220–L1227. [CrossRef] [PubMed]
4. Tufvesson, E.; Andersson, C.; Weidner, J.; Erjefält, J.S.; Bjermer, L. Inducible nitric oxide synthase expression is increased in the alveolar compartment of asthmatic patients. *Allergy* **2016**, *72*, 627–635. [CrossRef] [PubMed]
5. Radi, R. Immuno-spin trapping: A breakthrough for the sensitive detection of protein-derived radicals, a commentary on "Protein radical formation on thyroid peroxidase during turnover". *Free Radic. Biol. Med.* **2006**, *41*, 416–417. [CrossRef] [PubMed]

6. Bayable, S.D.; Melesse, D.Y.; Lema, G.F.; Ahmed, S.A. Perioperative management of patients with asthma during elective surgery: A systematic review. *Ann. Med. Surg.* **2021**, *70*, 102874. [CrossRef] [PubMed]
7. Petsky, H.L.; Kew, K.M.; Turner, C.; Chang, A.B. Exhaled nitric oxide levels to guide treatment for adults with asthma. *Cochrane Database Syst. Rev.* **2016**, *2016*, CD011440. [CrossRef] [PubMed]
8. Smith, A.D.; Cowan, J.O.; Brassett, K.P.; Herbison, G.P.; Taylor, D.R. Use of Exhaled Nitric Oxide Measurements to Guide Treatment in Chronic Asthma. *N. Engl. J. Med.* **2005**, *352*, 2163–2173. [CrossRef]
9. Saraiva-Romanholo, B.M.; Machado, F.S.; Almeida, F.M.; Nunes, M.D.P.T.; Martins, M.A.; Vieira, J.E. Non-Asthmatic Patients Show Increased Exhaled Nitric Oxide Concentrations. *Clinics* **2009**, *64*, 5–10. [CrossRef]
10. Berry, M.A.; Shaw, D.E.; Green, R.H.; Brightling, C.E.; Wardlaw, A.J.; Pavord, I.D. The use of exhaled nitric oxide concentration to identify eosinophilic airway inflammation: An observational study in adults with asthma. *Clin. Exp. Allergy* **2005**, *35*, 1175–1179. [CrossRef]
11. Warke, T.J.; Fitch, P.S.; Brown, V.; Taylor, R.; Lyons, J.D.M.; Ennis, M.; Shields, M.D. Exhaled nitric oxide correlates with airway eosinophils in childhood asthma. *Thorax* **2002**, *57*, 383–387. [CrossRef] [PubMed]
12. Liu, F.; Li, W.; Pauluhn, J.; Trübel, H.; Wang, C. Rat models of acute lung injury: Exhaled nitric oxide as a sensitive, noninvasive real-time biomarker of prognosis and efficacy of intervention. *Toxicology* **2013**, *310*, 104–114. [CrossRef]
13. Lee, R.P.; Wang, D.; Kao, S.J.; Chen, I.H. The Lung Is the Major Site That Produces Nitric Oxide to Induce Acute Pulmonary Oedema in Endotoxin Shock. *Clin. Exp. Pharmacol. Physiol.* **2001**, *28*, 315–320. [CrossRef] [PubMed]
14. Barnes, P.J.; Kharitonov, A.S. Exhaled nitric oxide: A new lung function test. *Thorax* **1996**, *51*, 233–237. [CrossRef] [PubMed]
15. Chen, R.-M.; Wu, G.-J.; Tai, Y.-T.; Sun, W.-Z.; Lin, Y.-L.; Jean, W.-C.; Chen, T.-L. Propofol reduces nitric oxide biosynthesis in lipopolysaccharide-activated macrophages by downregulating the expression of inducible nitric oxide synthase. *Arch. Toxicol.* **2003**, *77*, 418–423. [CrossRef]
16. Liu, M.-C.; Tsai, P.-S.; Yang, C.-H.; Liu, C.-H.; Chen, C.-C.; Huang, C.-J. Propofol significantly attenuates iNOS, CAT-2, and CAT-2B transcription in lipopolysaccharide-stimulated murine macrophages. *Acta Anaesthesiol. Taiwanica* **2006**, *44*, 73–81.
17. Chu, C.-H.; Liu, D.D.; Hsu, Y.-H.; Lee, K.-C.; Chen, I.H. Propofol exerts protective effects on the acute lung injury induced by endotoxin in rats. *Pulm. Pharmacol. Ther.* **2007**, *20*, 503–512. [CrossRef]
18. Gao, J.; Zeng, B.; Zhou, L.; Yuan, S. Protective effects of early treatment with propofol on endotoxin-induced acute lung injury in rats. *Br. J. Anaesth.* **2004**, *92*, 277–279. [CrossRef]
19. Krumholz, W.; Abdulle, O.; Knecht, J.; Hempelmann, G. Effects of i.v. anaesthetic agents on the chemotaxis of eosinophils in vitro. *Br. J. Anaesth.* **1999**, *83*, 333–335. [CrossRef]
20. Bedirli, N.; Demirtas, C.Y.; Akkaya, T.; Salman, B.; Alper, M.; Bedirli, A.; Pasaoglu, H. Volatile anesthetic preconditioning attenuated sepsis induced lung inflammation. *J. Surg. Res.* **2012**, *178*, e17–e23. [CrossRef]
21. Liu, R.; Ishibe, Y.; Ueda, M. Isoflurane–Sevoflurane Administration before Ischemia Attenuates Ischemia–Reperfusion-induced Injury in Isolated Rat Lungs. *Anesthesiology* **2000**, *92*, 833–840. [CrossRef]
22. Schulz, K.F.; Altman, U.G.; Moher, D.; CONSORT Group. CONSORT 2010 Statement: Updated guidelines for reporting parallel group randomised trials. *BMJ* **2010**, *340*, c332. [CrossRef] [PubMed]
23. American Thoracic Society. Recommendations for standardized procedures for the on-line and off-line measurement of exhaled lower respiratory nitric oxide and nasal nitric oxide in adults and children-1999. *Am. J. Respir. Crit. Care Med.* **1999**, *160*, 2104–2211. [CrossRef]
24. American Thoracic Society; European Respiratory Society. ATS/ERS recommendations for standardized procedures for the online and offline measurement of exhaled lower respiratory nitric oxide and nasal nitric oxide, 2005. *Am. J. Respir. Crit. Care Med.* **2005**, *171*, 912–930. [CrossRef] [PubMed]
25. Pisi, R.; Aiello, M.; Tzani, P.; Marangio, E.; Olivieri, D.; Chetta, A. Measurement of Fractional Exhaled Nitric Oxide by a New Portable Device: Comparison with the Standard Technique. *J. Asthma* **2010**, *47*, 805–809. [CrossRef]
26. Matthews, J.N.; Altman, D.G.; Campbell, M.J.; Royston, P. Analysis of serial measurements in medical research. *BMJ* **1990**, *300*, 230–235. [CrossRef]
27. Gustafsson, L.; Leone, A.; Persson, M.; Wiklund, N.; Moncada, S. Endogenous nitric oxide is present in the exhaled air of rabbits, guinea pigs and humans. *Biochem. Biophys. Res. Commun.* **1991**, *181*, 852–857. [CrossRef]
28. Alving, K.; Weitzberg, E.; Lundberg, J.M. Increased amount of nitric oxide in exhaled air of asthmatics. *Eur. Respir. J.* **1993**, *6*, 1368–1370. [PubMed]
29. Silkoff, P.E.; McClean, P.; Spino, M.; Erlich, L.A.; Slutsky, A.S.; Zamel, N. Dose-Response Relationship and Reproducibility of the Fall in Exhaled Nitric Oxide After Inhaled Beclomethasone Dipropionate Therapy in Asthma Patients. *Chest* **2001**, *119*, 1322–1328. [CrossRef]
30. Maniscalco, M.; Bianco, A.; Mazzarella, G.; Motta, A. Recent Advances on Nitric Oxide in the Upper Airways. *Curr. Med. Chem.* **2016**, *23*, 2736–2745. [CrossRef]
31. Harnan, E.S.; Tappenden, P.; Essat, M.; Gomersall, T.; Minton, J.; Wong, R.; Pavord, I.; Everard, M.; Lawson, R. Measurement of exhaled nitric oxide concentration in asthma: A systematic review and economic evaluation of NIOX MINO, NIOX VERO and NObreath. *Health Technol. Assess.* **2015**, *19*, 820. [CrossRef] [PubMed]
32. Fahy, J.V. Type 2 inflammation in asthma—Present in most, absent in many. *Nat. Rev. Immunol.* **2015**, *15*, 57–65. [CrossRef] [PubMed]

33. Kharitonov, S.; Barnes, P. Clinical aspects of exhaled nitric oxide. *Eur. Respir. J.* **2000**, *16*, 781–792. [CrossRef] [PubMed]
34. Soma, T.; Iemura, H.; Naito, E.; Miyauchi, S.; Uchida, Y.; Nakagome, K.; Nagata, M. Implication of fraction of exhaled nitric oxide and blood eosinophil count in severe asthma. *Allergol. Int.* **2018**, *67*, S3–S11. [CrossRef] [PubMed]
35. Logotheti, H.; Pourzitaki, C.; Tsaousi, G.; Aidoni, Z.; Vekrakou, A.; Ekaterini, A.; Gourgoulianis, K. The role of exhaled nitric oxide in patients with chronic obstructive pulmonary disease undergoing laparotomy surgery—The noxious study. *Nitric Oxide* **2016**, *61*, 62–68. [CrossRef]
36. Murphy, P.G.; Myers, D.S.; Davies, M.; Webster, N.R.; Jones, J.G. The antioxidant potential of propofol (2,6-DIISOPROPYLPHENOL). *Br. J. Anaesth.* **1992**, *68*, 613–618. [CrossRef]
37. Aarts, L.; Van Der Hee, R.; Dekker, I.; De Jong, J.; Langemeijer, H.; Bast, A. The widely used anesthetic agent propofol can replace α-tocopherol as an antioxidant. *FEBS Lett.* **1995**, *357*, 83–85. [CrossRef]
38. Chang, H.; Tsai, S.-Y.; Chang, Y.; Chen, T.-L.; Chen, R.-M. Therapeutic concentrations of propofol protects mouse macrophages from nitric oxide-induced cell death and apoptosis. *Can. J. Anaesth.* **2002**, *49*, 477–480. [CrossRef]
39. González-Correa, J.A.; Cruz-Andreotti, E.; Arrebola, M.M.; López-Villodres, J.A.; Jódar, M.; De La Cruz, J.P. Effects of propofol on the leukocyte nitric oxide pathway: In vitro and ex vivo studies in surgical patients. *Naunyn-Schmiedebergs Arch. Exp. Pathol. Pharmakol.* **2008**, *376*, 331–339. [CrossRef]
40. Chen, H.I.; Hsieh, N.-K.; Kao, S.J.; Su, C.-F. Protective effects of propofol on acute lung injury induced by oleic acid in conscious rats. *Crit. Care Med.* **2008**, *36*, 1214–1221. [CrossRef]
41. Wang, D.; Wei, J.; Hsu, K.; Jau, J.-C.; Lieu, M.-W.; Chao, T.-J.; Chen, H.I. Effects of nitric oxide synthase inhibitors on systemic hypotension, cytokines and inducible nitric oxide synthase expression and lung injury following endotoxin administration in rats. *J. Biomed. Sci.* **1999**, *6*, 28–35. [CrossRef] [PubMed]
42. Vincent, J.-L.; Zhang, H.; Szabo, C.; Preiser, J.-C. Effects of Nitric Oxide in Septic Shock. *Am. J. Respir. Crit. Care Med.* **2000**, *161*, 1781–1785. [CrossRef] [PubMed]
43. Li, Q.F.; Zhu, Y.S.; Jiang, H.; Xu, H.; Sun, Y. Isoflurane Preconditioning Ameliorates Endotoxin-Induced Acute Lung Injury and Mortality in Rats. *Anesthesia Analg.* **2009**, *109*, 1591–1597. [CrossRef] [PubMed]
44. Helmy, S.A.K.; Wahby, M.A.M.; El-Nawaway, M. The effect of anaesthesia and surgery on plasma cytokine production. *Anaesthesia* **1999**, *54*, 733–738. [CrossRef] [PubMed]
45. Li, H.-Y.; Meng, J.-X.; Liu, Z.; Liu, X.-W.; Huang, Y.-G.; Zhao, J. Propofol Attenuates Airway Inflammation in a Mast Cell-Dependent Mouse Model of Allergic Asthma by Inhibiting the Toll-like Receptor 4/Reactive Oxygen Species/Nuclear Factor κB Signaling Pathway. *Inflammation* **2018**, *41*, 914–923. [CrossRef]
46. Zhang, J.; Bai, C. Elevated Serum Interleukin-8 Level as a Preferable Biomarker for Identifying Uncontrolled Asthma and Glucocorticosteroid Responsiveness. *Tanafos* **2017**, *16*, 260–269.
47. Ogawa, Y.E.; Duru, A.E.; Ameredes, B.T. Role of IL-10 in the Resolution of Airway Inflammation. *Curr. Mol. Med.* **2008**, *8*, 437–445. [CrossRef]
48. Wilson, E.B.; Brooks, D.G. The Role of IL-10 in Regulating Immunity to Persistent Viral Infections. *Negat. Co-Recept. Ligands* **2011**, *350*, 39–65. [CrossRef]
49. Ke, J.J.; Zhan, J.; Feng, X.B.; Wu, Y.; Rao, Y.; Wang, Y.L. A Comparison of the Effect of Total Intravenous Anaesthesia with Propofol and Remifentanil and Inhalational Anaesthesia with Isoflurane on the Release of Pro- and Anti-Inflammatory Cytokines in Patients Undergoing Open Cholecystectomy. *Anaesth. Intensiv. Care* **2008**, *36*, 74–78. [CrossRef]
50. Wakabayashi, S.; Yamaguchi, K.; Kumakura, S.; Murakami, T.; Someya, A.; Kajiyama, Y.; Nagaoka, I.; Inada, E. Effects of anesthesia with sevoflurane and propofol on the cytokine/chemokine production at the airway epithelium during esophagectomy. *Int. J. Mol. Med.* **2014**, *34*, 137–144. [CrossRef]
51. Jin, Y.; Zhao, X.; Li, H.; Wang, Z.; Wang, D. Effects of sevoflurane and propofol on the inflammatory response and pulmonary function of perioperative patients with one-lung ventilation. *Exp. Ther. Med.* **2013**, *6*, 781–785. [CrossRef] [PubMed]
52. Tian, H.-T.; Duan, X.-H.; Yang, Y.-F.; Wang, Y.; Bai, Q.-L.; Zhang, X. Effects of propofol or sevoflurane anesthesia on the perioperative inflammatory response, pulmonary function and cognitive function in patients receiving lung cancer resection. *Eur. Rev. Med. Pharmacol. Sci.* **2017**, *21*, 5515–5522. [CrossRef]
53. Habre, W.; Matsumoto, I.; Sly, P.D. Propofol or halothane anaesthesia for children with asthma: Effects on respiratory mechanics. *Br. J. Anaesth.* **1996**, *77*, 739–774. [CrossRef] [PubMed]
54. Lauer, R.; Vadi, M.; Mason, L. Anaesthetic management of the child with co-existing pulmonary disease. *Br. J. Anaesth.* **2012**, *109*, i47–i59. [CrossRef]
55. Conti, G.; Dell'Utri, D.; Vilardi, V.; De Blasi, R.A.; Pelaia, P.; Antonelli, M.; Bufi, M.; Rosa, G.; Gasparetto, A. Propofol induces bronchodilation in mechanically ventilated chronic obstructive pulmonary disease (COPD) patients. *Acta Anaesthesiol. Scand.* **1993**, *37*, 105–109. [CrossRef] [PubMed]
56. Molliex, S.; Crestani, B.; Dureuil, B.; Bastin, J.; Rolland, C.; Aubier, M.; Desmonts, J.-M. Effects of Halothane on Surfactant Biosynthesis by Rat Alveolar Type II Cells in Primary Culture. *Anesthesiology* **1994**, *81*, 668–676. [CrossRef]
57. Puglisi, F.; Crovace, A.; Staffieri, F.; Capuano, P.; Carravetta, G.; De Fazio, M.; Lograno, G.; Lacitignola, L.; Troilo, V.L.; Martines, G.; et al. Comparison of hemodynamic and respiratory effects of propofol and sevoflurane during carbon dioxide pneumoperitoneum in a swine model. *Chir. Ital.* **2007**, *59*, 105–111.

58. Ouedraogo, N.; Roux, E.; Forestier, F.; Rossetti, M.; Savineau, J.-P.; Marthan, R. Effects of Intravenous Anesthetics on Normal and Passively Sensitized Human Isolated Airway Smooth Muscle. *Anesthesiology* **1998**, *88*, 317–326. [CrossRef]
59. Peratoner, A.; Nascimento, C.S.; Santana, M.C.E.; Cadete, R.A.; Negri, E.M.; Gullo, A.; Rocco, P.R.M.; Zin, W.A. Effects of propofol on respiratory mechanic and lung histology in normal rats. *Br. J. Anaesth.* **2004**, *92*, 737–740. [CrossRef]
60. Eames, W.O.; Rooke, A.G.; Wu, R.S.-C.; Bishop, M.J. Comparison of the Effects of Etomidate, Propofol, and Thiopental on Respiratory Resistance after Tracheal Intubation. *Anesthesiology* **1996**, *84*, 1307–1311. [CrossRef]
61. Yamakage, M.; Hirshman, C.A.; Croxton, T.L. Inhibitory Effects of Thiopental, Ketamine, and Propofol on Voltage-dependent Calcium sup 2+ Channels in Porcine Tracheal Smooth Muscle Cells. *Anesthesiology* **1995**, *83*, 1274–1282. [CrossRef] [PubMed]
62. Ginz, H.F.; Zorzato, F.; Iaizzo, P.A.; Urwyler, A. Effect of three anaesthetic techniques on isometric skeletal muscle strength. *Br. J. Anaesth.* **2004**, *92*, 367–372. [CrossRef] [PubMed]
63. Fagerlund, M.J.; Krupp, J.; Dabrowski, M.A. Propofol and AZD3043 Inhibit Adult Muscle and Neuronal Nicotinic Acetylcholine Receptors Expressed in Xenopus Oocytes. *Pharmaceuticals* **2016**, *9*, 8. [CrossRef]
64. Haeseler, G.; Störmer, M.; Bufler, J.; Dengler, R.; Hecker, H.; Piepenbrock, S.; Leuwer, M. Propofol Blocks Human Skeletal Muscle Sodium Channels in a Voltage-Dependent Manner. *Anesthesia Analg.* **2001**, *92*, 1192–1198. [CrossRef] [PubMed]
65. Zhang, X.-Y.; Simpson, J.L.; Powell, H.; Yang, I.; Upham, J.; Reynolds, P.N.; Hodge, S.; James, A.L.; Jenkins, C.; Peters, M.; et al. Full blood count parameters for the detection of asthma inflammatory phenotypes. *Clin. Exp. Allergy* **2014**, *44*, 1137–1145. [CrossRef] [PubMed]

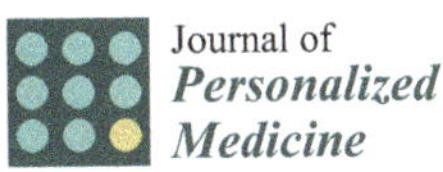
Journal of *Personalized Medicine*
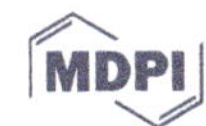

Article

Relationship between Mechanical Ventilation and Histological Fibrosis in Patients with Acute Respiratory Distress Syndrome Undergoing Open Lung Biopsy

Hsin-Hsien Li [1,2], Chih-Wei Wang [3], Chih-Hao Chang [4,5], Chung-Chi Huang [2,4], Han-Shui Hsu [1,6] and Li-Chung Chiu [4,7,*]

1 Institute of Emergency and Critical Care Medicine, School of Medicine, National Yang Ming Chiao Tung University, Taipei 11221, Taiwan; hsinhsien@mail.cgu.edu.tw (H.-H.L.); hsuhs@vghtpe.gov.tw (H.-S.H.)
2 Department of Respiratory Therapy, Chang Gung University College of Medicine, Taoyuan 33302, Taiwan; cch4848@cgmh.org.tw
3 Department of Pathology, Chang Gung Memorial Hospital, Chang Gung University College of Medicine, Taoyuan 33305, Taiwan; weger@cgmh.org.tw
4 Department of Thoracic Medicine, Chang Gung Memorial Hospital, Chang Gung University College of Medicine, Taoyuan 33305, Taiwan; ma7384@adm.cgmh.org.tw
5 Department of Thoracic Medicine, New Taipei Municipal TuCheng Hospital and Chang Gung University, Taoyuan 33302, Taiwan
6 Division of Thoracic Surgery, Department of Surgery, Taipei Veterans General Hospital, Taipei 112201, Taiwan
7 Graduate Institute of Clinical Medical Sciences, College of Medicine, Chang Gung University, Taoyuan 33302, Taiwan
* Correspondence: pomd54@cgmh.org.tw; Tel.: +886-3-328-1200 (ext. 8467)

Citation: Li, H.-H.; Wang, C.-W.; Chang, C.-H.; Huang, C.-C.; Hsu, H.-S.; Chiu, L.-C. Relationship between Mechanical Ventilation and Histological Fibrosis in Patients with Acute Respiratory Distress Syndrome Undergoing Open Lung Biopsy. *J. Pers. Med.* **2022**, *12*, 474. https://doi.org/10.3390/jpm12030474

Academic Editors: Ioannis Pantazopoulos and Ourania S. Kotsiou

Received: 1 February 2022
Accepted: 14 March 2022
Published: 16 March 2022

Abstract: Background: Mechanical ventilation brings the risk of ventilator-induced lung injury, which can lead to pulmonary fibrosis and prolonged mechanical ventilation. Methods: A retrospective analysis of patients with acute respiratory distress syndrome (ARDS) who received open lung biopsy between March 2006 and December 2019. Results: A total of 68 ARDS patients receiving open lung biopsy with diffuse alveolar damage (DAD; the hallmark pathology of ARDS) were analyzed and stratified into non-fibrosis (n = 56) and fibrosis groups (n = 12). The duration of ventilator usage and time spent in the intensive care unit and hospital stay were all significantly higher in the fibrosis group. Hospital mortality was higher in the fibrosis than in the non-fibrosis group (67% vs. 57%, p = 0.748). A multivariable logistic regression model demonstrated that mechanical power at ARDS diagnosis and ARDS duration before biopsy were independently associated with histological fibrosis at open lung biopsy (odds ratio 1.493 (95% CI 1.014–2.200), p = 0.042; odds ratio 1.160 (95% CI 1.052–1.278), p = 0.003, respectively). Conclusions: Our findings indicate that prompt action aimed at staving off injurious mechanical stretching of lung parenchyma and subsequent progression to fibrosis may have a positive effect on clinical outcomes.

Keywords: mechanical ventilation; acute respiratory distress syndrome; open lung biopsy; histology; diffuse alveolar damage; pulmonary fibrosis; idiopathic pulmonary fibrosis; outcomes

1. Introduction

Acute respiratory distress syndrome (ARDS) is a heterogeneous syndrome with complex pathophysiologic mechanisms characterized by severe hypoxemia and high mortality [1]. The pathogenesis of ARDS includes an exudative phase, a proliferative phase, and a fibrotic phase. Alveolar type II cell hyperplasia occurs after the initial exudative phase, resulting in the formation of resident fibroblasts and extracellular matrix. As disease progresses to the fibrotic phase, extensive basement membrane damage and inadequate or delayed reepithelialization can lead to the development of interstitial and intraalveolar fibrosis, which often requires prolonged mechanical ventilator support [2].

The typical histological hallmark of ARDS is diffuse alveolar damage (DAD) manifesting as hyaline membrane formation, lung edema, inflammation, and hemorrhage [3]. Roughly only half of the patients diagnosed with ARDS based on current criteria present evidence of DAD upon open lung biopsy (OLB) or autopsy [4–7]. Note, however, that not all ARDS patients progress to the fibrotic phase, as any imbalance in profibrotic or antifibrotic mediators could affect progression to the fibroproliferative phase [8]. In patients with ARDS, pulmonary fibrosis often leads to prolonged mechanical ventilation and poor clinical outcomes [9,10].

Idiopathic pulmonary fibrosis (IPF) is a chronic progressive fibrotic interstitial pneumonia with unknown etiology and poor prognosis. It is characterized by deterioration of the lung parenchyma structure and respiratory function [11]. Acute exacerbation of idiopathic pulmonary fibrosis (AE-IPF) has been defined as an acute clinically significant respiratory deterioration of unidentifiable cause, commonly leading to acute hypoxemia respiratory failure requiring mechanical ventilation [12]. The typical histological features of AE-IPF are DAD and/or organizing pneumonia superimposed on the usual interstitial pneumonia (UIP) pattern (i.e., acute lung injury occurring in an IPF/UIP lung), such that it shares many of the pathological features of ARDS [13,14].

A lung-protective ventilation strategy remains the cornerstone of treatment for ARDS patients and has been positively correlated with improved survival [2]; however, it brings with it the risk of ventilator-induced lung injury (VILI) and subsequent lung fibrosis [15]. Researchers have yet to establish optimal ventilator settings for patients with pulmonary fibrosis. Our objective in this study was to examine the association between serial changes in ventilator settings and histological fibrosis in ARDS patients with DAD based on OLB and compare clinical outcomes between fibrosis and non-fibrosis groups.

2. Materials and Methods

2.1. Study Design and Patients

This retrospective study was based on analysis of all ARDS patients who underwent OLB at Chang Gung Memorial Hospital (CGMH) in Taiwan between March 2006 and December 2019. CGMH is a tertiary care referral center with a 3700-bed general ward and 278-bed adult intensive care unit (ICU). The exclusion criteria included age of <20 years and histological findings not indicative of DAD.

At our institution, the decision to perform OLB was made by the treating intensivist in cases where the etiology of ARDS was unknown and the patient presented rapid pulmonary infiltration following a complete microbiologic examination including bronchoalveolar lavage. Surgical procedures were performed by a chest surgeon in an operating room or at the bedside in the ICU. Informed consent was obtained from the family prior to OLB. Under general anesthesia and mechanical ventilator support with adequate oxygenation, video-assisted thoracoscopic surgery or a 5-cm thoracotomy was used to secure the origins using an endoscopic stapler-cutter. The biopsy site was a new or progressive lesion identified via high-resolution computed tomography (HRCT) or chest X-ray. Every tissue specimen was examined by pathologists. The local Institutional Review Board for Human Research approved this study (CGMH IRB No. 202000760A3 and 202100595A3), and the need for informed consent was waived due to the retrospective nature of the study.

2.2. Definitions

ARDS was defined in accordance with the Berlin criteria [7]. Dynamic driving pressure (ΔP) was calculated as peak inspiratory pressure (Ppeak) minus positive end-expiratory pressure (PEEP) [16]. Mechanical power (MP) was calculated using the following equation [17,18]: MP (Joules/minutes) (J/min) = 0.098 × tidal volume (V_T) × respiratory rate (RR) × (Ppeak–1/2 × ΔP).

Ppeak is equivalent to plateau pressure in pressure-controlled ventilation, and Ppeak was used as a surrogate for plateau pressure to calculate MP if not specified [17]. Ventilator-free days was defined as the number of days between day 1 and day 28 or day 90 in which the patient breathed without assistance for at least 48 consecutive hours. Patients who did not survive to 28 days or 90 days were assigned zero ventilator-free days. Patients were stratified into the non-fibrosis group (DAD with exudative or proliferative phase) or the fibrosis group (DAD with fibrotic phase or chronic feature of honeycomb fibrosis).

2.3. Data Collections

Demographic data, comorbidities, and the etiologies of ARDS were recorded from hospital charts. The dates of hospital and ICU admission, mechanical ventilator initiation and liberation, date of ARDS diagnosis and OLB, ICU and hospital discharge, and time of death were collected. Arterial blood gas and mechanical ventilator settings parameters were recorded at approximately 10 a.m. daily after ARDS onset.

2.4. Histological Diagnosis

Based on analysis of hematoxylin- and eosin-stained lung tissue slices, a diagnosis of DAD (with or without fibrosis) was made independently by at least two pathologists who were blinded to the patients' clinical information. Any discrepancies were discussed by the pathologists with the aim of reaching a final consensus as to histological diagnosis. The presence of DAD indicated hyaline membrane formation, intra-alveolar edema, alveolar type I cell necrosis, alveolar type II cell proliferation, the interstitial proliferation of myofibroblasts and fibroblasts, or organizing interstitial fibrosis [3]. AE-IPF represents DAD and/or organizing pneumonia superimposed on the UIP pattern [13,14]. We defined fibrosis as the manifestation of collagenous fibrosis or chronic appearance of microcystic honeycombing, or both [19].

2.5. Statistical Analysis

Continuous variables are presented as mean ± standard deviation or median (interquartile range), and categorical variables are reported as numbers (percentages). A student's *t*-test or the Mann–Whitney *U* test were used to compare continuous variables among groups. Categorical variables were tested using the chi-square test for equal proportions or the Fisher's exact test. Risk factors associated with histological fibrosis at OLB day were initially analyzed using univariate analysis, followed by a multivariable logistic regression model with stepwise selection. The results are presented using odds ratios and 95% confidence intervals (CIs). All statistical analysis was performed using SPSS 26.0 statistical software, and statistical significance was considered when the 2-sided p value was less than 0.05.

3. Results

3.1. Study Populations

This study identified 89 ARDS patients who underwent OLB within the study period and screened for inclusion and exclusion criteria. All ARDS patients were deeply sedated and paralyzed during the initial phase, including the day of OLB, and most cases received pressure-controlled ventilation until attempts at weaning from the mechanical ventilator. After excluding 21 patients who did not fulfill the histological DAD, 68 patients with histological DAD were analyzed (Figure 1). Based on the histological findings, 56 patients were assigned to the non-fibrosis group, and 12 patients were assigned to the fibrosis group. In the fibrosis group, 7 patients had DAD with the fibrotic phase and 5 patients presenting the AE-IPF.

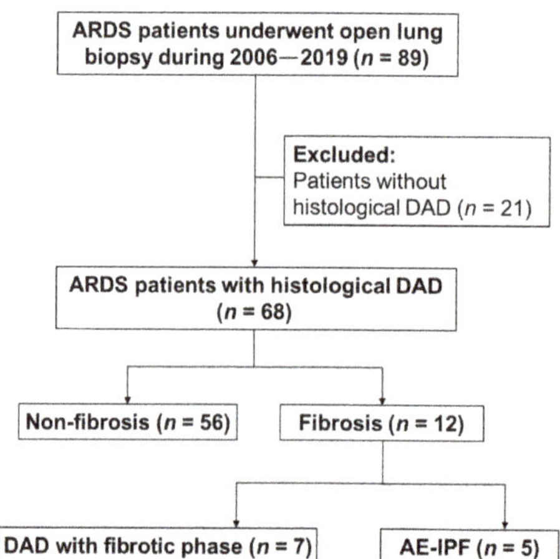

Figure 1. Flow chart of ARDS patients receiving open lung biopsy. ARDS: acute respiratory distress syndrome; DAD: diffuse alveolar damage; AE-IPF: acute exacerbation of idiopathic pulmonary fibrosis.

3.2. Histological Findings

Compared to normal lung tissue (Figure 2A), DAD in the initial stage was characterized by the formation of hyaline membrane (Figure 2B) and in the later stage by interstitial fibrosis (Figure 2C). The term honeycomb fibrosis refers to the typical appearance of cysts in scarred lung tissue (i.e., UIP pattern) (Figure 2D). Organizing pneumonia was deemed indicative of acute exacerbation of UIP (Figure 2E).

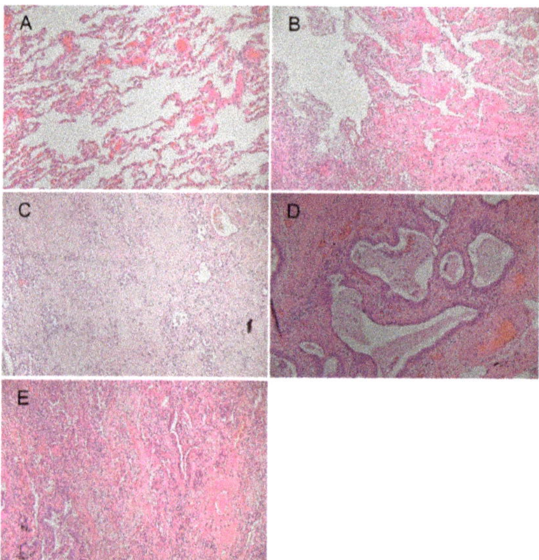

Figure 2. Human lung tissues samples from enrolled patients stained using hematoxylin and eosin. (**A**) Normal lung tissue defined as thin alveolar capillary membrane with clear alveolar space; (**B**) diffuse alveolar damage in which alveolar surfaces are lined with hyaline membranes; (**C**) lung tissue showing distinct indications of interstitial fibrosis; (**D**) UIP showing honeycomb fibrosis; (**E**) organizing pneumonia indicating acute exacerbation of UIP. 4X magnification. UIP: usual interstitial pneumonia.

3.3. Baseline Characteristics and Clinical Variables: Non-Fibrosis and Fibrosis Groups

As shown in Table 1, we observed no significant difference between non-fibrosis and fibrosis groups in terms of age, gender, body weight, body mass index, or comorbidities. In both groups, most of the ARDS cases were attributable to pulmonary causes (n = 58, 85%). The median interval between ARDS diagnosis and biopsy was significantly longer in the fibrosis group than the non-fibrosis group (18 (9–30) vs. 8 (5–12) days, $p = 0.024$). In terms of ventilator settings at the time of ARDS diagnosis, MP, Ppeak, and dynamic ΔP levels were significantly higher in the fibrosis group than in the non-fibrosis group (all $p < 0.05$). On the day of biopsy, Ppeak and dynamic ΔP values remained significantly higher in the fibrosis group than in the non-fibrosis group, and dynamic compliance was significantly lower (all $p < 0.05$).

Table 1. Background characteristics and clinical variables: non-fibrosis and fibrosis on histological findings.

Characteristics	All (n = 68)	Non-Fibrosis (n = 56)	Fibrosis (n = 12)	p
Age (years)	60.4 ± 16	59.4 ± 14.8	65.3 ± 20.8	0.255
Male (gender)	39 (57%)	31 (55%)	8 (67%)	0.472
Body weight (kg)	60.7 ± 11.7	61.0 ± 12.3	58.4 ± 6.1	0.566
Body mass index (kg/m^2)	23.7 ± 3.8	23.8 ± 3.9	22.8 ± 3.3	0.488
Comorbidities				
Diabetes mellitus	12 (18%)	9 (16%)	3 (25%)	0.432
Hypertension	20 (29%)	18 (32%)	2 (17%)	0.486
Chronic lung diseases	7 (10%)	6 (11%)	1 (8%)	1.0
Immunocompromised	18 (27%)	16 (29%)	2 (17%)	0.494
ARDS etiologies				
Pulmonary causes	58 (85%)	47 (84%)	11 (92%)	0.678
Extrapulmonary causes	10 (15%)	9 (16%)	1 (8%)	0.678
PaO_2/FiO_2 at day of ARDS diagnosis (mmHg)	135 (61–204)	136 (61–213)	118 (58–187)	0.613
Ventilator settings at day of ARDS diagnosis				
Mechanical power (J/min)	24.6 ± 9	23.5 ± 8.2	29.9 ± 10.8	0.023
Tidal volume (mL/kg PBW)	8.6 ± 1.9	8.7 ± 2	8.4 ± 1.6	0.764
PEEP (cm H_2O)	10.9 ± 2.4	11 ± 2.5	11 ± 2.1	0.566
Peak inspiratory pressure (cm H_2O)	31.7 ± 5.6	31.1 ± 4.9	36.1 ± 5.3	0.004
Mean airway pressure (cm H_2O)	17.6 ± 3.5	17.5 ± 3.4	18.5 ± 4	0.345
Dynamic driving pressure (cm H_2O)	20.9 ± 5.2	20.2 ± 4.4	24 ± 7.5	0.021
Total respiratory rate (breaths/min)	24.9 ±5	24.3 ± 4.9	27.3 ± 5.2	0.088
Dynamic compliance (mL/cm H_2O)	24.8 ± 10.5	24.8 ± 8.9	24.8 ± 16.5	0.989
Day from ARDS diagnosis to biopsy	8 (5–14)	8 (5–12)	18 (9–30)	0.024
PaO_2/FiO_2 at biopsy day (mmHg)	139 (104–194)	137 (103–199)	141 (98–191)	0.867
Ventilator settings at biopsy day				
Mechanical power (J/min)	23.8 ± 7.7	23.1 ± 6.9	27 ± 10.3	0.12
Tidal volume (mL/kg PBW)	7.7 ± 1.8	7.7 ± 1.7	7.6 ± 2.3	0.961
PEEP (cm H_2O)	12.3 ± 2.6	12.5 ± 2.5	11.3 ± 2.6	0.191
Peak inspiratory pressure (cm H_2O)	34.4 ± 6.9	33.6 ± 6.2	38.2 ± 9.1	0.037
Mean airway pressure (cm H_2O)	19.3 ± 3.8	19.4 ± 3.6	18.8 ± 5.1	0.567
Dynamic driving pressure (cm H_2O)	22.1 ± 6.8	21.1 ± 6.0	26.8 ± 8.2	0.007
Total respiratory rate (breaths/min)	25.2 ± 5	24.9 ± 4.7	26.3 ± 6.5	0.373
Dynamic compliance (mL/cm H_2O)	20.5 ± 7.6	21.3 ± 7.6	17.1 ± 6.7	0.017
Hospital mortality, n (%)	40 (59%)	32 (57%)	8 (67%)	0.748
Duration of mechanical ventilator (days)	22 (15–34)	21 (14–32)	35 (24–74)	0.028

Table 1. *Cont.*

Characteristics	All (n = 68)	Non-Fibrosis (n = 56)	Fibrosis (n = 12)	p
Length of ICU stay (days)	27 (17–37)	25 (16–34)	51 (32–80)	0.001
Length of hospital stay (days)	34 (22–56)	31 (20–46)	55 (32–81)	0.004
Ventilator-free days at day 28	0 (0–5)	0 (0–11)	0 (0–0)	0.036
ICU-free days at day 28	0 (0–7)	0 (0–8)	0 (0–0)	0.036
ICU-free days at day 60	0 (0–35)	0 (0–40)	0 (0–0)	0.008
Hospital-free days at day 90	51 (29–66)	54 (16–34)	25 (2–54)	0.01

Data is presented as mean ± standard deviation, count or median (interquartile range). ARDS: acute respiratory distress syndrome; PaO_2: partial pressure of oxygen in arterial blood; FiO_2: fraction of inspired oxygen; PBW: predicted body weight; PEEP: positive end-expiratory pressure; ICU: intensive care unit.

The overall hospital mortality rate was 59%, and the mortality was relatively higher in the fibrosis group than in the non-fibrosis group (67% vs. 57%, $p = 0.748$). The duration of mechanical ventilation, length of ICU stay, and length of hospital stay were significantly higher in the fibrosis group than in the non-fibrosis group (all $p < 0.05$).

3.4. Baseline Characteristics and Clinical Variables: DAD with a Fibrotic Phase and AE-IPF Groups

As shown in Table 2, the patients in the AE-IPF group were older than those in the DAD with a fibrotic phase group. There were no significant differences between the two groups in terms of age, gender, body weight, body mass index, or comorbidities. In terms of ventilator settings at ARDS diagnosis, we observed no significant differences between the two groups. The median interval between ARDS diagnosis and biopsy was longer in the DAD with a fibrotic phase group than the AE-IPF group (28 (17–53) vs. 7 (4–21) days). On the day of biopsy, patients in the AE-IPF group received higher MP, higher V_T, higher Ppeak, higher mean airway pressure, higher dynamic ΔP, and higher RR than patients in the DAD with a fibrotic phase group, although the difference did not reach the level of significance (Table 2 and Figure 3). Dynamic compliance was similar between the two groups on the day of biopsy.

Table 2. Background characteristics and clinical variables: DAD with a fibrotic phase and AE-IPF on histological findings.

Characteristics	DAD with a Fibrotic Phase (n = 7)	AE-IPF (n = 5)	p
Age (years)	59.3 ± 25.5	73.6 ± 8.36	0.204
Male (gender)	5 (71%)	3 (60%)	0.769
Body weight (kg)	60.5 ± 8.1	56.4 ± 3.2	0.379
Body mass index (kg/m^2)	23.4 ± 4.4	22.1 ± 1.7	0.657
Comorbidities			
Diabetes mellitus	1 (14%)	2 (40%)	0.31
Hypertension	1 (14%)	1 (20%)	0.793
Chronic lung diseases	1 (14%)	0 (0%)	0.377
Immunocompromised	2 (29%)	0 (0%)	0.19
ARDS etiologies			
Pulmonary causes	6 (86%)	5 (100%)	1.0
Extrapulmonary causes	1 (14%)	0 (0%)	1.0
PaO_2/FiO_2 at day of ARDS diagnosis (mmHg)	68 (39–138)	136 (118–176)	0.794
Ventilator settings at day of ARDS diagnosis			
Mechanical power (J/min)	30 ± 8.7	30 ± 14	0.987
Tidal volume (mL/kg PBW)	8.9 ± 1.9	7.8 ± 1.1	0.434
PEEP (cm H_2O)	10.6 ± 2.2	10.4 ± 2.2	0.897

Table 2. *Cont.*

Characteristics	DAD with a Fibrotic Phase (n = 7)	AE-IPF (n = 5)	p
Peak inspiratory pressure (cm H_2O)	34.6 ± 5.6	34.4 ± 5.7	0.971
Mean airway pressure (cm H_2O)	18.6 ± 4.1	18.4 ± 4.4	0.946
Dynamic driving pressure (cm H_2O)	24 ± 5.2	24 ± 10.7	1.0
Total respiratory rate (breaths/min)	27.1 ± 4.6	27.6 ± 6.6	0.889
Dynamic compliance (mL/cm H_2O)	21.2 (15–21.6)	15.9 (14.1–49)	0.755
Day from ARDS diagnosis to biopsy	28 (17–53)	7 (4–21)	0.242
PaO_2/FiO_2 at biopsy day (mmHg)	168 (95–192)	106 (89–141)	0.546
Ventilator settings at biopsy day			
Mechanical power (J/min)	25.2 ± 11.4	29.4 ± 9.2	0.851
Tidal volume (mL/kg PBW)	6.8 ± 2.7	8.8 ± 1.3	0.301
PEEP (cm H_2O)	11 ± 3.2	11.8 ± 1.8	0.394
Peak inspiratory pressure (cm H_2O)	37.4 ± 10	39.2 ± 8.8	0.757
Mean airway pressure (cm H_2O)	17.7 ± 5.3	20.4 ± 4.9	0.628
Dynamic driving pressure (cm H_2O)	26.4 ± 8.8	27.4 ± 8.3	0.663
Total respiratory rate (breaths/min)	25.3 ± 3.8	27.8 ± 9.5	0.537
Dynamic compliance (mL/ cm H_2O)	15.8 (11.7–18.6)	15.2 (10.1–27.6)	0.876

Data is presented as mean ± standard deviation, count, or median (interquartile range). DAD: diffuse alveolar damage; AE-IPF: acute exacerbation of idiopathic pulmonary fibrosis; ARDS: acute respiratory distress syndrome; PaO_2: partial pressure of oxygen in arterial blood; FiO_2: fraction of inspired oxygen; PBW: predicted body weight; PEEP: positive end-expiratory pressure.

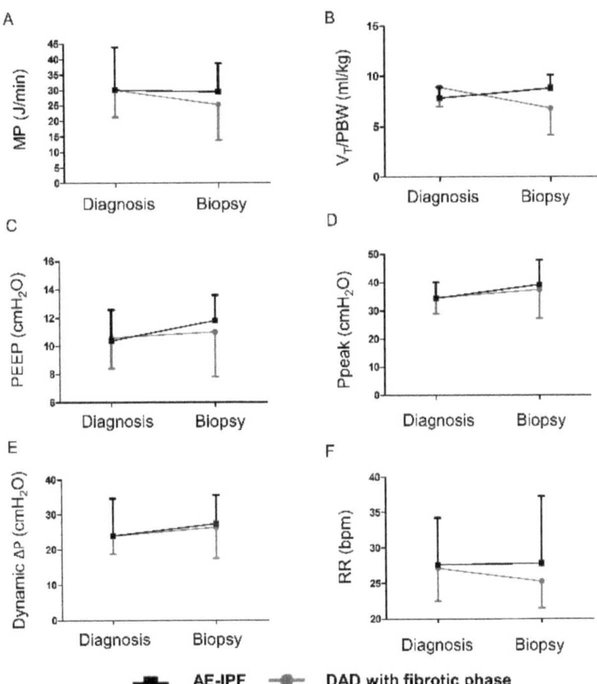

Figure 3. Serial changes in the ventilatory variables of (**A**) MP (**B**) V_T/PBW (**C**) PEEP (**D**) Ppeak (**E**) Dynamic ΔP (**F**) RR between ARDS diagnosis and open lung biopsy of patients in the DAD with a fibrotic phase and AE-IPF groups. ARDS: acute respiratory distress syndrome; DAD: diffuse alveolar damage; AE-IPF: acute exacerbation of idiopathic pulmonary fibrosis; MP: mechanical power; V_T: tidal volume; PBW: predicted body weight; PEEP: positive end-expiratory pressure; Ppeak: peak inspiratory pressure; ΔP: driving pressure; RR: respiratory rate; bpm: beats per minute.

3.5. Clinical Outcomes: DAD with a Fibrotic Phase and AE-IPF

As shown in Table 3 and Figure 4, 90-day hospital mortality was higher in the AE-IPF group than in the DAD with a fibrotic phase group (80% vs. 57%, $p = 0.242$). The duration of mechanical ventilation, length of ICU stay, and length of hospital stay were higher in the DAD with a fibrotic phase group than the AE-IPF group. The number of ventilator-free days at day 90, and ICU-free days at day 60 were also higher in the DAD with a fibrotic phase group than the AE-IPF group.

Table 3. Clinical outcomes as a function of DAD with a fibrotic phase and AE-IPF on histological findings.

Outcomes	DAD with Fibrotic Phase ($n = 7$)	AE-IPF ($n = 5$)	p
90-day hospital mortality, n (%)	4 (57%)	4 (80%)	0.242
Other outcomes			
Duration of mechanical ventilator (days)	46 (22–75)	42 (24–66)	0.84
Length of ICU stay (days)	72 (37–81)	48 (24–78)	0.319
Length of hospital stay (days)	82 (53–93)	57 (27–98)	0.364
Ventilator-free days at day 90	14 (0–23)	0 (0–0)	0.224
ICU-free days at day 60	1 (0–0)	0 (0–0)	0.424

Data is presented as a count or median (interquartile range). DAD: diffuse alveolar damage; AE-IPF: acute exacerbation of idiopathic pulmonary fibrosis; ICU: intensive care unit.

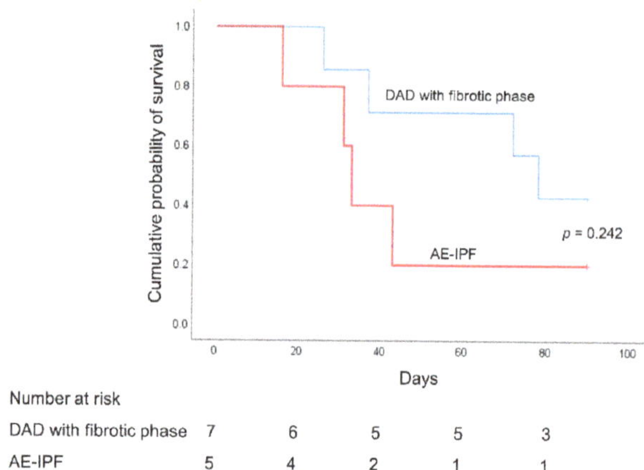

Figure 4. Kaplan–Meier 90-day survival curves of patients with acute respiratory distress syndrome undergoing open lung biopsy, as stratified by DAD with a fibrotic phase and AE-IPF. DAD: diffuse alveolar damage; AE-IPF: acute exacerbation of idiopathic pulmonary fibrosis.

3.6. Factors Associated with Histological Fibrosis at OLB

After adjusting for significant confounding variables, a multivariable logistic regression model revealed that patients who had higher MP at ARDS diagnosis and had a longer ARDS duration before biopsy were significantly associated with histological fibrosis at OLB (odds ratio 1.493 (95% CI 1.014–2.200), $p = 0.042$ and odds ratio 1.160 (95% CI 1.052–1.278), $p = 0.003$, respectively) (Table 4).

Table 4. Factors associated with histological fibrosis at open lung biopsy using a multivariable logistic regression model.

Characteristics	Odds Ratio (95% CI)	p
MP at day of ARDS diagnosis (J/min)	1.493 (1.014–2.200)	0.042
ARDS duration before biopsy (days)	1.160 (1.052–1.278)	0.003

CI: confidence interval; MP: mechanical power; ARDS: acute respiratory distress syndrome. The multivariable analysis model included continuous variables (age, body weight, body mass index, ventilatory variables at day of ARDS diagnosis, and day from ARDS diagnosis to biopsy) and categorical variables (gender, comorbidities, and ARDS etiologies). For the continuous variables, the odds ratio means that the risk of histological fibrosis at open lung biopsy increases or decreases per unit increase in these variables.

4. Discussion

The primary insight in this study was the fact that ARDS patients with histological DAD and fibrosis based on OLB received significantly higher airway pressures, and had significantly longer durations of mechanical ventilator use and longer ICU and hospital stays. Hospital mortality was higher in the fibrosis group than in the non-fibrosis group. In the fibrosis group, patients with AE-IPF received higher ventilator load and had higher hospital mortality than those in the DAD with a fibrotic phase group.

DAD is the pathological hallmark of ARDS. In the current study, we enrolled only ARDS patients with histological evidence of DAD using data from OLB, unlike previous studies that included ARDS patients with and without DAD using data from OLB or autopsy [6,20,21]. The pathogenesis or the time course of lung damage in ARDS proceeds through an exudative phase (for roughly the first week after ARDS onset), proliferative phase (between the first and third weeks following ARDS onset), and fibrotic phase (beyond 3 or 4 weeks after ARDS onset) [2,22]. In the current study, the median duration from ARDS diagnosis to OLB was 28 days in the DAD with a fibrotic phase group. Some of the patients had progressed to DAD with a fibrotic phase within 3 weeks of ARDS onset. This indicates that the diagnosis of ARDS depends on clinical criteria, and that the onset of lung damage and histological fibrosis may begin before all the criteria for clinical diagnosis of ARDS are met [19]. Patients in the fibrosis group had significantly longer ARDS duration before biopsy (i.e., could have a longer duration of lung damage) than patients in the non-fibrosis group. In a multivariable logistic regression model, longer ARDS durations before biopsy were independently associated with histological fibrosis at OLB. This indicates that mechanical ventilation, histological fibrosis at OLB, and clinical outcomes of ARDS patients were related to the onset of lung damage.

The causes of pulmonary fibrosis during ARDS progression are multifactorial (e.g., inflammation and VILI) [9,15]. The course and onset of lung fibrosis can be traced to persistent injury and repair in response to mechanical strain and stress on epithelial cell resulting from volutrauma and atelectrauma, which subsequently triggers the fibroproliferative cascade [15,23]. The mechanical force could cause numerous intracellular mediators directly or indirectly released into the lung, which induces further lung damage and the subsequent development of lung fibrosis [15]. The extent of the ventilator load needed to cause pulmonary fibrosis was unknown. However, mechanical ventilation, histological fibrosis at OLB, and the clinical outcomes of ARDS patients could be directly related to the onset of lung fibrosis. MP refers to the energy delivered by a ventilator to the respiratory system per unit of time, as determined by volume, pressure, flow, and RR. Researchers have established that MP is of higher predictive value than individual ventilator parameters in assessing the risk of VILI [17,18]. Excessive MP has been shown to promote VILI and appears to be strongly correlated with histology (DAD score) and the expression of interleukin-6, a marker of inflammation [24]. Driving pressure is inversely proportional to lung compliance and aerated remaining functional lung size and has been linked to mortality in ARDS patients [16,25].

Few studies have examined the correlation between serial changes in ventilator settings and the development of histological fibrosis in ARDS patients. Serial changes in the ventilator settings may reflect the severity of nonresolving lung damage. In the current study, the MP and airway pressures (Ppeak and dynamic ΔP) received by the fibrosis group were significantly higher than those received by the non-fibrosis group at ARDS diagnosis. Thus, it is likely that the formation of lung fibrosis can be attributed at least in part to energy load (i.e., MP). In a multivariable logistic regression model, higher MP at ARDS diagnosis was independently associated with histological fibrosis at OLB. Compliance of the respiratory system was associated with the severity of lung injury, duration of ARDS, extent of lung fibrosis, and clinical outcomes [19]. Dynamic compliance in the fibrosis group was significantly lower and dropped more rapidly than in the non-fibrosis group on biopsy day. This may be due to the presence of fibrosis and a longer interval between ARDS diagnosis and OLB in the fibrosis group.

IPF is a form of chronic fibrosing interstitial pneumonia characterized by a progressive decline in lung function with radiological and/or histopathological indications of UIP [11,26]. Note, however, that UIP is not synonymous with IPF. The UIP pattern of fibrosis has also been linked to other conditions, such as connective tissue disease (mostly rheumatoid arthritis), drug toxicity, chronic hypersensitivity pneumonitis, asbestosis, and Hermansky–Pudlak syndrome [26,27]. AE-IPF and ARDS are quite similar in terms of DAD, lung inflammation, and respiratory mechanics. AE-IPF can lead to severe acute hypoxemic respiratory failure, requiring mechanical ventilator support. Patients with AE-IPF face a higher risk of mortality (may reach 95%) [14], which may be related to the fact that IPF patients tend to be older. In our study, 5 of the 12 patients in the fibrosis group presented histological findings indicative of UIP, and none of these patients presented with connective tissue disease, drug toxicity, or asbestosis. A pathologist and radiologist agreed that the cause of respiratory failure in this group was primarily AE-IPF. Patients in the AE-IPF group were older than those in the DAD with a fibrotic phase group (mean age 73.6 vs. 59.3 years), and the mortality was higher than DAD with a fibrotic phase group (80% vs. 57%).

Impaired lung mechanics due to structural, biochemical, and anatomical aberrations render fibrotic lungs susceptible to VILI [28]. At present, there is no solid evidence indicating the optimal and personalized ventilator settings for fibrotic lungs, including AE-IPF; some concepts can be derived from the evidence regarding ARDS because both share some common features. A "lung resting strategy" to avoid high PEEP during expiration and thereby prevent further lung injury has been posited as an alternative to the "open lung approach" (for ARDS cases presenting only DAD) for patients with pulmonary fibrosis and UIP, due to the fact that the presence of fibrotic tissue renders the lung structure highly fragile and prone to VILI (i.e., the "squishy ball lung" concept) [28]. In our study, patients in the DAD with a fibrotic phase and AE-IPF groups received similar ventilator settings except for V_T at ARDS diagnosis. However, patients in the AE-IPF group received a higher energy load (i.e., MP), higher V_T, and higher airway pressures than in the DAD with a fibrotic phase group on the biopsy day. This indicates that intensivists may not recognize the disease status well and apply lung-protective ventilation at ARDS onset promptly; however, as disease progression, patients in the AE-IPF group received a higher ventilator load than those in the DAD with a fibrotic phase group on biopsy day due to underlying chronic fibrotic lungs, which contributed to a higher risk of VILI.

The strength of our study was that we investigated pulmonary fibrosis based on histological fibrosis from OLB. Previous studies examining the effect of pulmonary fibrosis on clinical outcomes in ARDS patients reported a link between HRCT scores indicative of fibroproliferative changes and clinical outcomes/mortality [10,29]. Nonetheless, thin-section CT scanning, including inspiratory, expiratory, and prone sequences, is the most important tool by which to evaluate pulmonary fibrosis. Serial images and quantitative estimates are also essential for differentiating fibrosis progression [27]. Overall, imaging alone cannot be relied upon to confirm destruction of the lung parenchyma, delineate active fibroproliferation, or assess the degree of lung fibrosis [8]. At present, there is no definitive biomarker for DAD, and HRCT findings are insufficient to differentiate DAD from DAD with organizing pneumonia, which was indicative of acute exacerbation of

UIP [30]. The only way to confirm the presence of DAD is to obtain lung tissues via OLB or autopsy [20]. Unfortunately, cases that end in autopsy are very likely to be more severe than live cases, and autopsy series are unable to differentiate clinical outcomes or effects on mortality [19,20]. In the current study, we investigated the effect of pulmonary fibrosis on clinical outcomes by enrolling ARDS patients with histological DAD and fibrosis who had undergone OLB.

This retrospective study was hindered by a number of limitations. First, all patients were from a single tertiary care referral center over a long enrollment period. Furthermore, we focused on only cases of ARDS that had undergone OLB who fulfilled the histological DAD with fibrosis (i.e., fibrotic phase or AE-IPF) or not, which limited the number of recruited patients. Note that we opted not to exclude the 5 patients with chronic fibrosis (i.e., UIP pattern) from the fibrosis group (n = 12), similar to that of a previous ARDS study based on autopsies in which half of the fibrosis group (15 of 30 patients) also presented with chronic microcystic honeycombing [19]. Besides, we further divided the fibrosis group into the DAD with a fibrotic phase or the AE-IPF group and compared clinical outcomes. Second, the causes of pulmonary fibrosis are complex and multifactorial, and the exact causal relationship between mechanical ventilation and pulmonary fibrosis was difficult to determine due to the retrospective nature of the study. It is important to emphasize that mechanical ventilation, histological fibrosis at OLB, and clinical outcomes of ARDS patients could be directly related to the onset of lung damage and fibrosis. Third, compliance with lung-protective ventilation with lower tidal volumes tends to decrease in real-world clinical practice [1]. Our study was conducted over a long study period from 2006 to 2019 with retrospective analysis, and there was no standard protocol for the ventilator settings among the enrolled ICUs. Therefore, the ARDS patients included in this study received a relatively high V_T than 6 mL/kg PBW of the current guidelines [2], which may make external validation to other ARDS cohorts difficult to perform and may have influenced the clinical outcomes. Finally, corticosteroids have anti-inflammatory and antifibrosis effects; however, we opted not to address the use of steroid therapy, due to a lack of evidence pertaining to the benefits of steroid treatment for persistent ARDS and fibrotic lungs.

5. Conclusions

Our findings revealed that ARDS patients with histological DAD and fibrosis received significantly higher airway pressures, underwent mechanical ventilation for a longer duration, and remained in the ICU and hospital for a longer period. Hospital mortality was higher in the fibrosis group than in the non-fibrosis group. In the fibrosis group, patients with AE-IPF received a higher ventilator load and faced higher mortality than those in DAD with a fibrotic phase.

Implementing optimal ventilator settings as early as possible may be necessary to reduce the risk of VILI and pulmonary fibrosis. Further large-scale studies are required to identify the mechanisms by which mechanical ventilation induces pulmonary fibrosis, and define safety standards aimed at minimizing the risk of VILI and fibrosis.

Author Contributions: Conceptualization, H.-H.L. and L.-C.C.; methodology, H.-H.L. and C.-W.W.; software, H.-H.L. and L.-C.C.; validation, C.-H.C. and C.-C.H.; formal analysis, H.-H.L. and L.-C.C.; investigation, H.-H.L. and H.-S.H.; resources, C.-H.C., C.-C.H. and L.-C.C.; data curation, H.-H.L., C.-W.W. and L.-C.C.; writing—original draft preparation, H.-H.L. and L.-C.C.; writing—review and editing, H.-H.L. and L.-C.C.; visualization, C.-H.C. and C.-C.H.; supervision, C.-C.H. and H.-S.H.; project administration, L.-C.C.; funding acquisition, L.-C.C. All authors have read and agreed to the published version of the manuscript.

Funding: This research was funded by grants CMRPG3K1151 and CMRPG3L0821 from Chang Gung Memorial Hospital.

Institutional Review Board Statement: The study was conducted in accordance with the guidelines of the Declaration of Helsinki, and approved by the Institutional Review Board of CGMH IRB No. 202000760A3 and 202100595A3 and waived the need for informed consent.

Informed Consent Statement: Patient consent was waived due to the retrospective and observational nature of the study.

Data Availability Statement: All data is available from the corresponding authors on reasonable request.

Acknowledgments: The authors would like to express their appreciation to the patients and staffs in the ICUs at Chang Gung Memorial Hospital. We thank Yu-Jr Lin in the Research Services Center for Health Information, Chang Gung University, for validating and confirming all statistics in this study.

Conflicts of Interest: The authors declare no conflict of interest.

References

1. Bellani, G.; Laffey, J.G.; Pham, T.; Fan, E.; Brochard, L.; Esteban, A.; Gattinoni, L.; van Haren, F.; Larsson, A.; McAuley, D.F.; et al. Epidemiology, Patterns of Care, and Mortality for Patients with Acute Respiratory Distress Syndrome in Intensive Care Units in 50 Countries. *JAMA* **2016**, *315*, 788–800. [CrossRef] [PubMed]
2. Thompson, B.T.; Chambers, R.C.; Liu, K.D. Acute Respiratory Distress Syndrome. *N. Engl. J. Med.* **2017**, *377*, 562–572. [CrossRef] [PubMed]
3. Katzenstein, A.L.; Bloor, C.M.; Leibow, A.A. Diffuse alveolar damage–the role of oxygen, shock, and related factors. A review. *Am. J. Pathol.* **1976**, *85*, 209–228. [PubMed]
4. Guerin, C.; Bayle, F.; Leray, V.; Debord, S.; Stoian, A.; Yonis, H.; Roudaut, J.B.; Bourdin, G.; Devouassoux-Shisheboran, M.; Bucher, E.; et al. OLB in nonresolving ARDS frequently identifies diffuse alveolar damage regardless of the severity stage and may have implications for patient management. *Intensive Care Med.* **2015**, *41*, 222–230. [CrossRef]
5. Kao, K.C.; Hu, H.C.; Chang, C.H.; Hung, C.Y.; Chiu, L.C.; Li, S.H.; Lin, S.W.; Chuang, L.P.; Wang, C.W.; Li, L.F.; et al. Diffuse alveolar damage associated mortality in selected acute respiratory distress syndrome patients with OLB. *Crit. Care* **2015**, *19*, 228. [CrossRef]
6. Lorente, J.A.; Cardinal-Fernández, P.; Muñoz, D.; Frutos-Vivar, F.; Thille, A.W.; Jaramillo, C.; Ballén-Barragán, A.; Rodríguez, J.M.; Peñuelas, O.; Ortiz, G.; et al. Acute respiratory distress syndrome in patients with and without diffuse alveolar damage: An autopsy study. *Intensive Care Med.* **2015**, *41*, 1921–1930. [CrossRef]
7. Ranieri, V.M.; Rubenfeld, G.D.; Thompson, B.T.; Ferguson, N.D.; Caldwell, E.; Fan, E.; Camporota, L.; Slutsky, A.S. Acute respiratory distress syndrome: The Berlin Definition. *JAMA* **2012**, *307*, 2526–2533.
8. Burnham, E.L.; Janssen, W.J.; Riches, D.W.; Moss, M.; Downey, G.P. The fibroproliferative response in acute respiratory distress syndrome: Mechanisms and clinical significance. *Eur. Respir. J.* **2014**, *43*, 276–285. [CrossRef]
9. Cabrera-Benitez, N.E.; Laffey, J.G.; Parotto, M.; Spieth, P.M.; Villar, J.; Zhang, H.; Slutsky, A.S. Mechanical ventilation-associated lung fibrosis in acute respiratory distress syndrome: A significant contributor to poor outcome. *Anesthesiology* **2014**, *121*, 189–198. [CrossRef]
10. Ichikado, K.; Muranaka, H.; Gushima, Y.; Kotani, T.; Nader, H.M.; Fujimoto, K.; Johkoh, T.; Iwamoto, N.; Kawamura, K.; Nagano, J.; et al. Fibroproliferative changes on high-resolution CT in the acute respiratory distress syndrome predict mortality and ventilator dependency: A prospective observational cohort study. *BMJ Open* **2012**, *2*, e000545. [CrossRef]
11. Raghu, G.; Remy-Jardin, M.; Myers, J.L.; Richeldi, L.; Ryerson, C.J.; Lederer, D.J.; Behr, J.; Cottin, V.; Danoff, S.K.; Morell, F.; et al. Diagnosis of Idiopathic Pulmonary Fibrosis. An Official ATS/ERS/JRS/ALAT Clinical Practice Guideline. *Am. J. Respir. Crit. Care Med.* **2018**, *198*, e44–e68. [CrossRef] [PubMed]
12. Collard, H.R.; Ryerson, C.J.; Corte, T.J.; Jenkins, G.; Kondoh, Y.; Lederer, D.J.; Lee, J.S.; Maher, T.M.; Wells, A.U.; Antoniou, K.M.; et al. Acute Exacerbation of Idiopathic Pulmonary Fibrosis. An International Working Group Report. *Am. J. Respir. Crit. Care Med.* **2016**, *194*, 265–275. [CrossRef] [PubMed]
13. Kim, D.S.; Park, J.H.; Park, B.K.; Lee, J.S.; Nicholson, A.G.; Colby, T. Acute exacerbation of idiopathic pulmonary fibrosis: Frequency and clinical features. *Eur. Respir. J.* **2006**, *27*, 143–150. [CrossRef] [PubMed]
14. Marchioni, A.; Tonelli, R.; Ball, L.; Fantini, R.; Castaniere, I.; Cerri, S.; Luppi, F.; Malerba, M.; Pelosi, P.; Clini, E. Acute exacerbation of idiopathic pulmonary fibrosis: Lessons learned from acute respiratory distress syndrome? *Crit. Care* **2018**, *22*, 80. [CrossRef]
15. Slutsky, A.S.; Ranieri, V.M. Ventilator-induced lung injury. *N. Engl. J. Med.* **2013**, *369*, 2126–2136. [CrossRef]
16. Chiu, L.C.; Hu, H.C.; Hung, C.Y.; Chang, C.H.; Tsai, F.C.; Yang, C.T.; Huang, C.C.; Wu, H.P.; Kao, K.C. Dynamic driving pressure associated mortality in acute respiratory distress syndrome with extracorporeal membrane oxygenation. *Ann. Intensive Care* **2017**, *7*, 12. [CrossRef]
17. Chiu, L.C.; Lin, S.W.; Chuang, L.P.; Li, H.H.; Liu, P.H.; Tsai, F.C.; Chang, C.H.; Hung, C.Y.; Lee, C.S.; Leu, S.W.; et al. Mechanical power during extracorporeal membrane oxygenation and hospital mortality in patients with acute respiratory distress syndrome. *Crit. Care* **2021**, *25*, 13. [CrossRef]
18. Gattinoni, L.; Tonetti, T.; Cressoni, M.; Cadringher, P.; Herrmann, P.; Moerer, O.; Protti, A.; Gotti, M.; Chiurazzi, C.; Carlesso, E.; et al. Ventilator-related causes of lung injury: The mechanical power. *Intensive Care Med.* **2016**, *42*, 1567–1575. [CrossRef]

19. Thille, A.W.; Esteban, A.; Fernández-Segoviano, P.; Rodriguez, J.M.; Aramburu, J.A.; Vargas-Errázuriz, P.; Martín-Pellicer, A.; Lorente, J.A.; Frutos-Vivar, F. Chronology of histological lesions in acute respiratory distress syndrome with diffuse alveolar damage: A prospective cohort study of clinical autopsies. *Lancet Respir. Med.* **2013**, *1*, 395–401. [CrossRef]
20. Cardinal-Fernández, P.; Bajwa, E.K.; Dominguez-Calvo, A.; Menéndez, J.M.; Papazian, L.; Thompson, B.T. The Presence of Diffuse Alveolar Damage on OLB Is Associated With Mortality in Patients With Acute Respiratory Distress Syndrome: A Systematic Review and Meta-Analysis. *Chest* **2016**, *149*, 1155–1164. [CrossRef]
21. Thille, A.W.; Esteban, A.; Fernández-Segoviano, P.; Rodriguez, J.M.; Aramburu, J.A.; Peñuelas, O.; Cortés-Puch, I.; Cardinal-Fernández, P.; Lorente, J.A.; Frutos-Vivar, F. Comparison of the Berlin definition for acute respiratory distress syndrome with autopsy. *Am. J. Respir. Crit. Care Med.* **2013**, *187*, 761–767. [CrossRef] [PubMed]
22. Tomashefski, J.F., Jr. Pulmonary pathology of acute respiratory distress syndrome. *Clin. Chest Med.* **2000**, *21*, 435–466. [CrossRef]
23. Albert, R.K.; Smith, B.; Perlman, C.E.; Schwartz, D.A. Is Progression of Pulmonary Fibrosis due to Ventilation-induced Lung Injury? *Am. J. Respir. Crit. Care Med.* **2019**, *200*, 140–151. [CrossRef] [PubMed]
24. Santos, R.S.; Maia, L.A.; Oliveira, M.V.; Santos, C.L.; Moraes, L.; Pinto, E.F.; Samary, C.D.S.; Machado, J.A.; Carvalho, A.C.; Fernandes, M.V.S.; et al. Biologic Impact of Mechanical Power at High and Low Tidal Volumes in Experimental Mild Acute Respiratory Distress Syndrome. *Anesthesiology* **2018**, *128*, 1193–1206. [CrossRef]
25. Amato, M.B.; Meade, M.O.; Slutsky, A.S.; Brochard, L.; Costa, E.L.; Schoenfeld, D.A.; Stewart, T.E.; Briel, M.; Talmor, D.; Mercat, A.; et al. Driving pressure and survival in the acute respiratory distress syndrome. *N. Engl. J. Med.* **2015**, *372*, 747–755. [CrossRef]
26. Wuyts, W.A.; Cavazza, A.; Rossi, G.; Bonella, F.; Sverzellati, N.; Spagnolo, P. Differential diagnosis of usual interstitial pneumonia: When is it truly idiopathic? *Eur. Respir. Rev.* **2014**, *23*, 308–319. [CrossRef]
27. Hobbs, S.; Chung, J.H.; Leb, J.; Kaproth-Joslin, K.; Lynch, D.A. Practical Imaging Interpretation in Patients Suspected of Having Idiopathic Pulmonary Fibrosis: Official Recommendations from the Radiology Working Group of the Pulmonary Fibrosis Foundation. *Radiol. Cardiothorac. Imaging* **2021**, *3*, e200279. [CrossRef]
28. Marchioni, A.; Tonelli, R.; Rossi, G.; Spagnolo, P.; Luppi, F.; Cerri, S.; Cocconcelli, E.; Pellegrino, M.R.; Fantini, R.; Tabbì, L.; et al. Ventilatory support and mechanical properties of the fibrotic lung acting as a "squishy ball". *Ann. Intensive Care* **2020**, *10*, 13. [CrossRef]
29. Kamo, T.; Tasaka, S.; Suzuki, T.; Asakura, T.; Suzuki, S.; Yagi, K.; Namkoong, H.; Ishii, M.; Morisaki, H.; Betsuyaku, T. Prognostic values of the Berlin definition criteria, blood lactate level, and fibroproliferative changes on high-resolution computed tomography in ARDS patients. *BMC Pulm. Med.* **2019**, *19*, 37. [CrossRef]
30. Chung, J.H.; Kradin, R.L.; Greene, R.E.; Shepard, J.A.; Digumarthy, S.R. CT predictors of mortality in pathology confirmed ARDS. *Eur. Radiol.* **2011**, *21*, 730–737. [CrossRef]

MDPI
St. Alban-Anlage 66
4052 Basel
Switzerland
Tel. +41 61 683 77 34
Fax +41 61 302 89 18
www.mdpi.com

Journal of Personalized Medicine Editorial Office
E-mail: jpm@mdpi.com
www.mdpi.com/journal/jpm

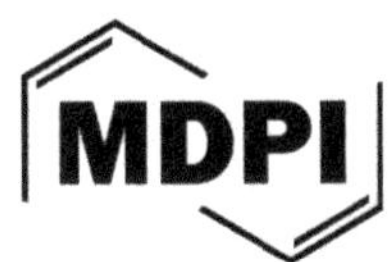